The GALE ENCYCLOPEDIA of ENVIRONMENTAL HEALTH

The GALE ENCYCLOPEDIA of ENVIRONMENTAL HEALTH

VOLUME
2

M–Z
ORGANIZATIONS
GLOSSARY
GENERAL INDEX

JACQUELINE L. LONGE, EDITOR

GALE
CENGAGE Learning

Detroit • New York • San Francisco • New Haven, Conn • Waterville, Maine • London

GALE CENGAGE Learning

Gale Encyclopedia of Environmental Health

Project Editor: Jacqueline L. Longe

Editorial: Laurie Fundukian, Kristin Key, Brigham Narins, Bodhan Romaniuk, Jeffrey Wilson

Product Manager: Anne Marie Sumner

Editorial Support Services: Andrea Lopeman

Indexing Services: Laura Doricott

Rights Acquisition and Management: Christine M. Myaskovsky, Robyn V. Young

Composition: Evi Abou-El-Seoud

Manufacturing: Wendy Blurton

Imaging: John Watkins

Product Design: Kristine Julien

© 2013 Gale, Cengage Learning

ALL RIGHTS RESERVED. No part of this work covered by the copyright herein may be reproduced, transmitted, stored, or used in any form or by any means graphic, electronic, or mechanical, including but not limited to photocopying, recording, scanning, digitizing, taping, Web distribution, information networks, or information storage and retrieval systems, except as permitted under Section 107 or 108 of the 1976 United States Copyright Act, without the prior written permission of the publisher.

For product information and technology assistance, contact us at
Gale Customer Support, 1-800-877-4253.
For permission to use material from this text or product,
submit all requests online at www.cengage.com/permissions.
Further permissions questions can be emailed to
permissionrequest@cengage.com

While every effort has been made to ensure the reliability of the information presented in this publication, Gale, a part of Cengage Learning, does not guarantee the accuracy of the data contained herein. Gale accepts no payment for listing; and inclusion in the publication of any organization, agency, institution, publication, service, or individual does not imply endorsement of the editors or publisher. Errors brought to the attention of the publisher and verified to the satisfaction of the publisher will be corrected in future editions.

Library of Congress Cataloging-in-Publication Data

The Gale encyclopedia of environmental health / Jacqueline L. Longe, editor. -- First edition.
 volumes cm
 Includes bibliographical references and index.
 ISBN-13: 978-1-4144-9880-5 (set : alk. paper)
 ISBN-10: 1-4144-9880-2 (set : alk. paper)
 ISBN-13: 978-1-4144-9881-2 (vol. 1 : alk. paper)
 ISBN-13: 978-1-4144-9882-9 (vol. 2 : alk. paper)
 [etc.]
 1. Environmental health--Encyclopedias. I. Longe, Jacqueline L., editor. II. Title: Encyclopedia of environmental health.
 RA565.G33 2013
 362.103--dc23
                                                                    2012051705

Gale
27500 Drake Rd.
Farmington Hills, MI, 48331-3535

ISBN-13: 978-1-4144-9880-5 (set)   ISBN-10: 1-4144-9880-2 (set)
ISBN-13: 978-1-4144-9881-2 (vol. 1)   ISBN-10: 1-4144-9881-0 (vol. 1)
ISBN-13: 978-1-4144-9882-9 (vol. 2)   ISBN-10: 1-4144-9882-9 (vol. 2)

This title is also available as an e-book.
ISBN-13: 978-1-4144-9883-6 ISBN-10: 1-4144-9883-7
Contact your Gale, a part of Cengage Learning sales representative for ordering information.

Printed in China
1 2 3 4 5 6 7 17 16 15 14 13

CONTENTS

Alphabetical List of Entries......................vii
Introduction..xiii
Advisory Board..xv
Contributors...xvii
Chronology..xxi
Entries
    Volume 1: A–L..1
    Volume 2: M–Z......................................501
Organizations..837
Glossary...851
General Index...883

ALPHABETICAL LIST OF ENTRIES

A

Acetone
Acid rain
Agency for Toxic Substances and Disease Registry
Agricultural chemicals
AIDS
Air pollution
Algal bloom
Altitude sickness
Ambient air
Amebiasis
American Public Health Association
Ammonia exposure
Anthrax
Antimicrobial resistance
Asbestos
Asbestosis
Aspergillosis
Asthma
Autism
Avian influenza

B

Background radiation
Bedbug infestation
Benzene
Benzene and benzene derivatives exposure
Benzo(a)pyrene
Berylliosis
Bhopal, India
Bioinformatics
Biomonitoring
Biosafety
Bioterrorism
Biotoxins
Bisphenol A
Black lung disease
Bronchitis
Brownfield sites
Brucellosis
Byssinosis

C

Cadmium
Cadmium poisoning
Campylobacteriosis
Cancer
Carbon monoxide poisoning
Cellular telephones
Centers for Disease Control and Prevention
Chartered Institute of Environmental Health
Chemical poisoning
Chernobyl nuclear power station
Child survival revolution
Chlorination
Chlorine exposure
Cholera
Chronic kidney disease
Chronic wasting disease
Clean Air Act
Clean Water Act
Climate change
Colony collapse disorder
Communicable diseases
Comprehensive Environmental Response, Compensation, and Liability (Superfund) Act (1980)
Creutzfeldt-Jakob disease
Cruise ship health
Cryptosporidiosis
Cutting oil exposure
Cyanosis

D

Dams
Decompression sickness
Dengue fever
Diphtheria
Disaster preparedness
Disease outbreaks
Drinking water supply
Drought
Dysentery

E

Earth day
Earthquakes
Ebola hemorrhagic fever
Electric shock injuries
Emergency Planning and Community Right-to-Know Act (1986)
Emergency preparedness
Emergent diseases
Emphysema

Endemic
Endocrine disruptors
Environmental Protection Agency
Epidemiology
Ergonomics
Escherichia coli
Explosives
Exposure science
Exxon Valdez

F

Famine
Federal Insecticide, Fungicide, and Rodenticide Act (1972)
Federal Water Pollution Control Act (1972)
Fibrosis
Flooding
Flu pandemics
Food additives
Food and Drug Administration
Food contamination
Food poisoning
Food safety
Foodborne illness
Fracking
Fukushima Daiichi nuclear power station
Fungal infections
Fungicide

G

Giardiasis
Global public health
Goiter
Guinea worm disease
Gulf oil spill
Gulf War syndrome

H

H1N1 influenza A
Haiti earthquake
Hantavirus
Hazardous waste
Healthy Cities
Heat disorders
Heat stress index
Heavy metals and heavy metal poisoning
Hemorrhagic fevers
High temperaure environments
Horn of Africa drought and famine
Housing
HPV vaccination
Human papilloma virus
Humanitarian aid
Hurricanes

I

Icelandic volcano eruption
Indoor air quality
Industrial hygiene
Insecticide poisoning
Ionizing radiation

J

Japanese earthquake 2011

K

Katrina

L

Land use
Lead
Lead poisoning
Legionnaire's disease
Leptospirosis
Leukemia
Levee
Listeriosis
Love Canal
Low temperature environments
Lyme disease

M

Malaria
Manganese exposure
Measles
Medical waste
Melanoma
Meningitis
Mercury
Mercury poisoning
Methemoglobinemia
Microbial pathogens
Mold
Multiple chemical sensitivity
Mumps

N

National Ambient Air Quality Standards
National Environmental Health Association
National Environmental Policy Act (1969)
National Institute for Occupational Safety and Health
National Institute of Environmental Health Sciences
National Parks
Nature deficit disorder
Necrotizing fasciitis
Neurotoxin
9/11 terrorist attacks
Noise pollution
Non-ionizing radiation
Norovirus

O

Occupational Safety and Health Act (1970)
Occupational Safety and Health Administration
Oil spills, health effects of
Omnibus Flood Control Act (1936)

One Health Initiative
Oxfam
Ozone
Ozone exposure

P

Pandemic
Parasites
Patch testing
Plague
Polio
Population and disease
Population pyramid
Posttraumatic stress disorder
Protein energy malnutrition
Public Health Service

R

Rachel Carson Council
Radiation
Radiation exposure
Radiation injuries
Red Cross
Resource Conservation and Recovery Act
Risk assessment (public health)
River blindness
Rivers and Harbor Act (1899)
Rodents

S

Safe Drinking Water Act (1972)
Sanitation
Save the Children
Schistosomiasis
Severe acute respiratory syndrome
Seveso, Italy
Shigellosis
Sick building syndrome
Sierra Club
Silicosis
Skin cancer
Sleeping sickness
Smallpox
Smog
Smoking
Soil Conservation Act (1935)
Sulfur exposure
Superfund Amendments and Reauthorization Act (1986)
Swimming advisories

T

Talcosis
Teratogens
Thesaurosis
Three Mile Island
Times Beach
Tornado and cyclone
Toxic sludge spill in Hungary
Toxic Substances Control Act (1976)
Toxicology
Traveler's health
Tropical disease
Tsunamis
Tuberculosis
Typhoid fever
Typhus

U

Ultraviolet radiation
UNICEF
U.S. Department of Health and Human Services

V

Vaccination
Vector (mosquito) control
Viruses
Volatile organic compound
Volcanic eruptions

W

Water fluoridation
Water pollution
Water quality
Water quality standards
Waterborne diseases
West Nile virus
Whooping cough
Wildfires
World Health Organization

XYZ

Yellow fever
Yokkaichi asthma
Zero population growth
Zoonoses

PLEASE READ—IMPORTANT INFORMATION

The *Gale Encyclopedia of Environmental Health* is a health reference product designed to inform and educate readers about a wide variety of environmental health issues affecting the world's population. Gale, Cengage Learning believes the product to be comprehensive, but not necessarily definitive. It is intended to supplement, not replace, consultation with a physician or other healthcare practitioner. While Gale, Cengage Learning has made substantial efforts to provide information that is accurate, comprehensive, and up-to-date, Gale, Cengage Learning makes no representations or warranties of any kind, including without limitation, warranties of merchantability or fitness for a particular purpose, nor does it guarantee the accuracy, comprehensiveness, or timeliness of the information contained in this product. Readers should be aware that the universe of medical knowledge is constantly growing and changing, and that differences of opinion exist among authorities. Readers are also advised to seek professional diagnosis and treatment for any medical condition, and to discuss information obtained from this book with their healthcare provider.

INTRODUCTION

The *Gale Encyclopedia of Environmental Health* is a one-stop source for information that covers all aspects of environmental health, including recent and historic natural and manmade environmental health events, environmentally related health conditions and diseases, important public health practices and initiatives, environmental terms, and significant organizations and legislation. It addresses environmental health concerns affecting the human population globally. The encyclopedia minimizes medical jargon and uses language that any reader can understand, while still providing thorough coverage of each topic.

SCOPE

Over 250 full-length articles are included in *The Gale Encyclopedia of Environmental Health*. Entries follow a standardized format that provides information at a glance. Categories include:

Environmental health crises
- Definition
- Description
- Demographics
- Causes and symptoms
- Common diseases and disorders
- Treatment
- Public health role and response
- Prognosis
- Prevention

Organizations and legislation
- Definition
- Purpose
- Demographics
- Description
- Results
- Research and general acceptance
- Interactions
- Aftercare
- Complications
- Parental concerns

Diseases and conditions
- Definition
- Demographics
- Description
- Causes and symptoms
- Diagnosis
- Treatment
- Public health role and response
- Prognosis
- Prevention

INCLUSION CRITERIA

A preliminary list of environmental health topics was compiled from a wide variety of sources, including professional medical guides and textbooks, consumer guides, and encyclopedias. An advisory board comprised of public health professionals and environmental scientists evaluated the topics and made suggestions for inclusion. The final selections were determined by Gale editors in conjunction with the advisory board.

ABOUT THE CONTRIBUTORS

The entries were written by experienced writers, including healthcare practitioners and educators, researchers, and other professionals. The essays were reviewed by advisors to ensure that they are appropriate, current, and accurate.

HOW TO USE THIS BOOK

The Gale Encyclopedia of Environmental Health has been designed with ready reference in mind:

- Straight **alphabetical arrangement** of topics allows users to locate information quickly.
- **Bold-faced terms** within entries direct readers to related articles.
- Lists of **key terms** are provided where appropriate to define unfamiliar terms or concepts. A **glossary** of key terms is also included at the back of Volume 2.
- **Cross-references** placed throughout the *Encyclopedia* direct readers to primary entries from alternate names and related topics.
- **Questions to Ask Your Doctor** sidebars provide sample questions that patients can ask their physicians.
- **Resources** at the end of every entry direct readers to additional sources of information on a topic.
- Approximately 30 **biographical and historic sidebars** are included with main topical essays. These sidebars are of particular relevance to the entries they accompany and highlight historic figures or events pertaining to the main topic.
- A **chronology** of significant events and discoveries in the field of environmental health helps give the reader a broad sense of the growth of environmental health through time and its importance as a public health discipline.
- Valuable **contact information** for organizations and support groups is included with each entry and compiled in the back of Volume 2.
- A comprehensive **general index** allows users to easily find areas of interest.

GRAPHICS

The Gale Encyclopedia of Environmental Health is enhanced with over 125 full-color images, including photographs, tables, and custom illustrations.

ADVISORY BOARD

A number of experts in public health, medicine, and environmental science have provided invaluable assistance with this encyclopedia. Several of the advisors listed have also acted as contributing advisors, writing various articles related to their fields of expertise and experience.

Peter Brimblecombe, PhD
Professor of Atmospheric Chemistry
School of Environmental Sciences
University of East Anglia
Norwich, United Kingdom

L. Fleming Fallon, MD, PhD, DrPH
Professor and Director of Public Health
College of Health and Human Services
Bowling Green State University
Bowling Green, Ohio

Brenda Wilmoth Lerner, RN
Writer and Managing Editor
LernerMedia
Paris, France

Melinda G. Oberleitner, DNS, RN, APRN, CNS
Associate Dean and Professor
College of Nursing and Allied Health Professions
University of Louisiana at Lafayette
Lafayette, Louisiana

CONTRIBUTORS

Margaret Alic, PhD
Science Writer
Eastsound, Washington

William G. Ambrose Jr., PhD
Department of Biology
Bates College
Lewiston, Maine

William A. Atkins
Science Writer
Atkins Research and
    Consulting
Pekin, Illinois

Howard Baker
Medical Writer
North York, Ontario,
    Canada

Julia R. Barrett
Science Writer
Madison, Wisconsin

Brian R. Barthel, PhD
Department of Community
    Health
Utah Valley University
Orem, Utah

Stuart Batterman, PhD
School of Public Health,
    University of Michigan
Ann Arbor, Michigan

Linda K. Bennington, MNS, RNC
Senior Lecturer
College of Health Sciences
Old Dominion University
Norfolk, Virginia

Paul R. Bloom, PhD
Soil Science Department
University of Minnesota
St. Paul, Minnesota

Gregory D. Boardman, PhD
Department of Civil
    Engineering
Virginia Polytechnic Institute and
    State University
Blacksburg, Virginia

Marci L. Bortman, PhD
The Nature Conservancy
Huntington, New York

Barbara Boughton
Health and Medical Writer
El Cerrito, California

Marie Bundy
Freelance Writer
Port Republic, Maryland

Rosalyn Carson-DeWitt, MD
Medical Writer
Durham, North Carolina

Paul Checchia, MD, FAAP
*Director, Pediatric Cardiac
Intensive Care Program*
St. Louis Children's Hospital
*Assistant Professor of Pediatric
    Critical Care and Cardiology*
Washington University School
    of Medicine
St. Louis, Missouri

Liane Clorfene Casten
Freelance Journalist
Evanston, Illinois

Stacy Chamberlin
Freelance Writer
Michigan

David Clarke
Freelance Journalist
Bethesda, Maryland

Helen Colby, MS

Terence H. Cooper, PhD
Soil Science Department
University of Minnesota
St. Paul, Minnesota

David A. Cramer, MD
Medical Writer
Chicago, Illinois

Rhonda Cloos, RN
Medical Writer
Austin, Texas

Arnold Cua, MD
Physician
Reno, Nevada

John Cunningham
Freelance Writer
St. Paul, Minnesota

Mary Ann Cunningham, PhD
Department of Geology and
    Geography
Vassar College
Poughkeepsie, New York

William P. Cunningham, PhD
Department of Genetics
    and Cell Biology
University of Minnesota
St. Paul, Minnesota

Tish Davidson, AM
Medical Writer
Fremont, California

Frank M. D'Itri, PhD
Institute of Water
    Research
Michigan State University
East Lansing, Michigan

Contributors

Teresa C. Donkin
Freelance Writer
Minneapolis, Minnesota

L. Fleming Fallon, Jr., MD, PhD, DrPH
Professor and Director of Public Health
College of Health and Human Services
Bowling Green State University
Bowling Green, Ohio

Gordon R. Finch, PhD
Department of Civil Engineering
University of Alberta
Edmonton, Alberta, Canada

Karl Finley
Medical Writer
Michigan

Paula Anne Ford-Martin, MA
Wordcrafts
Warwick, Rhode Island

Janie Franz
Freelance Writer
Grand Forks, North Dakota

Rebecca Frey, PhD
Research and Administrative Associate
East Rock Institute
New Haven, Connecticut

Ron Gasbarro, PharmD
Medical Writer
New Milford, Pennsylvania

Jill Granger, MS
Senior Research Associate
University of Michigan
Ann Arbor, Michigan

Laith F. Gulli, MD, MSc(MedSci), MSA, MscPsych, MRSNZ, FRSH, FRIPHH, FAIC, FZS, DAPA, DABFC, DABCI
Consultant Psychotherapist in Private Practice
Lathrup Village, Michigan

Kapil Gupta, MD
Medical Writer
Winston-Salem, North Carolina

Maureen Haggerty
Medical Writer
Ambler, Pennsylvania

Katherine Hauswirth
Freelance Writer
Roanoke, Virginia

Alyson C. Heimer, MA
International Affairs Consultant
New Haven, Connecticut

Malcolm T. Hepworth, PhD
Department of Civil and Mineral Engineering
University of Minnesota
Minneapolis, Minnesota

Fran Hodgkins

Alexander I. Ioffe, PhD
Senior Scientist
Geological Institute of the Russian Academy of Sciences
Moscow, Russia

Michelle L. Johnson, MS, JD
Portland, Oregon

Paul A. Johnson, EdM
Medical Writer
San Diego, California

David Kaminstein, MD
Medical Writer
West Chester, Pennsylvania

Christopher McGrol y Klyza, PhD
Department of Political Science
Middlebury College
Middlebury, Vermont

M. Elizabeth Kunkel

Monique Laberge, PhD
Research Associate
Department of Biochemistry and Biophysics
McGill University
Montreal, Quebec, Canada

Jeffrey P. Larson, RPT
Physical Therapist
Sabin, Minnesota

Jill Lasker
Medical Writer
Midlothian, Virginia

Brenda Wilmoth Lerner, RN
K. Lee Lerner
LernerMedia
Paris, France

Larry Lutwick, MD, FACP
Director, Infectious Diseases
VA Medical Center
Brooklyn, New York

Alair MacLean
Environmental Editor
OMB Watch
Washington, DC

Warren Maltzman, PhD
Consultant, Molecular Pathology
Demarest, New Jersey

Ruth E. Mawyer, RN
Medical Writer
Charlottesville, Virginia

Richard A. McCartney, MD
Fellow, American College of Surgeons
Diplomat, American Board of Surgery
Richland, Washington

Robert G. McKinnell, PhD
Department of Genetics and Cell Biology
University of Minnesota
St. Paul, Minnesota

Leslie Mertz

Melodie Monahan
Copyeditor
West Bloomfield, Michigan

Jeffrey Muhr

David E. Newton
Medical Writer
Ashland, Oregon

Andrea Nienstedt, MA

Melinda G. Oberleitner, DNS, RN, APRN, CNS
Associate Dean and Professor
College of Nursing and Allied Health Professions
University of Louisiana at Lafayette
Lafayette, Louisiana

Stephanie Ocko
Freelance Journalist
Brookline, Massachusetts

Teresa Odle
Medical Writer
Albuquerque, New Mexico

J. Ricker Polsdorfer, MD
Medical Writer
Redmond, Washington

Megan Porter, RD, LD
Research Dietitian and Weight Loss Instructor
Portland, Oregon

Stephen Randtke
Department of Civil Engineering
University of Kansas
Lawrence, Kansas

Lewis G. Regenstein
Author and Environmental Writer
Atlanta, Georgia

Linda Rehkopf
Freelance Writer
Marietta, Georgia

Paul E. Renaud, PhD
Department of Biology
East Carolina University
Greenville, North Carolina

Belinda Rowland, PhD
Medical Writer
Voorheesville, New York

Mark W. Seeley
Department of Soil Science
University of Minnesota
St. Paul, Minnesota

Judith Sims, MS
Science Writer
Logan, Utah

Jennifer Sisk
Medical Writer
Havertown, Pennsylvania

Douglas Smith
Freelance Writer
Dorchester, Massachusetts

Linda Wasmer Smith
Medical Writer
Albuquerque, New Mexico

Anna Rovid Spickler, DVM, PhD
Center for Food Security and Public Health
Iowa State University
Ames, Iowa

Carol Steinfeld
Freelance Writer
Concord, Massachusetts

Paulette L. Stenzel, PhD
Eli Broad College of Business
Michigan State University
East Lansing, Michigan

Liz Swain
Medical Writer
San Diego, California

Bethany Thivierge
Biotechnical Writer/Editor
Technicality Resources
Rockland, Maine

Carol A. Turkington
Medical Writer
Lancaster, Pennsylvania

Samuel Uretsky, PharmD
Medical Writer
Wantagh, New York

Usha Vedagiri
IT Corporation
Edison, New Jersey

Terry Watkins
Indianapolis, Indiana

Ken R. Wells
Freelance Writer
Laguna Hills, California

Angela Woodward
Freelance Writer
Madison, Wisconsin

CHRONOLOGY

165–180	The Antonine Plague, a suspected smallpox outbreak, kills upwards of 5,000 a day in Rome, Italy, possibly killing as many as five million in total.
541	The Plague of Justinian causes the death of one quarter of the Mediterranean population. It is most probably a bubonic plague.
1338–58	The Black Death spreads across Europe, Asia, and Africa, ultimately killing around 100 million people. The cause of this pandemic was bubonic plague.
1492–1900	Europeans spread typhoid, smallpox, measles, and other disease, killing approximately 95% of the Native American population.
1700	Bernardino Ramazzini (1633–1714) publishes first comprehensive occupational health treatise, which was the birth of occupational health.
1700–1800	In the United States, governmental agencies are created to address mounting health problems, sanitation and the protection of water supply, concerns that arose with the industrial revolution.
1779	The first recognized Dengue epidemics occur at about the same time in Asia, Africa, and North America in the 1780s. The disease is named dengue in 1779 with Benjamin Rush describing the first case report in 1789.
1796	Edward Jenner (1749–1843) publishes his first paper on the potential for inoculation, which leads to the development of the small pox vaccine.
1793	Yellow Fever appears in the United States in the late seventeenth century. In 1793, Philadelphia is the scene of one of the worst outbreaks.
1804	The first city water treatment plant is built in Scotland, initiating the idea that all people should have access to clean, safe drinking water.
1816–26	The first of seven cholera outbreaks kills over 100,000 British soldiers in Europe and Asia and is believed to have spread in Calcutta from infected rice. The total number of victims is unknown.
1829–51	A second cholera pandemic in the United States, Asia, and Europe kills over 100,000.
1842	Social reformer Edwin Chadwick, publishes his landmark report, *Report on the Inquiry into Sanitary Conditions of the Laboring Population of Great Britain*. This report outlines the major public health challenges facing England, leading to the beginnings of reform.
1852–60	A third cholera epidemic strikes Russia. One million people die.
1860	Louis Pasteur describes germ theory. He also develops pasteurization process to kill bacteria in liquids such as milk.
1863	New York City conducts the first sanitary survey. New York's Association for the Improvement of the Condition of the Poor (est. 1844) finds "dark, contracted, ill constructed, badly ventilated and disgustingly filthy" housing. Some 18,000 people live in cellar apartments whose floors are putrid mud.
1872	The American Public Health Association (APHA) founded by Dr. Stephen Smith, a physician, attorney and commissioner of New York City's Metropolitan Health Board, puts forth the concept of a national health service.
1879	The National Board of Health is established.

1881	The first anthrax vaccine is perfected by Louis Pasteur.
1881	The Red Cross is founded by Clara Barton.
1884	Sir Edwin Chadwick becomes the founding president of the Association of Public Sanitary Inspectors in England. The Association is now known as the Chartered Institute of Environmental Health.
1845–49	Famine in Ireland kills more than one million. One to two million Irish emigrate to escape the famine.
1880	Working at a military hospital in Constantine, Algeria, Dr. Alfonse Laveran discovers the parasite responsible for malaria.
1891	Bisphenol A is first synthesized by Russian chemist, Alexksandr Dianin.
1889–90	The Asiatic or Russian flu is first reported in Russia in May 1889. It spreads all over the world and within the course of a year kills over 250,000 in Western Europe alone.
1892	The Sierra Club is founded by John Muir.
1895	APHA publishes the *Standard Methods for the Examination of Water and Sewage*.
1900	Walter Reed reports at the APHA Annual Meeting that mosquitoes carry yellow fever.
1903	Typhoid fever in Ithaca, New York, causes 82 deaths that include 29 Cornell University students. Contamination is traced to a dam construction site.
1905	APHA publishes the *Standard Methods for the Examination of Milk*.
1906	The first Federal Food and Drug Act passes; APHA publishes the *American Journal of Public Hygiene*.
1906	A typhoid outbreak in New York is traced to a cook named Mary Mallon. "Typhoid Mary" is a carrier of the disease but refuses to stop working. She is quarantined for life on North Brothers Island. Total number of typhus deaths reach 600 in 1906, with three victims being attributed to Mary Mallon.
1911	Raw milk causes streptococcus outbreak in Boston, Massachusetts, that kills 48, when it is delivered door-to-door.
1911	*Journal of the American Public Health Association* is established, later becoming the *American Journal of Public Health*.
1916	A polio epidemic kills 6,000 in the United States.
1918–19	Also known as the Spanish Flu, the influenza pandemic spreads from the United States to other parts of the world, most likely exacerbated by the movement of soldiers during World War I. An estimated 50 to 100 million people die within six months.
1919	Eglantyne Jebb establishes the Save the Children fund in England to aid children affected by World War I in Europe.
1919	An outbreak of botulism is responsible for killing 19 in the United States and is traced to canned olives from California.
1922	Door-to-door-delivered raw milk contaminated by streptococcus kills 22 in Portland, Oregon.
1924–25	More than 1,500 from New York, Chicago, and Washington, DC, become ill with typhoid fever from consuming oysters from Long Island, New York. One hundred fifty die.
1928	Scottish physician Alexander Fleming (1881–1955) inadvertently discovers penicillin while studying molds.
1932	Save the Children spreads to the United States in order to aid children of the Great Depression.
1938	The Fair Labor Standards Act (FLSA) passes as part of President Roosevelt's New Deal. FLSA provides regulations for employers to improve conditions of workers.
1942	The Oxford Committee for Famine Relief (Oxfam) is founded in Britain to help get food to women and children starving in enemy-occupied Greece during World War II.
1944	The National Health Service is founded in Great Britain.
1946	Centers for Disease Control and Prevention (CDC) is established in 1946 in Atlanta as the Communicable Disease Center.
1948	United Nations establishes the World Health Organization.
1950	Jonas Salk (1914–1995) introduces Salk vaccine for polio.
1950	Mass TB immunization with the Bacille Calmette-Guerin (BCG) vaccine is under way to protect children from tuberculosis.

1952	The Great Smog of London kills as many as 12,000.
1952	In the United States, polio takes the lives of 3,000.
1953–87	Camp Lejeune water supply is contaminated with harmful chemicals that sicken military personnel and their families.
1955	The polio vaccine virtually eradicates polio from the United States.
1956	National Library of Medicine opens.
1961	The burning of petroleum and crude oil in Yokkaiichi, Japan, causes a toxic smog containing sulfur dioxide.
1962	President John F. Kennedy signs into law the Migrant Health Act, which provides for the establishment of health clinics across the nation designed to deal specifically with migrant health issues.
1963	Measles vaccine is developed.
1964	The Surgeon General's Report on Smoking and Health is published; President Johnson signs the Medicare/Medicaid Act.
1968	Noroviruses are named after the original strain that caused an outbreak of gastroenteritis in a Norwalk, Ohio school.
1969	Federal Coal Mine Health and Safety Act of 1969 passes in the United States.
1970	Congress establishes the Environmental Protection Agency(EPA); the Occupational Safety and Health Administration (OSHA); and the National Institute for Occupational Safety and Health (NIOSH).
1970	Amendments to the Clean Air Act greatly expand its effectiveness.
1972	The Clean Water Act passes.
1975	First cases of Lyme disease are discovered in Lyme, Connecticut, where the disease gets its name.
1976	Two hundred twenty-one attendees of the American Legion conference in Philadelphia fall ill and 34 die. The disease is called Legionaire's disease.
1976	In Seveso, Italy, a town near Milan, poisonous chemical dioxin is released into the air by an explosion at a Hoffman-LaRoche chemical plant, causing evacuation of 600 and hundreds of cases of chloroacne. Animal deaths are widespread.
1979	An anthrax outbreak in the Soviet Union is suspected to be caused by secret bioweapons lab.
1979	Three Mile Island nuclear power station suffers a heating of the core but not a full reactor meltdown. Thirteen million curies of radioactive gases are released. The INES rating is a 5, meaning it is an accident with wider consequences. No deaths are attributed to the accident.
1980	The Love Canal neighborhood near Niagara Falls, New York, is evacuated due to leakage of hazardous chemicals from a former dump site on which the neighborhood was built.
1980	The World Health Organization announces the eradication of smallpox.
1981	The CDC begins to report cases of rare pneumonia and cancers in young gay men. This marks the beginning of the AIDS/HIV epidemic though the virus was present previously.
1982	Acquired Immune Deficiency Syndrome (AIDS) becomes an established term.
1984	Salmonella used by cult to contaminate salad bars in rural Oregon causes 750 cases.
1984	The Union Carbide plant in Bhopal, India, leaks an estimated 32 tons of toxic gases, leading to approximately 20,000 deaths.
1984–85	Famine in Ethiopia gets worldwide attention that results in Live Aid concerts around the world.
1985	Listeria-contaminated Mexican cheese produced in Los Angeles sickens Hispanic women, many whom were pregnant. Twenty-eight die.
1985	Times Beach, Missouri, evacuates and becomes a ghosttown in the aftermath of EPA findings confirming years of DDT contamination.
1986	Chernobyl nuclear power station melts down during a safety check of the system. WHO estimates 9,000 victims of the meltdown. The International Nuclear and Radiological Event Scale (INES) ranks Chernobyl a 7, meaning it is a major long-term impact on humans and the environment.
1987	Global AIDS initiative is started by the World Health Organization.
1988	Congress passes the Medical Waste Tracking Act of 1988.

1989	The *Exxon Valdez* spills approximately 11 million U.S. gallons (38,000 m³) of oil into Prince William Sound.		2004	A fourth death is attributed to avian flu in Vietnam.
1989	The Kids in the Environment project in California launches children's environmental health (CEH) initiatives in the United States.		2005	Hurricane Katrina hits New Orleans, causing levees to break and widespread devastation creates an environmental health crisis. Approximately 2,000 people die.
1991	Approximately 250,000 military deployed during the Gulf War experience a multi-symptom illness of unexplained origin known as Gulf War syndrome.		2006	APHA launches Get Ready campaign, an all hazards preparedness initiative.
			2006	Former Soviet KGB agent tests positive for polonium and dies in London.
1991–92	Drought and civil war cause famine in Somalia. An estimated 300,000 deaths occur.		2006	E. coli O157:H7 outbreak involves bagged spinach grown at Paicines Ranch in San Benito County, California. Five die and 200 people become ill after eating bagged spinach.
1994	Medicine and Public Health Initiative is established by the APHA and American Medical Association.		2008	Babies in China are poisoned by melamine in Chinese-produced infant formula. At least three babies die. Melamine is the same chemical found to sicken and kill pets in 2007 Chinese-produced pet foods.
1995	Former President Bill Clinton proclaims the first full week of April as National Public Health Week.			
1995	Religious cult releases sarin gas in Tokyo subway killing 12.			
1997	Prior to her death, Diana, Princess of Wales, supports the cause to ban land mines. Her support brings public awareness to the health and safety problems caused by land mines left in conflict areas.		2008	Cyclone kills 22,000 in Myanmar.
			2008	An earthquake in Sichuan Province in China kills 50,000.
			2008–09	Cholera outbreak in Zimbabwe takes over 4,000 lives.
1998	Twenty-one people die from listeria-contaminated Ball Park brand hot dogs and Sara Lee deli meats processed at a Michigan plant.		2008–09	Contamination of peanut butter with salmonella typhimurium causes 714 to become ill across 46 states. Nine die.
			2009	Over 15,000 die worldwide from influenza.
2001	September 11th terrorist attacks result in almost 3,000 deaths. Subsequent illness and deaths associated with exposure during the attacks continue to be assessed.		2009	Swine flu victims reach 60 in Mexico as the world faces a possible pandemic with the H1N1 virus.
			2009	Australian bush fires claim 181 lives.
2001	Anthrax letters sent to 5 media outlets and 2 senators offices sicken 22 people and kill 5.		2010	An earthquake with a 7.0 magnitude strikes Haiti, killing over 300,000, injuring over 300,000, and displacing over 1 million people. An outbreak of cholera rises.
2002	Listeria-contaminated Pilgrim's Pride brand turkey meats sicken people in multiple states and cause eight deaths.			
2003	Severe acute respiratory syndrome (SARS) is a contagious and potentially fatal disease that first appears in the form of a multi-country outbreak in early February 2003.		2010	Deepwater Horizon oil spill leaks an estimated 155 million gallons of oil into the Gulf of Mexico. The initial explosion kills 11 people. Long-term health effects are unknown.
2004	Earthquake with 9.1 magnitude hits off the coast of Sumatra, causing catastrophic tsunami that hits 14 countries. Over 225,000 people die and 1.7 million are displaced.		2010	An industrial accident releases 35 million cubic feet (1 million cubic meters) of liquid alumina sludge in western Hungary. Approximately nine people die and 122 are injured.

2010	More than 1,100 die in Pakistan floods.
2011	Cantaloupes from Colorado spread listeria across 28 states, sickening 146 and killing 36.
2011	The Joplin, Missouri, tornado kills 117 and is one of the deadliest in U.S. history.
2011	Fukushima Daiichi nuclear power station meltdown rates an INES 7 and is one of the worst nuclear disasters. The nuclear meltdown occurs following an earthquake and devastating tsunami that hits the Japanese coast.
2011–12	Haiti fights cholera outbreaks since the 2010 earthquake. Over 6,500 people die.
2011–12	East Africa drought causes famine in Somalia.
2012	The United States experiences an outbreak of fungal meningitis that kills 15 and a rash of necrotizing fasciitis cases during the summer. Hantavirus causes deaths of campers at Yellowstone National Park.
2012	Eleven people die in Cuba from Hurricane Sandy. The United States sustains catastrophic flooding in the most populated areas of New York City and the East Coast. Forty people die as a result of the super storm.
2013	A Carnival cruise ship takes five days after a fire cuts power onboard to reach port. Passengers face questionable sanitary conditions and cruise ship health is brought to the attention of the public.
2013	A meteor injures at least 950 when it crashes in the Ural mountains near Chelyabinsk, Russia.

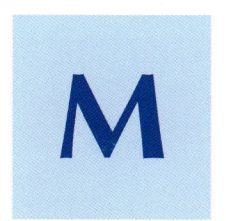

Mad cow disease *see* **Creutzfeldt-Jakob disease**

Malaria

Definition

Malaria is a serious infectious disease caused by a parasite called *plasmodium*, which is transmitted via bites of infected mosquitoes. In the human body, the **parasites** multiply in the liver and then infect red blood cells. The disease is most common in tropical climates. It is characterized by recurrent symptoms of chills, fever, and an enlarged spleen. The disease can be treated with medication, but it often recurs. Malaria is **endemic** (occurs frequently in a particular locality) in many developing countries. Isolated, small outbreaks sometimes occur within the boundaries of the United States. There are concerns that **climate change** might allow the disease to be more widespread if suitable breeding areas for the mosquitoes are present.

Description

Malaria is a growing problem in the United States. The **Centers for Disease Control and Prevention** (CDC) continues to conduct malaria surveillance in order to detect locally acquired cases. Since the Anopheles mosquito that carries the malaria parasite exists in the United States, there is a constant risk that malaria could be reintroduced. In 2007, CDC reported 1,505 cases of malaria among persons in the United States. All but one of these cases were acquired outside the United States; one was acquired through a blood transfusion. More than half of the cases were reported by New York, Florida, California, Texas, New Jersey, and Maryland. Although malaria can be transmitted in blood, the U.S. blood supply is not screened for malaria. Widespread malarial epidemics are far less likely to occur in the United States, but small localized epidemics could return to the Western world. As of 2012, primary care physicians were being advised to screen returning travelers with fever for malaria.

The picture is far more bleak, however, outside the territorial boundaries of the United States. In 2012, about 3.3 billion people, half of the world's population, were at risk of malaria, according to the **World Health Organization** (WHO). Every year, this situation leads to about 250 million malaria cases and nearly one million deaths. People living in the poorest countries are the most vulnerable, including Africa, India, Southeast Asia, the Middle East, Oceania, and Central and South America. Malaria is a extremely serious problem in Africa, where one in every five childhood deaths is due to the effects of the disease. An African child has on average between 1.6 and 5.4 episodes of malaria fever each year, and a child in Africa dies every 30 seconds from the disease.

As many as 500 million people worldwide are left with chronic anemia due to malaria infection. In some parts of Africa, people battle up to 40 or more separate episodes of malaria in their lifetime The spread of malaria is becoming even more serious as the parasites that cause malaria develop resistance to the drugs used to treat the condition.

Causes and symptoms

Human malaria is caused by four different species of a parasite belonging to genus *Plasmodium*: *Plasmodium falciparum* (the most deadly), *Plasmodium vivax*, *Plasmodium malariae*, and *Plasmodium ovale*. The last two are fairly uncommon. Many animals can get malaria, but human malaria does not spread to animals. Similarly, animal malaria does not spread to humans.

Individuals get malaria when bitten by a female mosquito that is looking for a blood meal and is infected with the malaria parasite. The parasites enter the blood stream and travel to the liver, where they

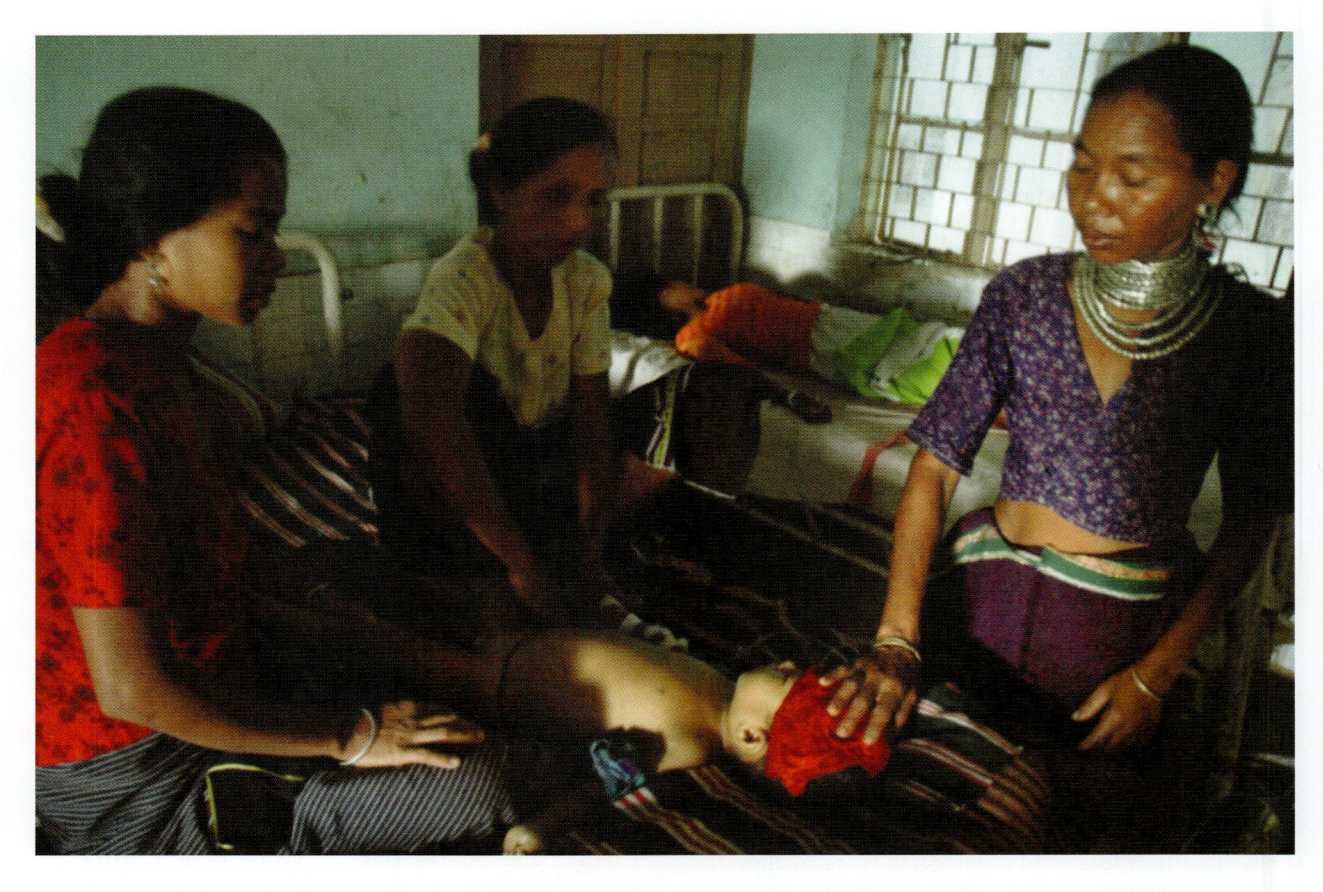

An eight-month-old child suffering from malaria in the Gandachara village in the Dhalai district of the northeastern state of Tripura in India. *(AP Images/Ramakanta Dey)*

multiply. When they re-emerge in the blood, symptoms appear. By the time patients show symptoms, the parasites have reproduced rapidly, clogging blood vessels and rupturing blood cells.

Malaria cannot be casually transmitted from one person to another. Instead, a mosquito bites an infected person and then passes the infection on to the next human it bites. Malaria also spreads via contaminated needles or in blood transfusions. Thus, all blood donors are carefully screened with questionnaires for possible exposure to malaria.

It is possible to contract malaria in nonendemic areas, although such cases are rare. Nevertheless, at least 89 cases of so-called airport malaria, in which travelers contract malaria while passing through crowded airport terminals, have been identified since 1969.

The amount of time between the mosquito bite and the appearance of symptoms varies, depending on the strain of parasite involved. The incubation period is usually between 8 and 12 days for falciparum malaria, but it can be as long as a month for the other types. Symptoms from some strains of *P.vivax* may not appear until 8–10 months after the mosquito bite occurred.

The primary symptom of all types of malaria is the malaria ague (chills and fever). In most cases, the fever has three stages, beginning with uncontrollable shivering for an hour or two, followed by a rapid spike in temperature (as high as 106°F), which lasts three to six hours. Then, just as suddenly, the patient begins to sweat profusely, which will quickly bring down the fever. Other symptoms may appear, including fatigue, severe headache, and nausea and vomiting. As the sweating subsides, the patient typically feels exhausted and falls asleep. In many cases, this cycle of chills, fever, and sweating occurs every other day, or every third day, and may last for between a week and a month. Those with the chronic form of malaria may have a relapse as long as 50 years after the initial infection.

Falciparum malaria is far more severe than other types of malaria because the parasite attacks all red blood cells, not just the young or old cells, as do other types. It causes the red blood cells to become sticky. A patient with this type of malaria can die within hours of the first symptoms. The fever is prolonged. So many red blood cells are destroyed that they block the blood vessels in vital organs (especially the kidneys), and the spleen becomes enlarged. There may be brain damage, leading to coma and convulsions. The kidneys and liver may fail.

Malaria in pregnancy can lead to premature delivery, miscarriage, or stillbirth.

Certain kinds of mosquitoes (called anopheles) can pick up the parasite by biting infected humans. (The more common kinds of mosquitoes in the United States do not transmit the infection.) This is true for as long as those individuals have parasites in their blood. Since strains of malaria do not protect against each other, it is possible for individuals to be reinfected with the parasites repeatedly. It is also possible for individuals to develop a chronic infection without developing an effective immune response.

Diagnosis

Malaria is diagnosed by examining blood under a microscope. The parasite can be seen in the blood smears on a slide. These blood smears may need to be repeated over a 72-hour period in order to make a diagnosis. Antibody tests are not usually helpful because many people develop antibodies from past infections, and the tests may not be readily available. A laser test to detect the presence of malaria parasites in the blood was developed in 2002.

Two new techniques to speed the laboratory diagnosis of malaria show promise. The first is acridine orange (AO), a staining agent that works much faster (3–10 min) than the traditional Giemsa stain (45–60 min) in making the malaria parasites visible under a microscope. The second is a bioassay technique that measures the amount of histadine-rich protein II (HRP2) in the patient's blood. It allows for an accurate estimation of parasite development. A dip strip that tests for the presence of HRP2 in blood samples appears to be more accurate in diagnosing malaria than standard microscopic analysis.

Individuals who become ill with chills and fever after being in an area where malaria exists must see a doctor and mention their recent travel to endemic areas. Individuals with the above symptoms who have been in a high-risk area should insist on a blood test for malaria. The doctor may believe the symptoms are just the common flu virus. Malaria is often misdiagnosed by North American doctors who are not used to seeing the disease. Delaying treatment of falciparum malaria can be fatal.

Malaria

Malaria caused an estimated 655,000 deaths in the world in 2010 (most recent year for which the World Health Organization [WHO] had statistics. These statistics represent a decline from 863,000 in 2008.

Estimated malaria cases and deaths by WHO Region, 2010

	Estimated cases	Estimated deaths
African Region	174 million	596,000
Americas Region	1 million	1,000
Eastern Mediterranean Region	10 million	15,000
European Region	200	0
South-East Asia Region	28 million	38,000
Western Pacific Region	2 million	5,000

(Table by PreMediaGlobal. © 2013 Cengage Learning.)

Treatment

Falciparum malaria is a medical emergency that must be treated in the hospital. The type of drugs, the method of giving them, and the length of the treatment depend on where the malaria was contracted and how sick the patient is.

For all strains except falciparum, the treatment for malaria is usually chloroquine (Aralen) by mouth for three days. Those falciparum strains suspected to be resistant to chloroquine are usually treated with a combination of quinine and tetracycline. In countries where quinine resistance is developing, other treatments may include clindamycin (Cleocin), mefloquin (Lariam), or sulfadoxone/pyrimethamine (Fansidar). Most patients receive an antibiotic for seven days. Those who are very ill may need intensive care and intravenous (IV) malaria treatment for the first three days.

Individuals who acquired falciparum malaria in the Dominican Republic, Haiti, Central America west of the Panama Canal, the Middle East, or Egypt can still be cured with chloroquine. Almost all strains of falciparum malaria in Africa, South Africa, India, and Southeast Asia are resistant to chloroquine. In Thailand and Cambodia, there are strains of falciparum malaria that have some resistance to almost all known drugs.

Patients with falciparum malaria need to be hospitalized and given antimalarial drugs in different combinations and doses depending on the resistance of the strain. Patients may need IV fluids, red blood cell transfusions, kidney dialysis, and assistance breathing.

The drug primaquine may prevent relapses after recovery from *P. vivax* or *P. ovale*. These relapses are caused by a form of the parasite that remains in the liver and can reactivate months or years later.

Another drug, halofantrine, is available abroad. While it is licensed in the United States, it is not marketed in the United States, and it is not recommended by the CDC.

Alternative treatment

The Chinese herb qiinghaosu (the Western name is artemisinin) has been used in China and Southeast Asia to fight severe malaria, and it became available in Europe in 1994. Because this treatment often fails, it is usually combined with another antimalarial drug (mefloquine) to boost its effectiveness. It is not available in the United States and other parts of the developed world due to fears of its toxicity, in addition to licensing and other issues.

The Western herb wormwood (*Artemesia annua*) that is taken as a daily dose can be effective against malaria. Protecting the liver with herbs such as goldenseal (*Hydrastis canadensis*), Chinese goldenthread (*Coptis chinensis*), and milk thistle (*Silybum marianum*) can be used as preventive treatment. Taking precautions to prevent mosquitoes from biting is another possible way to avoid malaria.

Prognosis

If treated in the early stages, malaria can be cured. Those who live in areas where malaria is epidemic, however, can contract the disease repeatedly, never fully recovering between bouts of acute infection.

Prevention

Malaria is an especially difficult disease to prevent by **vaccination** because the parasite goes through several separate stages. One vaccine appeared to protect up to 60% of people exposed to malaria. This was evident during field trials for the drug that were conducted in South America and Africa.

The World Health Association (WHO) worked to eliminate malaria between 1970 and 2000 by controlling mosquitoes. Their efforts were successful as long as the pesticide DDT killed mosquitoes and antimalarial drugs cured those who were infected. In the early 2000s, however, the problem returned a hundredfold, especially in Africa. Because both the mosquito and parasite were extremely resistant to the insecticides designed to kill them, governments tried to teach people to take antimalarial drugs as a preventive medicine and avoid getting bitten by mosquitoes.

Those who use the following preventive measures get fewer infections than those who do not:

- between dusk and dawn, remain indoors in well-screened areas
- sleep inside pyrethrin or permethrin repellent-soaked mosquito nets
- wear clothes covering the entire body

Individuals visiting endemic areas should take antimalarial drugs starting a day or two before they leave the United States. The drugs used are usually

---

KEY TERMS

Arteminisinins—A family of antimalarial products derived from an ancient Chinese herbal remedy. Two of the most popular varieties are artemether and artesunate, used mainly in Southeast Asia in combination with mefloquine.

Chloroquine—An antimalarial drug that began being used in the 1940s and stopped being used after evidence of quinine resistance appeared in the 1960s. In the early 2000s, it was considered ineffective against falciparum malaria almost everywhere. However, because it is inexpensive, it continued to be the antimalarial drug most widely in Africa. Native individuals with partial immunity may have better results with chloroquine than travelers with no previous exposure.

Mefloquine—An antimalarial drug that was developed by the U.S. Army in the early 1980s. By the early 2000s, malaria resistance to this drug had become a problem in some parts of Asia (especially Thailand and Cambodia).

Quinine—One of the first treatments for malaria, a natural product made from the bark of the Cinchona tree. It was popular until being superseded by chloroquine in the 1940s. In the wake of widespread chloroquine resistance, however, it became popular again. Quinine, or its close relative quinidine, can be given intravenously to treat severe *Falciparum* malaria.

Sulfadoxone/pyrimethamine (Fansidar)—An antimalarial drug developed in the 1960s. It was the first drug tried in some parts of the world where chloroquine resistance is widespread. It has been associated with severe allergic reactions due to its sulfa component.

chloroquine or mefloquine. This treatment is continued through at least four weeks after leaving the endemic area. However, even those who take antimalarial drugs and are careful to avoid mosquito bites can still contract malaria.

International travelers are at risk for becoming infected. Most Americans who have acquired falciparum malaria visited sub-Saharan Africa; travelers in Asia and South America are less at risk. Travelers who stay in air conditioned hotels on tourist itineraries in urban or resort areas are at lower risk than backpackers, missionaries, and Peace Corps volunteers. Some people in western cities where malaria does not usually exist may acquire the infection from a mosquito carried onto a jet. This is called airport or runway malaria.

Resources

BOOKS

Ashraf A. "Malaria." In *Ferri's Clinical Advisor 2010*. Philadelphia: Mosby Elsevier, 2010.

Beers, Mark H., and Robert Berkow, eds. "Extraintestinal Protozoa: Malaria." *The Merck Manual of Diagnosis and Therapy*. Whitehouse Station, NJ: Merck Research Laboratories, 2004.

Fairhurst, R. M., and T. E. Wellems. "Plasmodium Species (Malaria)." In *Principles and Practice of Infectious Diseases*, 7th ed. Edited by G. L. Mandell, J. E. Bennett, and R. Dolin. Philadelphia: Elsevier Churchill Livingstone, 2009.

Krogstad, D. J. "Malaria." In *Cecil Medicine*, 23rd ed. Edited by Lee Goldman, and D. Ausiello. Philadelphia: Saunders Elsevier, 2007.

Rocco, Fiammetta. *Quinine: Malaria and the Quest for a Cure That Changed the World*. New York: Harper Perennial, 2004.

World Health Organization. *World Malaria Report 2008*. Geneva: World Health Organization, 2008.

PERIODICALS

Van Lieshout, M., et al. "Climate Change and Malaria: Analysis of the SRES Climate and Socio-Economic Scenarios." *Global Environmental Change* 14 (2004): 87–99.

WEBSITES

Bill & Melinda Gates Foundation. "Malaria." http://www.gatesfoundation.org/GlobalHealth/Pri_Diseases/Malaria/ (accessed March 1, 2012).

Centers for Disease Control and Prevention (CDC). "Malaria." http://www.cdc.gov/malaria (accessed March 1, 2012)

World Health Organization (WHO). "Malaria: Global Malaria Programme (GMP)." WHO Programs and Projects. http://www.who.int/malaria (accessed March 1, 2012).

World Health Organization (WHO). "Malaria: Roll Back Malaria Partnership." WHO Programs and Projects. http://www.rbm.who.int/ (accessed March 1, 2012).

ORGANIZATIONS

Centers for Disease Control Malaria Hotline, (770) 332-4555

Centers for Disease Control Travelers Hotline, (770) 332-4559

Carol A. Turkington
Rebecca J. Frey, PhD
Karl Finley

Manganese exposure

Definition

Manganese exposure occurs when a person comes in contact with high levels of the metallic element manganese. This can happen through the intake of food and water with abnormally high manganese levels or by inhaling airborne manganese.

Description

Manganese is an essential mineral found in some rocks, soil, and foods. Although manganese is an important part in a person's everyday diet, exposure to too much manganese can pose a serious health threat.

Origins

Manganese is a metallic element. When comparing tonnage, manganese is the fourth most used metal in the world, behind iron, aluminum, and copper. Manganese plays an important role in the production of steel and in everyday health. It is an essential mineral, meaning manganese must be part of a person's everyday diet for optimal health and body function.

Manganese can be found naturally in many foods, such as nuts, legumes, seeds, whole grains, leafy green vegetables, and tea. People who do not get enough manganese from their everyday diet may take manganese supplements. Manganese is also found in low levels in soil and in ground and drinking water. Health organizations agree that the upper limit for daily manganese intake is 11 mg. Consuming more manganese than this daily can be very harmful to one's health.

Manganese is also found in some rocks and plays a vital role in the production of steel. It gives steel the ability to be harder, stiffer, and stronger. People with occupations that involve working with steel have a higher risk of being exposed to unsafe levels of manganese. Manganese particles enter the air when welding or steel production takes place. These particles can then be breathed in by workers. Manganese exposure is an important workplace safety issue and has been the subject of many lawsuits.

Causes and symptoms

There are three ways people are exposed to manganese. The first, and most common way, is through eating foods that contain manganese or by taking manganese-containing supplements. Drinking, swimming, or bathing in water containing manganese is the second way people are exposed to the mineral. Finally, people who work in factories that make steel or in occupations such as welding may be exposed to high levels of airborne manganese.

It is important that manganese-containing foods are part of one's everyday diet. However, being exposed to too high levels of manganese can create a serious health risk. Vegetarians who eat a diet high in grains, beans, and nuts may be exposed to higher levels of manganese than the average person. This is also true for people who drink a large amount of tea. Drinking, bathing, or swimming in water that has a high level of manganese will also expose a person to unsafe levels. People with impaired liver function may intake theoretically safe amounts of manganese but experience negative health effects because their livers are not able to properly remove the manganese from their system. Overall, it is uncommon for a person to be exposed to high levels of manganese these ways. Workers who have jobs that involve airborne manganese run the highest risk of manganese exposure.

The most common problem experienced by people who are exposed to high levels of manganese involves the nervous system. These people may show signs of behavioral changes, become slow and clumsy, and have trouble with movements. Symptoms of manganese exposure often are compared to the symptoms of Parkinson's disease, with noticeable tremors and other neurological symptoms. People exposed to lower, yet still unsafe, levels of manganese may show signs of slow movement, such as in the hands. Some studies have shown that manganese workers have fertility problems or a higher rate of low birth weight babies and greater likelihood of offspring with birth defects.

Children exposed to unsafe levels of manganese have shown abnormal brain development. This includes behavioral changes and difficulty learning and remembering. A 2010 study done in Canada found that children who were exposed to higher levels manganese at home through tap water averaged six points lower on IQ tests than children who had little or no manganese in their tap water. This was true even when all water in the study met Canada's guidelines for safe manganese concentrations.

Treatment

Testing for manganese exposure can be done through blood, urine, hair, or fecal exams. While low levels of manganese are always found within the body, these tests can allow physicians to see if a person has abnormal amounts of manganese in their system. Past exposures to manganese are hard to measure because in a healthy person, manganese is removed from the body within a few days. People who have been exposed to higher concentrations of manganese over a longer period will need medical treatment.

Chelation therapy, a treatment used for many types of heavy metal poisonings, may be used. The drug edetate calcium disodium is intravenously administered and travels through the blood stream gathering the manganese. This manganese will later be removed from the body through the urine. The entire process takes around 48 hours to complete and can only be performed by a professional who has been trained in chelation therapy. The use of chelation therapy has had very good results, but it may not be completely successful in the treatment of people who have had ongoing exposure to unsafe levels of manganese. By the time symptoms appear, it is often too late to just remove manganese from the body as treatment. As of 2012, there were no approved cures for the neurological and Parkinson's-like symptoms that go along with chronic manganese poisoning. Instead, focus is geared

---

KEY TERMS

Essential mineral—A mineral required in one's diet for optimal health and functioning of the body. Examples of essential minerals include manganese, iron, and zinc.

Fertility—The ability to conceive children.

Parkinson's disease—A neurological disorder caused by deficiency of dopamine, a neurotransmitter, that is a chemical that assists in transmitting messages between the nerves within the brain. It is characterized by muscle tremor or palsy and rigid movements.

Tremor—Shakiness or trembling.

> **QUESTIONS TO ASK YOUR DOCTOR**
>
> - How can I find out the manganese level of my tap water?
> - What can I do to reduce my exposure to manganese at work?
> - Is it safe for my child to take manganese supplements?

toward managing symptoms and slowing the progression of the disease.

Prognosis

Chelation therapy generally is very successful in the treatment of patients who have acute or short-term manganese exposure. People who have had chronic manganese exposure and have developed symptoms of severe neurological damage are unlikely to be cured using chelation therapy. Focus is on managing symptoms and the progression of the disease. Even with treatment, the symptoms of manganese poisoning are often irreversible.

Prevention

The best prevention against manganese exposure is through eating a healthy and well-balanced diet. By drinking, bathing, and swimming in water that meets health standards and not taking an unnecessary amount of manganese supplements, the average person should not be at risk for manganese exposure. People with liver disease should speak to their physician about the amount of manganese in their diet.

People whose occupation puts them at risk for being exposed to high levels of manganese should take precautions at their workplace. This includes removing work clothes that may be covered in manganese dust before returning home, wearing an appropriate mask at work to limit the amount of manganese breathed in, and doing work such as welding in well-ventilated areas. The United States **Food and Drug Administration** has set limits on the amount of manganese allowed in bottled water (0.05 mg/L) and the Occupational Health and Safety Administration has established a limit for manganese concentration in workplace air (5 mg/m^3). These limits have been establish to protect workers and everyday citizens from manganese exposure.

Resources

PERIODICALS

Menezes-Filho, Jose, et al. "Elevated Manganese and Cognitive Performance in School-Aged Children and Their Mothers." *Environmental Research*. (2011) 111(1): 156–163. http://www.ncbi.nlm.nih.gov/pmc/articles/PMC 3026060 (accessed October 15, 2012).

WEBSITES

Agency for Toxic Substances and Disease Registry. "Manganese." http://www.atsdr.cdc.gov/tfacts151.pdf (accessed October 15, 2012).
Agency for Toxic Substances and Disease Registry. "Public Health Statement." http://www.atsdr.cdc.gov/toxpro files/tp151-c1.pdf (accessed October 15, 2012).
U.S. EPA and Toxicity and Exposure Assessment for Children's Health. "Mangansese TEACH Chemical Summary." http://www.epa.gov/teach/chem_summ/ manganese_summary.pdf (accessed October 15, 2012).

ORGANIZATIONS

Agency for Toxic Substances and Disease Registry, 4770 Buford Hwy, NE, Atlanta, GA 30341, (800) 232-4636; TTY: (888) 232-6348, cdcinfo@cdc.gov, http://www. atsdr.cdc.gov/.
International Manganese Institute, 17 rue Duphot, Paris, France, +33 (0) 145 63 06 34, Fax: +33 (0) 1 42 89 42 92, http://www.manganese.org.
United States Environmental Protection Agency (EPA), Ariel Rios Building, 1200 Pennsylvania Avenue, N.W., Washington, DC 20460, (202) 272-0167; TTY (202) 272-0165, http://www.epa.gov.

Tish Davidson, AM

Measles

Definition

Measles is an infection caused by a virus, which displays a characteristic skin rash known as an exanthem. Measles is also sometimes called rubeola, 5-day measles, red measles, or hard measles.

There are two types of measles, each caused by a different virus. Although both produce a rash and fever, they are different diseases. When most people use the term measles they are referring to rubeola. The rubeola virus causes red measles, also known as hard measles or measles. Although most people recover without problems, rubeola can lead to pneumonia or inflammation of the brain (encephalitis). The second type of measles is called the rubella virus or German measles, also known as three-day measles. This type of measles is usually a milder disease. However, this virus can cause significant

Measles

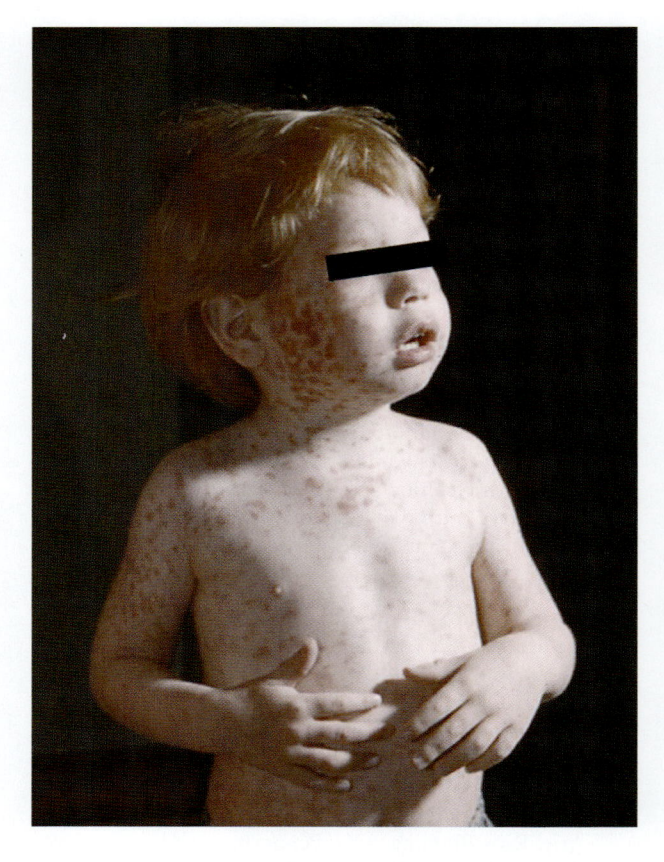

The young boy pictured here displays the characteristic maculopapular rash indicative of rubella, otherwise known as German measles or 3-day measles. *(CDC)*

birth defects if an infected pregnant woman passes the virus to her unborn child.

Description

Measles infections appear all over the world. Prior to the current effective immunization program, large-scale measles outbreaks occurred on a two to three-year cycle, usually in the winter and spring. Smaller outbreaks occurred during the off-years. Babies up to about eight months of age are usually protected from contracting measles, due to immune cells they receive from their mothers in the uterus. Once people have had a measles infection, they can never get it again.

One of the earliest known written descriptions of measles as a disease was provided by an Arab physician in the ninth century who described the differences between measles and **smallpox** in his medical notes. Later, a Scottish physician, Francis Home, demonstrated in 1757 that measles was caused by an infectious agent present in the blood of patients. In 1954 the virus that causes measles was isolated in Boston, Massachusetts, by John F. Enders and Thomas C. Peebles. Before measles vaccine was developed in 1963, nearly all children got measles by the time they were 15 years of age. Each year prior to 1963, about 450-500 people died because of measles, 48,000 were hospitalized, 7,000 had seizures, and about 1,000 suffered permanent brain damage or deafness. Today only about 50 cases a year are reported in the United States, and most of these originate outside the country.

Demographics

As a result of widespread immunization, the measles virus does not circulate in the United States. All reported cases of measles in the United States have been brought in from other countries, usually Europe and Asia. Travelers leaving the United States should be immune to measles. Although measles is usually considered to be a childhood disease, it can be contracted at any age by a person who never had the disease or been vaccinated. Unvaccinated individuals are 22 times more likely to get measles than are those who have two measles vaccines, usually given as measles, **mumps** and rubella vaccine (MMR).

Causes and symptoms

Measles is caused by a type of virus called a paramyxovirus. It is an extremely contagious infection, spread through the tiny droplets that may spray into the air when an individual carrying the virus sneezes or coughs. About 85% of those people exposed to the virus will become infected with it. About 95% of those people infected with the virus will develop the illness called measles. Once people are infected with the virus, it takes about 7–18 days before they actually becomes ill. The most contagious time period is the three to five days before symptoms begin through about four days after the characteristic measles rash has begun to appear.

The first signs of measles infection are fever, extremely runny nose, red eyes, and a cough. A few days later, a rash appears in the mouth, particularly on the mucous membrane lining the cheeks. This rash consists of tiny white dots (like grains of salt or sand) on a reddish bump. These are called Koplik's spots, and are unique to measles infection. The throat becomes red, swollen, and sore.

A couple of days after the appearance of the Koplik's spots, the measles rash begins. It appears in a characteristic progression, from the head, face, and neck, to the trunk, then abdomen, and next out along the arms and legs. The rash starts out as flat, red patches, but eventually develops some bumps. The rash may be somewhat itchy. When the rash begins to appear, the fever usually climbs higher, sometimes reaching as high as 105°F (40.5°C). There may be nausea, vomiting, diarrhea, and multiple swollen lymph nodes. The cough is usually more problematic at this point, and the patient feels very sick. The rash usually lasts about five days. As it fades, it turns a brownish color, and eventually the affected skin becomes dry and flaky.

Many patients (about 5–15%) develop other complications. Bacterial infections, such as ear infections, sinus infections, and pneumonia are common, especially in children. Other viral infections may also strike patients. These include croup, **bronchitis**, laryngitis, or viral pneumonia. Inflammation of the liver, appendix, intestine, or lymph nodes within the abdomen may cause other complications. Rarely, inflammations of the heart or kidneys, a drop in platelet count (causing episodes of difficult-to-control bleeding), or reactivation of an old **tuberculosis** infection can occur.

An extremely serious complication of measles infection is swelling of the brain. Called encephalitis, this can occur up to several weeks after the basic measles symptoms have resolved. About one out of every thousand patients develops this complication, and about 10–15% of these patients die. Symptoms include fever, headache, sleepiness, seizures, and coma. Long-term problems following recovery from measles encephalitis may include seizures and mental retardation.

A very rare complication of measles can occur up to 10 years following the initial infection. Called subacute sclerosing panencephalitis, this is a slowly progressing, smoldering swelling and destruction of the entire brain. It is most common among people who had measles infection prior to the age of two years. Symptoms include changes in personality, decreased intelligence with accompanying school problems, decreased coordination, involuntary jerks and movements of the body. The disease progresses so that affected individuals become increasingly dependent, ultimately becoming bedridden and unaware of their surroundings. Blindness may develop, and the temperature may spike (rise rapidly) and fall unpredictably as the brain structures responsible for temperature regulation are affected. Death is inevitable.

Measles during pregnancy is a serious disease, leading to increased risk of a miscarriage or stillbirth. In addition, the mother's illness may progress to pneumonia.

Risk factors

People who do not receive the vaccine for measles are much more likely to develop the disease. Unvaccinated people traveling to developing countries, where measles is more common, are also at higher risk of catching the disease., and people who do not have enough vitamin A in their diets are more likely to contract measles and to have more-severe symptoms.

Diagnosis

Measles infection is almost always diagnosed based on its characteristic symptoms, including Koplik's spots, and a rash which spreads from central body structures out toward the arms and legs. If there is any doubt as to the diagnosis, then a specimen of body fluids (mucus, urine) can be collected and combined with fluorescent-tagged measles virus antibodies. Antibodies are produced by the body's immune cells that can recognize and bind to markers (antigens) on the outside of specific organisms, in this case the measles virus. Once the fluorescent antibodies have attached themselves to the measles antigens in the specimen, the specimen can be viewed under a special microscope to verify the presence of measles virus.

Treatment

There are no treatments available to stop measles infection. Treatment is primarily aimed at helping the patient to be as comfortable as possible, and watching carefully so that antibiotics can be started promptly if a bacterial infection develops. Fever and discomfort can be treated with acetaminophen. Children with measles should never be given aspirin, as this has caused the fatal disease Reye's syndrome in the past. A cool-mist vaporizer may help decrease the cough. Patients should be given a lot of liquids to drink, in order to avoid dehydration from the fever.

Some studies have shown that children with measles encephalitis benefit from relatively large doses of vitamin A.

Alternative treatment

Botanical immune enhancement (with echinacea, for example) can assist the body in working through this viral infection. Homeopathic support also can be effective throughout the course of the illness. Some specific alternative treatments to soothe patients with measles include the Chinese herbs bupleurum (*Bupleurum chinense*) and peppermint (*Mentha piperita*), as well as a preparation made from empty cicada (*Cryptotympana atrata*) shells. The itchiness of the rash can be relieved with witch hazel (*Hamamelis virginiana*), chickweed (*Stellaria media*), or oatmeal baths. The eyes can be soothed with an eyewash made from the herb eyebright (*Euphrasia officinalis*). Practitioners of ayurvedic medicine recommend ginger or clove tea.

Prognosis

The prognosis for an otherwise healthy, well-nourished child who contracts measles is usually quite good. In developing countries, however, death rates may reach 15–25%. Adolescents and adults usually have a more difficult course. Women who contract the disease while pregnant may give birth to a baby with hearing impairment. Although only 1 in 1,000 patients with measles will develop encephalitis, 10–15% of those who do will die, and about another 25% will be left with permanent brain damage.

Prevention

Measles is a highly preventable infection. A very effective vaccine exists, made of live measles **viruses** which have been treated so that they cannot cause actual infection. The important markers on the viruses are intact, however, which causes an individual's immune system to react. Immune cells called antibodies are produced, which in the event of a future infection with measles virus will quickly recognize the organism, and kill it off. Measles vaccines are usually given at about 15 months of age; because prior to that age, the baby's immune system is not mature enough to initiate a reaction strong enough to insure long-term protection from the virus. A repeat injection should be given at about 10 or 11 years of age. Outbreaks on college campuses have occurred among unimmunized or incorrectly immunized students.

Measles vaccine should not be given to a pregnant woman, however, in spite of the seriousness of gestational measles. The reason for not giving this particular vaccine during pregnancy is the risk of transmitting measles to the unborn child.

Surprisingly, new cases of measles began being reported in some countries—including Great Britain—in 2001 because of parents' fears about vaccine safety. The combined vaccine for measles, mumps, and rubella (MMR) was claimed to cause **autism** or bowel disorders in some children. However, the **World Health Organization** (WHO) says there is no scientific merit to these claims. The United Nations expressed concern that unwarranted fear of the vaccine would begin spreading the disease in developing countries, and ultimately in developed countries as well. Parents in Britain began demanding the measles vaccine as a separate dose and scientists were exploring that option as an alternative to the combined MMR vaccine. Unfortunately, several children died during an outbreak of measles in Dublin because they had not received the vaccine. Child mortality due to measles is considered largely preventable, and making the MMR vaccine widely available in developing countries is part of WHO's strategy to reduce child mortality by two-thirds by the year 2015.

Public health role and response

According to the **Centers for Disease Control and Prevention** (CDC), worldwide, there are estimated to be 20 million cases and 164,000 deaths linked to measles each year. More than half of the deaths occur in India. In the United States, measles was declared eliminated in 2000 due to high **vaccination** coverage and effective public health response. That means measles no longer occurs year round in the United States. This effect is called "herd" immunity. But herd immunity may now be weakening a bit since some parents are choosing to not vaccinate their children. Measles is still common in some parts of Europe, Asia, the Pacific, and Africa. Travelers who have not been vaccinated are at risk of getting the disease and spreading it to their friends and family members who may not be up to date with vaccinations. Because of this risk, all travelers should be up

---

KEY TERMS

Antibodies—Cells made by the immune system which have the ability to recognize foreign invaders (bacteria, viruses), and thus stimulate the immune system to kill them.

Antigens—Markers on the outside of such organisms as bacteria and viruses, which allow antibodies to recognize foreign invaders.

Encephalitis—Swelling, inflammation of the brain.

Exanthem (plural, exanthems or exanthemata)—A skin eruption regarded as a characteristic sign of such diseases as measles, German measles, and scarlet fever.

Koplik's spots—Tiny spots occurring inside the mouth, especially on the inside of the cheek. These spots consist of minuscule white dots (like grains of salt or sand) set onto a reddened bump. Unique to measles.

MMR vaccine—The standard measles, mumps, and rubella (MMR) vaccine that is given to prevent measles, mumps and rubella (German measles). The MMR vaccine is now given in two dosages. The first should be given at 12-15 months of age. The second vaccination should be given at 4-6 years. There are some exceptions depending on a person's health condition.

> **QUESTIONS TO ASK YOUR DOCTOR**
>
> - What are the indications that I may have measles?
> - How contagious is this disease?
> - What treatment options do you recommend for me?
> - What kind of changes can I expect to see with the antibiotics you have prescribed for me?

to date on their vaccinations, regardless of where they are going. Measles is one of the most contagious diseases, and even domestic travelers may be exposed on airplanes or in airports.

Resources

BOOKS

Corrales-Medina, V.F, et al."Viral and Rickettsial Infections." *Current Medical Diagnosis & Treatment*, edited by S.J. McPhee, et al. 50th ed. New York: McGraw-Hill Companies; 2011.

Justin L. Kaplan, and Robert S. Porter, eds. *The Merck Manual of Diagnosis and Therapy*. 19th ed. Whitehouse Station, NJ: Merck Research Laboratories, 2012.

Parker, A.A., et al. "Measles (Rubeola)." *CDC Health Information for International Travel 2010*, edited by G.W. Brunette, et al. Philadelphia: Mosby Elsevier, 2009.

PERIODICALS

Chiba, M. E., M. Saito, N. Suzuki, et al. "Measles Infection in Pregnancy." *Journal of Infection* 47 (July 2003): 40–44.

"Measles—United States, 2011. (From the Centers for Disease Control and Prevention)." *Journal of the American Medical Association* 307, no. 22 (2012): 2363-2365.

Scott, L. A., and M. S. Stone. "Viral Exanthems." *Dermatology Online Journal* 9 (August 2003): 4.

Sur, D. K., D. H. Wallis, and T. X. O'Connell. "Vaccinations in Pregnancy." *American Family Physician* 68 (July 15, 2003): 299–304.

ORGANIZATIONS

American Academy of Pediatrics (AAP), 141 Northwest Point Boulevard, Elk Grove Village, IL 60007-1098, (847) 434-4000, Fax: (847) 424-8000, kidsdocs@aap.org, http://www.aap.org.

Centers for Disease Control and Prevention (CDC), 1600 Clifton Road, Atlanta, GA 30333, (800) 232-4636, cdcinfo@cdc.gov, http://www.cdc.gov.

Rosalyn Carson-DeWitt, MD
Rebecca J. Frey, PhD
Karl Finley

Medical waste

Definition

Medical waste is solid waste from medical or clinical uses at hospitals, clinics, physician offices, dental offices, blood banks, medical research facilities, and veterinary facilities. Medical waste is a form of **hazardous waste** that is stained or soaked with blood or includes body tissues or organs. Medical waste also can be deemed hazardous because it contains certain toxins or is radioactive.

Description

Waste from medical practices and facilities can include used needles, syringes, surgical gloves, surgical instruments, blood-soaked bandages, lab samples, or body parts. This type of waste can expose people who handle it, and in turn an entire community, to infection. Medical waste materials also can include toxic chemicals, pharmaceuticals, or radioactive materials that can cause health risks to people and pollute the environment.

The **Environmental Protection Agency** began to define and control the tracking and disposal of medical waste in 1989 after Congress passed the Medical Waste Tracking Act of 1988. The act came about mostly because medical waste washed up on several East Coast beaches. Congress directed the **EPA** to gather data on the sources, associated health hazards, and current procedures and regulations for management and disposal of the waste. The EPA also was to evaluate the health hazards associated with transporting, incinerating, and burying medical waste materials in a landfill, and disposing of them in a sanitary sewer system. Under the act, the EPA gathered a lot of data, and most states subsequently controlled medical waste under local regulations.

Infection control practices in hospitals were emphasized and improved following the HIV/AIDS epidemic in the 1980s to better control the spread of the infection to healthcare workers or patients. This work included new hospital policies and government regulations regarding using and disposing of needles and other medical waste. New policies and regulations have been used around the world to better control the spread of many infections, most notably HIV and hepatitis.

Effects on public health

Careless handling of hazardous medical waste can have several detrimental effects on public health. Medical waste containing blood and other body fluids or body parts can spread diseases. Waste with needles

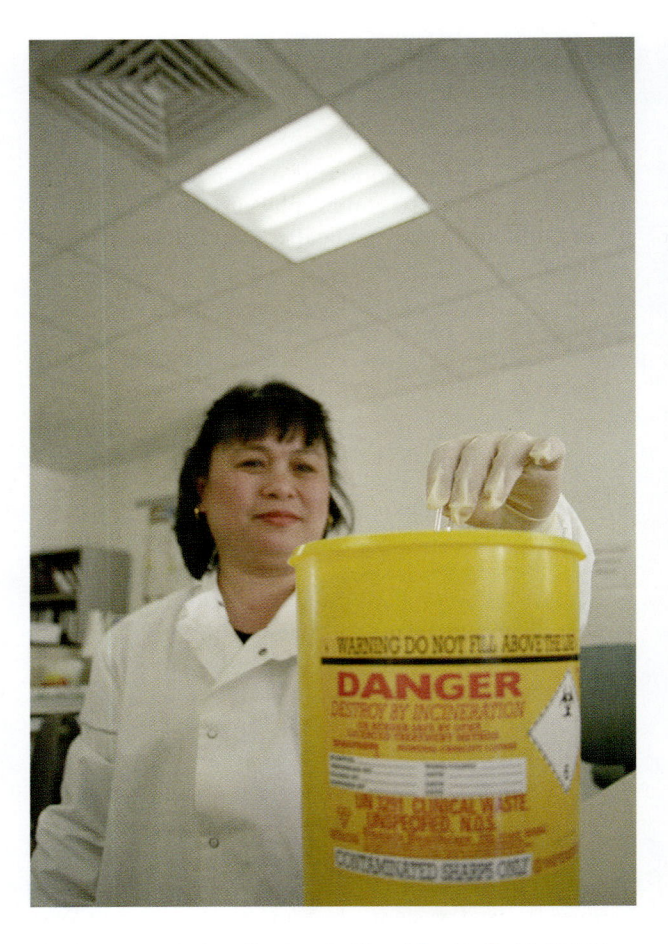

Medical waste being disposed of in a bin. (© Sotiris Zafeiris Photo Researchers, Inc.)

and other sharp objects presents physical hazards, and toxic or radioactive waste can harm individuals or the environment.

Risk factors

Medical waste use and disposal is not regulated everywhere in the world, and little research on public health effects from medical waste has been conducted in developing countries. What is more, there can be hazards associated with small, scattered sources of medical waste. It also can be impossible to enforce all medical waste management in spite of best efforts. As recently as September 2012, Volusia County, Florida, authorities reported medical waste washing ashore at Ormond Beach. The waste included hypodermic needles and medicine bottles that spread over a mile. The source of the waste was unknown.

Demographics

An EPA study reported that approximately 3.2 million tons of medical waste are produced in the United States each year. Not surprisingly, hospitals, long-term health care facilities, and physicians' offices are the major producers of medical wastes, which account for about 0.3% by weight of all municipal solid waste. However, facilities that produce less than 50 lb (23 kg) of medical waste per month are exempt from most requirements. More people are being treated at home, and many people with diabetes treat themselves with daily injections. In short, it is difficult to adequately measure all of the medical waste in the United States or elsewhere in the world.

In addition to ongoing concerns about the potential for medical waste to spread HIV/AIDs and hepatitis, other **disease outbreaks** can be caused or intensified by medical waste. In 2009, **World Health Organization** (WHO) officially recognized the 2009 H1N1 virus as the cause of influenza and noted that a **flu pandemic** was underway. This announcement caused increased attention to the role medical waste can play in spreading the virus through contaminated tissues, gloves, masks, and other waste.

Costs to society

There are potential health, pollution, and esthetic effects of unregulated medical waste. It is expensive for medical facilities to control biohazardous waste and ensure infectious and toxic materials do not enter the general waste stream or pollute communities' air and water. Healthcare facilities can spend five to 10 times as much to dispose of regulated medical waste as they do their general solid waste.

Common diseases and disorders

If not managed properly, medical waste can spread disease from hospital and other clinical settings to the general public. Occupational safety also is a concern because healthcare workers can become infected with diseases their patients have if they do not follow infection control procedures. Infections such as HIV and hepatitis can spread from patients to workers. In addition, some medical waste is toxic to humans and animals and can cause or add to pollution of water if not controlled properly.

Infectious disease

Many diseases can be spread by blood-borne pathogens, disease-causing microorganisms that exist in blood. Certain body fluids also carry blood or transmit pathogens that cause disease. Hepatitis B and HIV/AIDS are serious diseases that receive the most attention in healthcare facilities and the media. HIV is a virus that affects the immune system and can lead to

AIDS and many related conditions. Hepatitis B is an infection caused by the hepatitis B virus that affects the liver. The infection can be chronic and cause long-term damage to the liver. Other diseases that can spread through blood in medical waste are:

- brucellosis
- Creutzfeldt-Jakob disease
- malaria
- hepatitis C

Injuries

Certain types of medical waste can cause disease or injuries. For example, sharps, which include needles, scalpels, and other sharp medical instruments, can be coated with blood or fluids that spread disease but also can injure by cutting someone who comes in contact with them. Genotoxic waste includes highly toxic drugs and materials, such as chemotherapy medications used in treating cancer. Even waste from patients undergoing certain treatments can be highly toxic. These toxins can potentially contaminate municipal wastewater systems. Heavy metals, such as **mercury**, also can make their way to the environment. Mercury is used in thermometers. Its toxic effects vary, but mercury can cause poisoning and death. Its toxins can be released into the air during incineration, adding to **air pollution**. Finally, radioactive materials are used in medical imaging and to treat cancer. Ionizing **radiation** causes cancers. Exposure to high levels of radiation has been linked to birth defects, and direct exposure can cause serious radiation burns. The biggest problem with radioactive waste is the long half-life of the materials. Special management and disposal strategies are required to ensure the radiation is contained.

Public health role and response

The Medical Waste Tracking Act of 1988 was perhaps the most formal large response to managing medical waste and potential spread of disease resulting from medical waste. As a result of the participation of four states (New York, New Jersey, Connecticut, and Rhode Island), along with Puerto Rico, in the voluntary program, the EPA gathered data on the disease-causing potential of medical waste. The data helped the agency determine that the highest potential danger from medical waste existed at the occupational level. The **Occupational Safety and Health Administration** oversees a number of activities aimed at protecting healthcare workers from needlestick injuries and spread of blood-borne pathogens. Infection control practices are developed and monitored at health care facilities, by accrediting organizations, and by states.

> **KEY TERMS**
>
> **Biohazardous**—Describes biological agents or conditions and materials that pose potential hazards to people and the environment.
>
> **Creutzfeldt-Jakob disease**—A rare and progressive disease that targets certain brain tissue and causes early dementia and loss of muscle coordination.

Some states assess penalties for placing infectious waste materials into regular solid waste systems. These policies and regulations protect workers, patients, and communities.

WHO created the first comprehensive global publication to address the hazards and control of medical waste in 1999 and has since updated the information. The document addresses how countries can create regulations, improve planning, and minimize waste. It also suggests strategies for handling medical waste, such as how best to store, transport, and dispose of materials.

Prevention

Developing and adhering to proper controls of medical waste can help prevent threats to public health and safety. These threats might come in the form of infections that spread through blood-borne pathogens or because of health risks introduced by environmental exposure to medical waste products and toxins. Prevention includes proper management practices and knowing how to respond should an unexpected exposure occur. Proper management means that healthcare workers follow infection control policies and procedures promoted by their facilities and all regulations regarding infection control and medical waste management that are enforced by their states.

Efforts and solutions

Healthcare facilities, with the help of their states and consulting companies or agencies, have learned how to reduce the amount of regulated medical waste they produce. Doing so saves the facilities money by only paying for special handling of materials that are hazardous through careful sorting of wastes as employees use and discard them. Preventing the release of toxins such as mercury or dioxins from plastics during incineration has improved somewhat by hospitals packaging waste and shipping it to companies that can control emissions from commercial incinerators. A better solution is to increase use of reusable containers that

> **QUESTIONS TO ASK YOUR DOCTOR**
>
> - Does this facility follow sound infection control policies?
> - How can I safely dispose of medical waste I use in my home?
> - Are there any recent incidents of medical waste exposures in our community?

can be sterilized. An autoclave is equipment that uses steam heated to a temperature that destroys bacteria and pathogens. Materials then can be reused or added to general waste.

WHO asserts that awareness and training are the first steps toward creating change in many countries. The organization offers countries and facilities publications to help guide them in safe medical waste management on a daily basis or in emergencies.

Resources

WEBSITES

Centers for Disease Control and Prevention. "Biologic and Infectious Waste." http://www.cdc.gov/nceh/ehs/etp/biological.htm (accessed September 24, 2012).

Greenpeace International. "Alternatives to Incineration." http://www.greenpeace.org/international/en/campaigns/toxics/incineration/alternatives-to-incineration/ (accessed September 25, 2012).

HealthCare Waste Management. "The 10 Categories of HCRW." http://www.healthcarewaste.org/basics/categories/ (accessed September 25, 2012).

Miami Herald. "Medical Waste Washes Ashore in Ormond Beach." http://www.miamiherald.com/2012/09/15/3004081/medical-waste-washes-ashore-in.html (accessed September 25, 2012).

ORGANIZATIONS

Environmental Protection Agency, 1200 Pennsylvania Ave. NW, Washington, DC 20460, http://www.epa.gov/waste/comments.htm.

World Health Organization, Avenue Appia 20, 1211 Geneva 27, Switzerland, 41 22 791-2111, Fax: 41 22 791-3111, publications@who.int, http://www.who.int.

Teresa G. Odle

Medically unexplained illnesses *see* **Gulf War syndrome**

Melanoma

Definition

Malignant melanoma is a type of cancer arising from the melanocyte cells of the skin. The melanocytes are cells in the skin that produce the pigment melanin. Malignant melanoma develops when the melanocytes no longer respond to normal control mechanisms of cellular growth and are capable of invasion locally or spread to other organs in the body (metastasis), where again they invade and compromise the function of that organ.

Description

Melanocytes, embryologically derived from the neural crest, are distributed in the epidermis and thus are found throughout the skin. They produce a brown pigment known as melanin and are responsible for variation in skin color and also the color of moles. Malignant degeneration of the melanocyte gives rise to the tumor, melanoma, of which there are four subtypes. These are: superficial spreading, nodular, lentigo maligna, and acral lentiginous melanomas, accounting for 70%, 15%–30%, 4%–10%, and 2%–8% of cases, respectively. Malignant melanoma may develop anywhere on the body. In men, it is most common on the trunk. In women, it is most common on the back or legs. The subtype also may influence where the tumor develops; lentigo melanoma is more common on the face whereas acral lentiginous melanoma is more common on the palms of the hand, soles of the feet, or in the nail beds.

The locally invasive characteristic of this tumor involves vertical penetration through the skin and into the dermis and subcutaneous (under-the-skin) tissues of the malignant melanocytes. With the exception of the nodular variety of melanoma, there is often a phase of radial or lateral growth associated with these tumors. Since it is the vertical growth that characterizes the malignancy, the nodular variant of melanoma carries the worst prognosis. Fortunately, the superficial spreading type is most common.

The primary tumor begins in the skin, often from the melanocytes of a pre-existing mole. Once it becomes invasive, it may progress beyond the site of origin to the regional lymph nodes or travel to other organ systems in the body and become systemic in nature.

The lymph is the clear, protein-rich fluid that bathes the cells throughout the body. Lymph will work its way back to the bloodstream via small channels known as lymphatics. Along the way, the lymph is

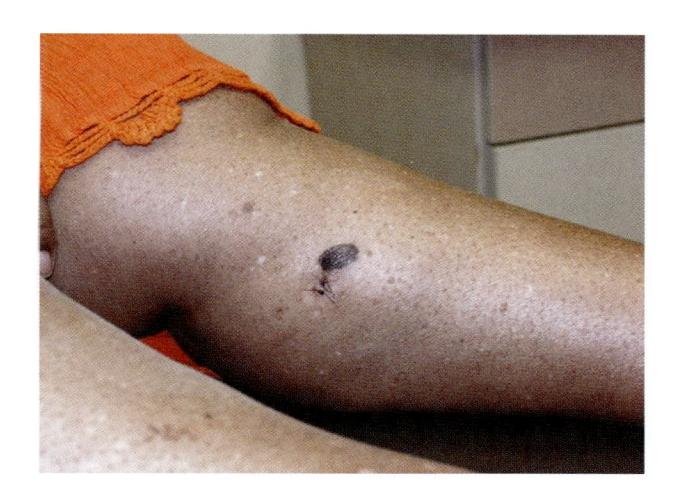

This image depicts the gross appearance of a cutaneous pigmented lesion located on a patient's left medial calf, which had been biopsied, evidenced by the presence of a stitched site of excision, and subsequently diagnosed as superficial spreading malignant melanoma (SSMM). *(CDC)*

filtered through cellular stations known as nodes, thus they are called lymph nodes. Nearly all organs in the body have a primary lymph node group filtering the tissue fluid, or lymph, that comes from that organ. Different areas of the skin have different primary nodal stations. For the leg, they are in the groin; for the arm, the armpit or axilla; for the face, it is the neck. Depending where on the torso the tumor develops, it may drain into one groin or armpit, or both.

Cancer, as it invades in its place of origin, may also work its way into blood vessels. If this occurs, it provides yet another route for the cancer to spread to other organs of the body. When the cancer spreads elsewhere in the body, it has become systemic in extent and the tumor growing elsewhere is known as a metastasis.

Untreated, malignant melanoma follows a classic progression. It begins and grows locally, penetrating vertically. It may be carried via the lymph to the regional nodes, known as regional metastasis. It may go from the lymph to the bloodstream or penetrate blood vessels, directly allowing it a route to go elsewhere in the body. When systemic disease or distant metastasis occurs, melanoma commonly involves the lung, brain, liver, or occasionally bone. The malignancy causes death when its uncontrolled growth compromises vital organ function.

Demographics

In the United States, melanoma accounts for less than 5% of all skin cancers, but the vast majority of deaths from **skin cancer**. Experts estimated that 76,250 new cases of melanoma would be diagnosed in 2012, with 9,180 of those cases eventually resulting in death. Of the seven most common cancers in the United States, only melanoma is becoming more common, with an annual increase of about 2% per year as of 2012. The incidence of melanoma has increased 800 percent over the past three decades for women, and 400 percent for men. Melanoma affects all age groups but is most commonly seen in individuals between 30 and 60 years of age.

Sun exposure is thought to be responsible for about 86% of all cases of melanoma. The melanocytes are part of the integument's photoprotective mechanism; in response to sunlight, they produce melanin that has a protective role from the sun's ultraviolet rays. For Caucasians, the amount of melanin present in the skin is directly related to sun exposure. However, it is not so much the total sun exposure that seems important, rather it is the history of sunburn (especially if severe or at an early age) that correlates with the increased risk. On this basis populations of fair-skinned people living in areas of high sun exposure such as the southwest United States or Australia are subject to increased risk. Malignant melanoma also affects non-Caucasians—though sun exposure probably does not play a role—at a rate of 10% that of Caucasians. The most common form of melanoma in African Americans is acral lentiginous melanoma.

Malignant melanoma may arise in the skin anywhere on the body. Experts estimate that 50% to 70% of all melanoma cases develop spontaneously while the remainder start in a pre-existing mole.

Causes and symptoms

The most common predisposing causes to the development of malignant melanoma are environmental and genetic. The environmental factor is excessive sun exposure. There are also genetically transmitted familial syndromes with alterations in the CDKN2A gene, which encodes for the tumor-suppressing proteins p16 and p19. In 2003, a group of Swedish researchers reported that 63 out of a group of 71 melanoma patients, or 89% of the group, had mutations in either the NRAS or the BRAF gene. The researchers found that these mutations occur at an early point in the development of melanoma and remain as the tumor progresses.

Some researchers think there may be two pathways to malignant melanoma, one involving exposure to sunlight and the other with melanocyte proliferation triggered by other factors. This hypothesis is based on the difference in distribution of moles on the body between patients who develop melanomas on the face and neck, and those who develop melanomas on the trunk.

A small percentage of melanomas arise within burn scar tissue. Researchers do not yet fully understand the relationship between deep burns and an increased risk of skin cancer.

Melanin production in fair-skinned people is induced by sun exposure. An exposure substantial enough to result in mild sunburn will be followed by melanin producing a tan that may last a few weeks. Both **ultraviolet radiation** and damaging oxygen radicals caused by sun exposure may damage cells, particularly their DNA. Researchers suspect that this damage induces mutations that result in the development of malignant melanoma. Though these mutations are alterations of the genome causing the melanoma, they are environmentally induced and account for sporadic or spontaneous cases of this disease.

A positive family history of one or two first-degree relatives having had melanoma substantially increases the risk on a genetic basis. A family tendency is observed in 8%–12% of patients. There is a syndrome known as the dysplastic (atypical) nevus syndrome that is characterized by atypical moles with bothersome clinical features in children under age ten. Such individuals have to be observed closely for the development of malignant melanoma. Chromosome 9p has been identified as being involved in familial predisposition. There are mutations in up to 50% of familial melanoma patients of the tumor-suppressing gene CDKN2A. The actual number of moles increases risk, but the size of the moles needs be considered. Those with ten larger moles of over 1 cm (0.4 in.) are at more risk than those with a higher number (50–99) of smaller moles. Finally, when a child is born with a large congenital mole, careful observation for change is appropriate because of increased risk.

An excellent way of identifying changes of significance in a mole is the ABCDE rule:

- asymmetry
- border irregularity
- color variegation
- diameter exceeding 6 mm (0.24 in.)
- elevation above surrounding tissue

Three of these criteria refer to variability of the lesion (color variegation refers to areas of light color and black scattered within the mole). Thus small, uniform regular lesions have less cause for concern. It is important to realize that change in a mole or the rapid development of a new one are very important symptoms.

Another summary of important changes in a mole is the Glasgow 7-point scale. The symptoms and signs below can occur anywhere on the skin, including the palms of the hands, soles of the feet, and also the nail beds:

- change in size
- change in shape
- change in color
- inflammation
- crusting and bleeding
- sensory change
- diameter more than 7 mm (0.3 in)

In this scheme, change is emphasized along with size. Bleeding and sensory changes are relatively late symptoms.

Symptoms related to the presence of regional disease are mostly those of nodules or lumps in the areas containing the lymph nodes draining the area. Thus nodularity can be found in the armpit, the groin, or the neck if regional nodes are involved. There is also a special type of metastasis that can occur regionally with malignant melanoma; it is known as an in-transit metastasis. If the melanoma is spreading through the lymph system, some of the tumor may grow there, resulting in a nodule part way between the primary site and the original lymph node. These in-transit metastasis are seen both at the time of original presentation or later after primary treatment has been rendered, the latter being a type of recurrence.

Finally, in those who either are diagnosed with or progress to widespread or systemic disease, symptoms and signs are related to the affected organ. Thus neurologic problems, lung problems, or liver problems develop depending on the organ involved.

Diagnosis

None of the clinical signs or symptoms is an absolute indication that a patient has malignant melanoma. The actual diagnosis is accomplished by biopsy, a procedure that removes tissue to examine under a microscope. It is important that the signs and symptoms are used to develop a suspicion of the diagnosis because the way the biopsy is performed for melanoma may be different than for other lesions of the skin.

When dealing with an early malignant melanoma, it is very important to establish the exact thickness of penetration of the primary tumor. Any biopsy that does not remove the full vertical extent of the primary is inadequate. Therefore, if a skin lesion is suspicious, full thickness excisional biopsy is the approach recommended. Shave biopsies and biopsies that remove only a portion of the suspect area are inappropriate. Often, in an early case, the excision involves just the suspicious lesion with minimal normal skin, but it should be a full vertical excision of the skin. If a melanoma is diagnosed, further treatment of this area will often be necessary but does not compromise outcome (prognosis). In some special areas of the body, minor modifications may be necessary about initial total excision, but full thickness excision should always be the goal.

Once the diagnosis is obtained, careful examination of the patient for regional lymph node involvement should be done. A careful review to uncover any symptoms of widespread disease is also appropriate.

The more common patient has an early melanoma, and extensive testing is not usually warranted. Routine testing in this situation involves a complete blood count, a chest x ray, and determinations of blood enzymes including lactic dehydrogenase and alkaline phosphatase.

If the patient has signs or symptoms of more advanced disease, or if the lesion's depth of penetration is sizeable, further imaging studies may be appropriate. These would involve CAT scans of the abdomen, the chest, or regional nodal areas, or a CT or MRI of the brain.

The treatment of malignant melanoma is primarily surgical. Newer, more effective protocols involving the medical oncologist are being developed for the patient with systemic disease. **Radiation** therapy has a limited role in the treatment of melanoma, primarily that of helping to ease the effects of metastasis to the brain or sometimes the skeleton.

Clinical staging, treatments, and prognosis

The key to successful treatment is early diagnosis. Patients identified with localized, thin, small lesions (typified by superficial spreading subtype) nearly always survive. For those with advanced lesions, the outcome is poor in spite of progress in systemic therapy.

Clinical staging

Malignant melanoma is locally staged based on the depth of penetration through the skin and its appendages. There are two ways of looking at the depth of penetration. The Clarke system utilizes the layers of the dermis and the skin appendages present at that layer to identify the depth of penetration. The Breslow system uses the absolute measurement of depth. Though useful conceptually, the Clarke system is used less frequently because skin is of different thickness in different regions of the body. The depth of penetration is much greater when the tumor reaches the subcutaneous fat when the skin involved is the back as opposed to the face. It turns out that the Breslow measurement is more reproducible and thus more useful; therefore, for purposes here, depth of penetration by absolute measurement (Breslow) is used in local staging.

Stage I and stage II have no involvement of the regional lymph nodes and are thus localized to the site of origin. These stages are subdivided on the basis of penetration. Stage Ia is 0.75 mm or less (1 mm = 0.04 in), and Stage Ib is 0.75 mm to 1.5 mm penetration. Stage IIa is 1.5 mm to 4.0 mm and Stage IIb is over 4.0 mm or into the subcutaneous fat. In stage III and IV, there is disease beyond the primary site. Stage III is defined by the presence of in-transit or regional nodal metastasis or both. Stage IV is defined by the presence of distant metastasis.

Treatment

Once the diagnosis of malignant melanoma has been established by biopsy and the stage has been identified using the results of the examination and studies, a treatment plan is developed. Melanoma is not cured unless it is diagnosed at a stage when it can be isolated and removed surgically. Considerations revolve around the extent of the local and regional nodal surgery for stages I through III. For stage IV patients, or those that are treated and then develop recurrence at distant sites, chemotherapy or immunotherapy is planned. Studies are in progress to improve the results from traditional chemotherapeutic regimens. Adjuvant therapy (auxiliary drug treatment used to make possibility of relapse less for those at high risk) is also considered.

Surgical therapy for the primary site is that of wide local removal of the skin, including subcutaneous tissue surrounding the lesion. In the past, wide excisions were large and encompassed 2 in of tissue in all directions wherever feasible. It has been shown that such wide local excisions are not necessary, and doctors seek to determine what the necessary width is. Studies from the **World Health Organization** Melanoma Group and by the Melanoma Intergroup Committee in the United States have provided general guidelines based on the depth of penetration of the melanoma. These guidelines and anatomic considerations need to be kept in mind by the surgeon.

The next issue in primary management is whether the patient needs to have the regional lymph nodes removed in addition to treatment of the primary tumor. The problems associated with the resection of regional lymph nodes are those of lifelong edema or swelling in the extremity. Though it does not occur in all patients (5%–20%, depending on the extremity and extent of the dissection), it can be a disabling symptom. Certainly, if it could be ascertained that there was disease in the nodes, resection (removal) would be appropriate. However, if there were no disease, the risk of edema should be avoided. In patients with no signs of regional disease, depth of penetration of the primary tumor helps guide the decision. If the tumor penetrates less than 1mm, dissection is not usually done. If it is 1–2 mm, node dissection may be done at the time of primary treatment or the patient may be observed and only undergo lymph node dissection if the area later shows signs of disease. If the patient has enlarged lymph nodes or the depth of the tumor has led to the evaluation by CAT scan showing enlarged nodes, resection of the nodes will be considered. In the latter case, more extensive imaging of the lung, liver, or brain may be appropriate to be sure the patient doesn't already have stage IV disease.

Questions related to which patients should have resection of regional lymph nodes have led to an intermediary procedure known as sentinel lymph node mapping and biopsy. Intermediate thickness melanomas 1–4 mm deep (0.04–0.2 in.) may have nodal involvement even if the exam and any other studies done are normal. If a radioisotope tracer or blue dye is injected into the area of the primary tumor, very shortly it will travel to the lymph nodes draining that area. These sentinel nodes are thus identifiable and are the most likely to harbor any regional metastatic disease. If these nodes alone are biopsied and are normal, the rest of the lymph node group can be spared. If they show microscopic deposits of tumor, then the full resection of the lymph node group may be completed. This procedure allows selection of those patients with intermediate thickness melanoma who will benefit from the regional lymph node dissection.

Patients with metastatic melanoma who do not respond well to other therapies may be candidates for treatment with aldesleukin (also called interleukin-2), a specific kind of biological response modifier that promotes the development of T cells. These cells are part of the lymphatic system and can directly interact with and fight cancer cells. Although interleukin is produced naturally in the body, its therapeutic form is developed via biotechnology in a laboratory setting. In some patients, this medication has helped shrink tumors. Side effects, however, can be severe and range from flu-like symptoms to whole-body infection (sepsis) and coma.

> ## KEY TERMS
>
> **Adjuvant therapy**—Therapy administered to patients who are at risk of having microscopic untreated disease present but have no manifestations.
>
> **Dermis**—The deeper portion or layer of the skin.
>
> **Dysplastic nevus syndrome**—A familial syndrome characterized by the presence of multiple atypical appearing moles, often at a young age.
>
> **Epidermis**—The superficial layer of the skin.
>
> **Genome**—Composed of DNA, the genetic makeup of the cell.
>
> **Immunotherapy**—Therapy using biologic agents that either enhance or stimulate normal immune function.
>
> **Integument**—The skin.
>
> **Lymph node dissection**—Surgical removal of an anatomic group of lymph nodes.
>
> **Lymphedema**—Swelling of an extremity following surgical removal of the lymph nodes draining that extremity.
>
> **Melanocyte**—Cells derived from the neural crest that are in the skin and produce the protein pigment melanin.
>
> **Metastasis**—A tumor growth or deposit that has spread via lymph or blood to an area of the body remote from the primary tumor.
>
> **Nevus**—A mole.
>
> **Resection**—The act of removing something surgically.
>
> **Skin appendages**—Structures related to the integument such as hair follicles and sweat glands.
>
> **Systemic disease**—Used to refer to a patient who has distant metastasis.
>
> **Variegation**—Patchy color variation.

Some patients, such as those with IIb or stage III melanoma, are at high risk for the development of recurrence after treatment. Although these patients are clinically free of disease after undergoing primary treatment, they are more likely to have some microscopic disease in the body that studies have not yet been able to identify. In an effort to decrease the rate of relapse, adjuvant therapy may be considered. Interferon alpha 2a is an agent that stimulates the immune system. This adjuvant therapy may slightly increase the duration of a patient's disease-free state and lengthen overall survival. However, interferon alpha 2a has high toxicity, and patients may not tolerate the side effects.

Unfortunately, treatment for those patients who have or go on to develop systemic disease usually fails; melanoma that has metastasized to the brain is particularly difficult to treat. The chemotherapeutic agent dacarbazine, or DTIC, seems to be the most active agent. Overall responses are noted in about 20% of patients, and they last only two to six months. Combination therapy may be an option. The regimen of DTIC + BCNU (carmustine) + cisplatin + tamoxifen delivers a response rate of 40%. Combining biologic or immunologic agents such as interferon with standard chemotherapeutic agents is under study and showing improved response rates, though toxicity is substantial and only the healthier, younger patients tolerate the treatment.

Some researchers are investigating the reasons why melanomas are so resistant to chemotherapy. One suggestion is that the genes ordinarily responsible for apoptosis (cell self-destruction) do not function normally in melanomas. The development of new drugs to treat melanoma depends on a better understanding of the complex processes involved in apoptosis.

Prognosis

Alternative and complementary therapies

Though radiation therapy has a minimal role in the primary treatment of malignant melanoma, for patients who have metastatic disease, radiation may be helpful. This is true in patients who have developed tumor deposits in areas such as the brain or the bone.

Almost all patients survive stage Ia malignant melanoma, and the suvivorship for stage I overall is more than 90%. Survival drops in stage IIa to about 65% at five years and is worse yet for stage IIb at slightly over 50%. Stage III has a survival rate at 5 years of 10% to 47%, depending on the size and number of regional nodes involved. Stage IV malignant melanoma is almost always fatal.

Coping with cancer treatment

For those with familial tendencies for malignant melanoma, genetic counseling may be appropriate.

QUESTIONS TO ASK YOUR DOCTOR

- What stage in my cancer?
- Has the cancer spread? What tests will be used to determine this?
- What are my treatment options?
- Is adjuvant therapy really necessary in my case?
- What are the risks and side effects of these treatments?
- What medications can I take to relieve treatment side effects?
- Are there any clinical studies underway that would be appropriate for me?
- What effective alternative or complementary treatments are available for this type of cancer?
- How debilitating is the treatment? Will I be able to continue working?
- How will the treatment affect my sexuality?
- Are there any local support groups for melanoma patients?
- What is the chance that the cancer will recur?
- Is there anything I can do to prevent recurrence?
- How often will I have follow-up examinations?

Psychological counseling may be appropriate for anyone having trouble coping with a potentially fatal disease. Local cancer support groups may be helpful and are often identified by contacting local hospitals or the American Cancer Society.

Clinical trials

Clinical trials are studies of new modes of therapy in an effort to improve results of treatment. A useful resource for those wishing to find a trial related to their particular situation can be found at http://www.emergingmed.com/networks/MRF/.

In an attempt to develop a new type of immunotherapy, melanoma-specific vaccines are being developed. Antigens specific to melanoma cells and other tumor-associated antigens are being used to stimulate the body's own natural immune system to attack and kill the cells of malignant melanoma. Though experimental, this type of therapy offers hope and clinical trials are underway. In 2003 a team of researchers in

New York reported that vaccines made from poxviruses show promise as a treatment for melanoma.

Prevention

Though it is difficult to prove that sunscreens statistically reduce the frequency of malignant melanoma, many authorities recommend use as protection from ultraviolet light (considered a major factor in the development of melanoma). Avoidance of severe sunburns is recommended.

Special concerns

Subungal melanoma is a type of acral lentiginous melanoma that occurs in the nail beds. Any pigmented lesion in these areas needs evaluation. They are commonly mistaken for bruises or infection. What matters most is knowing they exist so that proper evaluation can be performed as early as possible.

Malignant melanoma may also involve the eye, as melanin-producing cells exist there also. Again, familiarity with these spots is important so that pigmented growths are not ignored but evaluated early.

On rare occasions, a patient comes to the doctor with regional lymph node involvement, but the primary site of the tumor cannot be identified. The primary may not be producing pigment and is known as an amelanonic melanoma. Because these patients have stage III disease, they do less well as a group overall.

Resources

BOOKS

American Cancer Society. *QuickFACTS Melanoma Skin Cancer: What You Need to Know—NOW.* New York: American Cancer Society, 2012.

Ferrone, Soldano, ed. *Human Melanoma: From Basic Research to Clinical Application.* New York: Springer Verlag, 2012.

Gajewski, Thomas F., and F. Stephen Hodi, eds. *Targeted Therapeutics in Melanoma.* New York: Humana Press, 2011.

Wang, Steven Q. *Beating Melanoma: A Five-Step Survival Guide.* Baltimore: Johns Hopkins University Press, 2011.

PERIODICALS

Dori, J. F., and M. C. Chignol. "Tanning Salons and Skin Cancer." *Photochemical and Photobiological Sciences* 11, no. 1 (2012): 30–37.

Fernandez-Flores, A. "Prognostic Factors for Melanoma Progression and Metastasis: From Hematoxylin-Eosin to Genetics." *Romanian Journal of Morphology and Embryology* 53, no. 3 (2012): 449–59.

Levine, S. M., and R. L. Shapiro. "Surgical Treatment of Malignant Melanoma: Practical Guidelines." *Dermatologic Cllinics* 30, no. 3 (2012): 487–501.

WEBSITES

"Melanoma." National Cancer Institute. http://www.cancer.gov/cancertopics/types/melanoma (accessed on September 24, 2012).

"Melanoma." PubMed Health. http://www.ncbi.nlm.nih.gov/pubmedhealth/PMH0001853/ (accessed on September 24, 2012).

"Melanoma." Skin Cancer Foundation. http://www.skincancer.org/skin-cancer-information/melanoma (accessed on September 24, 2012).

Tan, Winston W. "Malignant Melanoma." http://emedicine.medscape.com/article/280245-overview (accessed on September 24, 2012).

ORGANIZATIONS

National Cancer Institute, 6116 Executive Blvd., Ste. 300, Bethesda, MD 20892-8322, (800) 422-6237, http://www.cancer.gov/global/contact/email-us, http://www.cancer.gov.

Richard A. McCartney, MD
Rebecca J. Frey, PhD

Meningitis

Definition

Meningitis is a potentially fatal inflammation of the meninges, the membranes that encase the brain and spinal cord.

Description

The brain and spinal cord are encased in three layers of membranes called the meninges. The space between the inner membranes contains cerebrospinal fluid (CSF), a lubricating and nutritive fluid that bathes the brain and the spinal cord and helps insulate the brain from trauma. Many blood vessels, as well as peripheral and cranial nerves, pass through this space. Swelling of the meninges, as occurs in meningitis, can damage and destroy brain tissue, compromise the blood supply to the brain, and interfere with CSF production and reabsorption.

Meningitis can be caused by viral, bacterial, and **fungal infections** that enter the bloodstream and are carried to the meninges. Non-infectious meningitis can be caused by some allergies, cancers, or autoimmune diseases. Outbreaks of viral and bacterial meningitis are

HATTIE ALEXANDER (1901–1968)

Hattie Alexander, a dedicated pediatrician, medical educator, and researcher in microbiology, won international recognition for deriving a serum to combat influenzal meningitis, a common disease that was nearly always fatal to infants and young children. Alexander subsequently investigated microbiological genetics and the processes whereby bacteria, through genetic mutation, acquire resistance to antibiotics. In 1964, as president of the American Pediatric Society, she became one of the first women to head a national medical association.

As an intern at the Harriet Lane Home of Johns Hopkins Hospital from 1930 to 1931, Alexander became interested in influenzal meningitis. The source of the disease was *Hemophilus influenzae*, a bacteria that causes inflammation of the meninges, the membranes surrounding the brain and spinal cord. In 1931, Alexander began a second internship at the Babies Hospital of the Columbia-Presbyterian Medical Center in New York City. There, she witnessed first-hand the futility of medical efforts to save babies who had contracted influenzal meningitis.

Alexander's early research focused on deriving a serum (the liquid component of blood containing antibodies) that would be effective against influenzal meningitis. Sera derived from animals that have been exposed to a specific disease-producing bacterium often contain antibodies against the disease and can be developed for use in immunizing humans against it. Alexander knew that the Rockefeller Institute in New York City had been able to prepare a rabbit serum for the treatment of pneumonia, another bacterial disease. Alexander therefore experimented with rabbit sera and, by 1939, was able to announce the development of a rabbit serum effective in curing infants of influenzal meningitis.

In the early 1940s, Alexander experimented with the use of drugs in combination with rabbit serum for the treatment of influenzal meningitis. Within the next two years, she saw infant deaths due to the disease drop by 80%.

---

not uncommon in childcare centers, college dormitories, and military bases. Viral meningitis, also called aseptic meningitis, is the most common type. It is a less severe infection than bacterial meningitis, is rarely fatal, and may not require any specific treatment. Bacterial meningitis is a medical emergency and has a high fatality rate if untreated.

Fungal meningitis is generally rare, although it sometimes develops as an opportunistic infection in HIV/AIDS patients. However, in 2012, a major fungal meningitis outbreak was linked to one or more contaminated drugs from a compounding pharmacy in Massachusetts. As of November 2012, 377 fungal meningitis cases had been reported from 19 states, with 23 deaths. Public health officials succeeded in contacting almost all of the estimated 14,000 patients in 23 states who had been injected with the potentially contaminated drug.

Risk factors

Children and young adults, especially those in group living situations, are most at risk for meningitis. Newborn boys are at three times the risk of newborn girls. Patients with a weakened immune system from HIV/AIDS, diabetes, or spleen removal are at greater risk, as are pregnant women. People who work with animals are at an increased risk for meningitis from *Listeria* infections. Unsafe sexual practices and a large number of sexual partners are risk factors for viral meningitis.

Demographics

There are approximately 1.5 cases of bacterial meningitis per 100,000 people in the United States each year. The introduction of the Hib vaccine against *Haemophilus influenzae* in 1990 shifted the median age for this type of meningitis from under two years to 39 years, and there was an increase in cases among adults over 60 in the 2000s. Viral meningitis usually develops in the late summer and early fall in children and adults under age 30. Most viral infections occur in children under the age of five.

Meningitis rates in developing countries are believed to be at least ten times higher than in the United States and Canada, with periodic epidemics occurring in sub-Saharan Africa and parts of India. The lack of access to vaccines is the major reason for these differences between developed and developing countries.

Causes and symptoms

Meningitis can result from the spread of an untreated infection elsewhere in the body, if there are enough disease-causing organisms to cross the blood-brain barrier or if the infected tissue is very near the meninges—as with a severe and poorly treated ear or sinus infection or a skull facture. Insect and animal bites can also inject disease-causing organisms directly into the bloodstream. Although uncommon, infections such as herpes simplex can spread along a nerve to the spinal cord and brain.

Disease agents

About 30% of viral meningitis cases in the United States are caused by enteroviruses that normally live in the human digestive tract, although the specific virus causing a meningitis case is often not identified. Enteroviruses are found in saliva, throat mucus, and feces, and they can be transmitted through direct contact with an infected person or a contaminated object or surface. Many other viruses—including those that cause **mumps**, **measles**, **polio**, and chickenpox, and West Nile, herpes simplex, and La Crosse viruses—can cause meningitis. Viral meningitis is usually a mild illness that often resolves without treatment within two weeks.

Bacterial meningitis can be transmitted by coughs, sneezes, and kisses. Most bacterial meningitis is caused one of four bacteria.

- *Streptococcus pneumoniae* causes pneumococcal meningitis, especially in young children.
- *Neisseria meningitidis* causes meningococcal meningitis. It is highly contagious and is often responsible for outbreaks and epidemics, especially in children and young adults.
- *H. influenzae* has been substantially reduced in the developed world due to the introduction of routine childhood vaccinations.
- *Listeria monocytogenes* is more likely to affect pregnant women and older adults and can cross the placenta and kill a developing fetus. Newborns can also develop meningitis from group B stretococci and *Escherichia coli* that are transmitted from the mother during labor and delivery.

Bacterial meningitis is often acute, developing in less than 24 hours. Subacute meningitis, caused by bacteria or **viruses**, develops over one to seven days. Chronic meningitis, which is rare, develops over a period of weeks. It may have a noninfectious cause and be due to a slow-growing fungus that invades the meninges and CSF. Cryptococcal meningitis is a life-threatening fungal disease that affects HIV/AIDS patients and others with immune system dysfunction. Most of the cases in the 2012 outbreak were caused by the fungus *Exserohilum rostratum*, although some were caused by *Aspergillus fumigatus*.

Symptoms

The symptoms of meningitis are almost always high fever, stiff neck, and severe headache, although the 2012 fungal outbreak caused variable symptoms. Some patients had only a mild headache and no fever; others suffered strokes. The debilitated elderly may not develop fever or other obvious meningitis symptoms. Meningitis symptoms in adults can also include:

- nausea and vomiting
- skin rash, especially with meningococcal meningitis
- drowsiness or difficulty awakening
- loss of appetite
- extreme light sensitivity
- difficulty concentrating and confusion
- seizures

Young infants may not develop a fever, and seizures may be their only symptom of meningitis. Other symptoms in infants and young children may include:

- bulging of the soft spot on top of an infant's skull
- constant crying
- poor feeding
- unusual sleepiness
- stiffness in the body and neck

Diagnosis

Diagnosis of the type of meningitis is essential for proper treatment. Recent exposure to disease agents through travel or contact with an infected person, animal, or insect may provide diagnostic clues. A patient with subacute meningitis may be examined for an ear, throat, or sinus infection. A neurological examination includes hearing and speech, vision, coordination and balance, reflexes, mental status, and recent changes in mood or behavior. There are several physical maneuvers that can indicate meningitis:

- Lowering the chin to the chest is difficult and painful.
- When raising one leg at the hip to a right angle from the examining table, the other leg cannot be straightened, or the maneuver causes neck pain.
- The knees and hips flex upward when bending a supine patient's neck forward.

A lumbar puncture or spinal tap is the insertion of a needle into the lower back to withdraw CSF for testing. The presence of infection-fighting white blood cells and excess protein in the CSF is an indication of meningitis. A low glucose level suggests bacterial meningitis. The CSF is cultured to grow and identify an organism. A throat swab may be cultured as well. A rapid CSF test detects viral DNA and can accurately identify about 90% of viral meningitis cases in less than three hours. If there is no virus, the disease is immediately treated with antibiotics against bacteria.

KEY TERMS

Aseptic meningitis—A term for meningitis not caused by bacteria.

Blood-brain barrier—The arrangement of blood vessels in the brain that prevents many substances from passing from the blood into brain tissues.

Cerebrospinal fluid (CSF)—Fluid produced within chambers in the brain that bathes the surfaces of the brain and spinal cord.

Enteroviruses—A family of viruses that normally live in the digestive tract and that can cause viral meningitis.

Hib—Conjugate vaccine; a vaccine that immunizes infants and children against *Haemophilus influenzae* that cause meningitis and pneumonia.

Lumbar puncture—Spinal tap; a procedure in which a very narrow needle is inserted between the vertebrae of the lower back to obtain a sample of cerebrospinal fluid for testing.

Meninges (singular, meninx)—The membranes that cover the brain and spinal cord.

Meningococcal meningitis—Highly contagious meningitis caused by the bacterium *Neisseria meningitidis*.

Opportunistic infection—An infection that usually occurs only in people with deficient immune systems.

Outbreak—A sudden increase in the incidence of a disease.

Pneumococcal meningitis—Meningitis caused by the bacterium *Streptococcus pneumoniae*.

Stroke—A sudden diminishing or loss of consciousness, sensation, or voluntary movement from a rupture or obstruction of a blood vessel in the brain.

A computed tomography (CT) scan may detect signs of inflammation of the meninges. A CT scan or magnetic resonance imaging (MRI) can also rule out head trauma, stroke, tumors, and blood clots in the brain.

Treatment

Bacterial meningitis is a life-threatening emergency that requires immediate hospital treatment, usually with intravenous penicillin or other broadspectrum antibiotic. One study found a 30% increase in death or neurological damage for every hour that antimicrobial treatment was delayed. Patients also may need treatment for shock, seizures, dehydration, and brain swelling. They may be given intravenous fluids and oxygen to assist breathing and have fluid drained from the sinuses or from the space between the meninges and the brain. Once the bacterial cause has been identified, treatment is usually with a combination of antibiotics. Fluoroquinolone-resistant *N. meningitidis* was first reported in the United States in 2007.

Viral meningitis is usually treated at home with a few weeks of bed rest. Patients can take over-the-counter pain relievers for muscle aches and pains and to reduce fever. Antiviral drugs may be used to treat a herpes infection.

Antifungal medications for meningitis can have harmful side effects, so treatment may be deferred until a fungal cause is definitively identified. Noninfectious meningitis from an allergic reaction or autoimmune disease may be treated with cortisone-type medications. Sometimes these conditions resolve without treatment.

Public health role and response

The U.S. **Centers for Disease Control and Prevention** (CDC) tracks outbreaks of meningitis; however, the U.S. **Food and Drug Administration** (FDA) was involved in the response to the 2012 outbreak of fungal meningitis because it involved contaminated drugs. Public health response was slowed because symptoms did not develop until one–six weeks or even longer after patients received spinal injections with the contaminated steroid. Furthermore, symptoms varied greatly and were unusual even for fungal meningitis. Some patients suffered strokes at the back of the brain, the area of the brain that the fungus reached first after traveling up the spinal cord. The strokes were caused by the fungus invading blood vessels and preventing oxygen from reaching brain cells.

The contaminated steroids, as well as contaminated products used in heart and eye surgery, were eventually traced to the New England Compounding Center, which had a history of problems, including inadequate contamination control. The center closed immediately and all of its products were recalled. A related facility was also closed and its products recalled when inspectors found sterility issues and that patients were receiving intravenous medication at the facility, in violation of state law.

The outbreak raised questions about the regulation of compounding pharmacies, which are licensed to fill nonstandard customized prescriptions for patients with special needs, such as a smaller dose or an ingredient removed. They are not subject to the same FDA regulations as drug manufacturers. A criminal investigation was launched because the New England Compounding Center had been functioning as a drug manufacturer and distributor. Some lawmakers called for increased regulation of compounding pharmacies, and congressional hearings were convened.

Meanwhile, public health officials were trying to advise doctors and patients. Because the meningitis symptoms were so delayed and varied, the FDA advised that all patients who were injected with drugs produced or sold by the pharmacy be followed for up to six months. In an outbreak of five cases of fungal meningitis from contaminated injections ten years previously, one patient did not become ill until 152 days after the injection. Meningitis patients were being treated with oral or intravenous voriconzole, but as of November 2012, it was not known whether the drug was effective or how long patients needed to continue it.

Prognosis

Prognosis depends on a variety factors, especially the cause of the meningitis. Patients usually recover from viral meningitis within two to four weeks. Complications are rare, and the mortality rate is less than 1%. Patients with bacterial meningitis typically improve within 48–72 hours following initial treatment; however, they are more likely to experience complications caused by the disease. Acute bacterial meningitis has a mortality rate of 10–15% even with treatment, and 10–20% of survivors have complications such as blindness, hearing loss, learning disorders, speech problems, memory problems, behavior problems, brain damage, or paralysis. The longer treatment is delayed, the greater the risk for seizures or permanent neurological damage.

Prevention

There are vaccines for all of the bacteria that usually cause meningococcal meningitis in the United States, except group B. The Hib vaccine for *H. influenzae* meningitis and pneumococcal conjugate vaccine (PCV7) are included in regular childhood immunization schedules in the United States. Pneumococcal polysaccharide vaccine (PPSV) is given to older children and adults. The meningococcal conjugate vaccine (MCV4) is recommended for all children at ages 11–12. Adults over 55 should be immunized with a similar vaccine called MPSV4. As of 2012, a new vaccine that is effective against group B meningococcal meningitis was expected to be licensed in Europe and elsewhere.

WHAT TO ASK YOUR DOCTOR

- Could I have meningitis?
- How will you test for it?
- How did I get meningitis?
- How will you treat my meningitis?
- Can I transmit meningitis to others?

Other preventive measures against contagious meningitis include:

- Keeping the immune system strong by getting enough sleep, exercising regularly, and eating a healthy diet.
- Washing hands regularly, particularly when living in a dormitory or shared housing situation.
- Avoiding sharing glasses, cups, food utensils, and similar items with others who may have been infected or exposed to infection.
- Covering the nose or mouth before sneezing or coughing.
- Taking prescribed antibiotics during a meningitis outbreak in one's school or workplace.

Resources

BOOKS

Engdahl, Sylvia. *Meningitis*. Farmington Hills, MI: Greenhaven, 2010.
Shannon, Joyce Brennfleck. *Brain Disorders Sourcebook*. 3rd ed. Detroit: Omnigraphics, 2010.
Shmaefsky, Brian, and Hilary Babcock. *Meningitis*. New York: Chelsea, 2010.

PERIODICALS

Brown, David. "Meningitis Outbreak Has Medical Researchers Delving into Unknown Territory." *Washington Post* (October 21, 2012): A4.
Dooren, Jennifer Corbett, and Timothy W. Martin. "Doctors Grapple with Best Meningitis Care—A Month into the Outbreak, Physicians Across the Country Struggle to Find Most Effective Way to Diagnose and Treat Cases." *Wall Street Journal* (October 29, 2012): A6.
Grady, Denise. "'Worried Sick': Meningitis Risk Haunts 14,000." *New York Times* (October 22, 2012): A1.
Martin, Timothy W., Thomas M. Burton, and Betsy McKay. "Meningitis Cases Rise Amid Hunt for Victims." *Wall Street Journal* (October 8, 2012): A1.
Morin, Monte. "Waiting Is Agony for Patients Warned of Meningitis." *Los Angeles Times* (October 26, 2012): A1.

WEBSITES

"Company with Links to Meningitis-Linked Pharmacy Recalls All Products." *HealthDay*. October 31, 2012.

http://www.nlm.nih.gov/medlineplus/news/fullstory_130865.html (accessed November 7, 2012).

Mayo Clinic Staff. "Meningitis." Mayo Clinic. April 29, 2011. http://www.mayoclinic.com/health/meningitis/DS00118 (accessed November 7, 2012).

"Meningitis." MedlinePlus. November 1, 2012. http://www.nlm.nih.gov/medlineplus/meningitis.html (accessed November 7, 2012).

"Meningococcal Disease." Centers for Disease Control and Prevention. October 4, 2012. http://www.cdc.gov/meningococcal/index.html (accessed November 7, 2012).

"NINDS Meningitis and Encephalitis Information Page." National Institute of Neurological Disorders and Stroke. February 16, 2011. http://www.ninds.nih.gov/disorders/encephalitis_meningitis/encephalitis_meningitis.htm (accessed November 7, 2012).

ORGANIZATIONS

Immunization Action Coalition, 1573 Selby Avenue, Suite 234, St. Paul, MN, USA 55104, 1(651) 647-9009, Fax: 1(651) 647-9131, admin@immunize.org, http://www.immunize.org.

National Institute of Allergy and Infectious Diseases, Office of Communications and Government Relations, 6610 Rockledge Drive, MSC 6612, Bethesda, MD, USA 20892-6612, 1(301) 496-5717, Fax: 1(301) 402-3573, (866) 284-4107, ocpostoffice@niaid.nih.gov, http://www.niaid.nih.gov.

National Meningitis Association, PO Box 725165, Atlanta, GA, USA 31139, 1(866) FONE-NMA (366-3662), Fax: 1(877) 703-6096, http://www.nmaus.org.

U.S. Centers for Disease Control and Prevention, 1600 Clifton Road, Atlanta, GA, USA 30333, (800) CDC-INFO (232-4636), cdcinfo@cdc.gov, http://www.cdc.gov.

U.S. Food and Drug Administration, 10903 New Hampshire Avenue, Silver Spring, MD, USA 20993-0002, (888) INFO-FDA (463-6332), http://www.fda.gov.

World Health Organization, Avenue Appia 20, 1211 Geneva, Switzerland 27, 41 22 791-2111, Fax: 41 22 791-3111, info@who.int, http://www.who.int/en.

Helen Colby, MS
Tish Davidson, AM
Margaret Alic, PhD

Mercury

Definition

Mercury (Hg) is a naturally occurring element in minerals, rocks, soil, water, air, plants, and animals.

Description

The predominant forms in the atmosphere, water, and aerobic soils and sediments are elemental and mercuric mercury; while cinnabar is commonly found in mineralized ore deposits and anaerobic soils and sediments. Mercury is present throughout the atmosphere because of its relatively high vapor pressure. It vaporizes from the earth's surface and is transported in a global cycle, sometimes for hundreds of kilometers, before being deposited again with particulates, rain, or snow. The background concentrations in rocks and soils typically range between 20 and 100μg Hg/kg with a worldwide average of about 50μg Hg/kg. Natural background concentrations in the uncontaminated atmosphere are in the order of between 1 and 10 ng/m^3 increasing to between 50 and 1,000,000 ng/m^3 or more over mineralized areas. Mercury is transported to aquatic ecosystems via surface runoff and atmospheric deposition. Airborne concentrations associated with anthropogenic activities such as coal burning, smelting, industry, and incineration range between 100 and 100,000 ng/m^3. These sources of mercury account for about 70 percent of anthropogenic mercury in the atmosphere.

The element can be divided into two major categories, organic and inorganic. Inorganic mercury includes the elemental (Hg^0) silvery liquid metal (mp, 38°C; bp, 357°C) as well as mercurous ion (Hg^+), mercuric ion (Hg^{++}), and their compounds. Organic mercury includes chemical compounds which contain carbon atoms that are covalently bound to a mercury atom, such as methylmercury (CH_3-Hg^+).

During the latter half of the twentieth century, inorganic mercury was used extensively to produce caustic soda and chlorine (Cl) as well as to manufacture batteries, switches, street lamps, and fluorescent lamps. Gold mining, dental amalgams, pharmaceuticals, and other consumer items also consume inorganic mercury. Organic mercury applications have mostly been eliminated in agricultural fungicides, slimicides in paper pulp production, bacteriostats in water-based paints, and industrial catalysts.

Risk factors

Over the centuries the symptoms of inorganic **mercury poisoning** were well documented by the exposure of miners and industrial workers as mercury accumulated in their brains, kidneys, and livers. Loose teeth, tremors, and psychopathological symptoms were common at low exposure, but removal from the source would often enable the victims to recover. However, the effects of organic alkyl mercurials, such asmethylmercury, were more severe. With a half-life in the human body of about seventy days, continued exposure elevates the levels. It also crosses the blood/brain and placental barriers, attacking the central nervous system and inducing teratogenic (causing developmental disruption) changes in the fetus. The neurological symptoms include: loss of coordination in walking; slurred speech; constriction of the field of vision; loss of sensation, especially in the fingers, toes, and lips; and loss of hearing. Severe poisoning can cause coma, blindness, and death.

The concentrations of mercury in the ocean and uncontaminated freshwater are generally believed to be less than 300 and 200 ng/l respectively. However, new ultra clean analytical techniques indicate that the actual concentrations may be three- to five-fold lower. In contaminated aquatic systems concentrations as high as 5μg Hg/l have been reported. In the water column, mercury readily adsorbs onto organic particulates, metal oxides, and clays and settles into the sediments. Historically, depending on their location, the natural background concentrations of mercury in sediments have ranged between 10 and 200μg/kg. However, most aquatic systems have received some mercury contamination, and the rate has increased during the past century. Among sites that have been measured, the total concentrations have usually been from five to ten times greater than background and ranged from less than 0.5 mg Hg/kg (dry weight) in remote areas to 2,010 mg Hg/kg (dry weight) in Minamata Bay, Japan where mercury was dumped for many years into the bay by an industrial company, leading to severe public health problems.

In the aquatic ecosystem inorganic mercury is converted to methylmercury by both biotic and abiotic processes. It is then released, and aquatic organisms bioaccumulate it easily and have difficulty with metabolism and excretion. The biological half-life in fish may be as long as one to three years. Exposed organisms at each level of the food chain bioconcentrate methylmercury and pass it on to animals at the higher trophic levels.

Depending on the species of fish and the type and amount of mercury being released from the sediments, it may be magnified biologically from one thousand and 100 thousand times or more. While background levels of total mercury in freshwater and marine fishes from unpolluted waters typically range from less than 0.1 to about 0.2 mg Hg/kg, higher concentrations are found in some pelagic top predator ocean fishes such as tuna and shark, sometimes exceeding 1.5 mg/ kg. Conversely, fish from contaminated waters typically contain levels between 0.5 and 5.0 mg Hg/kg and up to 35 to 50 mg Hg/kg in highly contaminated areas.

The annual worldwide production of mercury was over 1,600 tons (about 1,500 metric tons) in the early twenty-first century, with most coming from China and Kyrgyzstan. Annual output fluctuates, and the Kyrgyzstan mines have suffered problems in recent years. The U.S. Natural Resources Defense Council (NRDC) is coordinating with the Chemical Registration Center (CRC) of China's State Environmental Protection Administration to assess China's mercury supply and demand to develop a plan to stop the mining of mercury and decrease the input of mercury into the environment. The NRDC's plan focuses on eliminating export of mercury by industrialized nations and phasing out mercury mining as well as the promotion of alternatives to mercury-based production in industry. Their goal is to reduce mercury trade by 75 percent over a ten-year period.

Public health role and response

The **Environmental Protection Agency (EPA)** prepared a Mercury Study Report, which was published in 1997. This report includes sources of mercury emissions in the United Staters, environmental and human health impacts of mercury emissions, and discusses control methods. Mercury is considered a hazardous air pollutant according to the **Clean Air Act**. In 2005, the **EPA** issued the Clean Air Mercury Rule, which regulates mercury emissions from coal-firing plants. The Clean Air Mercury Rule and the Clean Air Interstate Rule are part of the Clean Air Rules of 2004, which focus on **ozone** and fine particle production, non-road diesel emissions, and power plant emissions. Several standards have been developed to protect the public's health from the threat of mercury poisoning. The maximum permissible concentration allowed by the United States **Environmental Protection Agency (EPA)** under its drinking water standards is 2μg Hg/l. The United States **Food and Drug Administration (FDA)** guideline for mercury in seafood is 1 mg Hg/kg freshweight; however, some states, such as Michigan, adhere to a more restrictive guideline of 0.5 mg Hg/kg freshweight. The Food and Agriculture Organization of the United Nations (FAO), on the other hand, recommends a provisional tolerable intake (PTI) of 0.3 mg mercury per week for a person weighing 154 pounds (70 kg), of which no more than 0.2 should be in the methylated form.

Resources

BOOKS

Atwood, David A. *Recent Developments in Mercury Science.* Berlin: Springer, 2006.

Eisler, Ronald. *Mercury Hazards to Living Organisms*. Boca Raton, FL: CRC/Taylor & Francis, 2006.

Hightower, Jane M. *Diagnosis Mercury: Money, Politics, and Poison*. Washington, DC: Island Press/Shearwater Books, 2009.

Lew, Kristi. *Mercury; Understanding the Elements of the Periodic Table*. New York: Rosen Publishing Group, 2009.

SETAC North America Workshop on Mercury Monitoring and Assessment, and Reed Harris. *Ecosystem Responses to Mercury Contamination: Indicators of Change: Based on the SETAC North America Workshop on Mercury Monitoring and Assessment, 14–17 September 2003, Pensacola, Florida, USA*. Pensacola, FL: SETAC, 2007.

PERIODICALS

DePalma, Anthony. "EPA Sued Over Mercury in the Air." *New York Times* (March 30, 2005).

WEBSITES

Centers for Disease Control and Prevention (CDC). "Mercury." http://emergency.cdc.gov/agent/mercury/index.asp (accessed August 11, 2012).

United States Environmental Protection Agency (EPA). "Air: Air Pollutants: Mercury." http://www.epa.gov/ebtpages/airairpollutantsmercury.html (accessed August 11, 2012).

United States Environmental Protection Agency (EPA). "Emergencies: Poisoning: Mercury Poisoning." http://www.epa.gov/ebtpages/emerpoisoningmercurypoisoning.html (accessed August 11, 2012).

United States Environmental Protection Agency (EPA). "Water: Water Pollutants: Mercury." http://www.epa.gov/ebtpages/watewaterpollutantmercury.html (accessed August 11, 2012).

Frank M. D'Itri

Mercury poisoning

Definition

Mercury poisoning is exposure to harmful amounts of the toxic element, usually by breathing mercury vapors or ingesting compounds containing mercury. Mercury poisoning can permanently damage the nervous system and immune system, as well as the brain, lungs, kidneys, heart, and liver. High–level exposure can be fatal. Developing fetuses are particularly sensitive to mercury poisoning.

Description

Two early descriptions of mercury poisoning were given by German-Swiss physician and botanist Paracelsus (1493–1541), who was also known as Philippus Aureolus Theophrastus Bombastus von Hohenheim, in 1550, who described symptoms of mercury miners in central Europe; and by Italian physician Bernardino Ramazzini, who wrote about the terrible health conditions of mercury miners, gilders (those who apply thin layers of gold to surfaces), and mirror makers. Before, during, and after these times, mercury was often used as an elixir by alchemists, supposedly to provide immortality to those who drank it.

One of the largest modern cases of mercury poisoning occurred in the 1970s when grain was treated with mercury, as a **fungicide**, and given to Kurdish peasants who were starving in northern Iraq. It is estimated that 6,000 died from ingesting mercury-infected grain while another 100,000 were sickened.

In the 2010s, the use of mercury has been banned by many industries throughout the world; however, it is still commonly used in the production of batteries, cement, **explosives**, gold, steel, and other products. Although the use of mercury has been phased out or banned in some industries, it is still widely used in the production of gold, tin, cement, steel, batteries, and explosives, and in laboratories and hospitals.

Mercury (Hg) is a naturally occurring element in air, water, and soil. Three forms of mercury pose different potential health hazards:

- Elemental or metallic mercury, also called quicksilver, is a shiny, silvery metal that is a liquid at room temperature but is easily vaporized to a colorless, odorless gas that can be inhaled. Elemental mercury is released into the air by natural processes such as volcanic activity and by various industrial processes, especially coal–burning power plants. It is extremely poisonous and 79–80% of inhaled mercury vapor is absorbed by the lungs. In the past, mercury vapors poisoned hat makers—hence the Mad Hatter of *Alice in Wonderland*. Elemental mercury is used in thermometers, compact fluorescent light bulbs (CFLs), electrical switches, and older–type dental fillings.

- Inorganic mercury compounds include mercuric oxide (HgO) and mercuric salts, such as mercuric chloride ($HgCl_2$). These compounds are usually white powders or crystals. Inorganic mercury is used in many industries and can be found in some skin ointments and creams, disinfectants, fungicides, folk medicines, red cinnabar pigment, and button batteries that power small electronic devices.

- Organic mercury compounds are carbon–containing substances, such as methylmercury, ethylmercury, and phenylmercury. Bacteria in soil and water convert inorganic mercury in the environment into

GALE ENCYCLOPEDIA OF ENVIRONMENTAL HEALTH

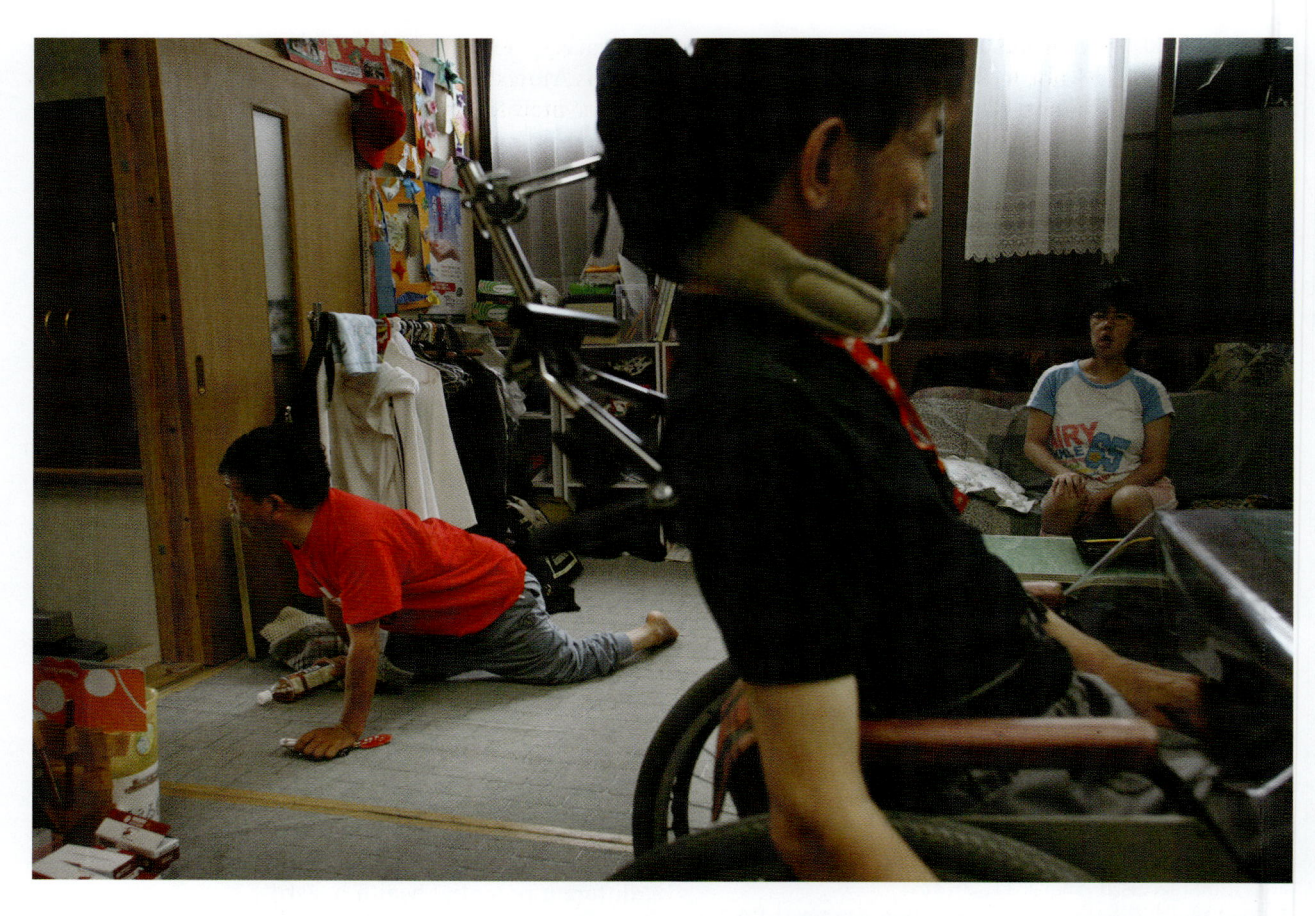

Unable to walk, Isamu Nagai crawls on the floor next to Youji Kaneko, center, at the Hotto Hausu vocational center for disabled people in Minamata, Japan. *(AP Images.)*

methylmercury, which accumulates in fish. Larger and older fish generally have the highest levels of methylmercury. In some parts of the world, organic mercury is used as an antifungal agent in seed grain fed to animals. It is also found in older antiseptics and in some medical preservatives, including trace amounts of thimerosal in some childhood vaccines.

Because the body cannot easily rid itself of mercury, repeated exposure results in its build up in tissues. Elemental mercury vapor and methylmercury are the most dangerous forms because they readily reach the brain. Most humans have trace amounts of methylmercury in their bodies. Methylmercury crosses the placenta to the developing fetus, whose red blood cells can have mercury concentrations that are 30% higher than those of the mother. It also passes to the newborn child through breast milk. Fetuses, infants, and young children are significantly more sensitive to the effects of mercury than are adults. During the 1950s, large amounts of organic mercury were dumped in Japan's Minamata Bay, killing some 1,000 people and causing severe nervous system damage in unborn children. Thus, mercury poisoning is sometimes called fetal Minamata Bay disease. Mercury poisonings have also occurred from eating meat from animals fed contaminated grain.

Risk factors

The major risk factor for mercury poisoning in children is the consumption of large amounts of contaminated fish and shellfish. Children who play with found or spilled mercury are also at risk. A CNN article in 2011 reported that eating large amounts of sushi (raw fish), such as Bluefin tuna, mackerel, yellowtail, swordfish, and sea bass, could cause neurological problems. The article *What the Yuck: Mercury Poisoning from Sushi* made the following recommendations: to not eat fish every day, to cut back on the types that contain the most mercury, and to avoid the worst ones if pregnant and nursing. In addition, the article advised parents to never feed children raw fish.

In 2012, the **Food and Drug Administration** (FDA) warned consumers not to buy skin products that contain mercury. Its report *Mercury Poisoning Linked to Skin Products*, published March 6, 2012, stated that certain skin creams, beauty and antiseptic soaps, and lotions, such as those that lighten the skin and anti-aging products that remove age spots, come into the country illegally or are brought into the United States from travelers to other countries. Many of these products contain mercury. The FDA states that it "does not allow mercury in drugs or in cosmetics, except under very specific conditions, which these products do not meet." The FDA recommends that consumers check the labels of such products for the words "mercurous chloride," "calomel," "mercuric," "mercurio," or "mercury." If labels or ingredients are not present on the product, then do not use it, and do not use products that are labeled in languages other than English.

Demographics

The prevalence of mercury poisoning in American children is hotly debated but is generally considered to be rare. Fish and shellfish contaminated with methylmercury are the major sources of mercury poisoning in the United States and around the world. A 2009 study by the U.S. **Centers for Disease Control and Prevention** (CDC) on the exposure of children to elemental mercury found that the largest exposures to mercury were from children stealing mercury from a school or industrial site. The vast majority of elemental exposures:

- were minimal or nontoxic
- occurred in homes or schools
- involved broken thermometers

Some of the most serious outbreaks of mercury poisoning have occurred in Japan and Iraq. For instance, large outbreaks of methylmercury poisoning (poisoning from mercury and chlorine) occurred in Japan between 1953 and 1965, Iraq from 1971 to 1972, and Ghana and Pakistan in 1969. The consumption of grains and fish contaminated with mercury are two high risk ways of getting mercury poisoning in these countries.

The risk of mercury poisoning also rises when gold rises in price as it has done for many years. This occurs because gold miners often have to separate mercury from ore in which gold is present in a process called gold-mercury amalgam. As the beginning of the 2010s, it was estimated that about 15 to 20 million gold prospectors are active in over 60 countries of the world, especially those of South America, Asia, and Africa. The January 3, 2011 Yale University report *Threat of Mercury Poisoning Rises with Gold Mining Boom* states: "Today's small-scale mining industry is motivated less by adventure than survival. Poverty-driven miners rely on inexpensive, outdated, polluting technologies and chemicals—chief among them mercury—with heavy costs for human health and the environment."

Causes and symptoms

The most common cause of mercury poisoning is eating fish and shellfish contaminated with high levels of methylmercury. Less common causes of mercury poisoning include:

- inhalation of vapors from spills, breakage of mercury–containing devices, off–gassing from polyurethane flooring containing a mercury catalyst, or mercury accumulation in poorly ventilated buildings
- breathing contaminated air from incinerators or industry
- inadequate remediation of toxic sites
- mercury used in cultural rituals or ceremonies
- mercury tracked home from workplaces
- mercury–based amalgams in dental fillings
- swallowing or inhaling mercury–containing batteries or their components
- direct skin contact with the element or its compounds

The same level of mercury vapor can result in higher mercury concentrations in children than in adults, because children have larger lung surface areas for their body weight. Furthermore, since mercury vapors are denser than air, there are higher levels closer to the ground where children breathe in the vapors. Although elemental mercury vapor is only slowly absorbed through the skin, it can irritate the skin and eyes and cause contact dermatitis. Touching or swallowing elemental liquid mercury is usually not harmful because it rolls off the skin and very little is absorbed by the gastrointestinal tract.

The effects of mercury exposure depend on a variety of factors including the

- form of mercury
- dose
- route of exposure—inhaled, ingested, or skin contact
- child's age, with fetuses and very young children being most susceptible
- child's health

Symptoms of elemental mercury poisoning appear within a few hours of exposure to high levels of vapor. Smaller amounts inhaled daily cause symptoms that develop over time. Symptoms can include:

- a metallic taste
- swollen, bleeding gums
- skin rashes
- eye irritation
- respiratory symptoms, especially in children, including severe coughing, shortness of breath, or difficulty breathing
- gastrointestinal symptoms, including nausea, vomiting, and diarrhea
- fever and chills
- high blood pressure or heart rate
- headaches
- neuromuscular symptoms, such as weakness, twitching, tremors, muscle atrophy, and impaired nerve responses
- emotional effects, such as mood swings, irritability, nervousness, or excessive shyness
- insomnia
- disturbed sensations
- cognitive impairment
- with high exposure, kidney impairment, respiratory failure, and death

Unlike elemental mercury, inorganic and organic mercury are absorbed through the intestinal tract, although a swallowed battery may pass harmlessly through a child. Symptoms of inorganic mercury poisoning include:

- skin rashes and dermatitis
- metallic taste
- drooling
- mouth lesions, severe mouth pain, and throat swelling
- severe abdominal pain
- vomiting
- bloody diarrhea
- decreased or absent urination
- severe breathing difficulty
- muscle weakness
- mood swings
- memory loss
- mental disturbances
- shock
- kidney failure
- death

Methylmercury can interfere with the neurological development of fetuses, infants, and children, causing the following:

- cerebral palsy
- brain damage and mental retardation
- language deficits
- attention deficits
- poor coordination
- growth retardation
- blindness
- seizures
- microcephaly (small head)

Symptoms of organic mercury poisoning most often develop over years or decades and include:

- "pins and needles" in the hands and feet and around the mouth
- numbness or pain on the skin
- poor coordination
- tremors
- muscle weakness
- impaired vision or blindness
- impaired speech and hearing
- impaired memory
- seizures and death with high–level exposure

Diagnosis

The diagnosis of people with mercury poisoning includes a complete physical examination, medical tests, and diagnostic procedures.

Examination

The child's vital signs—including temperature, pulse, breathing rate, and blood pressure—will be monitored. Important diagnostic information includes:

- the type and amount of exposure
- the time and duration of exposure
- the name of the product and its ingredients and strength

Tests

Blood or urine samples can be tested for exposure to elemental and inorganic mercury. Exposure to methylmercury is measured in whole blood or scalp hair. Mercury levels are often expressed as parts per million (ppm). For example, 1 parts per million (ppm) mercury in hair is equal to 1 milligram (mg) per kilogram (kg) of hair. The average mercury level in the hair of unaffected people is 2 ppm. Blood and urine

> ## MINAMATA, JAPAN (1956)
>
> When a chemical manufacturing plant discharged its industrial waste into the Minamata Bay, the Japanese town of Minamata experienced one of the worst cases of environmental contamination in history. The fish in the bay ingested this industrial waste, and the fish-eating Minamata citizens were poisoned after consuming large amounts of the methylmercury-contaminated seafood.
>
> Cats and birds were also affected and their strange behavior was noticed. The effects were so drastic, with cats jumping wildly and throwing themselves into the sea, the behavior was termed "dancing cat fever." Soon, the correlation between the contaminated fish and the odd behavior was made, with the first human victims reported in 1956.
>
> In 2004, Chisso, the chemical manufacturing plant responsible for the pollution, was forced to clean up the contamination. Chisso also financially compensated the victims, with the final financial settlement executed in March 2010.
>
> The town of Minamata lent its name to this disease. The term "Minamata disease" now encompasses all alkyl-mercury-poisoning cases.

tests may also be used to detect kidney damage from mercury poisoning.

Procedures

The following procedures are commonly used to diagnosis mercury poisoning:

- For swallowed inorganic mercury, an endoscope—a flexible instrument with a camera—may be inserted through the throat to look for burns in the esophagus or stomach.
- X rays are taken immediately to locate swallowed batteries and monitor their passing through the gastrointestinal tract.
- X rays may be taken to diagnose lung or kidney damage.

Treatment

Treatment can include traditional methods, including drugs and alternative methods.

Although inhaled elemental mercury poisoning can be difficult to treat, possibilities include:

- humidified oxygen or air
- a breathing tube inserted in the lungs
- suctioning mercury out of the lungs

Inorganic mercury poisoning is treated with supportive measures, including possibly intravenous fluids and electrolytes. Others include:

- Swallowed mercuric oxide may be treated by gastric lavage, in which a tube is inserted through the mouth to wash out the stomach.
- Swallowed mercuric chloride may be treated by making the child vomit.
- Endoscopy may be used to remove a swallowed battery from the esophagus or stomach.
- An inhaled battery is removed immediately from the larynx with a laryngoscope or from the lungs with a bronchoscope or by surgery.

Treatment for methylmercury poisoning depends on the severity and is similar to treatments for cerebral palsy. It may include fluids and electrolytes and kidney dialysis.

Drugs

Chelators—drugs that bind mercury and other heavy metals—may be required for weeks or months to remove mercury from the blood and protect the kidneys and brain. Other medications to treat mercury poisoning include:

- activated charcoal to absorb swallowed mercury in the stomach
- drugs to induce vomiting for mercuric chloride poisoning
- laxatives for mercuric oxide or mercuric chloride poisoning
- medications to treat symptoms

Alternative treatment

There are various alternative types of chelation therapy. These include bentonite clay baths and combinations of herbs, amino acids, and other nutritional supplements.

Public health role and response

The American Association of Poison Control Centers (AAPCC) should be called for instructions: (800) 222-1222. The AAPCC is a national voluntary health organization that represents 57 poison centers across the United States. According to the website of the AAPCC, the organization is "dedicated to actively advancing the health care role and public health mission of our members through information, advocacy, education and research." The AAPCC sets standards for poison center operations and certifies specialists in poison information. These professionals are available around the clock seven days a week to respond to all types of emergency requests relating to poisonings. In addition, the AAPCC maintains the only poison information and surveillance database in the United States, what is called the National Poison Data System.

Prognosis

The prognosis for mercury poisoning can include the following:

- A single low-level exposure to elemental mercury does not usually require treatment and is unlikely to have long-term effects.

- Untreated mercury poisoning can eventually cause pain, muscle weakness, vision loss, paralysis, or death.

- Severe elemental mercury poisoning can cause long-term damage to the lungs, kidneys, and central nervous system, including brain damage. Very large exposures are usually fatal.

- Swallowed batteries usually pass through the gastrointestinal tract without causing serious damage; however, the prognosis depends on the type of battery and how quickly the condition is treated.

- Severe inorganic mercury poisoning can cause massive blood and fluid loss, kidney failure, and probable death.

- Mercuric chloride is very toxic and even small swallowed doses can cause kidney failure and death. The prognosis depends on the amount of mercury, the symptoms within the first 10 to 15 minutes, and how quickly the poisoning is treated. Poisoning that occurs slowly over time may result in permanent brain damage.

- Mercuric oxide poisoning also can lead to organ failure and death.

- Damage from methylmercury is irreversible, although the symptoms do not usually worsen without additional exposure. Chronic brain damage from organic mercury poisoning is hard to treat and some children never recover. Methylmercury poisoning may also increase the risk for heart attacks.

- Both mercuric chloride and methylmercury are considered possible carcinogens.

KEY TERMS

Button batteries—Tiny, round batteries containing mercuric chloride that power items such as watches, hearing aids, calculators, cameras, and penlights.

Cerebral palsy—Brain damage before, during, or just after birth that results in lack of muscle coordination and problems with speech.

Chelators—Various compounds that bind to metals such as mercury.

Contact dermatitis—Skin inflammation from contact with an allergen or other irritating substance.

Elemental mercury (Hg)—Metallic mercury; quicksilver; a heavy, silvery, poisonous metallic element that is a liquid at room temperature but vaporizes readily.

Inorganic mercury—Inorganic compounds such as mercuric oxide (HgO) and mercuric chloride ($HgCl_2$).

Mercuric chloride; mercury(II) chloride ($HgCl_2$)—A poisonous crystalline form of inorganic mercury that is used as a disinfectant and fungicide.

Methylmercury—Any of various toxic compounds containing the organic grouping CH_3Hg. These compounds occur as industrial byproducts and pesticide residues; accumulate in fish and other organisms, especially those high on the food chain; and are rapidly absorbed through the human intestine to cause neurological disorders such as Minamata disease.

Organic mercury—Poisonous compounds containing mercury and carbon, such as methylmercury, ethylmercury, and phenylmercury.

Thimerosal—A crystalline organic mercury compound used as an antifungal and antibacterial agent and present in very small amounts in some vaccines.

Prevention

The U.S. Food and Drug Administration (FDA) and the **Environmental Protection Agency (EPA)** recommend that young children and women who are pregnant, may become pregnant, or are nursing:

- not eat swordfish, shark, king mackerel, or tilefish, all of which have high mercury levels

- eat up to 12 oz. (340 g; or two average portions) per week of a variety of low-mercury fish and shellfish,

> **QUESTIONS TO ASK YOUR DOCTOR**
>
> - Do I have mercury poisoning?
> - What are the short-term and long-term effects of mercury poisoning?
> - How will I be treated for mercury poisoning?
> - Will I completely recover from mercury poisoning?
> - How can I prevent being poisoned by mercury?
> - Are there other medical conditions with symptoms similar to mercury poisoning?

such as shrimp, canned light tuna, salmon, pollock, catfish, fish sticks, or fast-food fish
- eat no more than 6 oz. (170 g) per week of albacore ("white") tuna steak, which has higher levels of mercury
- check local advisories for fish caught by family and friends in local waters
- eat no more than 6 oz. (170 g.) per week of non-commercially caught fish from local waters if no advisories are available, and eat no other fish during the week
- feed young children smaller portions of fish

Other preventions for mercury poisoning include:
- teaching children never to touch mercury or any shiny, silver liquid
- carefully handling and properly disposing of mercury-containing products such as thermometers and fluorescent light bulbs
- following established procedures for mercury spills
- never vacuuming up spilled mercury, since this causes vaporization
- keeping children and pregnant women away from areas where liquid mercury is used
- contacting local health departments for large mercury spills

Resources

BOOKS

Groth, Edward. *Over the Limit: Eating Too Much High-Mercury Fish*. Montpelier, VT: Mercury Policy Project, 2008.

Shannon, Michael W., Stephen W. Borron, and Michael J. Burns, editors. *Haddad and Winchester's Clinical Management of Poisoning and Drug Overdose*. Philadelphia: Saunders/Elsevier, 2007.

Spaeth, Kenneth R., Antonios J. Tsismenakis, and Stefanos N. Kales. *Heavy Metals: A Rapid Clinical Guide to Neurotoxicity and Other Common Concerns*. New York: Nova Science, 2010.

PERIODICALS

Brennan, Richard J. "Nightmare of Mercury Poisoning Returns." *Toronto Star* (April 6, 2010): A1.

Daley, Beth. "Mercury Leaks Found as New Bulbs Break; Energy Benefits of Fluorescents May Outweigh Risk." *Boston Globe* (February 26, 2008): B2.

Haggart, Kelly. "Mercury Research Bears Fruit in the Amazon." *Women & Environments International* no. 76/77 (Fall 2008): 5–8.

Philibert, Aline, Maryse Bouchard, and Donna Mergler. "Neuropsychiatric Symptoms, Omega-3, and Mercury Exposure in Freshwater Fish-Eaters." *Archives of Environmental & Occupational Health* 63(3) (Fall 2008): 143–53.

WEBSITES

Besser, Richard E. *Children's Exposure to Elemental Mercury: A National Review of Exposure Events*. Agency for Toxic Substances and Disease Registry, Centers for Disease Control and Prevention, Mercury Workgroup. (February 2009). http://www.atsdr.cdc.gov/mercury/docs/MercuryRTCFinal2013345.pdf (accessed June 27, 2012).

"Major Methylmercury Outbreaks." Food and Drug Administration. (March 6, 2012). http://www.mercurydisabilityboard.com/facts/methylmercury-outbreaks/ (accessed June 27, 2012).

"Mercury." Environmental Protection Agency. (June 4, 2012). http://www.epa.gov/mercury/index.html (accessed June 27, 2012).

"Mercury." Medline Plus. (May 16, 2012). http://www.nlm.nih.gov/medlineplus/mercury.html (accessed June 27, 2012).

"Mercury Poisoning Linked to Skin Products." Food and Drug Administration. (March 6, 2012). http://www.fda.gov/ForConsumers/ConsumerUpdates/ucm294849.htm (accessed June 27, 2012).

"Mercury and Your Health." Agency for Toxic Substances and Disease Registry. (January 22, 2010). http://www.atsdr.cdc.gov/mercury/ (accessed June 27, 2012).

Siegel, Shefa. "Threat of Mercury Poisoning Rises With Gold Mining Boom." Yale University. (January 3, 2011). http://e360.yale.edu/feature/threat_of_mercury_poisoning_rises_with_gold_mining_boom/2354/ (accessed June 27, 2012).

"ToxFAQs^{TM} for Mercury." Agency for Toxic Substances and Disease Registry, Centers for Disease Control and Prevention. (March 3, 2011). http://www.atsdr.cdc.gov/toxfaqs/tf.asp?id=113&tid=24 (accessed June 27, 2012).

"What You Need to Know about Mercury in Fish and Shellfish." U.S. Food and Drug Administration and U.S. Environmental Protection Agency. http://www.fda.gov/downloads/Food/ResourcesForYou/Consumers/UCM182158.pdf (accessed June 27, 2012).

"What the Yuck: Mercury Poisoning from Sushi?" CNN Health. (2011). http://thechart.blogs.cnn.com/2011/04/08/what-the-yuck-mercury-poisoning-from-sushi/ (accessed June 27, 2012).

ORGANIZATIONS

Agency for Toxic Substances and Disease Registry, 4770 Buford Hwy., N.E., Atlanta, GA 30341, (800) 232-4636, http://www.atsdr.cdc.gov/.

Food and Drug Administration, 10903 New Hampshire Ave., Silver Spring, MD 20993, (888) 463-6332, http://www.fda.gov/.

National Institute of Neurological Disorders and Stroke, P.O. Box 5801, Bethesda, MD 20824, (301) 496-5751, (800) 352-9424, http://www.ninds.nih.gov/.

Occupational Safety and Health Administration, 200 Constitution Ave., Washington, D.C. 20210, (800) 321-6742, http://www.osha.gov/.

Margaret Alic, PhD
William A. Atkins, BB, BS, MBA

Methemoglobinemia

Definition

Methemoglobinemia is a blood disease where hemoglobin in the blood is converted to another form called methemoglobin, which cannot deliver oxygen to body tissues. Methemoglobinemia can either be congenital or acquired.

Description

The molecule hemoglobin in the blood is responsible for binding oxygen to provide to the body. When hemoglobin is oxidized to methemoglobin its structure changes and it is no longer able to bind oxygen. Hemoglobin is constantly under oxidizing stresses. However, normally less than 1% of a person's hemoglobin is in the methemoglobin state. This is due to the body's systems that reduce methemoglobin back to hemoglobin. Infants have a higher risk of acquiring methemoglobinemia because infant hemoglobin is more prone to be oxidized to methemoglobin.

Demographics

Methemoglobinemia occurs rarely throughout the world. Most cases of methemoglobinemia are acquired and result from exposure to certain drugs or other chemicals. However, the true incidence of acquired methemoglobinemia is unknown. Estimated incidence based on methylene blue use (the treatment of methemoglobinemia) reported to the American Association of Poison Control Centers is approximately 100 cases per year. This number is considered to be a underestimation due to underreporting of methemoglobinemia cases to U.S. poison control centers. One of the more common causes of acquired methemoglobinemia is exposure to topical benzocaine during medical procedures. An estimated 0.115% of patients undergoing transesophageal echocardiography (TEE) develop methemoglobinemia.

Hereditary methemoglobinemia has been classified as a rare disease, which is defined as one person or less affected per two thousand people.

Causes and symptoms

There are two causes of the congenital form of the disease. One cause is a defect in the body's systems to reduce methemoglobin to hemoglobin. The other cause is an inherited mutant form of hemoglobin called hemoglobin M that cannot bind to oxygen. Both of these forms are typically benign.

Acquired methemoglobinemia, which is more common than inherited forms, is caused by an external exposure to certain oxidizing chemicals or drugs, including anesthetics such as benzocaine, **benzene**, certain antibiotics (e.g., dapsone), and nitrites. These compounds can increase the formation of methemoglobin up to one thousand times.

Infants under six months of age are particularly susceptible to developing methemoglobinemia. They may acquire methemoglobinemia by drinking water containing nitrates (which are converted to nitrites in the digestive system of an infant), thereby developing a condition called blue baby syndrome. The nitrites react with hemoglobin in the blood, forming high amounts of methemoglobin. Nitrates may contaminate well waters from agricultural use of fertilizers or from septic systems. The U.S. **Environmental Protection Agency** drinking water standard of 10 milligrams per liter of nitrate-nitrogen is based on protecting infants from developing methemoglobinemia. Other causes of methemoglobinemia in infants are dehydration due to excessive diarrhea or from topical anesthetics containing benzocaine or prilocaine applied to their tissues (as may be done to gums to soothe the pain of teething).

With a methemoglobin level of 3-15% skin can turn to a pale gray or blue (**cyanosis**). With levels above 25% the following symptoms may be present:

- cyanosis unaffected by oxygen administration
- blood that is dark or chocolate in color that will not change to red in the presence of oxygen

- headache
- weakness
- confusion
- chest pain

When methemoglobin levels are above 70% death may result if not treated immediately.

Diagnosis

Diagnosis is based on the symptoms and history. If these are indicative of methemoglobinemia, blood tests are performed to confirm the presence and level of methemoglobin.

Treatment

For acquired methemoglobinemia, the typical treatment is with supplemental oxygen and with methylene blue. Methylene blue is administered with an IV over a five-minute period, followed by an IV flush with normal saline. Results are typically seen within 20 minutes. Methylene blue reduces methemoglobin to hemoglobin.

Though congenital methemoglobinemia is usually benign, the form due to a defective reducing system can be treated with ascorbic acid (vitamin C) taken daily. As of 2012 there was no treatment for the other congenital form due to hemoglobin M.

Alternative treatment

Alternative treatments include hyperbaric oxygen therapy and exchange transfusions. Hyperbaric oxygen therapy uses a special chamber, sometimes called a pressure chamber, to increase the amount of oxygen in the blood. The air pressure inside a hyperbaric oxygen chamber is about two and a half times greater than the normal pressure in the atmosphere, which helps the blood carry more oxygen to organs and tissues in the body. Exchange transfusion is a potentially lifesaving procedure that involves slowly removing the patient's blood and replacing it with fresh donor blood or plasma.

Public health role and response

In order to protect public health, in 2011, the U.S. **Food and Drug Administration** (FDA) alerted health care professionals that the agency continues to receive reports of methemoglobinemia associated with benzocaine sprays, with some cases resulting in fatalities. These sprays are used during medical procedures to numb the mucous membranes of the mouth and throat. However, as of 2012, labels of marketed benzocaine sprays were not yet required to warn about the risk of methemoglobinemia. The FDA was continuing to evaluate the safety of benzocaine.

Also, to protect infants from developing methemoglobinemia, the U.S. Environmental Protection Agency has set the Maximum Contaminant Level (MCL) for nitrate in drinking water at 10 milligrams per liter (mg/L). Since this standard takes available health effects information into account, infants are unlikely to develop methemoglobinemia caused by drinking water if the water contains nitrate at or below this level. In addition, community wells throughout the U.S. are required to be tested for nitrate contamination.

Prognosis

If found early, acquired methemoglobinemia can be easily treated with no side effects. After treatment with methylene blue the patient can expect a full recovery.

Prevention

If a person contracts methemoglobinemia from a specific medication or chemical, then that medication should be avoided in the future. For people with congenital methemoglobinemia, medications or other chemicals that are known to oxidize hemoglobin should not be used. Preventive measures are especially encouraged for pregnant women or women who are breast feeding.

Resources

BOOKS

Surhone, Lambert M., Mariam T. Tennoe, and Susan F. Henssonow, eds. *Methemoglobinemia*, Seattle, WA: Betascript, 2010.

> **KEY TERMS**
>
> **Congenital**—Existing at, and usually before, birth; referring to conditions that are present at birth, regardless of their causation.
>
> **Cyanosis**—The appearance of a blue or purple coloration of the skin or mucous membranes due to the tissues near the skin surface being low on oxygen
>
> **Oxidation**—When a chemical element or compound loses an electron.
>
> **Reduction**—When a chemical element or compound gains an electron.

WEBSITES

"Methemoglobinemia" http://www.ncbi.nlm.nih.gov/pubmedhealth/PMH0001588.

Judith L Sims

Microbial pathogens

Definition

Microbial pathogens are microorganisms that are capable of producing disease.

Description

Virtually all groups of bacteria have some members that are pathogens. Other disease-causing microbial agents are **viruses** and parasitic protozoa. Earlier methods of detecting and identifying microbial pathogens involved culturing and isolating bacterial colonies in growth media in the lab. With the advent of polymerase chain reaction (PCR) assays, identification of microorganisms became more definitive.

Treatment

Bacterial pathogens can be controlled antibiotics. However, these drugs are not effective against viruses or **parasites**, and indiscriminant use may increase the percentage of resistant strains of bacterial pathogens in any population. Antibiotic resistance has resulted in the reemergence of several disease. Many of the major bacteria causing disease in humans had at least one subtype or strain that is characterized by bacterial resistance to antibiotics. Viruses may also exhibit resistance to antiviral medications.

Marie H. Bundy

Mold

Definition

Mold refers to a large diverse group of fungal organisms that grow in filaments, resulting in a cottony, fuzzy appearance, and reproduce by forming spores. They grow on organic substances and other surfaces where moisture is present. They especially thrive in damp, warm environments. Molds that grow in shower stalls and bathrooms and that are white or gray in color are sometimes referred to as mildew.

Tiny mold spores are not visible to the naked eye. They are persistent, can be transported through the air, and can survive in conditions that molds cannot grow, such as dry environments. When mold spores land on a surface where moisture is present, the mold then starts to grow.

Molds are found both outdoors and indoors. Outdoors molds aid in the decomposition of organic matter such as dead trees, compost, and leaves. The most common types of indoor household mold include *Cladosporium*, *Penicillium*, *Stachybotrys*, *Alternaria*, and *Aspergillus*.

There are several diseases of animals and humans that can be caused by molds due to allergic sensitivity to their spores. In addition, molds can produce mycotoxins, which are toxic compounds that are produced as some types of molds grow. At this time there is not convincing evidence to link health effects to indoor exposure to airborne mycotoxins, although ingestion of moldy food with mycotoxins has been shown to result in illness.

Indoor molds can also destroy surfaces and objects on which they grow.

Description

Molds (fungi) are present almost everywhere. Molds can be many different colors and produce a musty odor. In an indoor environment hundreds of different kinds of mold are able to grow wherever there is moisture and an organic substrate, which serves as a food source. They can grow on building and other materials, including: the paper on gypsum wallboard (drywall), ceiling tiles, wood products, paint, wallpaper, carpeting, some furnishings, books/papers, clothes, and other fabrics. Mold can also grow on moist, dirty surfaces such as concrete, fiberglass insulation, heating and air conditioning ducts, and ceramic tiles. It is not possible to eliminate the presence of all indoor fungal spores and fragments; however, mold growth indoors can and should be prevented and removed as much as possible, for molds have been associated with human health effects in persons allergic to molds. Molds produce irritating substances that may act as allergens, and some molds produce toxic substances called mycotoxins.

Moisture in a building may come from a variety of sources, such as leakage or seepage through basement floors, showering, and cooking. The amount of moisture that air can hold is dependent on the temperature of the air, with colder air being able to hold less moisture than warmer air. This moisture can cause mold to grow. Mold can especially be troublesome after a building has been exposed to flooding.

Demographics

The prevalence of indoor dampness varies widely within and among countries, continents and climate zones. It is estimated to affect 10–50% of indoor environments in Europe, North America, Australia, India and Japan. In some areas, such as river valleys and coastal areas, the conditions of dampness can be substantially more severe.

Most people are not adversely affected by the presence of molds and other fungi. It has been estimated that about 10% of the population is allergic to one or more types of mold. Many of these people are affected by outdoor as well as indoor mold.

Except in buildings with extensive mold growth, the amount of mold found in indoor air is usually much less than what is found outdoors. For people with allergies to mold, however, there may be no practical level of exposure, either indoors or outdoors, that would not create discomfort or harm. It is therefore wise to remove and prevent indoor mold growth.

Causes and symptoms

For persons who are sensitive to molds, exposure may result in nasal stuffiness and sneezing, eye irritation, wheezing, coughing, sinus problems, fatigue, skin irritation, and headaches or migraines. Exposure to molds can trigger **asthma** episodes in persons with asthma. Allergic individuals vary in their degree of susceptibility to mold, with the severity of an allergic response depending on the extent and type of mold that is present.

Persons with chronic lung illnesses, such as obstructive lung disease or persons with severely weakened immune systems, including those with transplants, chemotherapy, **AIDS**, and newborn infants, may develop other diseases such as allergic bronchopulmonary **aspergillosis**, an allergic lung reaction to a type of fungus (most commonly Aspergillus fumigatus) that occurs in some people with asthma or cystic **fibrosis**, and hypersensitivity pneumonitis, an inflammation of the lung (usually of the very small airways) caused by the body's immune reaction to small air-borne particles, including molds, and resulting in fever, chills, coughing, shortness of breath, and body aches.

There is no consensus on how significant a threat that inhalation of molds in residential, school, or office settings are to human health, except to persons who are allergic to mold. Building-related illnesses are often difficult to diagnose and interpret, for symptoms are non-specific and often allergy-related, and it is difficult to make conclusive links to environmental factors.

Diagnosis

Diagnosis of mold infestations

The U.S. Environmental Protection Association (**EPA**) has stated that if visible mold is present, testing is usually unnecessary. No standards have been established for mold or mold spore levels, since tolerable or acceptable limits of mold exposure for humans have not been defined. Individuals vary in their susceptibility to mold, so testing and measurement of mold presence is not effective in predicting the degree of health risks from an occurrence of mold.

Therefore, a mold infestation is determined primarily on visual assessment, knowledge of the building structure, and the history of water damage in the building.

Diagnosis of diseases associated with mold infestations

To diagnose an allergy to mold or fungi, the medical practitioner must take a complete medical history. If mold allergy is suspected, the doctor may do skin tests, where extracts of different types of fungi will be used to scratch or prick the skin. If there is no reaction, allergy is not likely. In some people with allergy, irritation alone can cause a reaction, so it may not actually be an allergic reaction. Therefore the medical practitioner combines the patient's medical history, the skin testing results, and a physical examination to diagnose a mold allergy.

Treatment

Treatment of a mold infestation

Visible fungal growth represents unnecessary exposure and should not be present in indoor spaces. Visible fungus indicates improper moisture management in the building.

he first step in treatment of mold is to identify and repair the moisture problem. Mold will not grow unless sufficient moisture is present. Small amounts of mold growing on visible surfaces can usually be easily cleaned without professional assistance. Larger amounts of mold may require more extensive evaluation, repair or replacement, and dust control by professionals.

There are several methods available to clean up mold, depending on the size and type of surfaces affected. The work area can be cleaned using wet methods such as wet wiping with a detergent solution. In some cases, a dilute solution of chlorine bleach (no stronger than 1 cup of bleach in 1 gallon of water) or stronger commercial cleaners may be needed to kill the mold, for moldy surfaces should not be touched with bare hands. When washing with detergent and water, the use of rubber gloves is recommended. For bleach or harsher cleaning agents, nonporous gloves such as neoprene, nitrile, polyurethane, or PVC, should be worn along with protective eyewear. An N-95 respirator is recommended to limit exposure to airborne mold or spores during the cleaning process.

It is important to control dust associated with the clean-up activity. Dust should be controlled using damp cleaning methods and by using HEPA vacuuming. HEPA (High Efficiency Particulate Air) means that the vacuum filter is capable of removing particles that are 0.3 microns (one millionth of a meter) in diameter at 99.97% efficiency. Typical vacuum filters will not capture spores as efficiently and may disperse them in air. When the size of the area with visible mold growth is large or when sensitive people are present, the work area should be enclosed in plastic. The air inside the enclosure should be actively exhausted to the outdoors by placing the enclosed environment under negative pressure with respect to the rest of the room or building. If there are any leaks in the enclosure, that air will move from the cleaner areas outside the enclosure into the enclosure, and minimize air movement in the opposite direction.

When porous, cellulose-containing items such as drywall, clothing, carpets and carpet pads, textiles, upholstered furniture, leather, paper goods, and many types of artwork or decorative items get wet, they should be dried and disinfected within 48 hours or discarded. If sewage or gray water is involved, the materials should be discarded. These types of damp materials are usually the determining factor, rather than indoor humidity, are usually the primary determining factor whether mold growth will be excessive. Care should be taken to avoid that items not discarded become sources of re-infestation.

Treatment of diseases associated with mold

Since molds are common and it is difficult to avoid exposure, there are medications that may be used to alleviate allergic symptoms. These include:

- Nasal corticosteroid sprays to aid in the prevention and treatment of inflammation caused by an upper respiratory mold allergy;
- Antihistamines to help with itching, sneezing and runny nose by blocking histamine, an inflammatory chemical released by the immune system during an allergic reaction;
- Decongestants to relieve nasal congestion in the upper respiratory tract; and
- Montelukast to block the action of leukotrienes, which are immune system chemicals that cause allergy symptoms such as excess mucus.

Other treatments for mold allergy include:

- Immunotherapy to eliminate allergies through a series of allergy shots, although this therapy is only partially effective against mold allergies; and
- Nasal rinses to soothe nasal symptoms.

A doctor may recommend additional treatments if affected individuals have mold-induced allergic bronchopulmonary aspergillosis and hypersensitivity pneumonitis.

Public health role and response

The public health community in most cases does not recommend evacuation in response to a mold infestation. There is no established level of airborne mold that is accepted as unsafe for the general population. However evacuation may be warranted for sensitive populations, such as infants, elderly, the immune-suppressed, and those with medically confirmed symptoms related to mold exposure.

The presence of mold in a building does not in itself constitute a health threat. Although control of indoor mold growth is usually preferred, a health-based assessment of the indoor environment and its occupants is required to identify the extent of the health threat. Such a determination is especially critical in deciding upon an expensive course of action in a large commercial or public building. The health assessment should include:

- potential for exposure: an assessment of both the quantity and types of fungi present in bulk and air samples;
- diagnosis of exposure: a symptom survey of building occupants to determine if there are health complaints consistent with mold exposure. The pattern of symptom expression should be investigated, such as determining when did the symptoms start, end, and when were they the worst, and are most of the complaints confined to occupants of specific rooms; and
- verification of exposure: an exposure assessment (for example, an immuno-assay for immunoglobulin E (IgE) specific to molds present) to establish a link between the presence of molds with potential health

KEY TERMS

Allergen—A substance, such as mold, that causes an allergy.

Allergy—Extra sensitivity of the body to certain substances, such as pollens, foods, molds, or microorganisms, that produces an immune responses and that results in symptoms such as sneezing, itching, and skin rashes.

Alternaria—A group of fungi known as major plant pathogens and as common allergens in humans. They grow indoors and can cause hay fever or extra sensitive reactions that can lead to asthma. They can also cause infections in persons who are immunocompromised.

Aspergillus—A group of several hundred mold species found in various climates worldwide, some of which are important medically and commercially while others cause infection in humans and other animals.

Asthma—A chronic long-lasting inflammatory disease of the lung airways, where the inflammation causes the airways to spasm and swell periodically so that the airways narrow. The individual wheezes or gasp for airs until the obstruction to air flow either resolves spontaneously or responds to a wide range of treatments. Continuing inflammation makes the airways extra sensitive to stimuli such as cold air, exercise, dust mites, molds, pollutants in the air, and even stress and anxiety.

Cladosporium—A group of fungi that includes some of the most common indoor and outdoor molds. Their spores are wind-dispersed and are often extremely abundant in outdoor airs. They can grow on surfaces when moisture is present. The airborne spores are significant allergens and in large amounts they can severely affect asthmatics and people with respiratory diseases. Prolonged exposure may weaken the immune system.

Fungi—A group of organisms with a membrane-bound nucleus that derive their nourishment from dead or decaying organic matter. The group includes mushrooms, yeasts, mildew, and molds. They have rigid cell walls but lack chlorophyll.

Immunocompromised—Incapable of developing a normal immune response, usually as a result of disease, malnutrition, or immunosuppressive therapy.

Immunoglobulin E—A class of antibodies produced in the lungs, skin, and mucous membranes that are responsible for allergic reactions.

N-95 respirator—Most common of the types of particulate filtering face piece respirators. It filters at least 95 percent of airborne particles but is not resistant to oil.

Penicillium—A group of fungi of major importance in the natural environment as well as in food and drug production. Members of the genus produce penicillin, which is used as an antibiotic to kill or stop the growth of certain kinds of bacteria in the body. *Penicillium* is a common indoor mold, and its spores can cause mold allergy.

Stachybotrys—A group of molds with widespread distribution that inhabit materials high in cellulose. Certain species are known as "black mold" or "toxic black mold" in the U.S. and are frequently associated with poor indoor air quality arising from fungal growth on water-damaged building materials. Some species produce mycotoxins that are known to produce health symptoms, but it is not scientifically clear whether these mycotoxins affect human health during a mold infestation in a building.

---

effects and building occupants' health complaints. Strict criteria should be established for the diagnosis of mold exposure by qualified health professionals in order to make accurate health recommendations and to avoid unnecessary building remedies.

It is important that public health officials effectively communicate the effects of indoor mold exposure to the public. The key messages that should be conveyed are: the ubiquitous nature of fungi in the environment, the relative community of fungi found indoors compared to outdoors, the relative risk posed by the molds detected, and the range of options available to confront the problem.

Recent years have seen increased attention placed on mold-infested schools. Mold infestation in schools presents a special case in risk management and a challenge for public health officials, for parents usually have a low tolerance for either actual or perceived risk and are often organized and active in school issues.

Prognosis

Because people vary greatly in their immune response to environmental allergens, and because fungi are always present in the environment, it may not be possible to manage airborne fungal particles at a level protective of those individuals most sensitive to

> **QUESTIONS TO ASK YOUR DOCTOR**
>
> - Could my allergic symptoms be caused by molds?
> - What treatments are available to help alleviate symptoms?
> - What should I do to remediate the mold infestation in my home?
> - Should I stay in my home or should I evacuate during the remediation process?

their allergenic effects. Therefore, molds are categorized with pollen, dander, and mite excrement as allergens to be managed but cannot be eliminated. When people present with allergic hypersensitivity, health effects due to mold are due more to individual sensitivity than to the presence or absence of exposure. However, to reduce exposure, mold infestations should be treated.

Prevention

There is no practical way to eliminate mold and mold spores from an indoor environment. Therefore, to control or prevent the growth of mold, moisture levels within the building must be controlled. Methods of control include:

- fix leaks and seepage
- put plastic covers over dirt in crawl spaces
- direct ground water drainage away from a house
- use exhaust fans in kitchens and bathrooms to vent moisture to the outside
- vent clothes dryer to the outside
- scour sinks and tubs at least monthly
- clean garbage pails frequently
- clean refrigerator door gaskets and drip pans
- throw away or recycle old books, newspapers, clothing or bedding
- turn off humidifiers if moisture is condensing on windows
- use dehumidifiers and air conditioners, especially in hot, humid climates, but be sure to maintain them so mold does not grow in them
- raise the temperature of cold surfaces where moisture condenses by installing insulation or storm windows and by increasing air circulation in the home (opening doors, using fans, and moving furniture from wall corners

- use area rugs over concrete that can be taken up and washed frequently. If permanent carpet is installed on a concrete floor, consider using plastic sheeting as a vapor barrier and cover it with subflooring made of insulation covered with plywood
- use paints that contain mold inhibitors

After moisture control has been completed, it may be necessary to remove and discard the materials that were affected by the mold.

Resources

BOOKS

Billings, Kurt, and Lee Ann Billings. *Mold: The War Within.* Knoxville, TN: Partners Publishing LLC, 2010.

May, Jeffrey C., and Connie L. May. *The Mold Survival Guide: For Your Home and for Your Health.* Baltimore, MD: Johns Hopkins University Press, 2004.

Rosen, Gary. *Environmentally Friendly Mold Remediation Techniques that Significantly Reduce Childhood Asthma.* Naples, FL: Hope Academic Press, 2007.

Schaller, James, and Gary Rosen. *Mold Illness and Mold Remediation Made Simple.* Naples, FL: Hope Academic Press, 2006.

WEBSITES

"Mold." http://www.cdc.gov/mold/.

"Dampness and Mould" World Health Organization. http://www.euro.who.int/document/e92645.pdf.

ORGANIZATIONS

Allergy and Asthma Foundation of America, 8201 Corporate Drive, Suite 1000, Landover, Maryland, USA 20785, (800) 727-8462, Info@aafa.org, aafa.org.

Judith L. Sims

Multiple chemical sensitivity

Definition

Multiple chemical sensitivity (MCS) is a highly controversial disorder associated with unusually extreme sensitivity or allergy-like reaction in response to low-level exposure to chemicals, solvents, petroleum products, smoke, pollen, pet fur, perfumes, and volatile organic chemicals (VOCs) in particular. The disorder is also referred to as multiple chemical sensitivity syndrome, chemical injury, chemical sensitivity, environmental illness, multiple allergy, and total allergy syndrome, along with many other related terms.

Description

Unlike true allergies, MCS does not have an underlying cause that is relatively well understood. Consequently, it is generally regarded as idiopathic—meaning that it does not have a known mechanism of causation. As of 2012, MCS is not recognized as an "established organic disease" by the American Medical Association, the American Academy of Allergy and Immunology, the American College of Physicians, the International Society of Regulatory **Toxicology** and Pharmacology, and many other medical organizations.

In 1987, Dr. Mark R. Cullen defined MCS within the paper "The Worker with Multiple Chemical Sensitivities: An Overview" (2:655–661) within the journal *Occupational Medicine*. Cullen's definition states that MCS is a disorder:

- acquired after a documentable environmental exposure occurs that causes an objective evidence of health effects
- whose symptoms involve more than one organ system
- whose symptoms occur and go away repeatedly in response to predictable environmental stimuli
- whose symptoms occur in relation to measurable levels of chemicals
- where exposure is at levels so low that they are not known to cause harm to human health
- whose symptoms cannot be explained by any known test of organ function

In 2005, Dr. Michael Lacour and colleagues expanded the definition made by Cullen within the article "Multiple Chemical Sensitivity Syndrome (MCS)—Suggestions for an Extension of the U.S. MCS-case" (208, 141–151) in the journal *International Journal of Hygiene and Environmental Medicine*. Lacour includes these six fundamentals for MCS: (1) it is a chronic condition, (2) its symptoms recur reproducibly, (3) it occurs in multiple organ systems, (4) it occurs in response to low levels of exposure, (5) it occurs because of multiple unrelated chemicals, and (6) it improves or is resolved when incitants are removed. Lacour also adds the following symptoms:

- last at least six months, at which time they cause significant lifestyle or functional problems
- occur within the central nervous system in association with self-reported MCS symptoms
- must be present in the central nervous system with at least one symptom occurring within another organ system

> **KEY TERMS**
>
> **Somatoform disorders**—Any mental disorder characterized by symptoms that suggest physical illness or injury; however, with symptoms that cannot be completely explained by a medical condition, from exposure with a substance, or attributable to another mental disorder.
>
> **Toxicants**—Any type of poison made by humans or introduced into the environment by human activity, such as insecticides.
>
> **Volatile organic chemicals**—Any organic chemicals with a high vapor pressure at ordinary, room-temperatures.

Risk factors

MSC has been cited to occur due to a multitude of chemicals. Some of the more common include:

- agricultural chemicals such as pesticides, herbicides, and fertilizers
- air fresheners, deodorizers, and scented candles
- bleach, fabric softeners, and laundry detergents
- dishwashing liquid and detergent
- food-related products such as artificial dyes (FD&C Yellow #5), caffeine, monosodium glutamate (MSG)
- formaldehyde
- gasoline or diesel fuel
- glues, paint, paint thinners, polishes, solvents, and volatile organic compounds (VOCs)
- hair care products such as shampoos and hairsprays
- highlighters and various similar pens
- industrial cleaning chemicals such as fluid using in dry cleaning establishments
- petroleum-based products such as petroleum jelly and asphalt
- skin care products such as aftershave lotions, body and hand lotions, nail polishes, and perfumes

Demographics

Multiple chemical sensitivity has been described by numerous names since it was first studied in the 1940s. Patients who have MCS believe that their numerous symptoms are caused by low-level exposure to environmental chemicals—such low levels that average people cannot even detect such irritants. With used with MCS, chemicals refer generally to various natural and artificially made chemical agents. Medical professionals who treat MCS patients on a regular basis often refer to themselves as clinical ecologists.

Causes and symptoms

MCS has no uniform cause or consistent, measurable features. Insufficient medical evidence has yet to confirm a relationship between any of the various possible causes of MCS and the symptoms that individuals report. Individuals who have been diagnosed with MCS report widely varied symptoms. This makes it very difficult for MCS to be treated. Further, medical professionals contend it is a chronic condition identified by increased sensitivity to even slight exposure to chemicals, and that multiple symptoms occur in multiple organ systems. An episode of MCS is often caused by exposure to a newly introduced consumer product, such as new carpet. Proposed theories regarding the cause of MCS usually center around allergies, immune system dysfunction, neurobiological sensitization, and various psychological theories.

People with MCS often experience some of the following symptoms:

- burning, stinging eyes
- digestive ailments
- extreme fatigue, lethargy, malaise
- headache, migraine headache
- muscle and joint pain
- nausea
- poor (even loss of) memory and lack of concentration
- runny nose (rhinitis)
- sensitivity to light and noise
- sinus problems
- skin rashes and/or itching skin
- sleeping problems
- sore throat, cough
- vertigo, dizziness
- wheezing, breathlessness

Sometimes these symptoms are so disabled that the person cannot live or work except in an environment completely devoid of chemicals.

Critics argue that this condition should not receive clinical recognition as a disease, insisting that there is no conclusive scientific evidence to link the causes to the symptoms of the condition.

Diagnosis

Cases of MCS are usually diagnosed and evaluated based on the patient's description of symptoms and their connection to environmental exposures.

> **QUESTIONS TO ASK YOUR DOCTOR**
>
> - How common is multiple chemical sensitivity?
> - Is MCS real or imaginary?
> - Will I be taken seriously if I say I have MCS?
> - Where can I acquire more information about MCS?
> - Can you diagnosis my problem if I think I have MCS? If so, can you treat me?
> - What can I do to minimize my symptoms of MCS?
> - Will medicines help?
> - Are there tests to help better understand my problem with MCS?

Although it is clear that some people are very sensitive to various microorganisms, noxious chemicals, and common foods, there is little evidence that an immunologic basis exists for generalized allergy to environmental substances.

A medical professional will usually diagnosis MCS when observing all of the following:

- the patient exhibits an allergy-like reaction to extremely low levels of irritants, toxicants, or pollutants to which other people present at the time do not have any adverse reactions
- the patient is adversely affected by many different substances
- the problem is chronic; that is, it is not a single occurrence
- the same symptoms are repeated when the exact substance is re-introduced to the patient
- the patient improves when triggers are removed or are not present

Treatment

Because the diagnosis for MCS is difficult to make, treatment is also hard to determine. However, treatment measures can involve careful choices with regards to diet and living conditions. Patients with MCS normally have high rates of anxiety depression, and somatoform disorders. However, it is uncertain what relationship these psychiatric problems may have on the disorder. In some cases, counseling and psychotherapy have been useful. Medical professionals should earnestly evaluate and treat patients who have MCS.

Public health role and response

Because MCS is not recognized as a valid medical condition, little has been done with respect to a public response. The medical community treats MCS as best as it can under these limited circumstances.

Prognosis

For the most part, the prognosis for sufferers of MCS is best when they avoid pollutants and toxicants.

Prevention

One can prevent MCS by avoiding all chemicals that are known to adversely affect one's health. Although difficult at best, it is advised to live in an environment that is absent of pollutants and irritants of any kind—that is, a chemical-free environment.

Resources

BOOKS

Larsen, Laura, editor. *Environmental Health Sourcebook*. Detroit: Omnigraphics, 2010.

Matthews, Bonnye L. *Defining Multiple Chemical Sensitivity*. Jefferson, NC: McFarland, 2008.

Natelson, Benjamin H. *Your Symptoms Are Real: What to Do When Your Doctor Says Nothing Is Wrong*. Hoboken, NJ: John Wiley, 2008.

Pall, Martin L. *Explaining "Unexplained Illnesses": Disease Paradigm for Chronic Fatigue Syndrome, Multiple Chemical Sensitivity, Fibromyalgia, Post-Traumatic Stress Disorder, Gulf War Syndrome, and Others*. New York: Harrington Park Press, 2007.

Preston, Flora. *Convenient, "Safe" and Deadly: The True Costs of Our Chemical Lifestyle*. Lanark, ONT, Canada: Health Risk Navigation, 2006.

Sutton, Amy L. *Allergies Sourcebook: Basic Consumer Health Information About Allergic Disorders, such as Anaphylaxis*. Detroit: Omnigraphics, 2007.

Valkenburg, Els. *Understanding Multiple Chemical Sensitivity: Causes, Effects, Personal Experiences and Resources*. Jefferson, NC: McFarland, 2010.

WEBSITES

"Definitions of MCS." Danish Research Centre for Chemical Sensitivities. http://www.mcsvidencenter.dk/?site=2&side=13&id=341 (accessed September 18, 2012).

Magill, Michael K., and Anthony Suruda. "Multiple Chemical Sensitivity Syndrome." American Academy of Family Physicians. (September 1, 1998). http://www.aafp.org/afp/1998/0901/p721.html#afp19980901p721-b10 (accessed September 18, 2012).

"Multiple Chemical Sensitivity (MCS)." Ecos Organic Paints and Biosis Ltd. http://www.multiplechemical-sensitivi ty.org/ (accessed September 18, 2012).

"Multiple Chemical Sensitivities." Occupational Safety and Health Administration, U.S. Department of Labor. http://www.osha.gov/SLTC/multiplechemicalsensitivities/index.html (accessed September 18, 2012).

ORGANIZATIONS

Agency for Toxic Substances and Disease Registry, Centers for Disease Control and Prevention, 4770 Buford Hwy N.E., Atlanta, GA 30341, (800) 232-4636, http://www.atsdr.cdc.gov/.

American Academy of Environmental Medicine, 6505 E. Central Ave., #296, Wichita, KS 67206, 1(316) 684-5500, Fax: 1(316) 684-5709, administrator@aaemonline.org, http://aaemonline.org/.

American Medical Association, 515 N. State St., Chicago, IL 60654, (800) 621-8335, http://www.ama-assn.org/.

Environmental Defense Fund, 1875 Connecticut Ave. N.W., Ste. 600., Washington, D.C. 20009, (800) 684-3322, http://www.edf.org/.

Environmental Protection Agency, 1200 Pennsylvania Ave., N.W.; Ariel Rios Bldg., Washington, D.C. 20460, 1(202) 272-0167, http://www.epa.gov/.

Environmental Research Foundation, PO Box 160, New Brunswick, NJ 08908, 1(732) 828-9995, erf@rachel.org, http://www.rachel.org/.

National Institute of Occupational Safety and Health, Centers for Disease Control and Prevention, 1600 Clifton Rd., Atlanta, GA 30333, (800) 232-4636, cdcinfo@cdc.gov, http://www.cdc.gov/niosh/.

Occupational Safety and Health Organization, U.S. Department of Labor, 200 Constitution Ave., N.W., Washington, D.C. 20210, (800) 321-6742, http://www.osha.gov/.

William A. Atkins, BB, BS, MBA

Mumps

Definition

Mumps is a relatively mild short-term viral infection of the salivary glands that usually occurs during childhood. A contagious disease, mumps is characterized by a painful swelling of both cheek areas. The salivary glands are also called the parotid glands, therefore, *mumps* is sometimes referred to as an inflammation of the parotid glands (epidemic parotitis). The word *mumps* comes from an Old English dialect, meaning lumps or bumps within the cheeks.

Description

Mumps is a very contagious disease that spreads easily in such highly populated areas as day care centers and schools. Although not as contagious as **measles** or chickenpox, mumps was once quite common. Prior to the release of a mumps vaccine in the United States in

1967, approximately 92% of all children had been exposed to mumps by the age of 15. In these pre-vaccine years, most children contracted mumps between the ages of four and seven. Mumps epidemics came in two to five year cycles. The greatest mumps epidemic was in 1941 when approximately 250 cases were reported for every 100,000 people. In 1968, the year after the live mumps vaccine was released, only 76 cases were reported for every 100,000 people. By 1985, less than 3,000 cases of mumps were reported throughout the entire United States, which works out to about 1 case per 100,000 people. The reason for the decline in mumps was the increased usage of the mumps vaccine. However, 1987 noted a five–fold increase in the incidence of the disease because of the reluctance of some states to adopt comprehensive school immunization laws. Since then, state-enforced school entry requirements have achieved student immunization rates of nearly 100% in kindergarten and first grade. In 1996, the **Centers for Disease Control and Prevention** (CDC) reported only 751 cases of mumps nationwide, or, in other words, about one case for every five million people.

Risk factors

When the mumps virus is present in areas, such as schools, where close contact between people allows the virus to spread, outbreaks may occur. People who are not vaccinated against mumps are at higher risk of getting mumps and spreading the virus to others.

Although the risk of exposure to mumps for most travelers is be relatively low, travelers should be fully vaccinated or immune. This is especially important if traveling to states or countries experiencing mumps outbreaks.

Demographics

According to the CDC, before the introduction of a vaccine to protect against mumps, mumps was a common childhood disease in the United States, sometimes causing severe omplications, such as permanent deafness in children and, occasionally, swelling of the brain (encephalitis). There are normally only a few hundred cases of mumps every year in the United States. Mumps is most common in children 5 to 14 years of age who are not vaccinated, but the virus can infect a person at any age.

Causes and symptoms

The paramyxovirus that causes mumps is harbored in the saliva and is spread by sneezing, coughing, and other direct contact with another person's infected saliva. Once the person is exposed to the virus, symptoms generally occur in 14–24 days. Initial symptoms include chills, headache, loss of appetite, and a lack of energy. However, an infected person may not experience these initial symptoms. Swelling of the salivary glands in the face (parotitis) generally occurs within 12–24 hours of the above symptoms. Accompanying the swollen glands is pain on chewing or swallowing, especially with acidic beverages, such as lemonade. A fever as high as 104°F (40°C) is also common. Swelling of the glands reaches a maximum on about the second day and usually disappears by the seventh day. Once a person has contracted mumps, they become immune to the disease, despite how mild or severe their symptoms may have been.

While the majority of cases of mumps are uncomplicated and pass without incident, some complications can occur. Complications are, however, more noticeable in adults who get the infection. In 15% of cases, the covering of the brain and spinal cord becomes inflamed (**meningitis**). Symptoms of meningitis usually develop within four or five days after the first signs of mumps. These symptoms include a stiff neck, headache, vomiting, and a lack of energy. Mumps meningitis is usually resolved within seven days, and damage to the brain is exceedingly rare.

The mumps infection can spread into the brain causing inflammation of the brain (encephalitis). Symptoms of mumps encephalitis include the inability to feel pain, seizures, and high fever. Encephalitis can occur during the parotitis stage or one to two weeks later. Recovery from mumps encephalitis is usually complete, although complications, such as seizure disorders, have been noted. Only about 1 in 100 with mumps encephalitis dies from the complication.

About one-fourth of all post-pubertal males who contract mumps can develop a swelling of the scrotum (orchitis) about seven days after the parotitis stage. Symptoms include marked swelling of one or both testicles, severe pain, fever, nausea, and headache. Pain and swelling usually subside after five to seven days, although the testicles can remain tender for weeks.

Girls occasionally suffer an inflammation of the ovaries, or oophoritis, as a complication of mumps, but this condition is far less painful than orchitis in boys.

Diagnosis

When mumps reaches epidemic proportions, diagnosis is relatively easy on the basis of the physical symptoms. The doctor will take the child's temperature, gently palpate (touch) the skin over the parotid glands, and look inside the child's mouth. If the child has mumps, the openings to the ducts inside the mouth will be slightly inflamed and have a "pouty" appearance. With so many people vaccinated today, a case of mumps must be properly diagnosed in the event the salivary glands are swollen for reasons other than viral infection. For example, in persons with poor oral hygiene, the salivary glands can be infected with bacteria. In these cases, antibiotics are necessary. Also in rare cases, the salivary glands can become blocked, develop tumors, or swell due to the use of certain drugs, such as iodine. A test can be performed to determine whether the person with swelling of the salivary glands actually has the mumps virus.

Mumps tests may also be used to confirm that a person is immune to the virus due to previous infections or **vaccination**. Doctors however, most frequently diagnose current mumps infections based upon characteristic clinical findings.

Treatment

When mumps does occurs, the illness is usually allowed to run its course. The symptoms, however, are treatable. Because of difficulty swallowing, the most important challenge is to keep the patient fed and hydrated. The individual should be provided a soft diet, consisting of cooked cereals, mashed potatoes, broth-based soups, prepared baby foods, or foods put through a home food processor. Aspirin, acetaminophen, or ibuprofen can relieve some of the pain due to swelling, headache, and fever. Avoid fruit juices and other acidic foods or beverages that can irritate the salivary glands. Avoid dairy products that can be hard to digest. In the event of complications, a physician should be contacted at once. For example, if orchitis occurs, a physician should be called. Also, supporting the scrotum in a cotton bed on an adhesive-tape bridge between the thighs can minimize tension. Ice packs are also helpful.

Alternative treatment

Acupressure can be used effectively to relieve pain caused by swollen glands. The patient can, by using the middle fingers, gently press the area between the jawbone and the ear for two minutes while breathing deeply.

A number of homeopathic remedies can be used for the treatment of mumps. For example, belladonna may be useful for flushing, redness, and swelling. Bryonia (wild hops) may be useful for irritability, lack of energy, or thirst. Phytolacca (poke root) may be prescribed for extremely swollen glands. A homeopathic physician should always be consulted for appropriate doses for children, and remedies that do not work within one day should be stopped. A homeopathic preparation of the mumps virus can also be used prophylactically or as a treatment for the disease.

Several herbal remedies may be useful in helping the body recover from the infection or may help alleviate the discomfort associated with the disease. Echinacea (*Echinacea* spp.) can be used to boost the immune system and help the body fight the infection. Other herbs taken internally, such as cleavers (*Galium aparine*), calendula (*Calendula officinalis*), and phytolacca (poke root), target the lymphatic system and may help to enhance the activity of the body's internal filtration system. Since phytolacca can be toxic, it should only be used by patients under the care of a skilled practitioner. Topical applications are also useful in relieving the discomfort of mumps. A cloth dipped in a heated mixture of vinegar and cayenne (*Capsicum frutescens*) can be wrapped around the neck several times a day. Cleavers or calendula can

---

KEY TERMS

Asymptomatic—Persons who carry a disease and may be capable of transmitting the disease but who do not exhibit symptoms of the disease are said to be asymptomatic.

Autism—A severe developmental disorder that usually begins before three years of age and affects a child's social as well as intellectual development. Some researchers theorized that immunization with the MMR vaccine was a risk factor for autism.

Encephalitis—Inflammation of the brain.

Epidemic parotitis—The medical name for mumps.

Immunoglobulin G (IgG)—A group of antibodies against certain viral infections that circulate in the bloodstream. One type of IgG is specific against the mumps paramyxovirus.

Meningitis—Inflammation of the membranes covering the brain and spinal cord.

Orchitis—Inflammation or swelling of the scrotal sac containing the testicles.

Paramyxovirus—A genus of viruses that includes the causative agent of mumps.

Parotitis—Inflammation and swelling of the salivary glands.

also be combined with vinegar, heated, and applied in a similar manner.

Public health role and response

Mumps is a public health issue because it can be prevented by immunization. Thanks to successful vaccination programs, measles, mumps, and rubella (MMR) are now much less common in the United States and countries that have MMR immunization programs than they used to be. Finland reports complete eradication. The first vaccine against mumps was licensed in the United States in 1967, and by 2005, high two-dose childhood vaccination coverage reduced disease rates by 99%.

Prognosis

When mumps is uncomplicated, prognosis is excellent. However, in rare cases, a relapse occurs after about two weeks. Complications can also delay complete recovery.

Prevention

A vaccine exists to protect against mumps. The vaccine preparation (MMR) is usually given as part of a combination injection that helps protect against measles, mumps, and rubella. MMR is a live vaccine administered in one dose between the ages of 12–15 months, 4–6 years, or 11–12 years. Persons who are unsure of their mumps history and/or mumps vaccination history should be vaccinated. Susceptible health care workers, especially those who work in hospitals, should be vaccinated.

The mumps vaccine is extremely effective, and virtually everyone should be vaccinated against this disease. There are, however, a few reasons why people should *not* be vaccinated against mumps:

- Pregnant women who contract mumps have an increased rate of miscarriage, but not birth defects. As a result, pregnant women should not receive the mumps vaccine because of the possibility of damage to the fetus. Women who have had the vaccine should postpone pregnancy for three months after vaccination.
- Unvaccinated persons who have been exposed to mumps should not get the vaccine, as it may not provide protection. The person should, however, be vaccinated if no symptoms result from the exposure to mumps.
- Persons with minor fever-producing illnesses, such as an upper respiratory infection, should not get the vaccine until the illness has subsided.

QUESTIONS TO ASK YOUR DOCTOR

- What causes mumps?
- How long will my child be contagious?
- How are mumps treated?
- How can I help my child be more comfortable?
- Is there a risk of complications?

- Because mumps vaccine is produced using eggs, individuals who develop hives, swelling of the mouth or throat, dizziness, or breathing difficulties after eating eggs should not receive the mumps vaccine.
- Persons with immune deficiency diseases and/or those whose immunity has been suppressed with anticancer drugs, corticosteroids, or radiation should not receive the vaccine. Family members of immunocompromised people, however, should get vaccinated to reduce the risk of mumps.
- The CDC recommends that all children infected with human immunodeficiency disease (HIV) who are asymptomatic should receive the MMR vaccine at 15 months of age.

The mumps vaccine has been controversial in recent years because of concern that its use was linked to a rise in the rate of childhood **autism**. The negative publicity given to the vaccine in the mass media led some parents to refuse to immunize their children with the MMR vaccine. One result has been an increase in the number of mumps outbreaks in several European countries, including Italy and the United Kingdom.

In the fall of 2002, the *New England Journal of Medicine* published a major Danish study disproving the hypothesis of a connection between the MMR vaccine and autism. A second study in Finland showed that the vaccine is not associated with aseptic meningitis or encephalitis or autism. Since these studies were published, American primary care physicians have once again reminded parents of the importance of immunizing their children against mumps and other childhood diseases.

Resources

BOOKS

Colligan, L. H. *Measles and Mumps*. New York, NY: Benchmark Books, 2010.

Hecht, Alan. *Mumps*. New York, NY: Chelsea House Publications, 2012.

Temesgen, Z., ed. *Mayo Clinic Infectious Diseases Board Review*. New York, NY: Oxford University Press, 2011.

PERIODICALS

Adalja. A. A. "Vaccines, immunity, whooping cough, and mumps." *Biosecurity and Bioterrorism* 9, no. 1 (March 2011): 9–11.

Demicheli. V., et al. "Vaccines for measles, mumps and rubella in children." *Cochrane Database of Systematic Reviews* 15, no. 2 (February 2012): CD004407.

Eriksen, J., et al. "Seroepidemiology of mumps in Europe (1996-2008): why do outbreaks occur in highly vaccinated populations?" *Epidemiology and Infection* 12 (June 2012): 1–16.

Ruijs, W. L., et al. "The role of schools in the spread of mumps among unvaccinated children: a retrospective cohort study." *BMC Infectious Diseases* 11 (August 2011): 227.

Smith, S. D., and I. Gemmill. "Mumps: resurgence of a vanquished virus." *Canadian Family Physician* 57, no. 7 (July 2011): 786–790.

White, S. J., et al. "Measles, mumps, and rubella." *Clinical Obstetrics and Gynecology* 55, no. 2 (June 2012): 550–559.

Xu, P., et al. "The V protein of mumps virus plays a critical role in pathogenesis." *Journal of Virology* 86, no. 3 (February 2012): 1768–1776.

WEBSITES

"Fast Facts about Mumps." Centers for Disease Control. October 13, 2012. http://www.cdc.gov/mumps/about/mumps-facts.html

"Mumps." Mayo Clinic. October 5, 2012. http://www.mayo-clinic.com/print/mumps/DS00125/METHOD=print&DSECTION=all

"Mumps." Medline Plus, 28 September 2012. http://www.nlm.nih.gov/medlineplus/mumps.html

ORGANIZATIONS

American Academy of Pediatrics (AAP), 141 Northwest Point Boulevard, Elk Grove Village, IL 60007-1098, (847) 434-4000, Fax: (847) 424-8000, kidsdocs@aap.org, http://www.aap.org.

Centers for Disease Control and Prevention (CDC), 1600 Clifton Road, Atlanta, GA 30333, (800) 232-4636, cdcinfo@cdc.gov, http://www.cdc.gov.

National Foundation for Infectious Diseases, 4733 Bethesda Ave., Suite 750, Bethesda, MD 20814, (301) 656-0003, Fax: (301) 907-0878, (800) 232-4636, http://www.nfid.org.

Ron Gasbarro, PharmD
Rebecca J. Frey, PhD

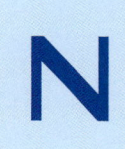

National ambient air quality standard (NAAQS)

Definition

The **Environmental Protection Agency (EPA)** established the National Ambient Air Quality Standards (NAAQSs) as a measure to control national **air pollution** in 1970 as part of the **Clean Air Act**. The NAAQSs was amended to include controls for six of the most common air pollutants, sometimes referred to as criteria pollutants, first in 1971 to include carbon monoxide (C0), nitrogen oxides (NO_X), ground-level **ozone**, particulate matter, and sulfur dioxide (SO_2) and in 1977 **lead** (Pb) was added. Hydrocarbons originally appeared on the list of pollutants, but were removed in 1978 because they were considered by legislators to be adequately regulated through the ozone standard established in newer sections of the Clean Air Act. The provisions of the law allow the **EPA** to identify additional substances as pollutants and add them to the list as needed.

Description

The NAAQSs were established based on the EPA's "criteria documents", which summarize the effect on human health caused by each pollutant, based on current scientific knowledge. The standards are usually expressed in parts of pollutant per million parts of air (ppm) and vary in the duration of time a pollutant can be allowed into the environment, so that only a limited amount of contaminant may be emitted per hour, week, or year, for example. The 1977 Clean Air Act amendments require the EPA to submit criteria documents to the Clean Air Scientific Advisory Committee and the EPA's Science Advisory Board for review. Although standards should be based on scientific evidence, politics often become involved as environmentalists and public health advocates battle industrial powers in setting standards.

For each of the criteria pollutants primary and secondary standard may be set. The primary standards are designed to protect human health. Secondary standards are to protect crops, forests, and buildings if the primary standards are not capable of doing so; presently the only pollutant without a secondary standard is carbon monoxide. These standards apply uniformly throughout the country, in each of 247 air quality control regions. All parts of the country were required to meet the NAAQSs by 1975, but this deadline was extended, in some cases, to the year 2011. The states monitor air pollution, enforce the standards, and can implement stricter standards than the NAAQSs if they desire. These standards are typically acceptable emission levels during a time period, not to be exceeded more than a certain number of times for a designated period of time. For instance, carbon monoxide emissions cannot exceed 9 ppm in an 8 hour time frame more than once per year.

The primary standards must be established at levels that would, "provide an adequate margin of safety—to protect the public—from any known or anticipated adverse effects associated with such air pollutant(s) in the ambient air." This phrase was based on the belief that there is a threshold effect of pollution: Pollution levels below the threshold are safe, levels above are unsafe. Although such an approach to setting the standards reflected scientific knowledge at the time, more recent research suggests that such a threshold probably does not exist. That is, pollution at any level is unsafe. The NAAQSs were also established without consideration of how much it will cost to achieve them; the standards are based on the best available control technology (BAT). The secondary standards are to "protect the public welfare from any known or anticipated adverse effects."

Pollutants

The six criteria pollutants come from a variety of sources and cause a host of health effects.

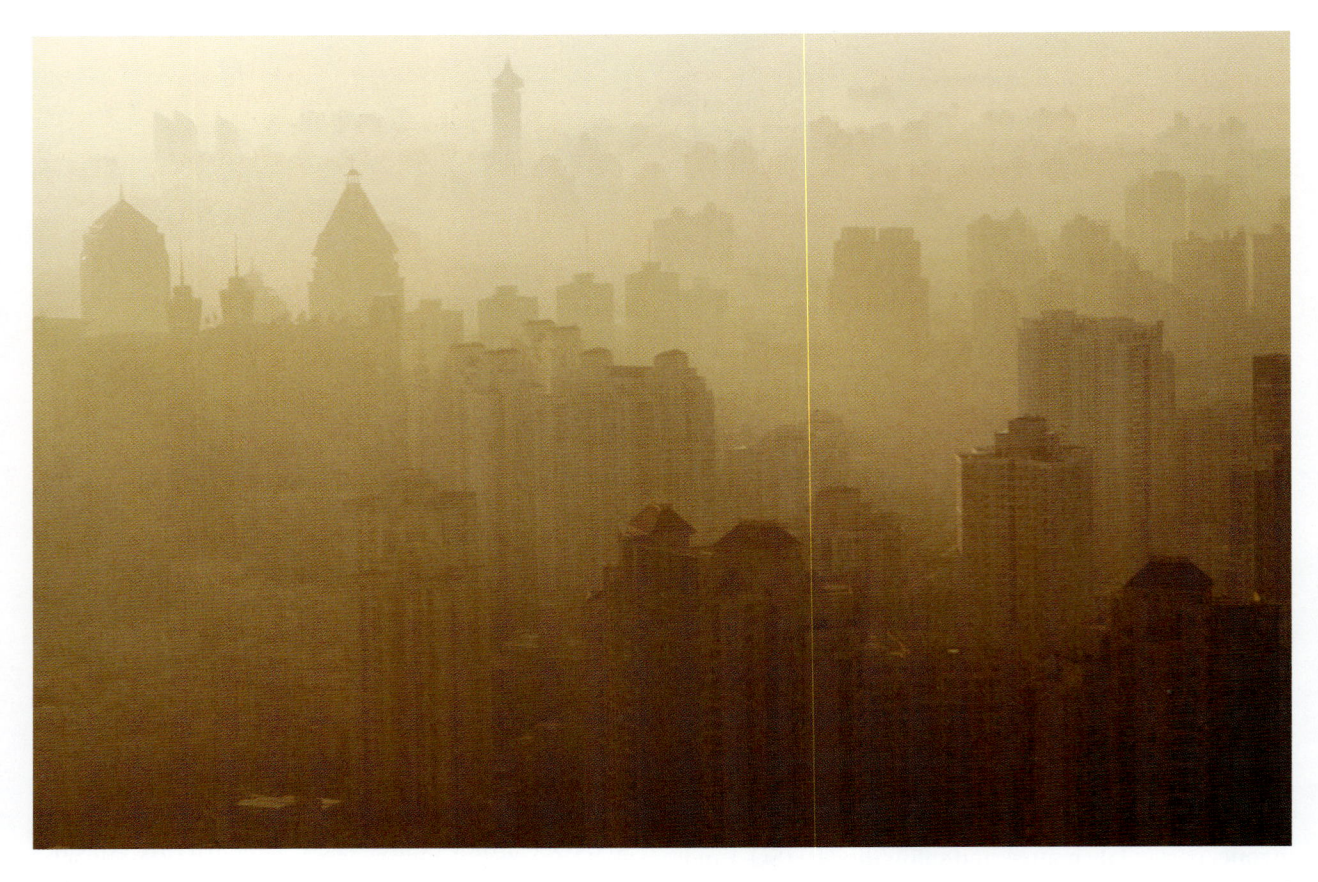

Smog at dawn, Shanghai, China, Asia. (© Robert Harding Picture Library Ltd Alamy)

- Carbon monoxide is a gas produced by the incomplete combustion of fossil fuels. It can lead to damage of the cardiovascular, nervous, and pulmonary systems, and can also cause problems with short-term attention span and sensory abilities.
- Lead, a heavy metal, has been traced to many health effects, mainly brain damage leading to learning disabilities and retardation in children. Most of the lead found in the air came from gasoline fumes until a 1973 court case, *Natural Resources Defense Council v. EPA*, prompted its inclusion as a criteria pollutant. Lead levels in gasoline were subsequently monitored.
- Nitrogen oxide is formed primarily by fossil fuel combustion. It not only contributes to acid rain and the formation of ground-level ozone, but it has been linked to respiratory illness.
- Ground-level ozone is produced by a combination of hydrocarbons and nitrogen oxides in the presence of sunlight, and heat. It is the prime component of photochemical smog, which can cause respiratory problems in humans, reduce crop yields, and cause forest damage. In 1979, the first revision of an original NAAQS slightly relaxed the photochemical oxidant standard and renamed it the ozone standard. Experts are currently debating whether this standard is low enough, and in 1991 the American Lung Association sued the EPA for failure to review the ozone NAAQS in light of new evidence.
- Particulate matter is composed of small pieces of solid and liquid matter, including soot, dust, and organic matter. It reduces visibility and can cause eye and throat irritation, respiratory ailments, and cancer. Through 1987, total suspended particulates were the basis of the NAAQS. In 1987, the standard was revised and based on particulate matter with an aerodynamic diameter of 10 micrometers or less (PM-10), which was identified as the main health risk.
- Sulfur dioxide is a gas produced primarily by coal-burning utilities and other fossil fuel combustion. It is the chief cause of acid rain and can also cause respiratory problems.

Results

To achieve the NAAQSs for these six pollutants, the Clean Air Act incorporated three strategies. First, the federal government would establish new source performance standards (NSPSs) for stationary sources such as factories and power plants and emission standards for mobile sources. Finally, the states would develop state implementation plans (SIPs) to address existing sources of air pollution. If the federal government determined that a SIP was not adequate to assure that the state would meet the NAAQSs, it could impose federal controls to meet them. According to the EPA, the SIPs must be designed to bring substandard air quality regions up to the NAAQSs, or to make sure any area already meeting the requirements continued to do so. The SIPs are intended to prevent increased air pollution in areas of noncompliance, either by preventing significant expansions of existing industries or the opening of new plants. The EPA faced press to allow economic development and growth in such non-attainment areas while still working to reduce air pollution. The 1977 amendments to the Clean Air Act required that new sources of pollution in non-attainment areas control emissions to the lowest achievable emission rate (LAER) for that type of source and pollution and demonstrate that the new pollution would be offset by new emission reductions from existing sources in the area, reductions that went beyond existing permits and compliance plans. New sources were allowed, but only if the additional pollution was offset by reductions at existing sources.

The 1990 amendments to the Clean Air Act dealt with the problem of such non-attainment areas. Six categories of ozone non-attainment were established, ranging from marginal to extreme, and two categories for both carbon monoxide and particulate matter were implemented. Deadlines to achieve the NAAQSs were extended from three to twenty years, and the EPA has allowed subsequent extensions. Increased restrictions were required in non-attainment areas; existing controls were tightened and smaller sources were made subject to regulation. Also, annual reduction goals were mandated to assist with reaching term goals. Areas considered to have made inadequate progress toward reaching attainment are subjected to stringent regulations on new plants and limited use of federal highway funds.

Resources

BOOKS

Schwartz, Joel. *Air Quality in America: A Dose of Reality on Air Pollution Levels, Trends, and Health Risks.* Washington, DC: AEI Press, 2008.

WEBSITES

Environmental Protection Agency. "Air: Air Quality." http://www.epa.gov/ebtpages/airairquality.html (accessed October 19, 2010).

Environmental Protection Agency. "Air: Air Quality: Monitoring." http://www.epa.gov/ebtpages/airairqualitymonitoring.html (accessed October 19, 2010).

Environmental Protection Agency. "Air: Air Quality: Nonattainment." http://www.epa.gov/ebtpages/airairqunonattainment.html (accessed October 1, 2012).

Environmental Protection Agency. "National Ambient Air Quality Standards (NAAQSs): Criteria." http://www.epa.gov/air/criteria.html (accessed October 1, 2012).

ORGANIZATIONS

Environmental Protection Agency, 1200 Pennsylvania Ave. NW, Washington, DC 20460, (202) 272-0167, http://water.epa.gov.

Christopher McGrory Klyza
Alyson C. Heimer, MA

National Environmental Health Association

Definition

The National Environmental Health Association (NEHA) originated in California, and was incorporated in 1937. The original impetus behind the creation of a national professional society for environmental health practitioners was "the desire by professionals of that day to establish a standard of excellence for this developing profession." This standard, or the Registered Environmental Health Specialist or Registered Sanitarian credential, signifies an environmental health professional who has mastered a body of knowledge (verified through the passing of an examination), and has "acquired sufficient experience, to satisfactorily perform work responsibilities in the environmental health field." The association founders believed that certification was necessary if the environmental health field was to grow as a legitimate and respected profession. The association is governed by a fourteen member board of directors that is chaired by the association's president. NEHA also employs 26 paid staff members.

Purpose

Following the initial purpose of the NEHA, this association presently operates as a strong professional society where members can network and learn from one another. NEHA's mission continues to be "to advance the environmental health and protection professional for the purpose of providing a healthful environment for all."

The association's activities derives its basis from the belief that a professional who is educated will be able to make the greatest contribution to healthful environmental goals. As is such, great emphasis is placed on NEHA's programs to provide both an educational and a motivational opportunity to members. NEHA's strategic directions are training and education, credentialing, advocacy, and increasing organizational capacity.

Programs and services

NEHA offers a variety of programs. Expanding beyond its original credential, today the association has seven national credential programs and maintains active partnerships with organizations nationwide for professional networking, and educational purposes.

NEHA publishes a peer-reviewed, the Journal of Environmental Health, which publishes articles covering all areas of the environmental health field, posts job openings, provides networking and committee participation opportunities, provides supplemental arguments to support positions on timely and serious environmental health concerns, and maintains an active online presence in serving as a constant resource for members.

Additionally, members may participate in the association through committees or as technical advisors which, for NEHA's purposes, essentially divide the environmental field by subject matter. Serving under the association's board of directors are numerous administrative and functional committees. The committees and advisory positions cover a variety of subject matter in the following areas: Air Quality, Children's Environmental Health, Disaster/Emergency Response, Drinking Water, Emerging Pathogens, Environmental Justice, Food (including Safety and Defense), Hazardous Materials/Toxic Substances, Healthy Homes and Healthy Communities, Injury Prevention, Institutions/Schools, International Environmental Health, Land Use Planning/Design, Legal, Meteorology/Weather/Global **Climate Change**, Occupational Health/Safety, Pools/Spas, Radiation/Radon, Recreational Water, Risk Assessment, Environmental Sustainability, Technology (including Computers, Software, GIS and Management Applications), Terrorism/All Hazards Preparedness, Wastewater, **Water Pollution** Control/Water Quality, and Workforce Development.

Membership

NEHA has over 4,500 members in the United States who practice their profession in the public and private sectors, academia and the uniformed services, with a majority being state and local county health department employees. NEHA's *Journal of Environmental Health* has subscribers in over 40 countries.

This single organization encompasses the entire environmental health profession and serves as "the forum for discussion of, and can address the broad spectrum of, environmental health issues." It is their fundamental belief that increased communication between professionals in the same field will increase the efficiency and efficacy of the work if it's members.

To further this goal NEHA hold an Annual Educational Conference (AEC) was designed to train, educate, and advance persons with an interest or career in environmental health and protection, and bring people together to build a professional network of environmental health colleagues, to exchange information, and discover new and practical solutions to environmental health issues. Imparting knowledge, presenting data, and providing inspiration to members are among the top priorities of the AEC and NEHA as a whole.

Resources

WEBSITES

National Environmental Health Association. "About." Denver: CO: 2012. http://www.neha.org/about/neha.html (accessed October 28, 2012).

NEHA AEC. "2012 NEHA AEC." Denver, CO: 2011. http://www.neha2012aec.org (accessed October 28, 2012).

The Healthy House Institute. "The Healthy House Institute (HHI) Supports 2013 NEHA Conference." Boise, ID: October 28th 2012. http://www.healthyhouseinstitute.com/information/media_center_news_room.php (accessed October 28, 2012).

Alyson C. Heimer, MA

National Environmental Policy Act (1969)

Definition

The National Environmental Policy Act (NEPA) of 1969 was signed into law on January 1, 1970, launching a decade marked by passage of key environmental legislation and increased awareness of environmental problems.

Purpose

The act established the first comprehensive national policies and goals for the protection, maintenance, and use of the environment. The act also established the Council on Environmental Quality (CEQ) to oversee NEPA and advise the president on environmental issues.

Demographics

Title I of NEPA declares that the U.S. federal government will use all practicable means and measures to create and maintain conditions under which people and nature can exist in productive harmony, while fulfilling the social and economic requirements of Americans. Included in this declaration are goals to attain the widest range of beneficial uses of the environment without undesirable consequences and to preserve culturally and aesthetically important features of the landscape. The declaration also commits each future generation of Americans to stewardship and preservation of the environment.

Description

To achieve the national environmental goals, the act directs all federal agencies to evaluate the impacts of major federal actions upon the environment. Before taking an action, each federal agency must prepare a statement describing (1) the environmental impact of the proposed action, (2) adverse environmental effects that cannot be avoided, (3) alternatives to the proposal, (4) short-term versus long-term impacts, and (5) any irreversible effects on resources that would result if the action were implemented. The act requires any federal, state, or local agency with jurisdiction over the impacted environment to take part in the decision-making process. The general public is given opportunities to take part in the NEPA process through hearings and meetings or by submitting written comments to agencies involved in a project.

Origins

Title II of NEPA created the CEQ, as part of the Executive Office of the President, to oversee implementation of NEPA and assist the president in preparing an annual environmental quality report. In 1993, President Clinton established the White House Office on Environmental Policy, with broad powers to coordinate national environmental policy. The CEQ issued regulations in 1978 that implement NEPA and are binding on all federal agencies. The regulations (40 CFR Parts 1500-1508) cover procedures and administration of NEPA, including preparation of environmental assessments and environmental impact statements. Many federal agencies have established their own NEPA regulations, following CEQ regulations, but customized for the particular activities of the agencies.

Results

Federal agencies must incorporate the NEPA review process early in project planning. A complete environmental analysis can be very complex, involving potential effects on physical, chemical, biological, and social factors of the proposed project and its alternatives. Various systematic methods have been developed to deal with the complexity of environmental analysis. There are three levels at which an action may be evaluated, depending on how large an impact it will have on the environment.

The first level is categorical exclusion, which allows an undertaking to be exempt from detailed evaluation if it meets previously determined criteria designated as having no significant environmental impact. Some federal agencies have lists of actions that have been thus categorically excluded from evaluation under NEPA.

Effects on public health

When an action cannot be excluded under the first level of analysis, the agency involved may prepare an environmental assessment to determine if the action will have a significant environmental effect. An environmental assessment is a brief statement of the impacts of the action and alternatives. If the assessment determines there will not be significant environmental consequences, the agency issues a finding of no significant impact (FONSI). The finding may describe measures that will be taken to reduce potential impacts. An agency can skip the second level if it anticipates in advance that there will be significant impacts.

An action moves to the third level of analysis, an environmental impact statement (EIS), if the environmental assessment determines there will be significant environmental impacts. An EIS is a detailed evaluation of the action and alternatives, and it is used to make decisions on how to proceed with the action. An agency preparing an EIS must release a draft statement for comment and review by other agencies, local governments, and the general public. A final statement is released with modifications based on the results of the public review of the draft statement. When more than one agency is involved in an action, a lead agency is designated to coordinate the environmental analysis. An agency also may be called upon to cooperate in an environmental analysis if it has expertise in an area of concern. The CEQ regulations describe a process for settling disagreements that arise between agencies involved in an environmental analysis.

In addition to having to prepare their own environmental assessments and environmental impact statements, the **Environmental Protection Agency (EPA)** is involved in all NEPA review processes of other federal agencies, as mandated by Section 309 of the **Clean Air Act**. Section 309 was added to the Clean Air Act in 1970, after NEPA was passed and the **EPA** formed, with the purpose of ensuring independent reviews of all federal actions impacting the environment. As a result, the EPA reviews and comments on all federal environmental impact statements in draft and final form, on proposed environmental regulations and legislation, and on other proposed federal projects the EPA considers to have significant environmental impacts. The EPA procedures for carrying out the Section 309 requirements are contained in the publication "Policies and Procedures for the Review of Federal Actions Impacting the Environment." The EPA is also responsible for many administrative aspects of the EIS filing process. The NEPA review process includes an evaluation of a project's compliance with other environmental laws such as the Clean Air Act. Federal agencies often integrate NEPA reviews with review requirements of other environmental laws to expedite decision-making and reduce costs and effort.

NEPA requires that previously unquantified environmental amenities be given consideration in decision-making along with more technical considerations. This stipulation means that the environmental analysis can be a subjective process, guided by the values of the particular players in any given project. The act does not define what constitutes a major action or what is considered a significant effect on the environment. Some agencies have developed their own guidelines for what types of actions are considered major. Examples of major actions include construction projects such as highway expansion and creek channelization. However, major actions do not always involve construction. For example, legislative changes that may affect the environment may come under NEPA review. When an action will be controversial or clearly violate a preset environmental standard, it also may be categorized as a major action with significant impacts. Actions that will have less measurable effects, such as disrupting scenic beauty, must be categorized more subjectively. The courts are frequently used to settle disputes about whether actions require compliance with NEPA.

Research and general acceptance

Although NEPA is targeted to federal agencies, its implementation has resulted in closer scrutiny of major environmental actions other than those sponsored by the government. Environmental analyses also are required for private developments that need federal pollution control permits such as water discharges, air emissions, waste disposal, and wetlands filling.

The level of effort that compliance with NEPA can require due to a new act of Congress can be seen in regards to the American Recovery and Reinvestment Act of 2009 (often simply referred to as the Recovery Act). The act directed that large government expenditures be made to create jobs (such as in public construction projects), encourage investment, and otherwise improve the U.S. economy during a time of recession. The large number of construction projects alone required a multitude of environmental reviews. Periodically, the CEQ has issued reports to the U.S. Senate and House of Representatives concerning compliance of the Recovery Act with NEPA. The ninth CEQ report concerning the Recovery Act was published in May 2011.

Resources

BOOKS

Johnson, Dennis W. *The Laws that Shaped America: Fifteen Acts of Congress and Their Lasting Impact.* New York: Routledge, 2009.

Stern, Marc J., and Michael J. Mortimer. *Exploring National Environmental Policy Act Processes Across Federal Land Management Agencies.* Portland, OR: U.S. Department of Agriculture, Forest Service, Pacific Northwest Research Station, 2009.

WEBSITES

Council of Environmental Quality, Department of Energy. "The NEPA Statute." http://ceq.hss.doe.gov/laws_and_executive_orders/the_nepa_statute.html (accessed August 13, 2012).

Teresa C. Donkin
Stacey Chamberlin

National Institute for Occupational Safety and Health

Definition

The National Institute for Occupational Safety and Health (NIOSH) is a research institute of the Centers for Disease Control (CDC). This federal government agency is charged with researching and making recommendations regarding prevention of work-related injuries and illnesses.

Purpose

The purpose of NIOSH is to gather data documenting incidence of occupational disease, exposure, and injury in the United States. After gathering and evaluating data, the agency develops criteria documents for specific hazards. By doing so, NIOSH helps create new knowledge about occupational health and safety. In addition, the agency acts as a leader in the United States and around the world in issues regarding workplace health and safety.

Demographics

In 2007, more than 5,400 workers in the United States died from occupational injuries, and nearly 49,000 deaths each year in the United States are attributed to work-related illnesses. NIOSH receives funding and helps fund programs to improve occupational safety. The agency is headquartered in Washington, DC, and Atlanta, but has staff in six other regional offices around the country. About 1,200 scientists work for NIOSH, and they come from a variety of backgrounds, including medicine, **epidemiology**, psychology, chemistry, **industrial hygiene**, and safety. NIOSH has 17 regional education and research centers at universities and eight agricultural disease research and training centers.

Description

NIOSH supports research and information gathering in a number of industries and occupations. In doing so, the agency tracks and publishes data on illnesses related to workplaces or occupations. These issues range from workers' allergies resulting from exposure to certain workplace materials to on-the-job traumatic injuries resulting from workplace dangers.

NIOSH staff also are involved in researching and publishing extensive data on how to make workplaces safer and how to prevent injuries. For example, the agency has several publications on safety in occupations such as mining, electrical and agricultural occupations, and how healthcare workers can handle patients without causing injury to themselves. To help identify and prevent accidents and illness, NIOSH researches hazards and exposures to workers in various industries. The agency also examines chemicals used in many occupations and the hazards associated with exposure to these chemicals. The agency participates in developing information used in determining standards for chemical exposure. NIOSH also conducts research and publishes documents to help employers and employees in response to emergencies that might arise from chemical hazards, along with other hazards that can occur in the workplace. These might include natural disasters such as flood, hurricanes, and **earthquakes** that could happen at any workplace, or potential emergencies more likely to occur in a certain area or industry.

NIOSH also participates in training and workforce development. This effort includes centers that focus on agricultural safety and health, hazardous substance training, and an emergency responder training program that helps teach emergency responders such as firefighters and paramedics about how to more safely respond to emergencies that involve hazardous chemicals or other materials. NIOSH conducts workplace evaluations to help assess workplaces for health hazards and recommend improvement to employers. The evaluations are free to employers and employees.

Origins

NIOSH was created by the **Occupational Safety and Health Act** of 1970, the same act that created the **Occupational Safety and Health Administration** (OSHA). Marcus Key was the first director of the agency. Since 1973, NIOSH has been a division of the CDC. NIOSH created its first list of toxic substances in 1971 and, along with OSHA, created a pocket guide to chemical hazards for the first time in 1978. The institute launched its website in 1996.

Results

In some cases OSHA has used NIOSH data and documents as the basis for specific legal standards to be followed by industry. NIOSH databases are available to other federal agencies, as well as state governments, academic researchers, industry, and private citizens. The organization also conducts seminars for those in the field of occupational safety and health, as well as for industry, labor, and other government agencies. NIOSH prepares various publications for sale to the public, and it provides a telephone hotline in its Cincinnati, Ohio, office for answering inquiries.

In April 1996, NIOSH and OSHA commemorated their twenty-fifth anniversary in an event that was jointly sponsored by the two agencies and by the Smithsonian Institute. In 2006, NIOSH celebrated ten years of the National Occupational Research Agenda (NORA), a public-private partnership that helps set priorities for research in occupational safety and health. In the first ten years of its existence, NORA helped advance knowledge in 21 areas of occupational science.

Resources

WEBSITES

Centers for Disease Control and Prevention. "About NIOSH." http://www.cdc.gov/niosh/about.html (accessed November 9, 2012).

Centers for Disease Control and Prevention. "About NORA." http://www.cdc.gov/niosh/nora/about.html (accessed November 9, 2012).

ORGANIZATIONS

National Institute for Occupational Safety and Health, Education and Information Division, 4676 Columbia Pkwy., Cincinnati, OH 45226, (800) 232-4636, Fax: (513) 533-8347, cdcinfo@cdc.gov, http://www.cdc.gov/niosh.

Teresa G. Odle

National Institute of Environmental Health Sciences (Research Triangle Park, North Carolina)

Definition

The National Institute of Environmental Health Sciences (NIEHS) conducts research on environment-related diseases. It is one of 27 components of the National Institutes of Health (NIH), which is part of the **U.S. Department of Health and Human Services** (DHHS).

Purpose

The mission of the NIEHS is to conduct research on environment-related diseases. The focus of research is on understanding how environmental factors, individual susceptibility, and age interrelate to cause human illness and on developing methods to reduce these illnesses. The NIEHS fulfills its mission through biomedical research programs, prevention and intervention activities, and communication strategies that include training, education, technology transfer, and community outreach.

Description

The National Institute of Environmental Health Sciences is one of 27 components of the National Institutes of Health, which is part of the DHHS. The NIEHS is located in Research Triangle Park, North Carolina. Research Triangle Park is located between Raleigh, Durham, and Chapel Hill, and is a hub for science and technology due to its proximity to large research universities.

Three divisions make up the NIEHS: the Division of Extramural Research and Training (DERT), the Division of Intramural Research (DIR), and the National **Toxicology** Program (NTP). Priority areas of these divisions include cancer, **autism**, nanomaterial, metal toxicity, and how substances such as pesticides, **air pollution**, and **endocrine disruptors** affect health. As of 2012, Linda S. Birnbaum was the director of the NIEHS.

Origins

In 1960, a study by the U.S. **Public Health Service** reported that environmental health problems required greater public and private effort and recommended that a central laboratory facility should be built. In 1964, Congress authorized planning funds for this facility. A site selection committee chose Research Triangle Park as the location where the facility should be built in 1965, and the NIEHS was established as the Division of Environmental Health Sciences within the NIH in 1966. In 1967, the Research Triangle Foundation in North Carolina presented the U.S. surgeon general with 509 acres (206 ha) in the Research Triangle Park to serve as a site for NIEHS. Two years later, the Division of Environmental Health Sciences was raised to institute status. The first edition of the NIEHS scientific journal, *Environmental Health Perspectives* was published in April 1972.

Research and general acceptance

Research is conducted through both onsite resources and an extramural science program. The Division of Extramural Research and Training supports a network of university-based environmental health-science centers and also provides research and training grants and contracts for research and development. Through DERT, the NIEHS supports the research of people such as Mexican chemist Mario J. Molina (1943–) of the Massachusetts Institute of Technology (MIT), who was a corecipient of the 1995 Nobel Prize in chemistry for work showing the loss of Earth's protective **ozone** shield.

The purpose of the Division of Intramural Research (DIR) is to provide research that addresses the environmental components of many different diseases. American biochemist Martin Rodbell (1925–1998), a NIEHS scientist in DIR, was a corecipient of the Nobel Prize in medicine for discoveries about the communication system that regulates cellular activity. DIR is organized into programs for clinical research, environmental biology, environmental diseases and medicine, and the Environmental Toxicology Program (the study of the effects of chemicals on organisms). The Clinical Research Laboratory conducts trials to assess the effects of environmental agents such as chemicals on diseases. The program for environmental biology includes the work of four laboratories: the Laboratory of Molecular Genetics studies the basic mechanisms of the mutational process, fundamental mechanisms of genomic stability, and the impact of environmental agents on the genetic apparatus; the Laboratory of Signal Transduction studies the effects of environmental agents on physiological processes and mechanisms; the Laboratory of Structural Biology studies environmentally associated diseases resulting from perturbations in biological processes; and the Laboratory of Neurobiology researches cellular and molecular processes in the nervous system and the vulnerability of these processes with respect to environmental toxins.

The second DIR program, for environmental diseases and medicine, includes six branches: **epidemiology** (study of the transmission and control of disease), biostatistics, reproductive and developmental toxicity, respiratory biology, molecular carcinogenesis, and comparative medicine. The epidemiology branch studies the impacts of environmental toxicants on human health and reproduction using sensitive health endpoints, susceptible subgroups, and highly exposed populations. The Laboratory of Reproductive and Developmental Toxicology develops an understanding of the basic mechanisms underlying normal and abnormal development and reproduction. The Laboratory of Respiratory Biology studies the respiratory tract system biology at the cellular, biochemical, and molecular level in order to develop an understanding of pathogenic mechanisms involved in the onset of diseases of the airways. The Laboratory of Molecular Carcinogenesis, comprised of eight interdisciplinary research groups, studies the mechanisms of environmental carcinogenesis by identifying the target genes in the process and by defining how chemicals act on these genes to influence cancer development. The biostatistics research groups conduct research in biomathematics and population genetics and in design and analysis of laboratory animal toxicology and carcinogenicity studies to develop methods for epidemiological and clinical studies, and also provides statistical and computational support to the NIEHS scientists. The sixth branch, comparative medicine, provides services and collaborative support to the NIEHS scientists in the areas of animal facilities management, animal procurement, health surveillance and disease diagnosis, clinical veterinary services, rodent breeding, technical and surgical assistance, and quality assurance support.

The third DIR program, the NTP, uses the research conducted at five laboratories. The Laboratory of Host Susceptibility is involved in all aspects of genetically modified animal model research with respect to chemical toxicity from planning studies to the analysis of results. In the cellular and molecular pathology branch (CMPB), researchers investigate the mechanisms involved in the formation of lesions, which arise spontaneously or in response to chemicals. Core laboratories for histology (the study of the structure of biological tissues at the microscopic level), electron microscopy, and clinical pathology (the study of disease) are operated through this laboratory. The CMPB is also responsible for all pathology data originating from the NTP studies on toxins and carcinogens. The programs operations branch provides the necessary information on new research technologies as well as supporting the information technology activities of the NTP research through development and maintenance of databases and websites. This branch also advises researchers on the implementation of their studies and provides quality control measures. The toxicology branch researches the effects of toxins and carcinogens on the immune and reproductive systems, development, and genetics of rodent models. This information is used for hazard identification and characterization, and ultimately in the establishment of regulations regarding toxins. Information on test substances is used by this branch to develop mathematical models for the prediction of the effects on organisms based on exposure to toxins as well as developing new technologies or methods of toxin assessment. The bio-molecular screening branch performs testing to study the biological effects of toxins and determine future research measures based on the level of toxicity.

Two laboratories aid the DIR environmental toxicology program. The Laboratory of Molecular Toxicology conducts studies utilizing genetics and genomics to characterize chemical toxic effects on biological mechanisms, including immune, reproductive, genetic, respiratory, and nervous system toxicities. This laboratory studies interactions of chemicals and metabolites with sub-cellular macromolecules and develops methods for characterizing toxicity of chemicals and other agents. The Laboratory of Pharmacology studies the exposure and disposition of environmental chemicals; the laboratory studies the enzyme systems involved in the metabolism of environmental chemicals and drugs; and it studies the mechanisms responsible for the toxic effects of xenobiotics (chemicals foreign to living organisms such as pesticides) and their metabolites, including photochemical and free radical mechanisms. The lab uses alternative model systems (from comparative and marine biology) to study the pharmacology and toxicology of chemicals and drugs; in addition, it provides chemical support for NIEHS scientists, including the assessment of chemical purity, stability, and biotransformation, which is the modification of a chemical through chemical processes in an organism.

The NIEHS sponsors research on the effects of environmental impacts in several areas. Some research topics include birth and developmental defects and sterility; women's health issues, including breast cancer susceptibility and osteoporosis; and Alzheimer's as well as other neurological disorders. The NIEHS sponsors research on hazards to the poor resulting from likely exposure to **lead** paint, hazardous chemicals at work, air and **water pollution**, and **hazardous waste** sites in their communities; some researchers focus on agricultural pollution, including natural materials (e.g., grain dust) and **agricultural chemicals**, whereas other researchers study signal error (i.e., whether environmental chemicals can mimic hormonal growth factors and contribute to the development of cancer or reproductive disorders). Still other

> **KEY TERMS**
>
> **Alzheimer's disease**—An incurable disease of older individuals that results in the destruction of nerve cells in the brain and causes gradual loss of mental and physical functions.
>
> **Autism**—A syndrome characterized by a lack of responsiveness to other people or outside stimulus, often in conjunction with a severe impairment of verbal and non-verbal communication skills.
>
> **Ecology**—The study of how organisms relate to one another and to their environment.
>
> **Epidemiology**—The study of the transmission and control of disease.
>
> **Histology**—The study of the structure of biological tissues at the microscopic level.
>
> **Osteoporosis**—A condition found in older individuals in which bones decrease in density and become fragile and more likely to break. It can be caused by lack of vitamin D and/or calcium in the diet.
>
> **Toxicology**—The study of the effects of chemicals on organisms.
>
> **Xenobiotics**—Chemicals that are foreign to living organisms, for example, pesticides.

research investigates alternatives to reducing the number of animals used in research, to refine the design of experiments to obtain more information at lower cost, and to replace animals with microbial and tissue cultures. Some research identifies biomarkers to measure the uptake and exposure to environmental toxins.

The NIEHS is the headquarters for the NTP, an interagency program within the DHHS. The NTP was established in 1978 to coordinate toxicology research and testing activities within the DHHS, to provide information about potentially toxic chemicals to regulatory and research agencies, and to strengthen the scientific basis of toxicology. The NTP coordinates toxicology activities of the NIEHS, the **National Institute for Occupational Safety and Health** of the Centers for Disease Control (NIOSH/CDC), and the National Center for Toxicological Research of the **Food and Drug Administration** (NCTR/FDA). The director of the NIEHS is also the director of the NTP. Primary research support within the NIEHS for the NTP is in the environmental toxicology program.

The Superfund Basic Research Program (SBRP), in coordination with the U.S. **Environmental Protection Agency (EPA)**, is also administered by the NIEHS. The **Superfund Amendments and Reauthorization Act** (SARA) of 1986 established a university-based program of basic research within the NIEHS. The SBRP receives funding from the **EPA** through an interagency agreement using Superfund trust monies. The funding is used to study human health effects of hazardous substances in the environment, especially those found at uncontrolled, leaking waste disposal sites. The primary objectives of the SBRP are to find methods, through basic research, to reduce the amount and toxicity of hazardous substances and to prevent resulting adverse human health effects. The SARA legislation specifically mandates that the basic research program administered by the NIEHS focus on methods and technologies to detect hazardous substances in the environment; developing advanced techniques for the detection, assessment, and evaluation of the effects on human health of hazardous substances; and basic biological, chemical, and physical methods to reduce the amount and toxicity of hazardous substances.

Given these mandates, the NIEHS supports projects in the areas of engineering, ecological, and hydrogeological research in conjunction with biomedically related components, thus encouraging collaborative efforts among researchers. Specific research areas in the SBRP include health effects, exposure or risk assessment, ecology, fate and transport, remediation, bioremediation, analytical chemistry, biomarkers, epidemiology, metals, and waste site characterization.

The NIEHS was also given responsibility for initiating a training grants program under the SARA. The major objective of the NIEHS worker education and training program, initiated in 1987, is to prevent work-related harm by assisting training so that workers know how to protect themselves and their communities from exposure to hazardous materials during hazardous waste operations, hazardous materials transportation, environmental restoration of nuclear weapons facilities, or chemical emergency response. Through this program, nonprofit organizations with a demonstrated record of providing occupational safety and health education develop safety and health curriculum for workers involved in handling hazardous waste or in responding to emergency releases of hazardous materials. Information concerning this program is disseminated through the National Clearinghouse for Worker Safety and Health Training.

The SBRP, through an interagency agreement, provides additional training by support of the NIOSH Hazardous Substance Continuing Education Program (HST), initiated in 1988 for hazardous substance professionals, and the NIOSH Hazardous Substance Academic

Training Program (HSAT), a graduate academic program initiated in 1993 allowing occupational safety and health professionals to specialize in the study of hazardous substances.

The NIEHS clearinghouse is an information service staffed with scientists who respond to questions concerning environmental health issues. Information on research is also provided through a NIEHS-sponsored journal, *Environmental Health Perspectives*.

Resources

WEBSITES

National Institute of Environmental Health Services. "2012–2017 Strategic Plan." http://www.niehs.nih.gov/health/materials/niehs_20122017_strategic_plan_frontiers_in_environmental_health_sciences_booklet_508.pdf (accessed October 27, 2012).

National Institute of Environmental Health Services. "The National Institute of Environmental Health Services." http://www.niehs.nih.gov/health/materials/niehs_overview.pdf (accessed October 27, 2012).

National Institute of Environmental Health Services. "Organizational Structure." http://www.niehs.nih.gov/about/orgchart/index.cfm (accessed October 27, 2012).

National Institute of Environmental Health Services. "Research at NIEHS." http://www.niehs.nih.gov/research/atniehs/index.cfm (accessed October 27, 2012).

ORGANIZATIONS

National Institute of Environmental Health Science, PO Box 12233, MD K3-16, Research Triangle Park, NC 27709, (919) 541-3345, Fax: (919) 541-4395, webcenter@niehs.nih.gov, http://www.niehs.nih.gov.

Judith Sims
Tish Davidson, AM

National park

Definition

National parks are areas that have been legally set apart by national governments because they have cultural or natural resources that are deemed significant for the country.

Purpose

National parks are developed in order to conserve nature, wildlife, and cultural heritage while allowing people to enjoy the land's natural beauty. They are managed to eliminate or minimize human disturbances, while allowing human visitation for recreational, educational, cultural, or inspirational purposes.

Description

National parks are typically large areas that are mostly undisturbed by human occupation or exploitation. They are characterized by spectacular scenery, abundant wildlife, unique geologic features, or interesting cultural or historic sites. Activities consistent with typical national park management include hiking, camping, picnicking, wildlife observation, and photography. Fishing is usually allowed, but hunting often is prohibited. In the United States, national parks are distinguished from national forests and other federal lands because timber harvesting, cattle grazing, and mining are, with a few exceptions, not permitted in national parks, whereas they are permitted on most other federal lands. As of 2012, over 7,000 national parks could be found worldwide in more than 120 countries. Fifty-eight of these national parks are in the United States.

Origins

The United States was the first country to establish national parks. The Yosemite Grant of 1864 was the first act that formally set aside land by the federal government for "public use, resort, and recreation." Twenty square miles (52 km^2) of land in the Yosemite valley in California and four square miles (10 km^2) of giant sequoia were put under the care of the state of California to be held "inalienable for all time." In 1872, President Ulysses S. Grant signed into law the establishment of Yellowstone National Park. Yellowstone differed from Yosemite in that it was to be managed and controlled by the federal government, not the state, and therefore has received the honor of being considered the first national park. Years later, Yosemite was turned over to the federal government for federal management. Since 1916, national parks in the United States have been administered by the National Park Service, an agency in the U.S. Department of the Interior.

The concept of national parks has been taken up by countries all over the world and continues to spread. Between 1972 and 1982, the number of national parks in the world increased by 47% and the area encompassed by the parks increased 82%.

Future outlook

Although parks consist of natural resources, they are conceived, established, maintained, and often threatened by humans. Many national parks in both developed and developing countries face threats. The most commonly reported threats are illegal removal of wildlife, destruction of vegetation, and increased erosion.

Often there is a lack of personnel to deal with these threats. Management problems also arise because demand for use of park resources is increasing. Many of these uses are conflicting, and virtually all would have significant impacts on the resources that characterize the parks. During the summer of 1962, the first World Conference on National Parks was held in Seattle, Washington. This historic conference and subsequent ones have given people of many nations a forum to discuss threats facing their parks and strategies for meeting the demand for conflicting uses. Additionally, hundreds of organizations around the world, such the International Union for Conservation of Nature and its World Commission on Protected Areas, work to get legislation passed and bring attention to the importance of protecting the world's national parks for future generations to enjoy.

Resources

BOOKS

Duncan, Dayton, and Ken Burns. *The National Parks—America's Best Idea.* New York: Alfred A. Knopf, 2009.

Oswald, Michael Joseph. *Your Guide to the National Parks: The Complete Guide to all 58 National Parks.* Whitelaw, WI: Stone Road Press, 2012.

WEBSITES

National Park Service. "Find a Park." http://www.nps.gov/findapark/index.htm (accessed October 29, 2012).

"National Parks Around the World." http://www.nationalparks.gov.uk/learningabout/whatisanationalpark/nationalparksareprotectedareas/nationalparksaroundtheworld.htm(accessed October 29, 2012).

Patry, Marc, and UNESCO World Heritage Centre. "World Heritage at the 5th IUCN World Parks Congress." http://unesdoc.unesco.org/images/0015/001508/150836e.pdf (accessed October 29, 2012).

ORGANIZATIONS

International Union for Conservation of Nature, Rue Mauverney 28, Gland, Switzerland 1196, 41(999) 0000, Fax: 41(999) 0002, http://www.iucn.org.

National Park Conservation Association, 777 6th St. NW, Ste. 700, Washington, DC 20001, (202) 223-6722, (800) NAT-PARK (628-7275), Fax: (202) 454-3333, npca@npca.org, http://www.npca.org.

National Park Foundation, 1201 Eye St. NW, Ste. 550B, Washington, DC 20005, (202) 354-6460, Fax: (202) 371-2066, ask-npf@nationalparks.org, http://www.nationalparks.org.

U.S. National Park Service, 1849 C St. NW, Washington, DC 20240, (202) 208-3818, http://www.nps.gov.

Ted T. Cable
Tish Davidson, AM

Nature deficit disorder

Definition

Nature deficit disorder (NDD) is a term coined by Richard Louv in his 2005 bestseller, *Last Child in the Woods: Saving Our Children from Nature-Deficit Disorder*. Louv's theory is that people, especially children, are disconnected from the natural world and spend far too little time outdoors in nature According to Louv, NDD contributes to a range of physical, mental, and behavioral conditions.

Description

Human beings evolved in nature. For almost all of human history, children and adults played and worked primarily in the open air. People were knowledgeable about the natural world. They got their vitamin D from sunlight rather than from supplements. But starting in the nineteenth century and increasingly throughout the twentieth century, millions of people became isolated from nature—and not just from forests and wilderness, but from farms and animals. Spending so much time indoors, especially for children, is new to the human race. The ramifications of this momentous change are beginning to be recognized by scientists, healthcare professionals, and the general public.

Until the mid-twentieth century, most children walked or rode bikes to school, played or did chores outside until dark, and spent their summers playing outdoors. However, with parents working ever-longer hours outside the home and the advent of electronic media geared to children and teens, that lifestyle began to disappear. In the early 2000s, the time children spend outside is likely to be on a manicured sports field in an organized activity that has little association with nature. Some experts warn that American children in the early 2000s may be the first in two centuries to have a shorter life expectancy than their parents, due to obesity and other health problems stemming from sedentary indoor lifestyles.

Sunlight is known to help relieve depression, especially seasonal affective disorder (SAD)—depression and anxiety that afflicts people in northern latitudes in the winter. A 2010 Japanese study of *shinrin-yoku* or "forest bathing" found that forest scenery, the smell of trees, or the sound of a stream lowered levels of the stress hormone cortisol, lowered pulse rate and blood pressure, reduced stress, and relaxed people. Studies have also found that children who participate in regular, unstructured play in nature are happier, calmer, more cooperative, more self-disciplined, and do better in school. Most of all, these children enjoy nature.

Origins

NDD is not a recognized medical or psychological condition. However, Louv's work garnered widespread attention, not just from outdoor enthusiasts and environmentalists, but from parents, educators, child and adolescent psychologists, public health officials, and others in the medical community. Louv followed up with a second book in 2011: *The Nature Principle: Human Restoration and the End of Nature-Deficit Disorder*.

In the United States and around the world, organizations such as The Nature Conservancy, the Audubon Society, and the National Wildlife Federation (NWF) have adopted the NDD concept to promote outdoor education and play. Outdoor schools and camps are proliferating. In the midst of urban decay, community groups are discovering nature in vacant lots. Overcoming NDD is a cornerstone of initiatives by the Obama administration and First Lady Michelle Obama for promoting outdoor physical activity to address the major health problems facing the nation: epidemics of obesity, diabetes, and heart disease.

Risk factors

Spending too little time outside in the natural world puts people at risk for NDD. Contributing factors include long hours spent at school and work and over-scheduling of children with enrichment classes, sports, and other organized activities. Above all, the hypnotic attraction of the screen—video games, Internet, texting, and television—draw children and adults away from outdoor activities. For the majority of American children who live in urban, sometimes even dangerous, neighborhoods, opportunities to be outside at all, much less in a natural environment, may be severely limited. Longer working hours and more household responsibilities keep adults inside, or, if outside, engaging in chores such as mowing the lawn, which is not exactly communing with nature. Medical conditions can also interfere with time spent outside.

Demographics

In the early 2000s approximately one-third of American children were overweight or obese, double or triple the number in 1990, and childhood obesity rates were highest in poor neighborhoods with few parks. More than one-third of American adults are obese and 66% are either overweight or obese. These children and adults are at significantly increased risk for type 2 diabetes, heart disease, high blood pressure, **asthma**, sleep apnea, some types of cancer, and various other medical conditions. They are also at increased risk for NDD.

A 2010 Kaiser Family Foundation study found that American children between eight and 18 spent an average of seven hours and 38 minutes every day consuming media—using a smart phone or computer, playing video games, or watching TV—while spending just 4–7 minutes daily in unstructured outdoor play. The amount of time American families spent visiting parks, camping, and fishing decreased by as much as 25% between 1987 and 2008. And these trends were increasing. Louv and others believe that attention deficit/hyperactivity disorder (ADHD) and other behavioral problems are often directly attributable to NDD. An estimated 4.5 million American children have been diagnosed with ADHD, and the diagnoses increased by 3% every year between 1997 and 2006. Prescriptions for ADHD medications and antidepressants for children have skyrocketed.

Causes and symptoms

Although NDD is widely attributed to the seductive influence of ever more stimulating and sophisticated electronic media and "screen time," these are not the only causes. Throughout the United States, many schools have curtailed or completely eliminated outdoor recess. Budget cuts and the demands of standards and testing have eliminated outdoor classroom experiences and field trips that do not fit into required curricula. Meanwhile, parents, inundated with media reports of child abductions, violence, and accidents, are keeping their children inside. Finally, natural areas are increasingly inaccessible in many urban environments. Parks and nature preserves may have restricted access and "stay on the trail" signs. Even environmental educators may limit children's direct experience of nature by telling them to "look, but don't touch." Louv argues that this disengagement from nature deprives children of essential experiences and reduces their respect for the natural world.

Symptoms ascribed to NDD include ADHD, depression, anxiety, stress, feelings of isolation and alienation, lack of creativity, poor physical fitness, and obesity. Poor school performance may also be a symptom of NDD, and studies have suggested that outdoor classrooms and experiences can contribute to significant gains in various academic subjects.

Poor eyesight and vitamin D deficiency may also be symptoms of NDD. Myopia (nearsightedness) is becoming increasingly common in young children, with time spent staring at electronic screens cited as one potential cause. Studies have suggested that children who play outside are less likely to be nearsighted and need eyeglasses. The human body produces vitamin D through exposure to sunlight. One study found that 9% of American children are vitamin D deficient, and 61% have insufficient vitamin D, potentially putting them at risk for various health problems.

Diagnosis

Since NDD is not a recognized disorder or syndrome, there is no specific diagnosis. Symptoms such as ADHD, depression, or anxiety, accompanied by a sedentary indoor lifestyle, may suggest NDD.

Treatment

The treatment for NDD is obvious: regular time spent outside in nature. Even if there is another underlying cause for the symptoms, time spent outside in the natural world benefits almost everyone and is unlikely to cause harm. More and more healthcare providers are prescribing nature time for their patients. So-called ecotherapy is used to improve mood and relieve depression, anxiety, and stress and can have physical as well as mental benefits. So-called nature prescriptions are used in the treatment of various chronic conditions, including obesity, high blood pressure, diabetes, and fatigue and other side effects of cancer therapy. Nature treatments for NDD are sometimes called "vitamin G" for "green time." Some healthcare practitioners write detailed park prescriptions, telling patients where to go, how often, for how long, and what to do when they get there. Treatments for obese children may include prescriptions for the entire family to get out in nature. Attention restoration theory for ADHD incorporates exposure to natural settings.

However, treatment for NDD is not always as simple as it sounds. It can require significant lifestyle changes for families and changes in school curricula, the establishment of accessible natural areas in inner cities, and societal investment in wild places. First and foremost, however, treating NDD requires a commitment from parents to unplug their kids and get them outside. The American Academy of Pediatrics suggests limiting children's screen time to no more than one or two hours per day. Such limits alone can encourage children to venture outside in search of something else to do. Parents need to set age-appropriate rules for sending their children out to play, including where they can go and for how long, and these rules will vary with the neighborhood. Connecting with other parents can help ensure safe unstructured neighborhood play. Prearranging outside time with other parents means that the children will have playmates when they venture out. Parents themselves need to set an example, by going for a hike or gardening rather than sitting in front of the TV or computer console. Spending time outside with their children has mental and physical health benefits for parents as well. The NWF's Be Out There Movement asks parents to take a pledge to get their children outside.

Above all, parents should not over-schedule prescribed activities for their children. The NWF recommends that young people be given a daily green hour for unstructured outside play and interaction with nature. They emphasize that the time and freedom to explore nature are important components of child development and advise overbooked families to prioritize play. There are numerous websites with creative ideas for more organized nature exploration and play.

Public health role and response

Most public health response to NDD has been at the grassroots level, with movements such as the Children & Nature Network and the No Child Left Inside Coalition, which lobbies for a federal No Child Left Inside Act to increase environmental education in schools. Environmental organizations are promoting antidotes for NDD, such as the NWF's Green Hour and Be Out There campaign. The program 100,000 Kids in the Outdoors asks adults to share outdoor time with children who would otherwise not be able to go out in nature.

The U.S. government has also begun to address NDD, with its America's Great Outdoors and Youth in the Great Outdoors programs. First Lady Michelle Obama's Let's Move campaign also encourages outdoor activities for counteracting NDD. The National

---

> **KEY TERMS**
>
> **Attention deficit/hyperactivity disorder (ADHD)**—Conditions characterized by age-inappropriate attention span, hyperactivity, and impulsive behavior.
>
> **Ecotherapy**—Psychotherapy that uses nature-based methods for treating anxiety and depression.
>
> **Myopia**—Nearsightedness.
>
> **Obesity**—An abnormal accumulation of body fat, usually 20% or more above ideal body weight or a body mass index (BMI) of 30 or above.
>
> **Overweight**—A body mass index (BMI) between 25 and 30.
>
> **Seasonal affective disorder (SAD)**—Depression that recurs in fall and winter as the hours of sunlight decrease.
>
> **Vitamin D**—A fat-soluble vitamin that is produced by the body through exposure to sunlight and can also be obtained from the diet and supplements.
>
> **Vitamin G**—A term used to describe green time—time spent outdoors in nature—that is essential for human health and well-being.

> **WHAT TO ASK YOUR DOCTOR**
>
> - Could my child be suffering from nature deficit disorder?
> - How can I tell if my child is not getting enough outdoor playtime?
> - Can adults suffer from nature deficit disorder?
> - Will more time outside in nature improve my child's attention deficit/hyperactivity disorder?
> - What are good ways for my family to increase our exposure to nature?

Environmental Education Foundation promotes outdoor education.

Prognosis

Research demonstrates that children are happier and healthier when they spend time outdoors. It appears that being out in nature may cause the brain to produce more beneficial chemicals. Research indicates that children who play outside are less likely to get sick, to suffer stress, or to be aggressive. They tend to be more adaptable and resilient. According to a 2010 NWF survey, a majority of educators report that children with regular unstructured outdoor playtime concentrate better, are more creative, and are better problem solvers. Studies have found that outdoor education improves attentiveness, focus, performance, and test scores.

Outdoor activities and play and exposure to nature may not cure ADHD, but they do appear to reduce symptoms. Unfortunately, children with ADHD may get less time outside than their peers, because they are more likely to be kept in during recess or after school because of behavior problems. Research indicates that schoolwork, ADHD, and depressive symptoms improve when children move to neighborhoods with more green space.

Nature therapy can be important for adult healing as well. Studies have shown that patients with a view of trees heal faster than those in windowless rooms or with views of city buildings. Even workers in windowless offices were healthier, happier, and more efficient with virtual windows—flat screens with nature views—although not as healthy, happy, or creative as workers with real windows with natural views.

Prevention

Although there is nothing new about recommending that children—especially overweight and obese children—get more physical exercise, the American Academy of Pediatrics and other organizations recommend that as much of that activity as possible be in the outdoors. In societies in which children are bombarded with electronic media, it is the responsibility of parents, schools, youth organizations, and society at large to combat NDD by getting youngsters outside in nature. Parents can organize walk-to-school groups. Schools can institute more environmental education. Combating NDD may contribute to better adjusted, smarter, and more creative children. Without a doubt, it will contribute to physically healthier children and adults. Ultimately however, children will play outside, not to reduce their stress or do better in school but because it is fun.

Resources

BOOKS

Christopher, Todd. *The Green Hour: A Daily Dose of Nature for Happier, Healthier, Smarter Kids.* Boston: Trumpeter, 2010.

Louv, Richard. *Last Child in the Woods: Saving Our Children from Nature-Deficit Disorder.* Chapel Hill, NC: Algonquin, 2005.

Louv, Richard. *The Nature Principle: Human Restoration and the End of Nature-Deficit Disorder.* Chapel Hill, NC: Algonquin, 2011.

Louv, Richard. *The Nature Principle: Reconnecting with Life in a Virtual Age.* Chapel Hill, NC: Algonquin, 2012.

Shalof, Tilda. *Camp Nurse: My Adventures at Summer Camp.* New York: Kaplan, 2010.

PERIODICALS

Abramovitz, Melissa. "Vitamin G for Your Mind." *Current Health Kids* 35, no. 8 (April/May 2012): 6–8.

Ackerman, Diane. "Nature: Now Showing on TV." *New York Times*, June 24, 2012.

Catchpole, Todd C., and Kimberly A. Catchpole. "Nature Play." *Parks & Recreation* 47, no. 4 (April 2012): 10, 12–13.

Louv, Richard. "Reconnecting to Nature in the Age of Technology." *Futurist* 45, no. 6 (November/December 2011): 41–45.

WEBSITES

"Be Out There." National Wildlife Federation. http://www.nwf.org/Get-Outside/Be-Out-There.aspx (accessed November 2, 2012).

"Be Out There—Whole Child: Developing Mind, Body and Spirit Through Outdoor Play." National Wildlife Foundation. http://www.nwf.org/~/media/PDFs/Be%20Out%20There/BeOutThere_WholeChild_V2.ashx (accessed November 2, 2012).

Coyle, Kevin. "Parents: 10 Reasons Kids Need Fresh Air." *National Wildlife*. National Wildlife Federation. January 1, 2010. http://www.nwf.org/News-and-Magazines/National-Wildlife/Outdoors/Archives/2010/Parents-10-Reasons-Kids-Need-Fresh-Air.aspx (accessed November 2, 2012).

Egan, Timothy. "Nature-Deficit Disorder." Opinionator. *New York Times*, March 29, 2012. http://opinionator.blogs.nytimes.com/2012/03/29/nature-deficit-disorder (accessed November 2, 2012).
"Kids' Health Issues 2011: Fighting Nature Deficit Disorder." KidsHealth. December 2010. http://kidshealth.org/parent/positive/issues_2011/2011_nature.html?tracking=P_RelatedArticle (accessed November 2, 2012).
Louv, Richard. "A Field Guide to the New Nature Movement: Applying the Nature Principle to Your Life and the Lives of Others." April 2012. http://richardlouv.com/books/nature-principle/field-guide (accessed November 5, 2012).
"Nature-Deficit Disorder: Do You Have It?" National Environmental Education Week. http://www.eeweek.org/resources/survey.htm (accessed November 2, 2012).
Sorgen, Carol. "Do You Need a Nature Prescription? Nature Therapy May Mean that Better Health Is Right Outside Your Door." WebMD. http://www.webmd.com/balance/features/nature-therapy-ecotherapy (accessed November 2, 2012).
Torgan, Carol. "8 Simple Tips to Grow Active, Healthy Kids: Trade in Screen Time for Green Time." *National Wildlife*. National Wildlife Federation. February 3, 2010. http://www.nwf.org/News-and-Magazines/National-Wildlife/Outdoors/Archives/2010/8-tips-to-grow-active-healthy-kids.aspx (accessed November 2, 2012).

ORGANIZATIONS

Children & Nature Network, 7 Avenida Vista Grande B-7, no. 502, Santa Fe, NM 87508, info@childrenandnature.org, http://www.cnaturenet.org.
National Environmental Education Foundation, 4301 Connecticut Ave., Ste. 160, Washington, DC 20008, (202) 833-2933, Fax: (202) 261-6464, http://www.outdoorfoundation.org.
National Wildlife Federation, PO Box 1583, Merrifield, VA 22116-1583, 1(703) 438-6000, (800) 822-9919, http://www.nwf.org.
The Nature Conservancy, 4245 North Fairfax Dr., Ste. 100, Arlington, VA 22203-1606, (703) 841-5300, (800) 628-6860, member@tnc.org, http://www.nature.org.
Outdoor Foundation, 1776 Massachusetts Ave. NW, Ste. 450, Washington, DC 20036, (202) 271-3252, info@outdoorfoundation.org, http://www.outdoorfoundation.org.

Margaret Alic, PhD

Necrotizing fasciitis

Definition

Necrotizing fasciitis (NF) is also called the flesh-eating disease. It is a rare condition in which bacteria destroy tissues underlying the skin. This tissue death, called necrosis or gangrene, spreads rapidly. This disease can be fatal in as little as 12 to 24 hours.

Demographics

The **Centers for Disease Control and Prevention** (CDC) estimates that there are between 650 and 800 cases each year in the United States. Necrotizing fasciitis mostly affects adults. The average age of patients is between 38 and 45 years. Males are three times more likely to be affected. About half of all patients diagnosed with NF were previously strong and healthy. Some people, however, are at greater risk of developing NF, including people with diabetes, heart disease, and other disorders that affect blood circulation; drug addicts and alcoholics; people with weakened immune systems, including those who have received organ transplants; and people with HIV infection are most at risk.

Most often the bacteria enter the body through an opening in the skin, quite often a very minor opening, even as small as a paper cut, a staple puncture, or a pin prick. It can also enter through weakened skin, such as a bruise, blister, or abrasion. It can also happen following a major trauma or surgery, and in some cases there appears to be no identifiable point of entry.

Description

Necrotizing fasciitis is an apt descriptor, meaning the infection appears to devour body tissue. Media reports increased in the middle and late 1990s, but the disease is not new. It first appeared between the 1840s to 1870s. Dr. B. Wilson, first termed the condition necrotizing fasciitis in 1952. However, the disease had been occurring for many centuries before it was described in the 1800s. Indeed, Hippocrates described it more than three millennia ago and thousands of reports exist from the Civil War. There are many terms used to describe necrotizing fasciitis, including flesh-eating bacterial infection or flesh-eating disease; suppurative fasciitis; dermal, Meleney, hospital or Fournier's gangrene; and necrotizing cellulitis.

Necrotizing fasciitis is divided into two types. Type I is caused by anaerobic bacteria, with or without the presence of aerobic bacteria. Type II, also called hemolytic streptococcal gangrene, is caused by group A streptococci; other bacteria may or may not be present. The disease may also be called synergistic gangrene.

Type I fasciitis typically affects the trunk, abdomen, and genital area. For example, Fournier's gangrene is a "flesh-eating" disease in which the infection encompasses the external genitalia. The arms and legs are most often affected in type II fasciitis, but the infection may appear anywhere.

Causes and symptoms

The two most important factors in determining whether a person will develop necrotizing fasciitis are the virulence (ability to cause disease) of the bacteria and the susceptibility (ability of a person's immune system to respond to infection) of the person who becomes infected with this bacteria.

In nearly every case of necrotizing fasciitis, a skin injury precedes the disease. As bacteria grow beneath the skin's surface, they produce toxins. These toxins destroy superficial fascia, subcutaneous fat, and deep fascia. In some cases, the overlying dermis and the underlying muscle are also affected.

Initially, the infected area appears red and swollen and feels hot. The area is extremely painful, which is a prominent feature of the disease. Over the course of hours or days, the skin may become blue-gray, and fluid-filled blisters may form. As nerves are destroyed the area becomes numb. An individual may develop dangerously low blood pressure. Multiple organ failure may occur, quickly followed by death.

Many different types of bacteria can cause this infection. A very severe and usually deadly form of necrotizing soft tissue infection is due to Streptococcus pyogenes, which is sometimes called flesh-eating bacteria. Necrotizing soft tissue infection develops when the bacteria enters the body, usually through a minor cut or scrape. The bacteria begin to grow and release harmful substances (toxins) that kill tissue and affect blood flow to the area. As the tissue dies, the bacteria enter the blood and rapidly spread throughout the body.

Symptoms of necrotizing fasciitis include skin that is red, swollen, and hot to the touch; fever; chills; nausea and vomiting; and diarrhea. The infection may spread rapidly and it can quickly become life-threatening. Affected individuals may also go into shock and have damage to skin, fat, and the tissue covering the muscle, referred to as gangrene. Necrotizing fasciitis can lead to organ failure and death.

Risk factors

Although necrotizing fasciitis is somewhat rare, some studies have indicated that about 25% of patients die from the progression of the condition. In general, patients with immune deficiency disorders such as diabetes, cancer, and kidney disease are at a greater risk for developing necrotizing fasciitis because of the compromised state of the immune system. Also, patients taking steroids for various different medical conditions should be aware of the elevated risk factor this causes.

The primary method of transfer for bacteria causing necrotizing fasciitis is through the skin. Therefore, open wounds are of particular concern for transmission. Wounds such as bedsores and postsurgical incisions also increase a patient's risk for developing necrotizing fasciitis.

Diagnosis

The appearance of the skin, paired with pain and fever raises the possibility of necrotizing fasciitis. An x ray, magnetic resonance imaging (MRI), or computed tomography (CT) scans of the area reveals a feathery pattern in the tissue, caused by accumulating gas in the dying tissue. Necrosis is evident during exploratory surgery, during which samples are collected for bacterial identification.

Treatment

Rapid, aggressive medical treatment, specifically, antibiotic therapy and surgical debridement, is imperative. Antibiotics may include penicillin, an aminoglycoside or third-generation cephalosporin, and clindamycin or metronidazole. Analgesics are employed for pain control. During surgical debridement, dead tissue is stripped away. After surgery, patients are rigorously monitored for continued infection, shock, or other complications.

Many doctors believe that multiple antibiotics should be used at the same time to protect the patient from methicillin-resistant staphylococcus aureus (MRSA), as well as infections with anaerobic bacteria, and polymicrobic infections. Treatments such as insertion of a breathing tube, intravenous administration of fluids, and drugs to support the cardiovascular system may be required. If available, hyperbaric oxygen therapy has also be used.

Prognosis

Necrotizing fasciitis has a fatality rate of about 25%. Diabetes, arteriosclerosis, immunosuppression, kidney disease, malnutrition, and obesity are connected with a poor prognosis. Older individuals and intravenous drug users may also be at higher risk. The infection site also has a role. Survivors may require plastic surgery and may have to contend with permanent physical disability and psychological adjustment.

Prevention

Necrotizing fasciitis, which occurs very rarely, cannot be definitively prevented. The best ways to lower the risk of contracting necrotizing fasciitis are:

KEY TERMS

Aerobic bacteria—Bacteria that require oxygen to live and grow.

Anaerobic bacteria—Bacteria that require the absence of oxygen to live and grow.

CT scan (computed tomography scan)—Cross-sectional x rays of the body are compiled to create a three-dimensional image of the body's internal structures.

Debridement—Surgical procedure in which dead or dying tissue is removed.

Dermis—The deepest layer of skin.

Fascia, deep—A fibrous layer of tissue that envelopes muscles.

Fascia, superficial—A fibrous layer of tissue that lies between the deepest layer of skin and the subcutaneous fat.

Gangrene—Dead tissue.

Hyperbaric oxygen therapy—A treatment in which the patient is placed in a chamber and breathes oxygen at higher-than-atmospheric pressure. This high-pressure oxygen stops bacteria from growing and, at high enough pressure, kills them.

Magnetic resonance imaging (MRI)—An imaging technique that uses a large circular magnet and radio waves to generate signals from atoms in the body. These signals are used to construct images of internal structures.

Necrosis—Abnormal death of cells, potentially caused by disease or infection.

Subcutaneous—Referring to the area beneath the skin.

- Take care to avoid any injury to the skin that may give the bacteria a place of entry.

- When skin injuries do occur, they should be promptly washed and treated with an antibiotic ointment or spray.

- People who have any skin injury should rigorously attempt to avoid people who are infected with streptococci bacteria, a bacteria that causes a simple strep throat in one person may cause necrotizing fasciitis in another.

- Have any areas of unexplained redness, pain, or swelling examined by a doctor, particularly if the affected area seems to be expanding.

Public health role and response

The news of flesh-eating bacteria incidents have heightened the awareness of the general public regarding their susceptibility to being infected with the deadly disease. Most cases of flesh-eating bacteria have been sporadic rather than associated with large outbreaks. But there are increasingly more reports from clinical centers. The disease is difficult to treat and immediate treatment is needed to prevent death. For this reason, the public health system's ability to contain a flesh-eating bacteria epidemic or similar outbreak remains somewhat questionable to many.

The CDC tracks specific infections in the United States, including necrotizing fasciitis caused by group A strep, with a special system called Active Bacterial Core surveillance (ABCs). ABCs is an important part of CDC Emerging Infections Programs network (EIP), a collaboration among CDC, state health departments, and universities. By sharing this kind of information in a timely way, public health professionals can look for trends in rising cases. Each year in the United States, there are about 650-800 cases of necrotizing fasciitis caused by group A strep; this is likely an underestimation as some cases are not reported. According to ABCs data, the number of annual infections does not appear to be rising.

Resources

BOOKS

Barie, P. S. "Eachempati SR." In *Conn's Current Therapy 2009*, edited by R. E. Rakel, and E. T. Bope, 835–39. Philadelphia: Saunders Elsevier, 2009.

Lewis Tilden, Thomasine E. *Help! What's Eating My Flesh? Runaway Staph and Strep Infections*. New York: Franklin Watts, 2008.

PERIODICALS

Hsu, H. E., et al. "Effect of Pneumococcal Conjugate Vaccine on Pneumococcal Meningitis." *New England Journal of Medicine* 360 (2009): 244–56.

WEBSITES

Centers for Disease Control and Prevention. "Group A Streptococcal (GAS) Disease." http://www.cdc.gov/ncidod/dbmd/diseaseinfo/groupastreptococcal_g.htm (accessed June 10, 2012).

ORGANIZATIONS

National Necrotizing Fasciitis Foundation, 2731 Porter SW, Grand Rapids, MI 49509, nnfffeb@aol.com, http://www.nnff.org.

Paul A. Johnson, EdM
Karl Finley

Neurotoxin

Definition

Neurotoxins are a special class of metabolic poison that attack nerve cells. Disruption of the nervous system as a result of exposure to neurotoxins usually is quick and destructive.

Description

Neurotoxins are categorized according to the nature of their impact on the nervous system. Anesthetics (e.g., ether, chloroform, halothane), chlorinated hydrocarbons (e.g., dichlorodiphenyltrichloroethane [DDT], Dieldrin, Aldrin), and heavy metals (e.g., **lead**, **mercury**) disrupt the ion transport across cell membranes essential for nerve action. Common pesticides, including carbamates such as Sevin, Zeneb, and Maneb, and the organophosphates such as Malathion and Parathion, inhibit acetylcholinesterase, an enzyme that regulates nerve signal transmission between nerve cells and the organs and tissues they innervate.

Neurotoxins are common in living organisms, including bacteria, fungi, plants, arachnids (e.g., spiders), marine life, and vertebrates. Botulinum neurotoxin, the cause of botulism, is produced by the bacterium *Clostridium botulinum*. Venomous snakes, spiders, and scorpions all paralyze their prey by injecting a neurotoxin. Parts of the Japanese puffer fish contain neurotoxins that can be fatal if eaten. Anesthetics are neurotoxins with beneficial medical uses. Botox, a form of botulinum toxin, has been approved by the U.S. **Food and Drug Administration** (FDA) for cosmetic and limited medical use.

Risk factors

Environmental exposure to neurotoxins can occur through a variety of mechanisms. These include improper use, improper storage or disposal of chemicals, inhalation during occupational use, or accidental spills during distribution or application. Neurotoxins also can be ingested in food and water. Because the identification and ramifications of all neurotoxins are not fully known, there is risk of exposure associated with this lack of knowledge.

Causes and symptoms

Cell damage associated with the introduction of neurotoxins occurs through direct contact with the chemical or a loss of oxygen to the cell. This results in damage to cellular components, especially in those required for the synthesis of protein and other cell components.

> **KEY TERMS**
>
> **Alzheimer's disease**—An incurable disease of older individuals that results in the destruction of nerve cells in the brain and causes gradual loss of mental and physical functions.
>
> **Amyotrophic lateral sclerosis (ALS)**—Also called Lou Gehrig's disease, a disease that causes degeneration of the nerves that control muscle movement. Eventually breathing muscles become paralyzed and the individual dies.
>
> **Chelation therapy**—A treatment used for many types of heavy metal poisonings in which edetate calcium disodium is administered intravenously. The drug attracts molecules of the heavy metal and binds with them in such a way that they can be eliminated in urine.
>
> **Lathyrism**—A disorder that affects humans and some domestic animals and results in degeneration of the nerves of the spinal cord. It is caused by eating legumes that contain the naturally occurring neurotoxin oxalyldiaminopropionic acid (ODAP).

The symptoms associated with pesticide poisoning include eye and skin irritation, blurred vision, headache, anorexia, nausea, vomiting, increased sweating, increased salivation, diarrhea, abdominal pain, slight bradycardia, ataxia, muscle weakness and twitching, and generalized weakness of respiratory muscles.

Symptoms associated with poisoning of the central nervous system include giddiness, anxiety, insomnia, drowsiness, difficulty concentrating, poor recall, confusion, slurred speech, convulsions, coma with the absence of reflexes, depression of respiratory and circulatory centers, paralysis, fall in blood pressure, and death.

Some links between environmental neurotoxin exposure and neuromuscular and brain dysfunction have been identified. Physiological symptoms of Alzheimer's disease, amyotrophic lateral sclerosis (ALS) or Lou Gehrig's disease, and lathyrism have been identified in populations exposed to substances containing known neurotoxins. For example, studies have shown that heroin addicts who used synthetic heroin contaminated with methylphenyltetrahydropyridine developed a condition that manifests symptoms identical to those associated with Parkinson's disease. On the island of Guam, the natives who incorporate the seeds of the false sago plant (*cycas circinalis*) into their

> **QUESTIONS TO ASK YOUR DOCTOR**
>
> - What test do I need to learn if my symptoms are caused by exposure to a neurotoxin?
> - Are my symptoms reversible or will the damage be permanent?
> - What can I do to protect myself against neurotoxin exposure in the workplace?

diet develop a condition very similar to ALS. The development of this condition has been associated with the specific nonprotein amino acid, B methyla-mino-1-alanine, present in the seeds.

Diagnosis

Diagnosis is made, usually by a neurologist, based on the patient's history and a variety of neurological and **toxicology** tests. Tests will vary depending on the type of neurotoxin suspected.

Treatment

Initial treatment consists of eliminating continued exposure to the neurotoxin. Beyond that, treatment varies depending on the type of neurotoxin to which the individual has been exposed. In many cases, supportive care is the only available treatment. Chelation therapy may be used as part of a comprehensive treatment for some heavy metal neurotoxins (e.g., lead). For a few neurotoxins such as rattlesnake venom, an antivenin can be administered. In many cases, neurological damage is irreversible.

Prevention

Prevention involves educating individuals about the potential neurotoxicity of chemicals used in the workplace and in hobbies. Organizations such as the U.S. **Environmental Protection Agency** (EPA) and the Occupational Health and Safety Administration (OSHA) set limits on the amount of many toxins, including neurotoxins, permitted in the environment and in the workplace.

Resources

BOOKS

Satoh, Tetsuo, ed. *Anticholinesterase Pesticides: Metabolism, Neurotoxicity, and Epidemiology.* Hoboken, NJ: Wiley, 2010.

Spaeth, Kenneth R. et al. *Heavy metals: A Rapid Clinical Guide to Neurotoxicity and Other Common Concerns.* New York: Nova Science, 2010.

WEBSITES

Camp, Allison. "Neurotoxins." Toxipedia.com. http://toxipedia.org/display/toxipedia/Neurotoxins (accessed October 17, 2012).
Centers for Disease Control and Prevention (CDC). "Organic Solvents." http://www.cdc.gov/niosh/topics/organsolv (accessed October 17, 2012).
National Center for Biotechnology Information. "Resources for Neurotoxins." http://www.ncbi.nlm.nih.gov/sites/ga?disorder=neurotoxins (accessed October 17, 2012).
National Geographic Society. "Pick Your Poison—12 Toxic Tales." http://science.nationalgeographic.com/science/health-and-human-body/human-body/poison-toxic-tales.html (accessed October 17, 2012).

ORGANIZATIONS

Agency for Toxic Substances and Disease Registry, 4770 Buford Hwy. NE, Atlanta, GA 30341, (800) 232-4636; TTY: (888) 232-6348, cdcinfo@cdc.gov, http://www.atsdr.cdc.gov/.
Centers for Disease Control and Prevention, 1600 Clifton Rd., Atlanta, GA 30333, (404) 639-3534, (800) CDC-INFO (800-232-4636); TTY: (888) 232-6348, inquiry@cdc.gov, http://www.cdc.gov.
Environmental Protection Agency (EPA), Ariel Rios Bldg., 1200 Pennsylvania Ave. NW, Washington, DC 20460, (202) 272-0167; TTY (202) 272-0165, http://www.epa.gov.

Brian R. Barthel
Tish Davidson, AM

9/11 terrorist attacks

Definition

On September 11, 2001, four planes were hijacked by 19 foreign-born terrorists with the intent of flying them into targets within the United States of America. Two planes, American Airlines Flight 11 and United Airlines Flight 175, originated from Logan Airport in Boston, MA and were flown into the World Trade Center (WTC), or twin towers, in the financial district of lower Manhattan, New York City. The first hit the North tower at 8:46 A.M., the second hit the south tower at 9:03 A.M. American Airlines flight 77 left Washington Dulles International Airport in Virginia at 8:42 A.M. and crashed into the Pentagon in Washington, DC at 9:37 A.M. A fourth plane, United Airlines Flight 93, originating from Newark International Airport, crashed landed in a field in Shanksville, Pennsylvania, at 10:03 A.M. after passengers overtook the hijackers.

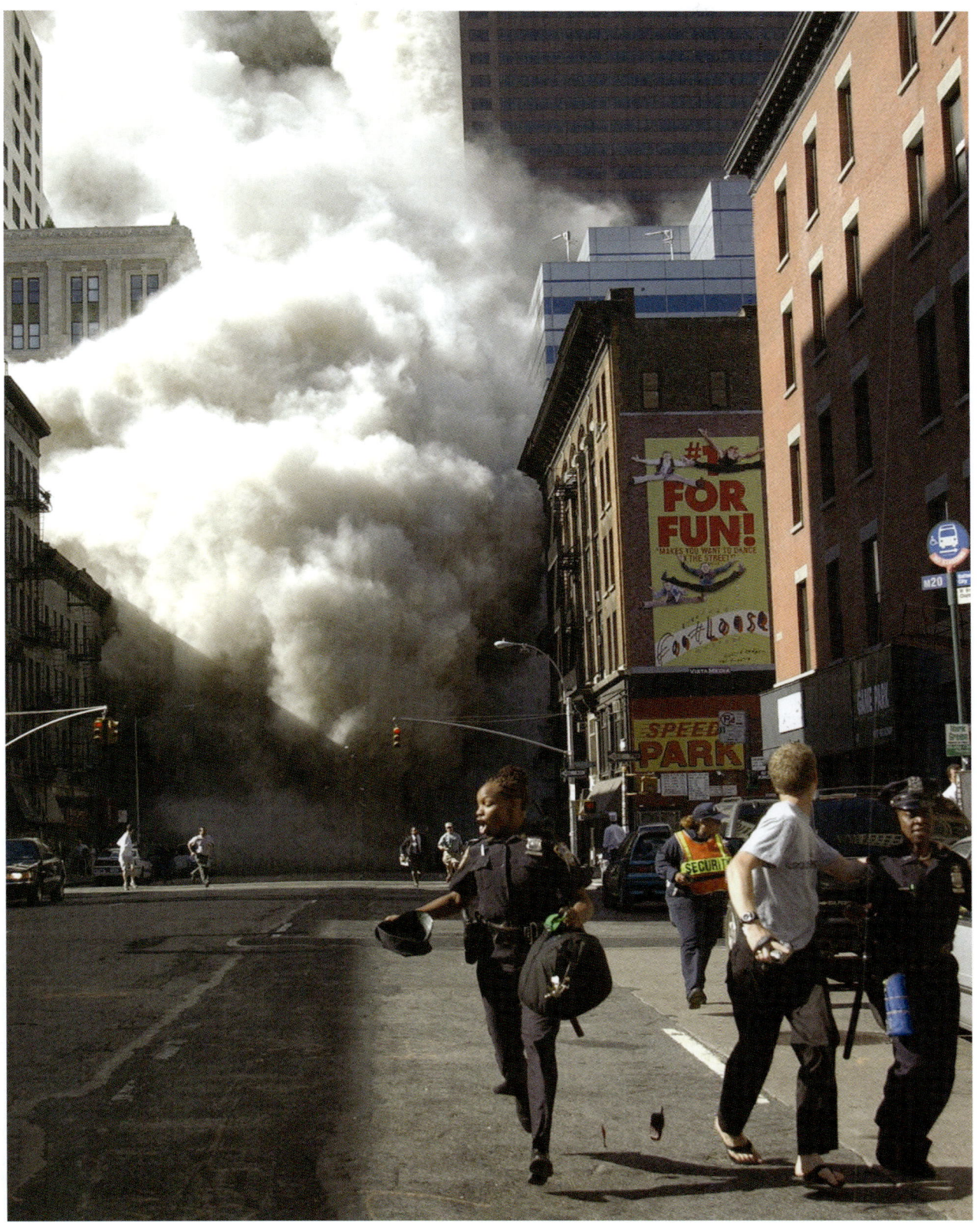

Police officers and civilians run away from New York's World Trade Center after an additional explosion rocked the buildings Tuesday morning, Sept. 11, 2001. *(AP Photo/Louis Lanzano)*

Description

The coordinated attack caused the collapse of the towers in New York (also referred to as "ground zero"), and the destruction of one wing of the pentagon, resulting in a total cost of more than $21.7 billion in government assistance and reconstruction aid and an additional $27.3 billion from economic decline for New York City alone. 2,996 lives were lost, (including the 227 passengers and crew on the planes and 19 terrorists), and thousands were injured.

The hijackers originated from a group called al-Qaeda, indirectly organized through a terrorist cell by it's leader, Mohamed Atta of Egypt. In addition to Atta, fifteen of the attackers were from Saudi Arabia, two from the United Arab emirates and one from Lebanon. The cell was quickly linked to Osama bin Laden, who claimed direct responsibility for the tack on September 9, 2001, in a video on an Arabic TV station. The attack had been planned for 5 years between Osama bin Laden and Khalid Sheikh Mohammed. The cell that perpetrated the attack included some experienced jihadists, a commercial pilot, and three Hamburg cell members who trained to fly in South Florida. In the spring of 2001 final targets were selected. It is commonly understood that the attack occurred as part of bin Laden's fatwa against the United States. Al-Qaeda disapproves of the U.S. foreign policies regarding the Middle East, including it's presence in Saudi Arabia, allegiance to Israel, and at that time the sanctions against Iraq.

Aftermath

The attacks were used as the rationale for U.S. engagement in Afghanistan starting October 7, 2001 and lasting until present day. These attacks were also used in part to justify a pre-emptive invasion into iraq on March 20, 2003, starting the Second Iraq War, which officially ended December 18, 2011. There remains a segment of the population that questions the validity of the events that occurred on 9/11, and consider the attack to be coordinated by the United States government perpetrated against it's own citizens. These claims are widely disregarded.

Economically, 9/11 caused a devastating blow to New York City's GDP. The Dow Jones Industrial Average dropped 14.3% the first week following the attack. 18,000 small businesses were displaced following the attack due to debris and the massive destruction to office and commercial space in lower Manhattan. North American air space was closed for days affected hundreds of thousands of flights.

The 9/11 Commission was established on November 27, 2002 to investigate and provide a complete report on the circumstances of the attack and provide a guide to response, preparedness and prevention. The report highlighted failures of both the Central Intelligence Agency and the Federal Bureau of Investigation. THe final report was published on August 21, 2004, after hearing testimony from members of various bureaus and departments, the executive cabinet, President George W. Bush, and past government officials. The Department of Homeland Security was established on January 24, 2003 to protect American citizens and coordinate between state and federal bodies to protection of infrastructure, transportation hubs, ports, and other potential targets of terrorism.

In October of 2012, a New York federal judge found Iran, the Taliban and al-Qaida culpable in the September 11 terrorist attacks and approved a $6 billion default judgment awarded to 47 victims, despite Iran's consistent denial of any connection to the attack. The James L. Zadroga 9/11 Health & Compensation Act, was signed into law by President Obama in early 2011, establishing the World Trade Center (WTC) Health Program and ensuring health care treatment for those affected by 9/11 through at least 2015.

Effects on public health

The most widespread health effect stemming from the 9/11 attacks was post traumatic stress disorder (PTSD). The Commissioner of the New York City Department of Health and Mental Hygiene reported that 19% of those in the immediate vicinity of the attack who sought medical treatment were still suffering from PTSD 506 years following the attack. In many instances these individuals lost friends and colleagues in the attack, suffered from respiratory or other illness caused by the debris cloud contaminants, witnessed the events first hand, or were involved in rescue operations.

In New York City, the dust cloud unleashed from the collapse of the towers contained hundreds of thousands of toxins which settled throughout lower Manhattan. Environmental reports did not return to normal until a year following the event. The debris also settled in the East and Hudson rivers. The first responders and clean up crews who operated in the vicinity during and following the attack have reported significant health effects as a result of inhaling foreign particulate matter after working in the debris field without adequate protective gear. In 2002 and 2009, two more people lost their lives as a result of the 9/11 attacks from dust, smoke, and contamination related illnesses. The city's medical examiner concluded that the ground zero dust was "harmful and even deadly."

Within the first ten years following the 9/11 terrorist attack, the following health effects were disproportionately experienced by those in the WTC Health Registry: **asthma**, persistent abnormal pulmonary function, sarcoidosis (inflammation) of the lungs, increased risk of some cancers, sinus and lung problems, depression and high risk of suffering from PTSD.

Most city workers did not have health coverage before the attack. A number of suits were filed against the City of New York and the federal government by firefighters, policemen and other first responders with health claims, demanding health care coverage for costs associated with 9/11-related medical issues. While some were compensated by the federal government for a period of a few years following the attack, concerns remained about coverage continuation until the Zadroga Act was enacted in 2011. The law set aside $2.775 billion dollars to compensate claimants for lost wages and other damages related to their illnesses, but as of October 2012, those funds had yet to be dispersed. The September 11 Victim Compensation Fund (2001–2003) was replaced by the 9/11 Fund, which was established to assist those 40,000–90,000 workers suffering from illnesses caused by being at ground zero during search and rescue. The fund covers 50 different kinds of cancer, respiratory and lung diseases, and PTSD therapy, in addition to other medical and health problems.

Effect on the environment

The destruction of the World Trade Center is the greatest acute environmental distort in the history of New York City. The fires caused toxic gases to be emitted from the rubble in a plume of airborne combustion that burned for months. The collapsed buildings created debris that contained **asbestos**, polycyclic aromatic hydrocarbons (PCBs), dioxins, crystalline silica, pulverized glass shards, heavy metals, and thousands of other toxins resulting in dangerous chemical combinations in the air. While these contaminants certainly affected those in lower manhattan for the first year, as of 2010, sampling by the **Environmental Protection Agency** and independent studies showed no or low levels of contamination.

Public Health role and response

National security threats remain despite the extensive amount of protections taken following the event. The Intelligence Reform and Terrorism Prevention Act of 2004 established the National Counterterrorism Center and required the Department of Homeland Security to take over pre-flight screenings of passengers from the Transportation Security Administration (TSA), closing security holes at airports and reducing the future risk of a similar attack.

The Departments of Homeland Security, Federal Emergency Response Agency, Environmental Protection Agency, and Center for Disease Control, among others, now have extensive guidelines for handling emergency repines, especially for terrorist attacks.

Resources

BOOKS

Government Publication Office (GPO). "The 9/11 Commission Report: Final Report of the National Commission on Terrorist Attacks Upon the United States." Washington, D.C.: GPO, July 22, 2004. http://www.gpo.gov/fdsys/pkg/GPO-911REPORT/pdf/GPO-911REPORT.pdf

PERIODICALS

DePalma, A. *For the first time, new York links death to 9/11 dust* New York: New York Times, May 24, 2007. Accessed: October 15, 2012. http://www.nytimes.com/2007/05/24/nyregion/24dust.html?pagewanted=print

The City of New York. "What we know about the health effects of 9/11." New York: Commissioner of the New York City Department of Health and Mental Hygiene. Updated: 2012. Accessed: October 19, 2012. http://www.nyc.gov/html/doh/wtc/html/know/know.shtml

Henry, S. and Jones, A. "9/11 responders wait for compensation for their illnesses." CNN, September 11, 2012. http://www.cnn.com/2012/09/10/us/september-11-zadroga-act/index.html

WEBSITES

9/11 Memorial. Updated: 2012. Accessed: October 19, 2012. http://www.911memorial.org/

The September 11 Digital Archive. Center for History and New Media and American Social History Project/Center for Media and Learning. Updated: 2011. Accessed: October 16, 2012. http://911digitalarchive.org/

Alyson C. Heimer, MA

Noise pollution

Definition

There are many definitions of noise, some technical and some philosophical. A common definition for noise is any loud, irritating, surprising, or unwanted sound made by humans, animals, nature, or machines. However, what is music to one person's ears might be noise to someone else and music along with parties can be a problem in crowded residential areas. For the most part, noise pollution is any unwanted sound or any sound that interferes with hearing, causes stress, or disrupts one's life. The source of most outdoor noise comes from construction and transportation systems,

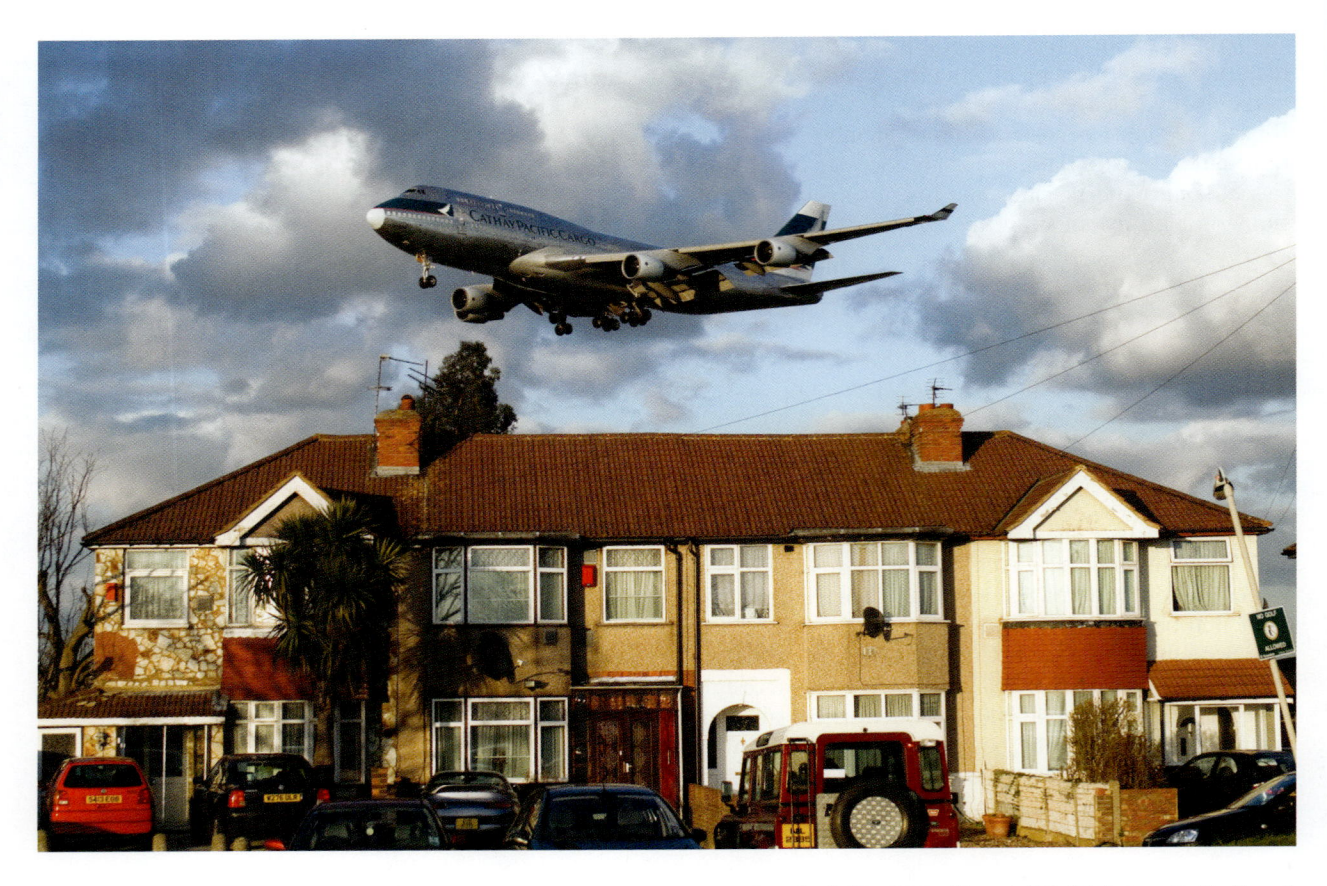

A Boeing 747 operated by Cathay Pacific Cargo on approach for landing at London's Heathrow Airport, UK. (© Antony Nettle Alamy)

including the noise from motor vehicles, aircraft, and railroads. For instance, a commercial jet preparing to land and flying over a residential area may likely produce noise pollution to these residents. Sound is measured either in dynes, watts, or decibels. Usually 80 decibels (db) is the level at which sound becomes physically painful; thus, it is often denoted as noise. Note that decibels are logarithmic; that is, a ten decibel (db) increase represents a doubling of sound energy.

Description

Humans detect sound by means of a set of sensory cells in the inner ear. These cells have tiny projections (called microvilli and kinocilia) on their surface. As sound waves pass through the fluid-filled chamber within which these cells are suspended, the microvilli rub against a flexible membrane lying on top of them. Bending of fibers inside the microvilli sets off a mechanico-chemical process that results in a nerve signal being sent through the auditory nerve to the brain where the signal is analyzed and interpreted.

The sensitivity and discrimination of one's hearing is remarkable. Normally, humans can hear sounds between 16 and 20,000 hertz (hz). A young child whose hearing has not yet been damaged by excess noise can hear the whine of a mosquito's wings at the window when less than one quadrillionth of a watt per square centimeter is reaching the eardrum.

The sensory cell's microvilli are flexible and resilient, but only up to a point. They can bend and then spring back up, but they die if they are smashed down too hard or too often. Prolonged exposure to sounds above about 90 decibels can flatten some of the microvilli permanently, and their function will be lost. By age thirty years, most Americans have lost five decibels of sensitivity and cannot hear anything above 16,000 hertz; by age sixty-five, the sensitivity reduction is 40 decibels for most people, and all sounds above 8,000 hertz are lost. By contrast, in the African country of Sudan, where the environment is very quiet, even 70-year-olds have insignificant hearing loss.

Risk factors

Noises come from many sources. Traffic is generally the most omnipresent noise in the city. Cars, trucks, and buses create a roar that permeates nearly everywhere. Around airports, jets thunder overhead, stopping conversation, rattling dishes, sometimes even cracking walls. Jackhammers rattle in the streets; sirens pierce the air; motorcycles, lawn mowers, snow blowers, and chain saws create an infernal din; and music from radios, televisions, and loudspeakers fill the air everywhere.

Demographics

Every year since 1973, the U.S. Department of Housing and Urban Development has conducted a survey to find out what city residents dislike about their environment. Every year the same factor has been near or at the top of the list as most objectionable. It is not crime, pollution, or congestion; it is noise—something that affects every person every day.

The U.S. Census Bureau stated that based on its 2009 American Housing Survey about 25.4 million people in the United States—out of a total of about 111.8 million households,—reported being upset or irritated by street noise or heavy traffic. A study by the **World Health Organization** found that environmental noise in Western Europe caused annoyance in many people, but it also caused much more serious medical conditions such as cardiovascular disease, cognitive impairment, sleep disturbances, and tinnitus.

It has been known for a long time that prolonged exposure to noises, such as loud music or the roar of machinery, can result in hearing loss. Evidence now suggests that noise-related stress also causes a wide range of psychological and physiological problems, ranging from irritability to heart disease. An increasing number of people are affected by noise in their environment. By the age of 40, nearly everyone in the United States has suffered hearing deterioration in the higher frequencies. An estimated 10% of Americans (30 million people) suffer serious hearing loss, and the lives of at least another 80 million people are significantly disrupted by noise.

Causes and symptoms

Extremely loud sounds—above 130 decibels, the level of a loud rock band or music heard through earphones at a high setting—actually can rip out the sensory microvilli, causing aberrant nerve signals that the brain interprets as a high-pitched whine or whistle. Many people experience ringing ears after exposure to very loud noises. Coffee, aspirin, certain antibiotics, and fever also can cause ringing sensations, but they usually are temporary.

Noise pollution can contribute to degrade health and abnormal behavior. Specifically, it can lead to physiological and psychological problems. When it becomes intolerable, noise pollution can cause aggression, annoyance, hypertension (high blood pressure), high stress levels, tinnitus, hearing loss, sleep disturbances, and other degrading health problems. Noise pollution can over the long-term cause cardiovascular problems in humans. For instance, if noise is persistently a part of one's work environment, then an increased incidence of coronary artery disease may occur.

One of the symptoms of noise pollution is hearing loss and related problems. For instance, a persistent ringing is called tinnitus. It has been estimated that 94% of the people in the United States suffer from some degree of tinnitus. For most people, the ringing is noticeable only in a very quiet environment, and they rarely are in a place that is quiet enough to hear it. About 35 out of 1,000 people have tinnitus severe enough to for it to interfere with their lives. Sometimes the ringing becomes so loud that it is unendurable, resembling the shrieking brakes on a subway train. Unfortunately, there is not yet a treatment for this distressing disorder. One of the first charges to the **Environmental Protection Agency (EPA)** when it was founded in 1970 was to study noise pollution and to recommend ways to reduce the noise in one's environment. Standards have since been promulgated for noise reduction in automobiles, trucks, buses, motorcycles, mopeds, refrigeration units, power lawnmowers, construction equipment, airplanes, and many other noise-producing devices and machines. The **EPA** has considered ordering that noise warnings be placed on power tools, radios, chain saws, and other household equipment. The **Occupational Safety and Health Administration** (OSHA) also has set standards for noise in the workplace that have considerably reduced noise-related hearing losses.

Common diseases and disorders

Whether self-inflicted or just part of everyday living noise can cause temporary or permanent deafness. When one is around noise for long periods of time, the risk of deafness is increased. For instance, train engineers, automobile mechanics, and construction workers are at increased risk for being hearing impaired, as are musicians in musical bands or listeners of their music. The most dangerous noise is that to which people voluntarily subject themselves while listening to music. In-ear headphones commonly used with portable media devices may reduce noise pollution for others but cause negative health problems in the wearer at volumes over 50 decibels.

Another problem caused by noise is decreased efficiency at work. Medical research has proven that the efficiency of a worker decreases as more noise is introduced. Most workers are disturbed by noise, which can

KEY TERMS

Logarithmic—Pertaining to the logarithm of a number, which is the exponent by which another fixed value, the base, has to be raised to produce that number; for example, the logarithm of 100 to base 10 is 2, because 100 is 10 to the power 2.

Mechanico-chemical—Relating to both mechanical and chemical processes.

Tinnitus—A condition characterized by ringing in the ears.

---

affect their concentration at performing their jobs. The first and foremost effect of noise is a decrease in the efficiency in working. Research has proved that human efficiency increases with noise reduction. Fatigue is another problem caused by noise. Because people are adversely affected by noise, they often take more time to complete their tasks, which leads to fatigue.

Stress levels are usually higher for people working around noise. Continued stress can lead to such medical conditions as anxiety, high blood pressure (hypertension), depression, and other such problems. If noise continues for long periods, it can eventually lead to mental illness and damage to the nervous system.

Treatment

Treatment for temporary or reversible hearing loss from noise pollution may be as simple as removing the source of the noise. However, permanent hearing loss may require hearing devices or hearing implants. Hearing aids help to make sounds louder by amplifying the sound waves that enter the ear. Although they do not restore hearing, they may help a person to function and communicate more easily. Hearing implants are devices that are worn outside or inside the ear. A cochlear implant is a type of implantable hearing device.

An audiologist can help to determine whether one's hearing has been compromised by noise pollution. Such a visit should be the first step to diagnosing and treating hearing loss. This medical professional will assist in determining the extent of hearing loss through a comprehensive hearing evaluation. If hearing loss is found, the audiologist may recommend various aids such as a change in lifestyle, hearing aids or other assistive listening devices, or surgery.

Public health role and response

Under the U.S. **Clean Air Act** of 1963 (with subsequent amendments in 1967, 1970, 1977, and 1990), the **Environmental Protection Agency** (EPA) established the Office of Noise Abatement and Control (ONAC) to pursue studies and investigations on noise and its effect on the public health and welfare. Through the ONAC, the EPA coordinated all federal noise control activities in 1981. In that year, the White House concluded that noise issues were best handled at the state and local level and primary responsibility for noise issues was transferred to state and local governments. However, as of 2012, the EPA retained authority to investigate and study noise and its effect, respond to inquiries on matters related to noise, disseminate information to the public regarding noise pollution and its adverse health effects, and evaluate the effectiveness of existing regulations for protecting the public health and welfare.

Prognosis

It is difficult to totally eliminate noise from busy society, but it can be reduced to more tolerable levels. Noises can be reduced by using white noise machines that play soothing sounds such as raindrops falling on a roof. Music at comfortable levels can also be played on a music device (such as an iPod) or a stereo in order to drown out irritating noises. White noise is also helpful when irritating noises in the night make it difficult to sleep. Meditation can also help to reduce stress levels caused by noise pollution.

Prevention

Noise can be prevented, or at least reduced, by the use of devices, laws, materials, and technology. Devices such as noise barriers can reduce roadway noise that occurs next to residential neighborhoods. Tees planted along busy roads, for instance, can block much of the noise that can otherwise impinge on people living nearby. Another solution for reducing road noise is limiting vehicle speeds on roads and highways, along with improving the texture of roadway surfaces, limiting the movement of heavy vehicles, improving tire design, and the use of traffic control systems that reduce the amount of braking and acceleration. Computer models are often designed to consider such factors when building new roads or making improvements on existing ones. These models take into account local topography, meteorological conditions, and population densities, to name a few.

For aircraft, engines are developed so they run more quiet than in the past. In addition, computer models are run to find the flight path than interferes the least with residential communities.

> **QUESTIONS TO ASK YOUR DOCTOR**
>
> - What can I do to prevent further hearing loss?
> - What can be done to treat my current hearing loss?
> - Where can I learn more about hearing loss?
> - What are my options to improve my hearing?

Resources

BOOKS

Hansen, Colin H. *Noise Control: From Concept to Application.* London; New York: Taylor & Francis, 2005.

Le Prell, Colleen G., et al, eds. *Noise-induced Hearing Loss, Scientific Advances.* New York: Springer, 2012.

National Academy of Engineering of the National Academies. *Technology for a Quieter America.* Washington, DC: National Academies Press, 2010.

Peters, R. J., B. J. Smith, and Margaret Hollins. *Acoustics and Noise Control.* Harlow, Essex, England: Pearson Education, 2011.

Wang, Lawrence K., Norman C. Pereira, and Yung-Tse Hung, eds. *Advanced Air and Noise Pollution Control.* Totowa, NJ: Humana Press, 2005.

WEBSITES

Centers for Disease Control and Prevention. "Noise and Hearing Loss Prevention." http://www.cdc.gov/niosh/topics/noise/ (accessed September 28, 2012).

Environmental Protection Agency. "Noise Pollution." http://www.epa.gov/air/noise.html (accessed September 18, 2012).

Healthy Living. "Shhh! Give Noise Pollution the Silent Treatment." http://shine.yahoo.com/healthy-living/shhh-give-noise-pollution-the-silent-treatment-2508243.html (accessed September 18, 2012).

WebMD Staff. "Hearing Loss." WebMD. http://www.webmd.com/a-to-z-guides/hearing-loss-treatment-overview (accessed September 18, 2012).

World Health Organization. "Noise Pollution." http://www.who.int/topics/noise/en (accessed September 18, 2012).

ORGANIZATIONS

Better Hearing Institute, 1444 I St. NW, Ste. 700, Washington, D.C. 20005, (202) 449-1100, Fax: (202) 216-9646, mail@betterhearing.org, http://www.betterhearing.org.

Environmental Protection Agency, 1200 Pennsylvania Ave. NW, Washington, DC 20460, (202) 272-0167, http://water.epa.gov.

National Hearing Conservation Association, 3030 W 81st Ave., Westminster, CO 80031, (303)224-9022, Fax: (303) 458-0002, nhcaoffice@hearingconservation.org, http://www.hearingconservation.org.

William P. Cunningham
William A. Atkins, BB, BS, MBA

Non-ionizing radiation

Definition

Non-ionizing **radiation** is radiation in that part of the electromagnetic spectrum that lacks sufficient energy to cause the ionization of an atom or molecule.

Description

The electromagnetic spectrum is the range of all possible electromagnetic radiation. Electromagnetic (EM) radiation is a form of energy consisting of oscillating electrical and magnetic waves that travel in conjunction with each other. EM radiation takes a variety of forms depending on the wave nature with which they travel. This is described by two variables, wavelength and frequency. The wavelength (λ) is the distance between adjacent peaks or troughs of the wave. The frequency (f) of a wave is the number of wavefronts that pass some given point in a designated period of time. Any unit of linear measure can be used to express the wavelength of a wave: for example, meter (m), centimeter (cm), nanometer (nm), or Ångström (Å). The choice of units depends to some extent on the type of wave being discussed. Radio waves, for example, typically have wavelengths ranging from a few millimeters to more than 100 kilometers, whereas gamma rays have wavelengths of less than 10 picometers (pm; a trillionth of a meter). The frequency of a wave is most commonly expressed in hertz (Hz), defined as one cycle per second. According to that definition, any given point on a wave with a frequency of 1 Hz passes some point in space once every second. As with wavelengths, the frequencies of waves varies significantly across the electromagnetic spectrum from a minimum of less than 10 Hz for extremely low frequency (ELF) radio waves to a maximum of more than 10^{24} (1 followed by 24 zeroes) for gamma radiation.

The energy of a wave is directly proportional to its frequency and inversely proportional to its wavelength. Thus, gamma radiation and X rays, both of which have very high frequencies, have high energies, whereas radio waves and microwaves, with relatively low frequencies, have relatively low energies. The particle that carries energy in an electromagnetic wave is the photon, whose symbol is the Greek letter gamma, γ. The energy of a photon is given by the $\lambda = hf$, where h is a constant known as Planck's constant. This expression illustrates the point that the greater the frequency of a wave, the greater its energy.

The atoms and molecules that make up matter are always in motion. That motion can take any one of three forms: translational, rotational, or vibrational. Translational motion involves the movement of a particle from one place to another, whereas rotational motion involves the spinning of a particle around a central axis. Vibrational motion is the back-and-forth motion of the components of a particle similar to the stretching and relaxation of a spring. The electrons present in atoms are also in motion; they spin around the nucleus, travel back and forth between atomic nuclei, or move to higher or lower energy levels in an atom. When radiation passes through matter, it has a tendency to increase the energy of particles that make up the matter. If incoming radiation carries a large amount of energy, as is the case with gamma radiation or x rays, it may be sufficient to expel one or more electrons from its normal atomic orbit, creating an ion. An ion is a particle that has gained or lost an electron. Radiation with sufficient energy to ionize atoms is called ionizing radiation. Other types of radiation may carry too little energy to actually expel electrons from an atom. They may, however, produce other effects in matter, such as increasing the translational, rotational, or vibrational energy of particles. Radiation with insufficient levels of energy to produce ionization is called non-ionizing radiation.

The boundary between ionizing and non-ionizing radiation in the electromagnetic spectrum is not clear. Generally speaking, radiation with frequencies higher than about 10^{15} Hz are regarded as ionizing, whereas radiation frequencies below that point are regarded as non-ionizing. The dividing point between the two types of radiation, then, is somewhere within the ultraviolet range of the electromagnetic spectrum.

Effects on public health

Ionizing radiation is universally recognized as a serious risk to human health since it destroys molecules of protein and DNA on which the body depends for its normal growth and function. The range of potential health problems resulting from exposure to ionizing radiation includes radiation burns and radiation sickness, blood disorders, reproductive problems, and cancers of most body organs. The effects of non-ionizing radiation on human health are somewhat less well known and the subject of ongoing research. These effects result not from the destruction of essential biochemical molecules, as is the case with ionizing radiation, but with temporary and less intensive effects of atoms and molecules. For example, exposure to an intense beam of low frequency radiation may, under somewhat unusual circumstances, increase the motion of molecules in the body to a point where body damage may occur.

The form of non-ionizing radiation of most frequent health concern is so-called near ultraviolet (UV) radiation. That term refers to UV radiation with energies too low to produce ionization in the body, but sufficiently high to produce other health results. In particular, near UV radiation has sufficient energy to produce burn-like effects on the skin and in the eyes. The sunburn that is typically associated with overexposure to sunlight is one such health effect, whereas inflammation of the eye is another. Sunburn is eventually responsible for the development of skin cancers which can be fatal, whereas inflammation of the eye may eventually evolve to become cataracts. The **World Health Organization** (WHO) estimates that exposure to near UV radiation may be responsible for between two and three million cases of basal cell and squamous cell carcinomas annually and 130,000 cases of malignant **melanoma**. Overall, WHO estimates that 66,000 people die each year worldwide from one or another form of **skin cancer**. It also suggests that up to 20 percent of the 12 to 15 million cases of cataracts around the world each year can be attributed to near UV **radiation exposure**.

Radiation with somewhat less energy than that of near UV radiation includes light and infrared (IR) radiation, sometimes grouped together as *optical radiation*. Health effects similar to those found with near UV radiation are also found for optical radiation, but to a significantly lesser degree. Such effects include skin reactions, mild skin burns, and damage to the cornea. These health effects are likely to be found only among individuals who are exposed to unusually high intensity levels of optical radiation for extended periods of time.

The last category of radiation, which includes microwave and radio radiation, is sometimes called *EM field radiation*. The health effects resulting from exposure to EM field radiation consists primarily of modest heating effects on the body, as well as possible effects from exposure to electrical and magnetic fields. These effects may include disruption of nervous and muscular responses and feelings of disorientation and nausea.

Probably the most contentious issue about the health effects of exposure to non-ionizing radiation in the early 2000s has to do with cell phone use. Cell phones use a technology that involves radiation in the EM field radiation range and given the intensity with which some people use cell phones, concern has arisen about the possible health effects of long-term exposure to EM radiation. A large number of studies have been conducted on this question with, thus far, no clear results. Some research has shown a moderate increase in the rate of cancer among cell phone users, whereas other studies have been unable to replicate these

> **KEY TERMS**
>
> **Electromagnetic field radiation**—Microwaves and radio waves.
>
> **Electromagnetic radiation**—A form of energy consisting of oscillating electrical and magnetic waves that travel in conjunction with each other.
>
> **Electromagnetic spectrum**—The range of all possible electromagnetic radiation.
>
> **Frequency**—The number of wavefronts that pass some given point in a designated period of time.
>
> **Optical radiation**—Light and infrared radiation.
>
> **Wavelength**—The distance between adjacent peaks or troughs of a wave.

findings. No other health effects related to cell phone use has been confirmed. Researchers have some hope that one large-scale study, the Cohort Study of Mobile Phone Use and Health (COSMOS), will answer a number of fundamental questions about the relationship of cell phone use and health effects. The study was initiated in March 2010 and is expected to continue for at least 20 years. For the present, a number of national and international organizations have said that the forms of EM field radiation used in cell phone technology should be considered a possible carcinogen, suggesting that evidence is not yet convincing for the role of cell phones in cancer production but that due caution should be relevant to the use of these devices.

Resources

BOOKS

Biddle, Wayne. *A Field Guide to Radiation*. New York: Penguin, 2012.

Leszczynski, Dariusz, ed. *Radiation Proteomics: The Effects of Ionizing and Non-ionizing Radiation on Cells and Tissues*. New York: Springer, 2013.

Podgorsak, Ervin B. *Radiation Physics for Medical Physics*, 2nd ed. New York: Springer, 2010.

PERIODICALS

Bellieni, C. V., et al. "Exposure to Electromagnetic Fields from Laptop Use of Laptop Computers." *Archives of Environmental & Occupational Health* 67, no. 1 (2012): 31–36.

Burch, J. B., et al. "Radio Frequency Nonionizing Radiation in a Community Exposed to Radio and Television Broadcasting." *Environmental Health Perspectives* 114, no. 2 (2006): 248–53.

Izmerov, N. F. "Current Problems of Nonionizing Radiation." *Scandanavian Journal of Work, Environment & Health* 11, no. 3 (2012): 223–27.

Manzetti, S., and O. Johansson. "Global Electromagnetic Toxicity and Frequency-induced Diseases: Theory and Short Overview." *Pathophysiology* 19, no. 3 (2012): 185–91.

WEBSITES

National Cancer Institute. "Cell Phones and Cancer Risk." http://www.cancer.gov/cancertopics/factsheet/Risk/cellphones (accessed October 19, 2012).

Radiation Answers. "Let's Talk about Radiation: Answering Your Questions." http://www.radiationanswers.org/ (accessed October 19, 2012).

World Health Organization. "Non-Ionizing Radiations: Sources, Biological Effects, Emissions, and Exposures." http://www.who.int/peh-emf/meetings/archive/en/keynote3ng.pdf (accessed October 19, 2012).

ORGANIZATIONS

Health Physics Society, 1313 Dolley Madison Blvd., Ste. 402, McLean, VA 22101, (703) 790-1745, Fax: (703) 790-2672, hps@BurkInc.com, http://hps.org.

David E. Newton, EdD

Noroviruses

Definition

Noroviruses are a group of related, single-stranded RNA (ribonucleic acid) viruses that cause infection resulting in acute gastroenteritis in humans. Gastroenteritis, also commonly called stomach flu, involves an inflammation of the gastrointestinal tract, which results in diarrhea, abdominal **pain**, and vomiting. The infection caused by noroviruses is very highly contagious, being commonly spread through **water** or food that has been contaminated with fecal matter; or through contact with an infected person. Norovirus infections occur frequently in closed, and often-times crowded, environments where the viruses can quickly spread. Such places include hospitals and medical facilities, schools, nursing/retirement homes and day-care facilities, and cruise ships.

Demographics

Anyone can become infected with a norovirus. During norovirus outbreaks there are high rates of infection among people of all ages. There are a large number of genetically distinct strains of noroviruses. Immunity appears to be specific for the norovirus strain and lasts for only a few months. Therefore, norovirus infection can recur throughout a person's lifetime. Because of genetic (inherited) differences among humans, some people appear to be more susceptible to norovirus infection and may suffer more severe illness. People with type O blood are at the highest risk for severe infection.

Percentages of outbreaks of Norovirus in 2010 by location

Location	Count	Percentage
Long-term care facility	889	59%
Restaurant	123	8%
Party & event	99	7%
Hospital	65	4%
School	64	4%
Cruise ship	55	4%
Other & unknown	223	14%

Source: Centers of Disease Control and Prevention

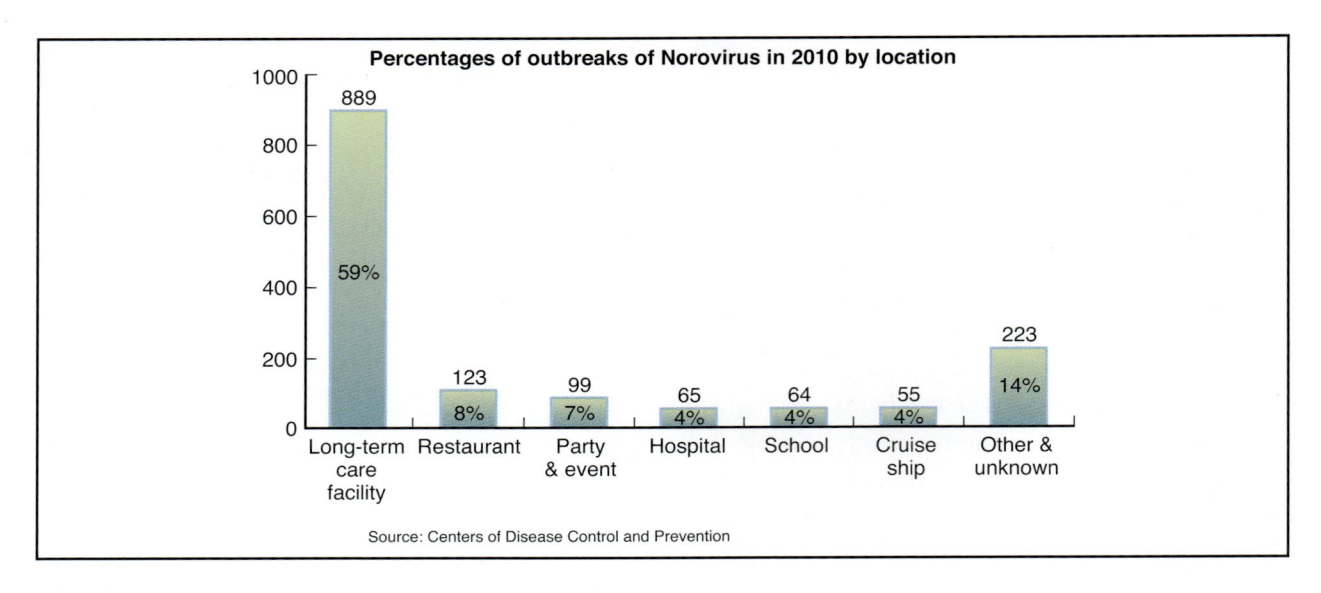

(Illustration by Electronic Illustrators Group. © 2013 Cengage Learning.)

Description

Norovirus infection is caused by a variety of viruses. All such viruses cause acute gastroenteritis, an inflammation of the stomach and intestines. The illness is highly contagious, and usually requires professional medical care to treat the most serious of the symptoms, which often times include dehydration, bloody stool, abdominal pain, and vomiting. Noroviruses are difficult to eliminate in the environment because they can withstand very high and low temperatures, along with being able to resist most disinfectants.

Noroviral infection

Noroviruses are a major cause of viral gastroenteritis—an inflammation of the linings of the stomach and small and large intestines that causes vomiting and diarrhea. Viruses are responsible for 30 to 40% of all cases of infectious diarrhea, and viral gastroenteritis is the second most common illness in the United States, exceeded only by the **common cold**.

Infected individuals are contagious from the first onset of symptoms until at least three days after full recovery. Some people may remain contagious for as long as two weeks after recovery.

Gastroenteritis

Gastroenteritis often is referred to as the stomach flu even though the flu is a respiratory illness caused by an **influenza** virus. Other common names for viral gastroenteritis include:

- food poisoning
- winter-vomiting disease
- non-bacterial gastroenteritis
- calicivirus infection

The U.S. **Centers for Disease Control and Prevention (CDC)** estimate, in 2012, that noroviruses are responsible for some 20 million cases of acute gastroenteritis in the United States every year. Epidemiologists estimate that about 50,000 Americans are hospitalized annually and about 400 people die each year because of norovirus infection. However, the **CDC** points out that many cases of acute gastroenteritis go unreported. Consequently, the U.S. health organization suggests that up to 300,000 hospitalizations occur annually and about 5,000 deaths occur each year, all due to noroviruses. In developing countries, noroviruses are a major cause of human illness. The CDC estimate that about 900,000 visits to clinics and other medical facilities by children in developed countries of the world result in about 64,000 hospitalizations. Even worse, about 200,000 children under the age of five years die from noroviruses each year in developing countries of the world.

Gastroenteritis caused by infection with a norovirus is rarely a serious illness. Typically an infected person suddenly feels very ill and may vomit many times in a single day. The symptoms, although quite unpleasant, usually last only 24 to 60 hours.

Transmission

Noroviruses are ubiquitous in the environment. They are highly contagious and are considered to be among the most infectious of viruses. The reasons for this include:

- Only a small number of viral particles—as few as 10—are required for infection.
- Although noroviruses cannot reproduce outside of their human hosts, they can remain viable for weeks or even months on objects and surfaces.
- Human immunity to norovirus is short-lived and strain-specific.

Noroviruses are transmitted among people by a fecal-oral route, either by ingestion of food or water contaminated with feces or by contact with the vomit or feces of an infected person. Norovirus infection can occur by:

- consuming contaminated food or liquids
- hand contact with contaminated objects or surfaces, followed by hand contact with the mouth
- contact with an infected person, including caring for the sick person or sharing food or utensils
- aerosolized vomit that is swallowed or that contaminates surfaces

Environmental contamination or contact with infected clothing or linen also may be a source of transmission. Although evidence is not available that norovirus infection can occur via the respiratory system, the sudden and violent vomiting of noroviral gastroenteritis can lead to contamination of the surroundings and of public areas. Particles laden with virus can be suspended in the air and swallowed.

FOODBORNE TRANSMISSION. Noroviruses account for at least 50% of food-related outbreaks of gastroenteritis. A European study, published in 2010, showed that 21% of all norovirus outbreaks are caused by foodborne transmission. In addition, 25% of the outbreaks were initially reported to be "food handler-associated." This was later found to be caused from contamination of the food source. In addition, restaurant or catered foods are common sources of norovirus transmission, with subsequent infection of household members. The majority of norovirus outbreaks occur via contamination by a food handler immediately before the food is consumed.

Foods that frequently are associated with norovirus outbreaks include:

- foods that are eaten without further cooking, including sandwiches, salads, and bakery products
- liquids such as salad dressing or cake icing in which the virus becomes evenly distributed
- food that is contaminated at its source, including oysters and clams from contaminated waters and raspberries irrigated with sewage-contaminated water
- food that becomes contaminated before distribution, including salads and frozen fruit.

- Shellfish, including oysters and clams, concentrate norovirus from contaminated water in their tissues. Steaming shellfish may not completely inactivate the virus.

WATERBORNE TRANSMISSION. There is widespread norovirus contamination of rivers and seas, often with more than one strain of the virus. Waterborne outbreaks of norovirus have been associated with:

- sewage-contaminated wells
- contaminated municipal water systems
- stream and lake water
- swimming pools and spas
- commercial ice

Outbreaks

Norovirus infection can spread rapidly through daycare centers, schools, prisons, hospitals, nursing homes, camps, and other confined spaces. Norovirus is responsible for about 40% of group- or institution-related outbreaks of diarrhea. Outbreaks usually peak during the winter months.

In 2008, it was reported that outbreaks of the norovirus occurred on several university campuses in California, Michigan, and Wisconsin. The CDC, along with state and local **health departments**, found that approximately 1,000 cases of illness resulted from these outbreaks, including 10 hospitalizations. In addition, one college campus was closed temporarily due to an outbreak. In February 2012, an outbreak of norovirus at a basketball tournament in Kentucky was responsible for 242 cases of acute gastroenteritis, although no source for the disease was ever identified.

Cruise ships have become notorious for norovirus outbreaks among passengers and staff. Cruise ships and naval vessels are at increased risk for contamination when docking in regions that lack adequate **sanitation** and where contaminated food or water may be brought onboard. Close living quarters and the arrival of new, susceptible passengers every one to two weeks exacerbate outbreaks on cruise ships. Norovirus outbreaks have been reported to continue through more than 12 successive cruises on a single ship.

Noroviruses are relatively rare on cruise ships but they do happen. In 2006, the CDC reported that 34 cases of norovirus were reported, while 27 were reported in 2007, 15 in 2008, and 13 in 2009—all from cruises originating from U.S. ports. In 2010, for instance, the Celebrity Cruises company had about 15% of its passengers come down with norovirus-like symptoms on its cruise ship that departed from Charleston, South

Carolina, on February 15, 2010. A year before the incident, a paper published in the medical journal *Clinical Infectious Diseases* found that a large number of norovirus outbreaks on cruise ships were the result of dirty public restroom facilities. However, in 2010, the CDC reported that the trend was down for contracting a norovirus on a cruise ship sailing from a U.S. port. In fact, the incidence of noroviruses on a cruise ship was at a decade-long low as of January 2010. The International Council of Cruise Lines reported that less than 1% of passengers become infected with norovirus each year. As reported by the CDC the outbreaks on cruise ships during the 2000s were on the decline. However, it is too early in the 2010s to tell if the trend will continue.

Generally, outbreaks of norovirus appear on the increase. Near the end of the 2000s, the CDC reported that norovirus outbreaks were increasing in many closed, crowded facilities across the country.

Risk factors

Humans are at increased risk from contracting noroviruses if they:

- travel frequently on cruise ships or stay at lodging establishments where many people are living in close surroundings
- live with children that attend school or day care
- have a weakened immune system
- live in nursing homes, retirement centers, or other such facilities

Causes and symptoms

Norovirus strains

Noroviruses lack outer envelopes and their genetic material is carried as single-stranded RNA rather than DNA (deoxyribonucleic acid). Although noroviruses are not new, the extent of norovirus infection was not recognized until the 1990s. This has led to increased research on noroviruses and more monitoring of outbreaks.

Until 2004 noroviruses were commonly referred to as:

- Norwalk virus
- Norwalk-like viruses (NLVs)
- caliciviruses
- small, round-structured viruses (SRSVs)

Noroviruses are named after the original strain—the Norwalk virus—that caused an outbreak of gastroenteritis in a Norwalk, Ohio, school in 1968. The virus was identified in 1972. Since then many related viruses have been identified. In 2004, these viruses were grouped together in the genus *Norovirus* within the Caliciviridae family of viruses. Eight to 10 distinct genogroups of norovirus have been found in various parts of the world. There are five common genogroups and, of those, three (GI, GII, and GIV) affect humans. Each of these groups can be further differentiated into at least 20 genetic clusters. Evidence suggests that noroviruses in different genetic clusters can recombine to form new, genetically distinct noroviruses. As of 2012, GII strains, especially GII4, are the most prevalent, and have caused the most norovirus outbreaks since 2002. However the most common method of identifying noroviruses—the reverse transcription-polymerase chain reaction (RT-PCR)—may not always identify GII genetic clusters correctly.

The increased number of norovirus outbreaks in European countries in the early 2000s—occurring in the spring and summer rather than in winter—were found to be associated with the emergence of a new variant of the GII4 strain. Increased international outbreaks in 2003 and 2004 also were caused by a GII4-related norovirus that was found to mutate rapidly. Mutations in the viral capsid—the virus' outer protective layer—were used to determine the predominant routes of norovirus transmission.

Then, in the first quarter of 2010, 334 cases of norovirus were reported at 65 different locations within the United Kingdom, Norway, France, Sweden, and Denmark. All of the cases were associated with the eating of raw oysters. The International Society of Infectious Diseases reports that the Rapid Alert System for Food and Feed (RASFF) database contained 19 reports of norovirus in oysters between March 2006 and March 2010—all within the European Union.

Symptoms

Symptoms of norovirus infection usually appear within 24–48 hours after exposure, with a median incubation period during outbreaks of 33–36 hours. However symptoms can occur as early as 12 hours or less after exposure.

Typical symptoms of norovirus infection are:

- nausea
- vomiting
- fever
- malaise (general feeling of sickness)
- watery or loose diarrhea without blood
- abdominal cramping and pain
- bloody stool

- dehydration
- weight loss

Among children, vomiting is the predominant symptom, whereas diarrhea is more common in adults. Vomiting can be frequent and violent and may occur without warning.

Additional symptoms of norovirus infection may include:

- low-grade fever
- chills
- headache
- muscle aches
- fatigue

Dehydration is the major risk from gastroenteritis caused by norovirus, particularly among infants, young children, the elderly, and those with underlying health conditions. Symptoms of dehydration include:

- dry mouth
- increased or excessive thirst
- low urine output
- nausea
- dizziness or faintness
- sunken eyes
- sunken fontanelle—the soft spot on an infant's head
- confusion

As many as 30–50% of norovirus infections do not produce symptoms. It is not known whether individuals with asymptomatic infections can transmit the virus.

Diagnosis

Identifying noroviruses

Viral gastroenteritis usually is diagnosed on the basis of the symptoms. Many types of viruses cause gastroenteritis. Rotoviruses are a leading cause of gastroenteritis in children who then transmit the virus to adults. In addition to noroviruses, viral gastroenteritis in humans can be caused by another genus of viruses within the Caliciviridae family. Formerly known as the Sapporo-like virus, or classic or typical calicivirus, these now are grouped in the genus *Sapovirus*. Other genera in the Caliciviridae family are not pathogenic in humans. Some bacteria and **parasites** also cause illnesses that are similar to norovirus infection.

The cloning and sequencing of noroviruses in the early 1990s made it easier to identify norovirus outbreaks. RT-PCR is the most commonly used method for identifying norovirus. With this technique the virus' RNA is used as the template for transcribing the corresponding DNA using the enzyme reverse transcriptase. The DNA is amplified into many copies using the polymerase chain reaction. Many state public health laboratories use this method to detect norovirus in vomit and stools. The best identification usually comes from stool samples taken within 48–72 hours after the onset of symptoms; however norovirus can be detected in stool samples taken five days after the onset of symptoms and sometimes even in samples taken up to two weeks after recovery.

Norovirus from fecal samples can be visualized using electron microscopy. With immune electron microscopy (IEM), antibodies against norovirus are collected from blood serum and used to trap and visualize the virus from fecal samples. However these methods require high concentrations of norovirus in the stool, as well as a fourfold increase in norovirus-specific antibodies in blood samples taken during the acute or recovery phases of gastroenteritis.

Enzyme-linked immunosorbent assays may be used to detect noroviruses in fecal samples. In these assays noroviral-specific antibodies bound to the virus are detected by the reaction of an enzyme that is attached to the antibody. Nucleic acid probes that hybridize with noroviral RNA also can be used for virus detection in feces.

Research continues on commercial devices for detecting noroviruses. For example, scientists at the Department of Infectious Diseases, Osaka Prefectural Institute of Public Health (Osaka, Japan) are developing modified reagent kits for norovirus genogroups I and II. They reported their advancement in the *Journal of Medical Virology* (December 2009).

Investigating outbreaks

Epidemiological studies often involve sequencing the norovirus RNA. This can help to determine whether outbreaks in different geographical locations are connected to each other and can help trace the source of the norovirus to contaminated food or water. CaliciNet is a database that stores the RNA sequences of all norovirus strains that cause gastroenteritis in the United States.

Criteria that are sometimes used to determine whether an outbreak of gastroenteritis is caused by a norovirus include:

- a mean incubation period of 24–48 hours
- a mean duration time for illness of 12–60 hours
- vomiting in more than 50% of patients
- failure to find a bacterial cause for the illness

During investigations of norovirus outbreaks, food handlers may be asked to provide a stool sample and possibly a blood sample. Food rarely is tested for norovirus since each type of food requires a specific assay. However, tests are used to detect the virus in shellfish. When large amounts—1–25 gallons (5–100 liters)—of water are processed through specially designed filters, the norovirus can be concentrated and assayed by RT-PCR.

Treatment

Gastroenteritis caused by noroviruses usually resolves itself without treatment within a very few days. As of 2012, medications or vaccines are not available that are effective against the norovirus. Viruses are not affected by **antibiotics** and antidiarrheal medications may prolong the infection.

Norovirus infections should be treated by:

- drinking plenty of fluids, such as water and juice, to prevent dehydration caused by vomiting and diarrhea
- intravenous fluids if severe nausea prevents drinking, particularly in small children
- drinking oral rehydration fluids (ORFs) to prevent dehydration and to replace electrolytes (salt and minerals) and glucose
- avoiding alcohol and caffeine which can increase urination

Commercially available ORFs include Naturalyte, Pedialyte, Infalyte, and Rehydralyte.

Juice, soda, and water do not replace lost electrolytes; nor do sports drinks replace nutrients and minerals lost through vomiting and diarrhea. In fact, drinks containing sugar may make diarrhea worse. Those taking diuretics should ask their healthcare provider whether to stop taking the medication during acute diarrhea.

Since the risk of dehydration is higher for infants and young children, the number of wet diapers per day should be closely monitored. Severely dehydrated children may receive rapid intravenous rehydration in a hospital or emergency-room setting.

A health care provider should be consulted if:

- symptoms of dehydration appear
- diarrhea persists for longer than a few days
- there is blood in the stool

Alternative treatment

An infusion of meadowsweet (*Filipendula ulmaria*) may reduce nausea. Once the symptoms are reduced, slippery elm (*Ulmus fulva*) may calm the digestive system. Castor oil packs placed on the abdomen can reduce inflammation and discomfort.

Homeopathic remedies for gastroenteritis include *Arsenicum album*, ipecac, and *Nux vomica*. Chinese patent herbal remedies include Po Chai and Pill Curing.

During recovery from viral gastroenteritis, live cultures of *Lactobacillus acidophilus*, found in live-culture yogurt or as powder or capsules, may be useful for restoring the native flora of the digestive tract. Scientific evidence for the safety and efficacy of most herbal, Chinese, alternative and other complementary medicines is often lacking, so they should be used only with caution.

Public health role and response

Public health responses to norovirus outbreaks pose distinctly difficult problems for public health agencies. Since the virus can not be cultured in the laboratory, a great deal of basic information is not readily available about the virus or the diseases it causes. Thus far, most guidelines for public health responses to outbreaks of gastroenteritis caused by noroviruses have been developed based on experiences in hospitals, cruise ships, and adult care facilities. The first step in the public health response to a suspected norovirus outbreak consists of data collection on reported cases that includes information such as the number of individuals affected, the time at which the outbreak occurred, the environmental conditions involved, especially the type of food that may have been involved, and the results of any laboratory tests that may have been conducted.

These items of information allow a public health agency to develop a plan of action that focuses on identifying and eliminating the suspected cause of the epidemic (such as the type of food involved) and initiate clean-up programs to eliminate that causative agent. Efforts to provide palliative care for those affected by the epidemic are also initiated. On a long term basis, information obtained about any specific outbreak of norovirus infection can be used to bolster and improve existing programs of education for the general public as well as for professionals in the field or, if such programs do not exist, to plan, develop, and implement such programs.

Prognosis

Norovirus infection is usually followed by complete recovery. Any long-term health effects are not known. Infected persons do not become long-term carriers of the virus. However, in some cases dehydration can become a very serious possible consequence of noroviral infection and can be fatal, particularly among young children, older people, and anyone with debilitating medical conditions or impaired immune systems.

Prevention

Noroviruses are difficult to destroy. They can survive freezing as well as temperatures as high as 140°F (60°C). Noroviruses can survive chlorine levels as high as 10 parts per million (ppm), far higher than the levels present in most public water systems. A 2004 study from the Netherlands found that inactivation of norovirus with 70% ethanol was inefficient and that **sodium** hypochlorite solutions were effective only at concentrations above 300 ppm.

The best **prevention** against noroviral infection is frequent, thorough hand washing with soap and water. All soaped hand surfaces should be rubbed vigorously for at least 10 seconds. The hands should be thoroughly rinsed under a stream of water. In particular hands always should be washed before handling food and after using the toilet or changing diapers.

Other important measures for preventing norovirus infection include:
- proper handling of cold foods
- careful washing of fruits and vegetables
- steaming oysters before eating, although even this may be insufficient for destroying norovirus
- taking particular care when handing the diapers of children with diarrhea
- properly disposing of sewage and diapers
- excluding sick infants and children from food preparation areas

To prevent further transmission of norovirus:
- All surfaces exposed to vomit or otherwise contaminated should be immediately cleaned and disinfected with a solution of between 5 to 10% bleach, followed by rinsing.
- Contaminated clothing and linens should be removed immediately and washed with hot water and detergent on the maximum machine cycle and with a minimum of handling, followed by machine drying.
- Vomit and feces should be discarded or flushed immediately and the toilet area should be kept clean.
- Exposed or contaminated food should be discarded.
- Masks may be worn while cleaning areas that have been badly contaminated with vomit or feces, such as in hospitals or nursing homes.
- Stay home and do not go to work or school in order to prevent further passing on of the virus.

KEY TERMS

Antibody—A blood protein produced in response to foreign material such as a virus; the antibody attaches to the virus and destroys it.

Calicivirus—A member of the Caliciviridae family of viruses that includes noroviruses.

Capsid—The outer protein coat of a virus.

Gastroenteritis—An inflammation of the lining of the stomach and intestines, usually caused by a viral or bacterial infection.

Genetic cluster—A group of viral strains with very similar, yet distinct, nucleic acid sequences.

Genogroup—Related viruses within a genus; may be further subdivided into genetic clusters.

Reverse transcription-polymerase chain reaction (RT-PCR)—A method of polymerase-chain-reaction amplification of nucleic acid sequences that uses RNA as the template for transcribing the corresponding DNA using reverse transcriptase.

Scientific studies have found that detergent-based cleaning with a cloth consistently fails to eliminate norovirus contamination. With fecal contamination, detergent-based cleaning, followed by cleaning with a combination hypochlorite/detergent formula containing 5,000 ppm of available chlorine significantly reduced contamination. However, norovirus still could be detected on as much as 28% of the surfaces. When this procedure failed to eliminate contamination, the virus was transmitted to the cleaner's hands. Contaminated fingers consistently transferred norovirus to up to seven different surfaces including doorknobs and telephones. However the contamination was diluted during secondary transmission and treatment with the combined bleach/detergent eliminated the virus without prior cleaning.

In situations where there is a periodic renewal of susceptible people, such as on cruise ships and at camps, the facility may have to be closed until cleaning is complete. Although many state and local health departments require that food handlers with gastroenteritis not return to work until two to three days following recovery, this may not be an adequate length of time to prevent noroviral transmission.

The prevention of norovirus outbreaks include reducing contamination of water supplies with human waste and using high-level chlorination—at least 10 ppm for more than 30 minutes. Surveillance

> **QUESTIONS TO ASK YOUR DOCTOR**
>
> - If we are planning to take a cruise, are there steps we can follow to reduce our risk of being infected with a norovirus?
> - What can we do to reduce the risk of our children's being infected by a norovirus in the school environment?
> - What types of palliative care can we provide to elderly parents in a nursing home who have contracted a noroviral infection?

of shorelines for potential sources of fecal contamination and for boats that are dumping human waste may help prevent shellfish-associated norovirus outbreaks.

In 2004, researchers at Washington University (St. Louis, Missouri) became the first to grow a norovirus in a laboratory setting. They grew a mouse norovirus, with the goal of studying the virus and developing a vaccine against it. Research is ongoing in the early 2010s. New surveillance systems also are being developed to detect norovirus outbreaks at an early stage.

Resources

BOOKS

Hall, Aron J. *Updated Norovirus Outbreak Management and Disease Prevention Guidelines*. Atlanta, GA: Centers for Disease Control and Prevention, 2011.

Vildevall, Malin. *The Norovirus Puzzle: Characterization of Human and Bovine Norovirus Susceptibility Patterns*. Linköping: Linköping University, Faculty of Health Sciences, 2011.

PERIODICALS

Verhoef, L., et al. "Use of Norovirus Genotype Profiles to Differentiate Origins of Foodborne Outbreaks." *Emerging Infectious Diseases* 16 4 (2010): 610–24.

WEBSITES

Manning, Anita. *Nasty, Contagious Norovirus Is 'Everywhere' Now*. USA Today. http://www.usatoday.com/news/health/story/health/story/2012-02-22/Nasty-contagious-norovirus-is-everywhere-now/53211908/1 (accessed August 23, 2012).

Norovirus. Centers for Disease Control and Prevention. http://www.cdc.gov/norovirus/ (accessed August 23, 2012).

Norovirus Infection. Mayo Clinic. http://www.mayoclinic.com/health/norovirus/DS00942 (accessed August 23, 2012).

Purdy, Michael C. *Scientists Grow Norovirus in Lab*. http://news.wustl.edu/news/Pages/4418.aspx (accessed August 23, 2012).

Norovirus: Symptoms and Treatment. WebMD. http://children.webmd.com/norovirus-symptoms-and-treatment (accessed August 23, 2012).

ORGANIZATIONS

Centers for Disease Control and Prevention, 1600 Clifton Rd., NE, Atlanta, GA 30333, (800) 232-4636, cdcinfo@cdc.gov, http://www.cdc.gov.

National Health Information Center. Office of Disease Prevention and Health Promotion. U.S. Department of Health and Human Services, P. O. Box 1133, Washington, DC 20013-1133, (847) 434-4000, http://www.health.gov/nhic/.

Margaret Alic, PhD

"What is OSHA?" *All About OSHA* http://www.allaboutosha.com (accessed October 2, 2012).

ORGANIZATIONS

U.S. Department of Labor, Occupational Safety & Health Administration–Room N3641, 200 Constitution Ave., Washington, DC 20210, (800) 321-OSHA (6742), http://www.osha.gov.

Oil spills, health effects of

Definition

Along with fouling marine and coastal ecosystems, offshore oil spills pose potential health hazards for humans, both as workers respond to spills and as oil impacts the environments where people live. After the 1989 **Exxon Valdez** oil spill that occurred in Prince William Sound off the coast of Alaska, one study published in the *American Journal of Psychiatry* showed that residents living in areas affected by the spill were more likely to suffer mental health problems than the general population, even years after the spill. (Few studies were conducted, however, on the health impacts of workers who were exposed to the oil during clean-up efforts.) In the wake of the 2010 BP (formerly British Petroleum) *Deepwater Horizon* oil spill in the Gulf of Mexico, information remains inconclusive on the actual human health hazards that could derive from the spill.

At a gathering of public health experts in late June 2010, U.S. surgeon general Regina Benjamin (1956–) noted some scientists' predictions that little or no toxic effects would result from short-term exposure to the oil, while indicating that "other scientists express serious concerns about the potential short-term and long-term impacts the exposure to oil and dispersants could have on the health of responders and [the local] communities." However, near the end of April 2011, the U.S. National Institutes of Health (NIH) began what was called a "massive, long-range health study" of the workers and volunteers who helped clean up the **Gulf oil spill**. Without clear medical indications concerning the long-term health consequences of about 55,000 workers and volunteers in Alabama, Florida, Louisiana, and Mississippi, the study intended to examine many of these people for ten years, looking for possible mental and physical health problems from their direct participation in the cleanup of Gulf of Mexico oil spill.

Demographics

Virtually everyone who lives near a coastline could be affected by an oil spill, as more than 38,000 oil tankers traverse the world's oceans and seas, delivering oil in its various stages from ports near the extraction site to ports where it is refined and later consumed. Offshore drilling fields are located primarily in the North Sea, the Gulf of Mexico, the South China Sea, and off the coasts of Nigeria, Angola, Brazil, the Canadian provinces of Nova Scotia and Newfoundland, and eastern Russia. Large land-based oil fields are located in the Middle East, the United States, Russia, Mexico, and Venezuela. Persons especially at risk to the potentially harmful effects of oil exposure include those with existing respiratory problems, pregnant women, and children. Potential adverse health problems for such people include respiratory ailments, such as those associated with the lower respiratory tract, and nausea. Developing fetuses and small children may also develop neurological problems and hereditary mutations.

Description

Although its composition varies somewhat depending on its source, crude oil is a naturally occurring brown or black liquid that is composed of a mixture of hydrocarbons and other organic compounds. Crude oil is toxic, flammable, and contains volatile organic compounds (VOCs) that have known adverse effects on human health, such as **benzene** (a carcinogen) and polycyclic aromatic hydrocarbons (PACs), which are toxic to the central nervous system. VOCs evaporate easily, moving from the oil into the air, and can be carried by prevailing winds miles from the source of a spill and into coastal communities. There is evidence that some dispersants, solvents, and collecting agents used to manage the spill can enhance some of the toxic effects of crude oil alone. Harmful airborne pollution released by burning the oil on the surface of a spill is also a health concern for both responders and local on-shore populations.

Causes and symptoms

People are exposed to oil-spill toxins through direct contact with oil on the skin; by breathing VOCs and other chemicals released into the air; or through oil-contaminated sand, soil, water, or food. Multiple exposure paths can occur simultaneously. All adverse reactions to oil are dependent upon both the duration of the exposure and a person's susceptibility to the particular toxins in the oil.

Hundreds of workers cleaning Alaskan shores, marshes, and oiled waterways after the *Exxon Valdez* spill complained of skin rashes, dizziness, headaches, and nausea during their work and for a short time afterward. Some experienced longer-lasting symptoms, including shortness of breath, muscle aches, and neurological problems, such as numbness and tingling of the extremities.

Public health officials along the Gulf Coast are monitoring for these symptoms in communities affected by the Deepwater Horizon spill, as well as establishing data-collection methods to document possible longer-term consequences of oil exposure, such as kidney damage, birth defects, and cancer. As of 2012, complaints among coastal residents, along with workers cleaning the oil both on land and at sea, included skin rashes, headaches, nausea, and irritation in the throat and eyes. Several workers also experienced heat stress due to working in hot and humid weather.

Although high levels of mental and emotional stress are expected during a natural or technological disaster, the Deepwater Horizon oil spill impacted an area whose vulnerable population was still recovering from hurricanes Ivan, Katrina, and Rita. Benjamin Springgate, a physician and public health researcher at Tulane University in New Orleans, Louisiana, estimated that over 30% of people in the impact zone of **Hurricane Katrina** experienced symptoms of anxiety, depression, or other mental illness after the storm, and also predicted that the impacts of the Deepwater Horizon oil spill on the mental health of coastal residents will be long term. The most frequent symptoms of stress-related mental disorders include feelings of hopelessness, disturbances in sleep patterns, lack of concentration, mood swings, irritability, inability to make productive decisions, nightmares or persistent memories of disturbing or frightening events, and general anxiety.

Common diseases and disorders

The most frequent mental disorders diagnosed among people affected by an oil spill include post-traumatic stress syndrome, anxiety disorders, and depression. A psychiatrist or other mental health professional diagnoses these disorders, mostly after a careful discussion of the symptoms. Other oil-spill-related illnesses are diagnosed according to the nature of symptoms, physical examination, and additional diagnostic or laboratory tests. For example, respiratory irritation from exposure to VOCs or other chemicals, followed by inflammation and decreased lung function, causes chemical pneumonia. It is most often diagnosed by history and physical examination, especially auscultation of (listening to) the lungs, examination of the sputum, and x rays, as are other types of pneumonia.

KEY TERMS

Carcinogen—An agent that is known to cause cancer.

Dispersant—A chemical that breaks up spilled oil into small particles that can be further scattered and broken down by water and wind, thus theoretically sparing oil damage to marine and coastal environments.

Deoxyribonucleic acid (DNA)—The twisted double-strand double-helix substance that provides genetic information inside an organism.

Mousse oil—Crude oil that has emulsified or weathered, mixed with dispersants, water, and marine material to form a spongy, light brown, mousse-like material.

Post-traumatic stress syndrome (PTSS)—A type of severe anxiety disorder that can develop after individuals experience traumatic events or situations.

Teratogen—An agent that is known to disturb the development of an embryo or fetus.

Volatile organic compounds (VOCs)—A large class of carbon-based chemicals that release gases into the air as they evaporate at room temperature. Found both in natural sources such as living trees, decomposing vegetation, and crude oil, and in human-made sources such as solvents, adhesives, and gasoline, VOCs help form ozone at ground levels and are major air contaminants.

Treatment

Mousse oil or tarballs on the skin can be cleaned with soap and water or mineral oil. Treatment of more serious illnesses of various body systems and organs exposed to oil depends on the system affected, the nature and length of the exposure, and the symptoms present. The **U.S. Department of Health and Human Services** created a $10 million fund to track Deepwater Horizon-related illnesses in order to develop a clear picture of their nature and to devise the most effective treatments. In addition, more than 14,000 oil spill workers volunteered to participate in a similar study for the U.S. **Centers for Disease Control and Prevention** (CDC). After that, the Gulf Long-term Follow-up (GuLF) Study was implemented to study the medical consequences of the Gulf of Mexico oil spill. Funded by the U.S. National Institutes of Health (NIH), along with a $10 million gift from BP, the Gulf Study will examine whether exposure to crude oil and

KEN SARO-WIWA (1941–1995)

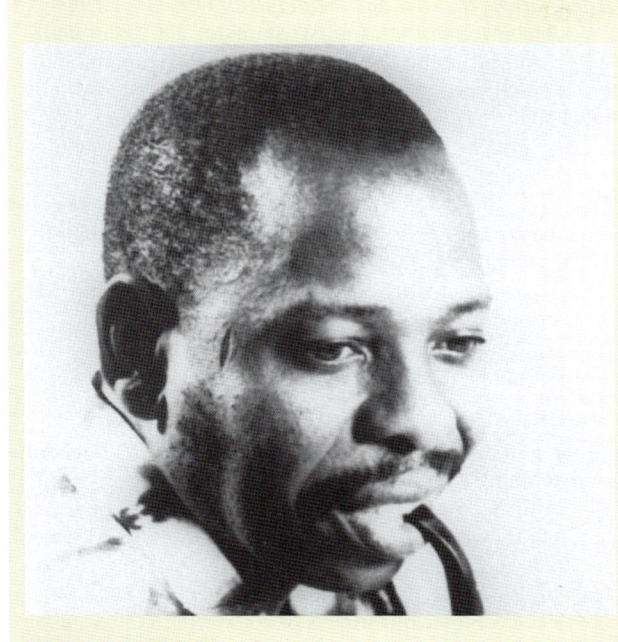

Oil was discovered in the Niger Delta in 1958, and garnered over $100 billion over the next 35 years. The Ogoni citizens saw none of this money, yet the oil extraction forced them to endure terrible air and water quality.

In 1991, Nigerian businessman Ken Saro-Wiwa dedicated himself to peacefully protesting the Ogoni people's situation. Saro-Wiwa joined the Movement for the Survival of the Ogoni People (MOSOP), and painstakingly worked as an advocate for Ogoni human and environmental rights. He travelled extensively and internationally to raise awareness and gain support, speaking out against the Royal Dutch Shell company and the oil extraction industry, as well as expressing his frustration in the lack of environmental regulations. Throughout his protests, he was detained and arrested many times. But some considered Saro-Wiwa an environmental hero. He was awarded the Right Livelihood Award and the Goldman Environmental Foundation of Califonia prize.

Saro-Wiwa and eight additional Ogoni elders were convicted of murdering four Ogoni governmental leaders in May 1994. They were not given a chance to obtain legal counsel or file an appeal. The nine of them were hanged on November 10, 1995.

(© Reuters/Corbis.)

---

dispersant chemicals had an adverse affect on the physical and mental health of workers and volunteers directly exposed to such substances involved in the oil spill.

Prognosis

The full effects of the Deepwater Horizon oil spill on the health and well-being of people living in communities along the northern Gulf of Mexico was not anticipated to be fully known until the oil was cleaned and the physical, ecological, and economic environments were restored, a process that was expected to take years. Scientists anticipated that the information gained from careful study of the detrimental effects of the oil spill on the physical and mental health of spill responders and Gulf coast residents would help identify both short- and long-term health issues related to the spill and allow for an effective response now and during future technological disasters.

Prevention

Avoiding contact with the oil is the most effective way to prevent negative health effects from an oil spill. Beaches along the northern Gulf Coast had no-swimming signs and flags posted in locations where oil from the Deepwater Horizon spill had affected the shore. Workers both offshore and at the spill site used a variety of personal protective equipment, including gloves, white plastic protective (hazmat) suits, respirators, and other barrier methods designed to prevent exposure to oil. (Hazmat is short for hazardous materials.)

Over the months that followed the Gulf Coast oil spill, authorities closed more than 30% of Gulf Coast federal fishing waters to both commercial and personal fishing in order to prevent oil-contaminated fish and shellfish from entering the food supply. Increased inspection of allowable catches helped ensure that Gulf fish making its way to the market were uncontaminated and of the usual high quality. As of March 20, 2011, most of the closed federal fishing waters had been reopened. Only those federal fishing waters surrounding the BP Deepwater Horizon oil spill remained closed, about 1,041 square miles (2,697 sq km), or approximately 0.4% of the Gulf of Mexico federal waters.

When winds bring onshore fumes from the spill, residents with existing respiratory problems are advised to remain indoors with recirculating air. Pregnant women should avoid oil-contaminated

> **QUESTIONS TO ASK YOUR DOCTOR**
>
> - I am pregnant and a coastal resident living near an oil spill. Should I leave the area?
> - Will my children be affected by the oil if they do not touch it?
> - Does smelling oil mean the air quality is unhealthy?
> - Where can I learn if the air is unsafe to breathe and the locally grown food unsafe to eat?
> - What specific symptoms should I be concerned about if I am in direct contact with an oil spill?
> - What are the health problems associated with pets and other domesticated and wild animals?

beaches and air, as components of crude oil are known teratogens and exposure to crude oil can result in decreased fetal survival. Children are also particularly vulnerable to DNA (deoxyribonucleic acid) damage from long-term exposure to airborne toxins emanating from oil spills. The U.S. **Environmental Protection Agency** set up more than 100 monitoring stations along affected areas of the Gulf Coast to detect unhealthy levels of VOCs, overall **ozone**, and particulate matter in the air and to issue regular air quality reports.

Innovative approaches were taken along the Gulf Coast to reach people who might be experiencing symptoms of stress but were unlikely to seek help. Peer listeners were trained to identify signs of distress during conversation, to offer encouragement that help is available, and to provide referrals to nearby mental health services. Personnel with knowledge of and sensitivities to local cultures, including those who speak Vietnamese and Spanish, were also made available to hear the needs and concerns of fishermen and other close-knit communities.

Resources

BOOKS

California Environmental Protection Agency. *San Francisco Bay Oil Spill Health Questions and Answers.* Sacramento: Office of Environmental Health Hazard Assessment, California Environmental Protection Agency, 2007.

Caputo, Christine A. *Oil Spills.* Mankato, MN: Capstone Press, 2011.

Freudenburg, William R., and Robert Gramling. *Blowout in the Gulf: The BP Oil Spill Disaster and the Future of Energy in America.* Cambridge: MIT Press, 2011.

The Gulf Oil Disaster and the Future of Offshore Drilling: Report to the President. Washington, DC: National Commission on the BP Deepwater Horizon Oil Spill and Offshore Drilling, 2011.

Ott, Riki. *Not One Drop: Betrayal and Courage in the Wake of the Exxon Valdez Oil Spill.* White River Junction, VT: Chelsea Green, 2008.

Ott, Riki. *Sound Truth and Corporate Myth$: The Legacy of the Exxon Valdez Oil Spill.* Cordova, AK: Dragonfly Sisters Press, 2005.

The Use of Surface and Subsea Dispersants During the BP Deepwater Horizon Oil Spill. Washington, DC: National Commission on the BP Deepwater Horizon Oil Spill and Offshore Drilling, 2010.

PERIODICALS

Arata, C. M., J. S. Picou, G. D. Johnson, and T.S. McNally. "Coping with Technological Disaster: An Application of the Conservation of Resources Model to the Exxon Valdez Oil Spill." *Journal of Traumatic Stress* 13, no. 1 (2000): 23–39.

Ha, M., W. J. Lee, S. Lee, and H. K. Cheong. "A Literature Review on Health Effects of Exposure to Oil Spill." *Journal of Preventive Medicine and Public Health* 41, no. 5 (2008): 345–54.

Palinkas, L. A., J. S. Petterson, J. Russell, and M. A. Downs. "Community Patterns of Psychiatric Disorders after the Exxon Valdez Oil Spill." *American Journal of Psychiatry* 150, no. 10 (1993): 1517–23.

WEBSITES

"Deepwater Horizon/BP Oil Spill: Federal Fisheries Closure and Other Information." NOAA Fisheries Service, National Oceanic and Atmospheric Administration. http://sero.nmfs.noaa.gov/deepwater_horizon_oil_spill.htm (accessed March 21, 2011).

"Deepwater Horizon Response: Gulf of Mexico Oil Cleanup." Centers for Disease Control and Prevention, National Institute for Occupational Safety and Health. http://www.cdc.gov/niosh/topics/oilspillresponse/ (accessed March 21, 2011).

"Interim Guidance for Protecting Deepwater Horizon Response Workers and Volunteers." Centers for Disease Control and Prevention, National Institute for Occupational Safety and Health. http://www.cdc.gov/niosh/topics/oilspillresponse/protecting/default.html (accessed March 21, 2011).

"Poison Centers and the Gulf Oil Spill." American Association of Poison Control Centers. http://www.aapcc.org/dnn/NewsandEvents/PoisonCentersandtheGulfOilSpill.aspx (accessed March 21, 2011).

"U.S. to Study Health Impact of BP Oil Spill." Reuters. http://af.reuters.com/article/energyOilNews/idAFN019813120110301 (accessed March 21, 2011).

Brenda Wilmoth Lerner, RN

Omnibus Flood Control Act (1936)

Definition

The Flood Control Act of 1936 was signed into law on June 22, 1936 by President Franklin Delano Roosevelt. The act authorized the United States Army Corps of Engineers to construct civil engineering projects such as dams, **levees**, flood gates, and other flood control measures throughout the United States.

Purpose

This was one of the first pieces of American legislation that established the responsibility of the federal government to protect people and property as long as the economic benefit did not outweigh the cost. Additionally, the legislation caused the federal government to have the War Department (precursor to the Department of Justice) run investigations and provide recommended improvements for rivers and waterways to increase flood control infrastructure. The Act places sill erosion, watershed, and water flow retardation under the purview of the Chief of Engineers.

Description

Origins

Prior to 1936, three prior Flood Control Acts had been passed (1917, 1920, and 1928) in response to several devastating floods in the 1800's and early 1900's. Following the Great Depression, several pieces of legislation were enacted to help put Americans back to work as part of The New Deal. Several versions of this bill have since been enacted.

Follow-on legislation in 1937, the Water Resources Development Act, and the Rivers and Harbors Act built on this initial legislation. The act was amended in 1977 to "appraise the status and trends of soil, water, and related resources on non-Federal land and assesses their capability to meet present and future demands, evaluate current and needed programs, policies, and authorities; and develop a national soil and water conservation program to give direction to USDA soil and water conservation activities."

Outcome

Between 1936 and 1937, $360 million was spent on these projects with the proviso that local communities would be responsible for maintaining the completed projects over time. Congress has since 1936 authorized the Corps of Engineers to construct hundreds of miles of artificial levees and flood control constructs including 375 large reservoirs and **dams**. The projects resulting from this act have fundamentally changed the physical plant status of the United States. These measures have saved the U.S. an incalculable amount of money by preventing property damage, and protecting millions of citizens from worry, injury and death.

Resources

BOOKS

Arnold, Joseph L. "The Evolution of the Flood Control Act of 1936." United States Army Corps of Engineers, 1988.

PERIODICALS

Altherr, T. "Review: The Evolution of the Flood Control Act of 1936." *Environmental History Review*: Spring 1991.

WEBSITES

74th CONGRESS. SESS. II. CHS. 651, 688. *Flood Control Act of 1936*. June 22, 1936. http://www.ccrh.org/comm/cottage/primary/1936.html (accessed October 17, 2012).

Alyson C. Heimer, MA

Onchocerciasis *see* **River blindness**

One Health Initiative

Definition

The One Health Initiative (OHI) is a collaborative effort of a number of health, medical, dental, and related organizations to study problems associated with humans and other animals.

Purpose

The purpose of the One Health Initiative is to learn more about diseases that exist primarily or exclusively in animals, but that may also be transmitted to humans, and to develop policies and mechanisms for controlling the spread of these diseases.

Origins

The principles on which OHI are based are as old as medicine itself. As early as the fourth century BCE, the Greek physician Hippocrates (c. 460 – c. 370 BCE) argued for an environmental origin of many human diseases. That idea was reborn many centuries later in the research of Italian physician Giovanni Maria Lancisi (1654–1720), whose work notably involved studies of the mechanisms by which influenza was spread through animal and human populations and the transmission of **malaria** from mosquito-infested swamps to human populations. A number of other physicians and medical researchers have further developed the theme that certain human diseases either have their origin in or are transmitted by way of nonhuman animals. German physician Rudolf Virchow (1821–1902), for example, coined the term *zoonosis* to describe diseases associated with animals (from the Greek, *nosos*, for "disease," and *zoo*, for "animal"). Virchow argued that "between animal and human medicine there are no dividing lines – nor should there be." One of Virchow's students, Canadian physician William Osler (1849–1919) brought Virchow's ideas to North America, where he put into practice those principles in his research on an outbreak of swine typhoid in Quebec in 1878.

The modern One Health (originally called One Medicine) movement is sometimes credited at least in part to the work of American veterinarian and Assistant Surgeon General James H. Steele who, in the 1940s, encouraged the health and medical communities to incorporate OHI thinking into their programs. He developed the first Veterinary Public Health Program in the Centers for Disease Control (now the **Centers for Disease Control and Prevention**) and was responsible for the inclusion of veterinarians in the U.S. **Public Health Service** for the first time in 1947. In April 2007, the Executive Board of the American Veterinary Medical Association (AVMA) appointed a committee, the One Health Initiative Task Force (OHITF) to consider the creation of a campaign to facilitate the collaboration of professionals in a variety of health-related fields to study diseases transmitted across species lines and non-transmitted diseases with similar characteristics in different species. A report issued by that committee in 2008 forms the basis for the present-day One Health Initiative campaign.

Description

The relevance of the One Health movement to modern medicine is based on the fact that nearly 60 percent of the 1,461 diseases now recognized in humans are transmitted by pathogens that move across species lines. In addition about three quarters of new infectious diseases in humans identified in recent years are zoonotic. A partial list of some of the zoonotic diseases of greatest concern in the early twenty first century are:

- anthrax, from domestic and wild animals
- avian influenza, from domestic and wild ducks and birds
- bovine tuberculosis, from cattle
- brucellosis, from cattle, goats, sheep, and pigs
- cat scratch fever, from cats
- cryptosporidiosis, from cattle, sheep, and domestic pets
- giardiasis, from other humans and from wild animals
- hantavirus syndrome, from rodents
- lyme disease, from ticks, rodents, sheep, deer, and small mammals
- pasteurellosis, from dogs, cats, and a variety of other mammals
- Q fever, from cattle, sheep, goats, and domestic cats
- rabies, from foxes, bats, and domestic dogs and cats
- streptococcal sepsis, from cattle and horses
- toxocariasis, from domestic cats and dogs
- trichinellosis, from domestic pigs and wild boars
- west Nile fever, from mosquitoes and wild birds

As the world's population continues to increase in size and extends its demand for meat protein, the risk of cross-species infections in humans will almost certainly increase. Proponents of the One Health philosophy argue that these data suggest that the next generation of human population may be the first one in recent history to experience a decrease in life expectancy because of the spread of new infectious diseases, many zoonotic in character. They suggest that one of the best approaches for dealing with this growing problem is to develop health programs that brings together professionals from a wide range of fields, including many specialized fields of medicine, veterinary medicine, osteopathy, nursing, dentistry, public health, and environmental health to solve the spread of zoonotic diseases.

The authors of the 2008 OHITF report point out that the early twenty first century may be about to experience a "perfect microbial storm" with which the world's medical community may not be prepared to deal and for which a One Health approach may be required. That "perfect storm" consists of a number of elements, including

- The spread of microbes that have adapted to existing treatments for infectious diseases;
- A significant increase in the amount and extent of global travel;
- An increasing susceptibility of groups of humans to infectious diseases;
- A rise in terrorist efforts to produce harm through the intentional release of pathogens;
- Global climate changes;
- Economic developments and changes in land use patterns in nations around the world;

> **KEY TERMS**
>
> **Pathogen**—A disease-causing organism.
>
> **Vector**—An organism capable of transferring an infectious disease from one organism to a different organism.
>
> **Zoonosis**—Having to do with diseases associated primarily with nonhuman animals.

- Changing patterns in human demographics and behaviors;
- Breakdowns in both public human and animal infrastructures;
- An increase and spread in poverty; and
- Pervasive patterns of social inequality throughout the world.

Proponents of a One Health approach to health and medical issues point to a number of examples of the issues with which they are concerned that have already occurred in recent years. These examples include

- The spread of HIV/AIDS infection, a zoonotic disease thought to have had its origins in non-human primates in the second half of the twentieth century in Africa;
- The arrival of the West Nile virus, severe acute respiratory syndrome (SARS), and monkeypox in the Western Hemisphere in the late twentieth and early twenty-first centuries, diseases that had previously not existed in the region;
- The emergence of bovine spongiform encephalopathy (BSE), "mad-cow disease" in parts of North America and Europe in the late twentieth century;
- The potential risk of the spread of highly contagious foot-and-mouth disease from cattle to humans in the United States in recent years;
- A similar risk of the spread across species lines of the highly potent porcine reproductive and respiratory syndrome (PRRS) from pigs to humans.

It is the primary goal of the One Health Initiative to deal with issues such as these. The mission statement of OHI outlines the methods by which the organization hopes to achieve its goals. It calls for joint efforts among professionals from all fields of health and medicine to

- Coordinate educational programs among human medical, veterinary medical, and public health institutions;
- Promote joint communication through journals, conferences, and allied health networks;
- Develop joint clinical programs for the assessment, treatment, and prevention of cross-species disease transmission;
- Encourage programs for the surveillance and control of cross-species disease;
- Promote research on cross-species disease transmission;
- Develop new diagnostic methods, vaccines, medicines, and prevention technology for cross-species diseases;
- Create programs for the education of decision-makers and the general public about zoonotic diseases.

One Health Initiative publishes a quarterly newsletter containing information about recent advances in the field of zoonotic diseases and related issues. It also provides links on its website to articles in peer-reviewed publications on the topic. Perhaps its most important activity is the sponsorship and co-sponsorship of a number of seminars, symposiums, conferences, conventions, and other meetings on topics related to cross-species disease transmission. Examples of the topics covered in those meetings include emerging infectious diseases, antimicrobial use and resistance, the human-animal bond in veterinary medicine, neglected influenza, building bridges between animal and human health, and the ongoing threat of **smallpox**.

Resources

BOOKS

Carter, Craig Nash. *One Man, One Medicine, One Health: The James H. Steele Story*. Charleston, SC: BookSurge, 2011.

Chorrnes, Eileen R., et al., eds. *Improving Food Safety Through a One Health Approach: Workshop Summary*. Washington, DC: National Academies Press, 2011.

Fox, Michael W. *Healing Animals & The Vision of One Health: Earth Care & Human Care*. North Charleston, SC: CreateSpace, 2011.

PERIODICALS

Coker, R., et al. "Towards a Conceptual Framework to Support One-health Research for Policy on Emerging Zoonoses." *Lancet Infectious Diseases* 11, 4. (2011): 326–31.

Day, M. J. "One Health: The Importance of Companion Animal Vector-borne Diseases." *Parasites and Vectors* 13, 4. (2011): 49.

Narrod, C., J. Zinsstag, and M. Tiongco. "A One Health Framework for Estimating the Economic Costs of Zoonotic Diseases on Society." *Ecohealth* 9, 2. (2012): 150–62.

Zinsstag, J., et al. "Mainstreaming One Health." *Ecohealth* 9, 2. (2012): 107–10.

WEBSITES

American Veterinary Medical Association. "One Health Initiative Task Force: Final Report." https://www.avma.org/KB/Resources/Reports/Documents/one-health_final.pdf (accessed on October 19, 2012).

"One Health: It's All Connected." American Veterinary Medical Association. https://www.avma.org/KB/Resources/Reference/Pages/One-Health.aspx (accessed on October 20, 2012).

"One Health Initiative." http://www.princeton.edu/sgs/publications/articles/OneHealth-article-June-2010.pdf (accessed on October 20, 2012).

"One Health Office." Centers for Disease Control and Prevention. http://www.cdc.gov/ncezid/dhcpp/one_health/index.html (accessed on October 20, 2012).

ORGANIZATIONS

American Veterinary Medical Association (AVMA), 1931 North Meacham Rd., Suite 100, Schaumburg, IL, USA 60173–4360, (800) 248–2862, Fax: 1(847) 925–1329, https://www.avma.org/About/WhoWeAre/Pages/contact.aspx, https://www.avma.org/.

David E. Newton, EdD

Oxfam

Definition

Oxfam is a confederation of 17 nation-based nongovernmental organizations (NGOs) that work directly with local communities and partner organizations in 92 countries. Oxfam provides disaster relief and develops programs to overcome poverty and promote sustainable development and social justice.

Purpose

Oxfam is one of the major deliverers of emergency relief for both manmade and natural disasters around the world. Because of its network of local community partners, Oxfam is sometimes able to provide disaster relief in regions where foreign-aid workers have been expelled, such as during the 2011 **drought** and **famine** in southern Somalia.

Although Oxfam's initial focus was providing food aid for the relief of famine, over the years its focus has grown to encompass strategies for combating the causes of hunger and famine. Thus, in addition to providing food and medicines to the poorest people on Earth, Oxfam works with other organizations and communities around the world for the implementation of sustainable development programs to overcome global poverty and social injustice. In particular, where possible, Oxfam follows up humanitarian disaster relief with programs to provide communities with sources of clean water and **sanitation**. It also works to provide the tools that enable communities to become financially self-supporting and to open national and international markets to produce and other products from poverty-stricken regions.

Because of its long-term goals for worldwide sustainable development, Oxfam is often viewed as having a more politically oriented agenda than many other international humanitarian organizations, with strong advocacy and lobbying arms and popular campaigns for influencing policy decisions at local, national, and international levels. In addition to preventing and relieving famine, malnutrition, and preventable diseases caused by poverty, Oxfam advocates for health care and education for all, an end to gender inequalities, an end to unfair trade rules and practices, and the combating of **climate change**.

Along with its local partner organizations and communities, Oxfam's work focuses on:

- emergency humanitarian response, including immediate life-saving relief from natural disasters and conflicts, as well as helping communities build resilience for coping with future disasters
- development through long-term programs to eliminate poverty and fight injustice
- campaigns to raise public awareness about the causes of worldwide poverty and encourage citizen action for social justice
- lobbying of governments and other decision-makers to overturn policies and practices that perpetuate poverty and injustice
- research and analysis, combined with the on-the-ground experiences of its partners in developing countries, to determine and promote best practices for overcoming poverty and injustice

Demographics

Oxfam International is headquartered in Oxford, England. It has advocacy offices in Brussels, Belgium; Geneva, Switzerland; Brasilia, Brazil; and New York City and Washington, DC. Its semiautonomous NGOs include:

- Oxfam America: http://www.oxfamamerica.org
- Oxfam Australia: http://www.oxfam.org.au
- Oxfam Canada: http://www.oxfam.ca
- Oxfam France: http://www.oxfamfrance.org

- Oxfam GB (Great Britain): http://www.oxfam.org.uk
- Oxfam Germany: http://www.oxfam.de
- Oxfam Hong Kong: http://www.oxfam.org.hk
- Oxfam-in-Belgium: http://www.oxfamsol.be
- Oxfam India: http://www.oxfamindia.org
- Oxfam Ireland: http://www.oxfamireland.org
- Oxfam Italy: http://www.oxfamitalia.org
- Oxfam Japan: http://www.oxfam.jp
- Oxfam Mexico: http://www.oxfammexico.org
- Oxfam New Zealand: http://www.oxfam.org.nz
- Oxfam Novib (Netherlands): http://www.oxfamnovib.nl
- Oxfam Québec: http://www.oxfam.qc.ca

Description

Origins

Oxfam originated in Oxford, England, in 1942, as the Oxford Committee for Famine Relief. Its purpose was to campaign for food relief for the starving people of World War II Axis-occupied Greece, which meant shipping food through the Allied naval blockade. The original Oxford organization was expanded in 1963 by a Canadian affiliate. In 1965, the organization adopted its telegraph address, OXFAM, as its name. In 1995, a group of independent NGOs formed Oxfam International, with the goals of more effective delivery of emergency relief and a more significant impact on reducing global poverty and injustice.

Principles

Oxfam operates on the principle that all people have certain basic human rights:

- The right to a earn a decent living. With a strong emphasis on the livelihoods of women, Oxfam campaigns for better working conditions, protection of natural resources that are crucial to the livelihoods of poor communities, and national and global fair-trade rules.
- The right to basic services—health care, education, and safe water. Oxfam funds schools and teacher training, provides health training and clean water supplies, and campaigns for aid that focuses on basic services.
- The right to be safe from harm. Oxfam provides emergency shelter, clean water, and sanitation and works with local communities to rebuild and better prepare for future disasters.
- The right to be heard. Oxfam supports its partners and communities in understanding their rights and voicing their concerns and campaigns for those in power to listen and act on those concerns.
- The right to equal treatment. Oxfam works to combat discrimination, especially against women, the disabled, and religious and ethnic minorities.

Humanitarian aid, security, and development issues

Every year 500,000 people are killed in wars and more than 30 million are driven from their homes by conflict and natural disasters. Oxfam responds to emergencies in more than 30 countries, with the immediate goals of reducing death and disease by providing access to food, shelter, and hygiene, and the longer-term goal of helping communities rebuild. Oxfam lobbies governments and other NGOs for more and faster relief aid in humanitarian crises, as well as for more effective international aid focusing on preventing death during pregnancy and childbirth, childhood vaccinations, and access to quality education. Oxfam advocates for international aid that supports local and national programs for eradicating poverty, rather than aid that imposes conditions such as spending cuts, opening up markets, privatization, or deregulation. Oxfam campaigns for cancellation of debt repayment by developing countries, so that the countries can focus on healthcare and educational services. It demands the honest, accountable, and transparent use of aid by recipient communities and governments.

Oxfam addresses issues of peace and security primarily through working with local communities to identify and root out the causes of conflict. It provides funding to train local people, especially women, in resolving conflict and preventing violence; for example, by easing ethnic tensions around water and grazing rights. Oxfam has also worked on developing systems to track the origin and trade of resources, such as "blood diamonds," that promote conflict, and it campaigns for an end to global trade in arms.

Agriculture and climate change are major Oxfam issues. Oxfam lobbies governments and NGOs to invest in agriculture to promote food security through crop diversification and sustainable water management and to counteract environmental degradation, climate change, and soaring energy costs. Oxfam is particularly concerned with issues of land distribution and access to agricultural markets. Poor people in developing countries are expected to be particularly affected by climate change. Changing rainfall patterns will exacerbate water problems, both droughts and floods, encourage new pests, and lead to more serious natural disasters, an inequality known as "climate poverty." In addition to calling for global reductions in climate-warming greenhouse gases, Oxfam is working with communities to better adapt and build resilience to climate change, as well as to protect their natural resources, through environmentally and socially responsible development.

Issues of equality

Oxfam has demanded that transnational corporations improve their policies and practices for the benefit of the developing countries in which they operate. Oxfam successfully lobbied the World Trade Organization to stop subsidizing the dumping of cheap exports on developing countries. In 2007, Oxfam was instrumental in brokering an agreement between Starbucks Coffee and the Ethiopian government for fairer prices for Ethiopian coffee-bean farmers.

Oxfam uses youth outreach to fight inequalities throughout the world, with programs to develop youth leadership, foster youth involvement in initiatives, and develop local and international networks. The Oxfam International Youth Partnership is a global network of youth in 150 countries working for initiatives to fight poverty and injustice.

Other major Oxfam issues include:

- promotion of active citizenship among people living in poverty
- education for every child, including its active participation in the Global Campaign for Education, making education accessible to all girls and lobbying for the training of two million new teachers for developing countries
- incorporation of the equal treatment of women into all of its work
- establishment of free quality health care for all, including clean drinking water, sanitation, access to doctors, and affordable medicines
- reduction of racism and discrimination and promotion of respect for indigenous people and minority rights around the world

Campaigns

As of 2012, Oxfam International's major campaigns included:

- Grow, a global movement to attack the root causes of hunger around the world
- agriculture, to combat rising food prices, biofuel crops that compete with food crops for land, and climate change, and promote agriculture for food security and jobs in poverty-stricken regions
- climate change
- conflicts and disasters, including controlling arms trafficking, the food crisis in East Africa and the Sahel region of West Africa, crises in Sudan and South Sudan, and ongoing conflict in the Democratic Republic of Congo
- health and education for all, including the Robin Hood Tax Campaign to tax bankers, the Millennium Development Goals of the United Nations, effective aid, and canceling debt repayment for developing countries
- fair trade, including Big Noise and the Make Trade Fair campaigns

Land grabs

In October 2012, Oxfam issued a major report on the global land rush. Although the world's farms produce enough food to feed 12 billion people, nearly one billion people are going hungry because of lack of access to land to grow food or lack of income to buy food. Rising food prices and competition for available resources are making the situation worse. Wealthy countries are currently buying or leasing large swaths of productive farmland in poor countries—the so-called land grab—and exporting the crops for profit. The land that has been sold off in the past decade could feed the one billion people who go hungry. A large proportion of these land sales have been to European and U.S. hedge funds and sovereign wealth funds from countries such as China and Saudi Arabia. Because of these land sales, poor farmers are being evicted. Oxfam has called on the World Bank to freeze its own land investments and to review its lending policies to prevent these land grabs.

Oxfam America

National Oxfam organizations have their individual issues and priorities. Oxfam America, headquartered in Boston, Massachusetts, maintains a policy and campaign office in Washington, DC, as well as seven regional offices around the globe. As of 2012, Oxfam America's issues included community finance, private sector engagement, access to medicines, fair trade, equality for women, water, worker' rights, insurance and rural resilience, and hunger and food security. The CHANGE initiative trains college students to become active in Oxfam America's social justice initiatives, developing leaders and inspiring global awareness.

Oxfam America's campaigns include:

- the campaign called Grow, Food, Justice, and Planet
- current emergencies, including food crises in the Sahel and East Africa, conflict in the Sudans, the

KEY TERMS

Biofuels—Liquid fuels from biomass, especially ethanol made from corn or sugarcane, and biodiesel from vegetable oils and animal fats.

Climate change—The ongoing increase in average global temperatures due to the release of carbon dioxide and other greenhouse gases, primarily from the burning of fossil fuels for energy production.

Famine—A humanitarian crisis defined as the most severe stage of food insecurity.

Food security—Access for all people at all times to the food required to lead a healthy and active life.

Nongovernmental organizations (NGOs)—Relief and development organizations that work independently of governments.

2011 El Salvador floods, the 2010 earthquake in Haiti, Pakistani floods, the war in Afghanistan, and conflict in the Democratic Republic of Congo
- U.S. Gulf Coast recovery from hurricanes and the BP oil spill
- the campaign called Saving Lives 24/7
- disaster risk reduction
- reform of development aid and relief
- oil, gas, and mining

The organization Charity Navigator has awarded Oxfam America four stars overall, with 60.31 points out of a possible 70. Oxfam America also received four stars for accountability and transparency with a score of 67.00 and three stars for financial performance with a score of 56.64.

Resources

BOOKS

Berry, Craig. *Globalisation and Ideology in Britain: Neoliberalism, Free Trade and the Global Economy*. Manchester, UK: Manchester University Press, 2011.

Cornwall, Andrea, and Deborah Eade. *Deconstructing Development Discourse: Buzzwords and Fuzzwords*. Oxford, UK: Oxfam, 2010.

Ilcan, Suzan, and Anita Lacey. *Governing the Poor: Exercises of Poverty Reduction, Practices of Global Aid*. Montreal, ONT: McGill-Queen's University Press, 2011.

Merino, Noël. *Health Care*. Farmington Hills, MI: Greenhaven, 2012.

Oxfam International. "Climate Change Adaptation and Disaster Risk Protection Will Be Challenges." In *Are Natural Disasters Increasing?*, edited by Stefan Kiesbye. Farmington Hills, MI: Greenhaven, 2010.

Tomalin, Emma. *Gender, Faith, and Development*. Oxford, UK: Oxfam, 2011.

Wilson, David, Kirsty Wilson, and Claire Harvey. *Small Farmers, Big Change: Scaling Up Impact in Smallholder Agriculture*. Oxford, UK: Oxfam, 2011.

Wilson, Kim, Malcolm Harper, and Matthew Griffith. *Financial Promise for the Poor: How Groups Build Microsavings*. Sterling, VA: Kumarian, 2010.

PERIODICALS

Strom, Stephanie. "Oxfam Urges U.S. Women to Pursue Efficiency in Food Use." *New York Times*, July 18, 2012.

WEBSITES

Geary, Kate. "'Our Land, Our Lives' Time Out on the Global Land Rush." Oxfam Briefing Note. http://www.oxfamamerica.org/files/our-land-our-lives.pdf (accessed October 11, 2012).

Philpott, Tom. "How Not to 'Feed the World.'" *Mother Jones*, October 10, 2012. http://www.motherjones.com/tom-philpott/2012/10/want-feed-world-first-stop-land-grabs (accessed October 11, 2012).

ORGANIZATIONS

Charity Navigator, 139 Harristown Rd., Ste. 201, Glen Rock, NJ 07452, (201) 818-1288, Fax: (201) 818-4694, info@charitynavigator.org, http://www.charitynavigator.org.

Oxfam America, 226 Causeway St., 5th Fl., Boston, MA 02114-2206, (617) 482-121, Fax: (617) 728-2594, (800) 77-OXFAM (776-9326), http://www.oxfamamerica.org.

Oxfam International Secretariat, 266 Banbury Rd., Ste. 20, Oxford, UK OX2 7DL, 44 865 339 100, Fax: 44 865 339 101, http://www.oxfam.org.

Margaret Alic, PhD

Ozone

Definition

Ozone is a toxic, usually colorless gas (that can be blue when in high concentration) with a characteristic acrid odor. A variant of normal oxygen, it has three oxygen atoms per molecule rather than the usual two.

Description

Ozone strongly absorbs **ultraviolet radiation** at wavelengths of 220 through 290 nm with peak absorption at 260.4 nm. Ozone will also absorb infrared **radiation** at wavelengths in the range 9–10 μg. Ozone occurs naturally in the ozonosphere (ozone layer), which surrounds the earth, protecting living organisms at the earth's surface from ultraviolet radiation. The ozonosphere is located in the stratosphere from 6–31 miles (10–50 km) above the earth's surface, with the highest concentration between 7.5 and 12 miles (12 and 20 km). The concentration of ozone in the ozonosphere is 1 molecule per 100,000 molecules, or if the gas were at standard temperature and pressure, the ozone layer would be 0.12 inch (3 mm) thick. However, the ozone layer absorbs about 90 percent of incident ultraviolet radiation.

Ozone in the stratosphere results from a chemical equilibrium between oxygen, ozone, and ultraviolet radiation. Ultraviolet radiation is absorbed by oxygen and produces ozone. Simultaneously, ozone absorbs ultraviolet radiation and decomposes to oxygen and other products. Ozone layer depletion occurs as a result of complex reactions in the atmosphere between organic compounds that react with ozone faster than the ozone is replenished. Compounds of most concern include the byproducts of ultraviolet degradation of chlorofluorocarbons (CFCs), chlorine and fluorine.

Effects on public health

Ozone is also a secondary air pollutant at the surface of the earth as a result of complex chemical reactions between sunshine and primary pollutants, such as hydrocarbons and oxides of nitrogen. Ozone can also be generated in the presence of oxygen from equipment that gives off intense light, electrical sparks, or creates intense static electricity, such as photocopiers and laser printers. Human olfactory senses are very sensitive to ozone, being able to detect ozone odor at concentrations between 0.02 and 0.05 parts per million. Toxic symptoms for humans from exposure to ozone include headaches and drying of the throat and respiratory tracts. Ozone is highly toxic to many plant species and destroys or degrades many building materials, such as paint, rubber, and some plastics. The threshold limit value (TLV) for air quality standards is 0.1 ppm or 0.2 mg O_3 per m^3 of air.

Industrial uses

Industrial uses of ozone include chemical manufacturing and air, water, and waste treatment. Industrial quantities of ozone are typically generated from air or pure oxygen by means of silent corona discharge. Ozone is used in water treatment as a disinfectant to kill pathogenic microorganisms or for oxidation of organic and inorganic compounds. Combinations of ozone and hydrogen peroxide or ultraviolet radiation in water can generate powerful oxidants useful in breaking down complex synthetic organic compounds. In wastewater treatment, ozone can be used to disinfect effluents, or to decrease their color and odor. In some industrial applications, ozone can enhance biodegradation of complex organic molecules. Industrial cooling tower treatment with ozone prevents transmission of airborne pathogenic organisms and can reduce odor.

Resources

BOOKS

Gillespie, Alexander. *Climate Change, Ozone Depletion and Air Pollution.* Leiden, UK, and Boston, MA: Nijboff/Brill, 2005.

WEBSITES

United States Environmental Protection Agency (EPA). "Air: Air Pollutants: Ground Level Ozone." http://www.epa.gov/ebtpages/airairpollutantsgroundlevelozone.html (accessed November 12, 2010).

United States Environmental Protection Agency (EPA). "Pollutants/Toxics: Ozone." http://www.epa.gov/ebtpages/pollozone.html (accessed November 12, 2010).

Gordon R. Finch

Ozone exposure

Definition

Ozone exposure is the breathing in of ground-level, or tropospheric, ozone.

Description

Ozone is a gas found both above and on Earth. Ozone found 10–30 miles (16–48 km) above Earth's surface is important in protecting Earth from the sun's ultraviolet rays. Ozone found at ground level is considered a health threat. Although ozone is everywhere, the concentration depends on various factors, including the amount of **smog** and pollution in a particular area. Warm weather also increases the level of ozone in the air. Ozone levels indoors often are between 20–80% of the level found outdoors, depending on whether windows are open or closed and if air conditioning is used.

The air quality index ranges from 0–500. Ozone is one component of this index. An air quality index between 0–50 is considered good, and **air pollution** poses little or no health risk. Other air quality index ranges include: moderate (51–100), unhealthy for sensitive groups (101–150), unhealthy (151–200), very unhealthy (201–300), and hazardous (301–500). At the level hazardous, everyone may experience serious health effects. Ozone concentration itself is measured in parts per million (ppm) or parts per billion (ppb).

Origins

Ground-level or tropospheric ozone, is the so-called "bad ozone" found at Earth's surface. This ozone is formed when air containing nitrogen oxide and volatile organic compounds react with sunlight. The major sources of these compounds come from the combustion of fossil fuels, such as pollutants from motor vehicles, gasoline vapors, factories, and chemical solvents. Ozone forms smog and is usually at its highest level during hot sunny days. Wind can transport ozone for long distances, meaning even rural areas may experience high levels of ozone concentration.

Risks

People who live in areas with high levels of ozone, such as large cities with heavy industry and many cars, are at the highest risk of developing symptoms of ozone exposure. Additionally, those who spend large amounts of time outdoors, especially exercising or doing manual labor, are at risk of developing symptoms due to ozone exposure, especially in areas where there is heavy smog. Children are at highest risk of ozone exposure because they often spend hours outdoors during the warm season. People with chronic respiratory diseases, such as **asthma** and chronic obstructive pulmonary disease (COPD), are more vulnerable to the effects of ozone than healthy adults. Scientists also have found that some people are more sensitive to the ozone than others, but they have not found a particular reason why these otherwise healthy people are so sensitive.

Causes and symptoms

Symptoms associated with ozone exposure are dependent on the concentration and length of the exposure. Even short-term exposure at low concentrations can be harmful to the upper respiratory tract and the lungs. Shortness of breath, tight chest, dry throat, coughing or wheezing, headaches, nausea, and feeling unable to breathe are other symptoms of short and low-concentration ozone exposure (0.25–0.75 ppm). Even exposure at relatively low concentrations has been associated with severe lung injury and in some cases death.

As the length and concentration of exposure increases, symptoms may become more severe. Extreme fatigue, reduced lung function, the inability to sleep or concentrate, dizziness, and discoloration of the skin have been seen in people who experience intermittent exposure (9 ppm) between 3–14 days. Ozone exposure can irritate the eyes within minutes at intermittent levels.

Near unconsciousness and severe respiratory irritation were seen in one study of 15 minutes of exposure to levels at 11 ppm. Researchers believe that 30 minutes of exposure to 50 ppm can be lethal. Other research has linked ozone exposure to a particular type of cardiac arrhythmia that is associated with a risk of premature death and stroke.

> ### KEY TERMS
>
> **Arrhythmia**—Abnormal heart rhythm.
>
> **Asthma**—A disease in which the air passages of the lungs become inflamed and narrowed.
>
> **Bronchitis**—A respiratory disorder caused by a viral or bacterial infection. Bronchitis is characterized by inflamed bronchi, excessive mucus production, and coughing.
>
> **Emphysema**—A lung disease in which there is an abnormal accumulation of air in the tissues. Symptoms often include trouble breathing and a cough. Emphysema is frequently caused by long-term smoking.
>
> **Smog**—A type of smoky fog that contains large amounts of air pollutants.

Treatment

For most people, no specific treatment is needed for ozone exposure. People who experience symptoms related to ozone exposure should move indoors where the concentration of ozone is lower. Symptoms will typically lessen and disappear on their own after a few hours. People with chronic respiratory problems or who continue to experience symptoms hours after moving to an area with a low ozone concentration may need to seek medical treatment for the specific symptoms they are experiencing.

Prognosis

Symptoms that are associated with low levels of ozone exposure usually disappear within 18 hours after the exposure has ended. Long-term effects due to higher concentrations of exposure or a longer exposure period may include headaches, irritation of the nose and throat, accelerated aging of the lungs, a decreased lung capacity and function of the lungs, and may worsen asthma, **emphysema**, and **bronchitis**. Not yet studied in humans but seen in animal populations, ozone exposure may lead to increased susceptibility to bacterial infections of the respiratory system. Studies also have associated increased mortality, especially in older adults and during the warm season, with ozone exposure. The **World Health Organization**

> **QUESTIONS TO ASK YOUR DOCTOR**
>
> - Where can I find out the ozone levels in my city?
> - Is it safe for my child to play outdoors during unhealthy air quality index levels?
> - How quickly should my symptoms of ozone exposure go away?

(WHO) estimated that two million people worldwide died in 2012 because of continued exposure to air pollution. The same year, the U.S. **Environmental Protection Agency (EPA)** attributed 40,000–50,000 deaths to air pollution exposure.

Prevention

People can protect themselves from dangerous levels of ozone exposure by reducing the amount of time spent outdoors when the air quality index in their area is listed as unhealthy. Ozone levels are often at their highest during warm months (April to October) and during the afternoon and evening hours. Limiting the amount of strenuous exercise during unhealthy air quality index periods will also reduce the amount of ozone exposure experienced. Ozone levels are usually lowest indoors when air-conditioning is used and air turnover rate is low.

Many governments and organizations are working to lower the amount of ground-level ozone. Regulations regarding the combustion of fossil fuels and other pollutants can help limit the amount of nitrogen oxide and volatile organic compounds released into the air. The United Nations Environment Programme, **EPA**, and many state and national governments all play an important role in working to reduce the formation of ground-level ozone. For example, the EPA **Clean Air Act** has set health-based standards for ozone in the air.

Resources

PERIODICALS

Devlin, Robert B., et al. "Controlled Exposure of Healthy Young Volunteers to Ozone Causes Cardiovascular Effects." *Circulation* 126 (2012): 104–111. http://circ.ahajournals.org/content/126/1/104.full (accessed October 12, 2012).

WEBSITES

AIRNow. "Air Quality Index (AQI)—A Guide to Air Quality and Your Health." http://airnow.gov/index.cfm?action=aqibasics.aqi (accessed October 13, 2012).

Canadian Centre for Occupational Health and Safety. "2 Health Effects of Ozone." http://www.ccohs.ca/oshanswers/chemicals/chem_profiles/ozone/health_ozo.html (accessed October 13, 2012).

Environmental Protection Agency. "Health Effects of Ozone in the General Population." http://www.epa.gov/apti/ozonehealth/population.html (accessed October 12, 2012).

Environmental Protection Agency. "Ozone and Your Health." http://www.epa.gov/airnow/ozone-c.pdf (accessed October 12, 2012).

ORGANIZATIONS

American Lung Association, 1301 Pennsylvania Ave. NW Suite 800, Washington, DC 20004, (202) 785-3355, (800) LUNGUSA (586-4872), Fax: (202) 202 452 1805, http://www.lungusa.org.

Environmental Protection Agency, Ariel Rios Bldg., 1200 Pennsylvania Ave. NW, Washington, DC 20460, (202) 272-0167; TTY (202) 272-0165, http://www.epa.gov.

United Nations Environment Programme, United Nations Avenue, Gigiri, PO Box 30552, 00100, Nairobi, Kenya, 254(20) 76-1234, Fax: 254(20) 76-448990, unepinfo@unep.org, http://www.unep.org.

Tish Davidson, AM

P

Pandemic

Definition

A pandemic is the outbreak of a disease on a global scale.

Description

When a disease occurs in higher numbers than expected, it often is referred to as a disease outbreak. Epidemiologists and other public health officials continuously monitor disease incidence to watch for outbreaks. If an infectious disease outbreak spreads to a high number of people in a given region, it might be termed an epidemic. A pandemic differs from an epidemic in that a pandemic spreads beyond a geographic region, affecting different areas around the world. The pandemic might involve a number of separate epidemics around the globe or a progressive, systematic spread of the disease throughout the world.

Perhaps the most well-known example in the twentieth century is the HIV/AIDS pandemic, which reached 65 million infections and 2.5 million deaths at its peak. Probably the first recorded pandemic was the Antonine **Plague**, which occurred sometime between 165–180 B.C.E. In this plague, soldiers from Asia might have brought **measles** or **smallpox** to Europe. The pandemic eventually killed as many as 5 million people.

A **cholera** outbreak in London was an important contributor to the advancement of public health and how people study infectious disease. But cholera can be traced to India in 1816. The disease spread through Bengal, China, and Europe.

Progress in science and public health efforts has eradicated or slowed many of the diseases that used to result in pandemics. Influenza, or flu, pandemics have caused many health problems throughout past and recent history, however. Between 1918 and 1920 the Spanish influenza probably killed more than 40 million people worldwide and 100,000 people in the United States. However, by the time the Asian flu struck in the 1950s, identification and response methods had improved.

Effects on public health

A pandemic can have major effects on community health, social structures, and economies. The effects might be felt more strongly in certain parts of the world or in certain people who are more vulnerable. For example, some countries are not as well equipped to handle massive immunizations and other practices to stem pandemics. Plus some people, such as the elderly, are more vulnerable to severe illness or death from diseases such as the flu than are others. Though most pandemics now can be predicted and often averted with actions such as immunizations, there remains the chance that a flu virus could emerge to which humans have little or no immunity. In that case, there would be serious health ramifications, and communities and countries might have to resort to travel restrictions and other methods to prevent transmission of the virus.

Cost to society

Influenza pandemics caused millions of deaths around the world in the twentieth century. The outbreak of **severe acute respiratory syndrome (SARS)** in 2003 caused economic losses and social disruption that reached far outside the borders of the affected countries. Pandemics can cause enormous healthcare costs and disrupt normal services that are essential to communities and regions.

Public health role and response

Public health entities such as the **World Health Organization** (WHO) and the **Centers for Disease Control and Prevention** (CDC), along with state and local organizations, walk a fine line in responding to possible pandemics as seen in 2009, when many of the world's governments responded strongly to an outbreak of H1N1 flu. WHO labeled H1N1 a pandemic and later received criticism for acting more aggressively than required in response to the flu outbreak. It was further complicated by a change in the description of pandemic that WHO had made a few years earlier. Critics called the change made on the WHO website a change in the definition of pandemic. WHO says the confusion comes from information that describes the stages of a pandemic.

Public health professionals should prepare for a pandemic in advance and with a comprehensive pandemic preparedness guide or checklist. The planning includes preparing for emergencies and disease surveillance. Also involved is determining how cases will be investigated and treated and how further spread of the disease in the community can be prevented. Determining how to maintain essential community services during the pandemic is essential. Surveillance should assist with early warning and prevention strategies at the time the pandemic occurs. Case management might include improved hygiene, immunizations, distancing of social groups, and even travel restrictions and quarantines.

If public health professionals are involved in helping a community during a pandemic, they often will study and evaluate the response that occurred after the pandemic has passed. This evaluation helps to improve response in that community and in other areas in the event of a future pandemic. Public health professionals also learn from response to epidemics and **disease outbreaks** and any mistakes made.

Resources

PERIODICALS

Doshi, Peter. "The Elusive Definition of Pandemic Influenza." *Bulletin of the World Health Organization.* 89 (2011): 532–38.

WEBSITES

National Council of Teachers of Mathematics. "The History of Pandemics." http://www.nctm.org/resources/content.aspx?id=10826 (accessed October 14, 2012).

World Health Organization. "WHO Checklist for Influenza Preparedness Planning." http://whqlibdoc.who.int/hq/2005/WHO_CDS_CSR_GIP_2005.4.pdf (accessed October 14, 2012).

ORGANIZATIONS

Centers for Disease Control and Prevention—Bioterrorism Preparedness & Response Program (CDC), 1600 Clifton Rd., Atlanta, GA 30333, (404) 639-3534, (888) 246-2675, cdcresponse@ashastd.org, http://www.bt.cdc.gov.

World Health Organization, Avenue Appia 20, 1211 Geneva 27, Switzerland, 2241 791 21 11, Fax: 2241 791 31 11, info@who.int, http://www.who.int.

Teresa G. Odle

Parasites

Definition

Parasites are organisms that live in or on the body of a host organism and are dependent on the host for completion of their life cycle, to the detriment of the host.

Demographics

Because of sanitary living conditions in the developed world, parasites do not cause widespread life-threatening infections. In the developing world, however, parasitic infections are epidemic. They kill and disable millions of people every year. Although parasites do not target individuals of any particular age, race, or gender, people living where there is poor **sanitation**, limited water treatment, and overcrowded conditions are more likely to be infected, as are recent immigrants or travelers who have been exposed to

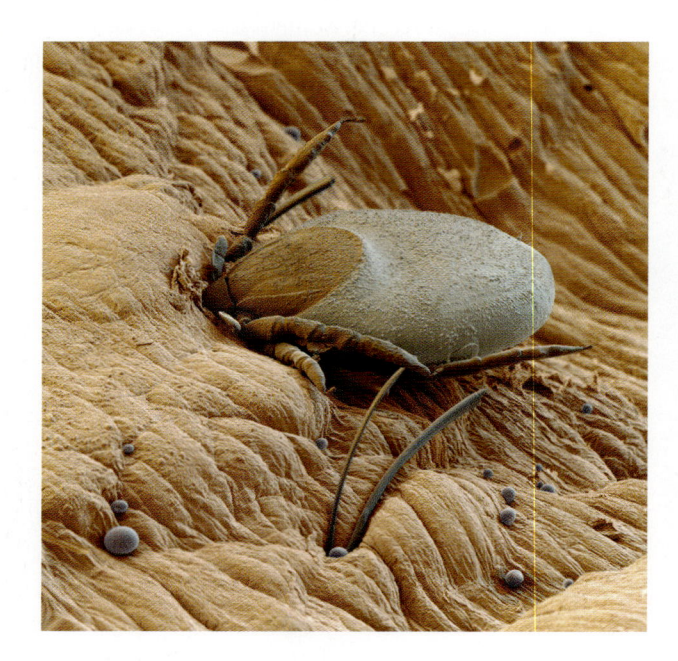

A tick. *(Eye of Science/Photo Researchers, Inc.)*

those conditions. In addition, people with compromised immune systems, such as individuals with HIV/AIDS infection or those receiving cancer treatments, are more likely to become severely ill from a parasitic infection.

Because parasites can live inside the human body for years without making their presence known, they are more common than one might think. According to one study, approximately half of all Americans carry at least one parasite that may or may not cause symptoms, depending on the type of parasite and the individual's health status.

The U.S. **Centers for Disease Control and Prevention** (CDC) requires that five parasitic diseases be reported: Chagas disease, cystericercosis, toxocariasis, toxoplasmosis, and trichomoniasis. Trichomoniasis is the most common parasite in the United States with about 7.4 million cases reported annually.

Description

Parasites may be plants, animals, **viruses**, bacteria, or fungi. They feed either on their host directly or upon its surplus fluids. They harm their hosts because they consume food, damage tissues and cells, and eliminate toxic wastes that can make the host sick. Some parasites, known as endoparasites, live inside their host, whereas ectoparasites live on the outside of their host. Organisms in which parasites reach maturity are called definitive hosts, and hosts harboring parasite stages are called intermediate hosts. Organisms that spread parasite stages between hosts are called vectors. Parasites can spread through the ingestion of contaminated food or water, from contact with infected animals, including pets (zoonotic parasites), through the bite of an infected insect, through transmission of infected blood, by inhaling dust containing eggs of parasites, or by direct contact through a cut or the skin.

Full-time, or obligatory, parasites have an absolute dependence on their hosts. Examples of this type are viruses, which can only live and multiply inside living cells, and tapeworms, which can only live and multiply inside other species. Part-time, or facultative, parasites, such as wood ticks, have parasitic and free-living stages in their life cycle and are only temporary residents of their hosts.

Parasites can generally be divided into large or macroparasites and small or microparasites. Large parasites can be seen with the naked eye. They include internal parasites such as roundworms, flukes, and tapeworms and external parasites such as ticks, lice, and fleas. Some large internal parasites lay eggs on the intestinal walls. As the eggs hatch, the young larvae feed on the food in the intestinal tract. Then they grow, reproduce, and start the cycle all over again. They sometimes dig through the digestive tract to get into the bloodstream, muscles, and other organs. These types of parasites can cause malnutrition and anemia because they tend to rob the body of essential nutrients; however, macroparasites that employ one or more intermediate hosts, such as flukes, tapeworms, or roundworms, have highly effective transmission stages but usually have only a limited effect on the population of the host.

Microparasites include viruses, bacteria, protozoa can only be seen with a microscope. Microparasites can migrate virtually anywhere in the body (into the bloodstream, muscles, and even vital organs such as the brain, the lungs, or the liver) and do substantial damage. Microparasites that are transmitted directly between infected hosts, such as rabies or distemper, target herd animals with a high host density and can significantly reduce population levels.

Risk factors

Risk factors that increase the chance for becoming infected with a parasite:

- an immune system weakened by disease or long-term exposure to toxic chemicals or environmental pollution

Disease	Parasite	Insect (vector)
African trypanosomiasis (sleeping sickness)	Trypanosoma brucei gambiense, Trypanosoma brucei rhodesiense	Tsetse flies
Babesiosis	Babesia species	Ixodes (hard-bodied) ticks
Chagas disease	Trypanosoma cruzi	Triatomine ("kissing") bugs
Leishmaniasis	Leishmania species	Phlebotomine sand flies
Malaria	Plasmodium species	Anopheles mosquitoes
Toxoplasmosis	Toxoplasma gondii	No insect vector

(Table by PreMediaGlobal. © 2013 Cengage Learning.)

- prolonged antibiotic use
- alcohol and/or drug abuse
- smoking
- prolonged emotional and/or physical stress
- malabsorption syndrome
- compromised immune system

Causes and symptoms

People can acquire a parasitic infection in many ways, including:

- being bitten by insects
- walking barefoot
- eating raw or undercooked pork, beef, or fish
- eating contaminated raw fruits and vegetables
- eating foods prepared by infected handlers
- drinking contaminated water
- having contact with infected persons (including sexual contact, kissing, sharing drinks, shaking hands, or sharing toys)
- inhaling dust that contains parasitic eggs or cysts
- playing with or picking up pet litter contaminated with parasitic eggs or cysts

In 2002, the Centers for Disease Control and Prevention (CDC) announced the first documented cases of transplant patients contracting a dangerous parasitic disease from infection with T. cruzi from organs harvested from a Central American donor. The infection caused Chagas disease, and two of the three donor recipients died. After that, the CDC identified several additional cases of Chagas diseased in transplant patients.

Causes

There are more than 100 types of human parasites. The following describe some of the most common species in the United States.

ARTHROPODS. Common arthropods such as ticks, mites, fleas, and lice may cause intense itching in affected areas. Ticks are particularly able to transmit serious disease such as **Lyme disease** and Rocky Mountains potted fever. Other parasites, spread by mosquitoes, cause more serious diseases such as western and eastern equine encephalitis, **malaria**, **Dengue fever**, and **yellow fever**.

INTESTINAL PARASITES. Some of the most common intestinal parasites include:

- Pinworms. This is the most common parasitic infection in the United States. The worm resides in the colon, yet it lays eggs outside the body, usually near the anus, a process that causes severe itching. The disease can be transmitted from one individual to another through dirty hands, clothing, bedclothes, and toys.
- Tapeworms. The two most common tapeworms are *Taenia solium* (pork tapeworm) and *Taenia saginata* (beef tapeworm). *Taenia solium* infestation is caused by eating undercooked pork, whereas *Taenia saginata* (pork tapeworm) infestation is caused by consuming raw beef. Adult tapeworms may become quite large, some as long as 20 feet (6.1 m). Of the two, pork tapeworm is the more harmful. It often causes anemia and weight loss. More seriously, when adult pork tapeworm eggs, excreted in human feces, are ingested by other people (which can happen with poor hygiene and sanitation), the parasitic life cycle that occurs in pigs and cattle takes place in the human host. Once in the human digestive system, the tapeworm eggs, called proglottids, develop into an embryonic form of the parasite called onchospheres that burrows through the intestinal wall and enters the bloodstream. From there it migrates into the muscles, eyes, and the brain, causing a condition called cysticercosis. Cysts in the brain often cause epileptic seizures.
- Protozoa. These include *Giardia lamblia*, *Entamoeba histolytica*, and *Cryptosporidium*. These organisms are some of the most common and infectious parasites in the world. They can be transmitted through contaminated food and water. They can also be spread from one person to another. Protozoa may spread throughout the body, causing abscesses in the lungs, liver, heart, and brain. Cramps, watery diarrhea, abdominal pain, and serious weight loss are common symptoms of Giardia infection. *Entamoeba histolytica* can cause dysentery, a severe form of intestinal infection, as well as liver and lung damage. Cryptosporidia can cause severe diarrhea in HIV/AIDS or cancer patients who have weakened immune systems.

CENTRAL NERVOUS SYSTEM PARASITIC INFECTIONS. *Toxoplasma gondii* is the most common parasite that invades the central nervous system (CNS). Humans become infected with this organism by eating raw or undercooked meat or by handling infected cat litter, which can contain eggs. Pregnant women who are infected may miscarry or deliver stillborn babies. Infected babies are born with congenital toxoplasmosis and have symptoms that include eye inflammation, blindness, jaundice, seizures, abnormally small or large heads, and mental retardation. In people with weakened immune systems, such as people with **AIDS**, toxoplasmosis can affect the whole body, causing inflammation, convulsions, trembling, headache, confusion, paralysis in half of the body, or coma.

Symptoms

The effects of parasites on their hosts depend on the health of the host, as well as the severity of the infestation. In diseased, old, or poorly fed individuals, parasite infestations can be fatal, but parasites do not typically kill their hosts, although they can slow growth and cause weight loss. Some plant parasites kill their hosts and then live on its decomposing remains, and certain species of hymenopteran insects are parasitoids, whose larva feeds within the living body of the host, eventually killing it.

Parasitic infections are difficult to diagnose because many individuals exhibit only vague symptoms or no symptoms at all. The following symptoms, although not unique to parasitic infections, may suggest that the individual is infected:

- diarrhea with foul-smelling stool that becomes worse in the later part of the day
- sudden changes in bowel habits (e.g., constipation that changes to soft and watery stool)
- constant rumbling and gurgling in the stomach area unrelated to hunger or eating
- heartburn or chest pain
- flu-like symptoms such as coughing, fever, and nasal congestion
- nonspecific food allergies
- itching around the nose, ears, and anus, especially at night
- weight loss with constant hunger

Other symptoms of parasitic infections include anemia, blood in the stool, bloating, diarrhea, gas, loss of appetite, intestinal obstruction, nausea, vomiting, sore mouth and gums, excessive nose picking, grinding teeth at night, chronic fatigue, headaches, muscle aches and pains, shortness of breath, skin rashes, depression, and memory loss.

Diagnosis

The following tests may be used to help doctors diagnose parasitic infections:

- Ova and parasite (O & P) test. Three to six stool samples are collected every one or two days to look for eggs and parasites.
- Cellophane tape (applied to the anal area). Ova (eggs) that stick to the tape prove pinworm infestation.
- Endoscopy. This procedure is used to obtain samples from the duodenum (the upper part of the small intestine), which are then analyzed for the presence of parasites.
- Urine sample and vaginal swab to detect *Trichomonas*, a parasite that causes vaginitis.
- Blood tests. High levels of eosinophils (a type of white blood cell) indicate infections. Antibodies against the parasites may also be detected. A study released in 2008 found that blood testing is often necessary to obtain a specific diagnosis. An increase in eosinophils, in particular, is associated with parasitic infections.
- X ray, MRI, and CT scans. X rays detect lesions in internal organs. Computed axial tomography (CT) scans and magnetic resonance imaging (MRI) are used to diagnose CNS parasitic infections.

Infected patients who are treated with anti-parasitic drugs or herbal remedies ought to be retested twice at the end of the treatment program; the tests should be given one month apart.

Treatment

Insect infestations

Infestations with lice, ticks, or fleas can be controlled by insecticides and attention to hygiene and household or environmental contact.

Intestinal parasites

Treatment for intestinal parasites usually involves anti-parasitic drugs. Depending on the severity of the condition and the species involved, treatment may include one (or more) of the following drugs: albendazole, furazolidone, iodoquinol, mebendazole, metronidazole, niclosamide, nitrazoxinide, paromomycin, pyrantel pamoate, pyrimethamine, quinacrine, sulfadiazine, or thiabendazole.

To prevent re-infection and transmission of disease, thorough cleaning of hands, clothes, sheets, and toys is recommended. Treatments should involve all members of the family and repeated treatments may be necessary.

CNS parasitic infections

Babies or HIV-infected individuals with toxoplasmosis are often given spiramycin or sulfadiazine plus pyrimethamine. Treatment may be continued indefinitely for HIV/AIDS patients to prevent recurrence.

Alternative treatment

Alternative and complementary therapies for parasitic infections reduce parasitic infections by improving nutrition and strengthening the immune system through herbal therapy and Ayurvedic medicine. Some herbal remedies are directly anti-parasitic and actually eliminate the organisms that cause disease. Patients who want to take allopathic anti-parasitic remedies should consult their doctor before using any of these herbs. Care should be taken before giving these remedies to children as they are rarely tested on children and adult dosage can cause overdose in children.

Nutritional therapy

The following dietary changes may help prevent or treat parasitic infections:

- Eating a well-balanced diet with lots of fiber, vegetables, fruits, whole grains, nuts, and seeds. Fiber helps eliminate worms from the intestines; good nutrition improves immune function and protects the body against parasitic invasion.
- Limiting dairy foods, sugar, and fat. Parasites thrive on these foods.
- Avoiding raw or undercooked fish, pork, or beef.
- Taking daily multivitamin/mineral supplements to prevent malnutrition and improve immune function.
- Supplementing the diet with probiotics such as *Lactobacillus acidophilus, Bifidobacteria*, and other beneficial intestinal bacteria that cultivate normal intestinal flora and suppress the spreading of parasites.

Herbal therapy

Herbal treatment should be given in combination with supportive dietary treatment and continued until the worms are completely eradicated. The following herbs are helpful in treating parasitic infestations:

- *Melaleuca alternifolia* (tea tree) oil. First discovered by Australian aborigines, tea tree oil has many uses, including treating intestinal parasites, lice, and ticks.
- *Artemisia annua* (wormwood herb) and citrus seed extract. These can be used together to help eliminate intestinal parasites such as *Giardia lamblia*.
- Berberine-containing herbs. Berberine is an antimicrobial alkaloid that can prevent parasites from attaching to the intestinal walls of human hosts. One study found that berberine was as effective against amoebal *Giardia lamblia* as metronidazole, the standard treatment. Herbs that contain berberine include goldenseal (*Hydrastis canadensis*), barberry (*Berberis vulgaris*), Oregon grape (*Berberis aquifolium*), and goldthread (*Coptis chinensis*).

> ## KEY TERMS
>
> **Eosinophil**—A type of white blood cell that increases in number in response to certain medical conditions, such as allergy or parasitic infection.
>
> **Intestines**—Also called the bowels and divided into the large and small intestine. They extend from the stomach to the anus, where waste products exit the body. The small intestine is about 20 ft (6.1 m) long and the large intestine, about 5 ft (1.5 m) long.
>
> **Protozoa**—Single-celled microorganisms belonging to the subkingdom Protozoa that are more complex than bacteria. About 30 protozoa cause diseases in humans.
>
> **Zoonotic**—Any disease or parasite of animals that can be transmitted to humans under natural conditions. Lyme disease and rabies are examples.

Ayurvedic medicine

Momordica charantia (bitter melon) is a safe remedy for pinworm infection. The melon is a vegetable shaped like a cucumber with a bitter taste. It can be found in most Oriental markets. It should be sliced thinly and eaten raw with other vegetables to reduce its bitter taste. Daily consumption of one to two bitter melons for seven to 10 days can eliminate pinworm infection. Patients may want to repeat the regimen after several months to prevent re-infection. Chinese herbal combinations also help treat parasitic infections by supporting the gastrointestinal system, stimulating immune response, and killing parasites.

Results

Though parasitic infections are difficult to diagnose, complete recovery from infestation can be achieved with appropriate therapy. Because re-infestation is common, multiple treatments may be necessary.

Prevention

The following measures can help prevent parasitic infections:

- Washing hands before eating and after using the toilet.
- Wearing gloves when gardening or working with soil or sand because soil can be contaminated with eggs or cysts of parasites.
- For pregnant women, avoiding handling cat litter.

> **QUESTIONS TO ASK YOUR DOCTOR**
>
> - If I am traveling to an underdeveloped country, how can I protect myself against parasite infection?
> - What side effects can I expect from the anti-parasitic drugs you have prescribed?
> - Are alternative therapies effective against parasite infection?
> - I have several symptoms that suggest a parasitic infection. What else might be causing those symptoms?
> - Can the type of parasite I am infected with be transmitted directly to other people?

- Not allowing children to be licked by pets; not allowing children to kiss pets that are not dewormed regularly.
- Washing fresh vegetables carefully. Many people get *Entamoeba histolytica* by eating contaminated raw fruit and vegetables.
- Avoiding eating raw meat, which may contain *Giardia lamblia*.
- Wearing long-sleeved shirts, long pants, and boots when walking in the woods. In addition, spraying insect repellent on clothing to prevent tick bites.

Resources

BOOKS

Drisdelle, Rosemary. *Parasites: Tales of Humanity's Most Unwelcome Guests*. Berkeley: University of California Press, 2010.

Dunn, Rob R. *The Wild Life of Our Bodies: Predators, Parasites, and Partners That Shape Who We Are Today*. New York: Harper, 2011

McGuire, Robert A. *Parasites, Pathogens, and Progress: Diseases and Economic Development*. Cambridge, MA: MIT Press, 2011.

Zuk, Marlene. *Riddled with Life: Friendly Worms, Ladybug Sex, and the Parasites That Make Us Who We Are*. New York: Mariner Books, 2008.

WEBSITES

American Academy of Family Physicians. "Pets and Parasites." Familydoctor.org http://familydoctor.org/familydoctor/en/prevention-wellness/staying-healthy/pets-animals/pets-and-parasites.printerview.all.html (accessed October 29, 2012).

MedlinePlus "Parasitic Disease." http://www.nlm.nih.gov/medlineplus/parasiticdiseases.html (accessed October 29, 2012).

Centers for Disease Control and Prevention. "Parasites." http://www.cdc.gov/parasite (accessed October 29, 2012).

Merck Manual Staff. "Approach to Parasitic Infections." http://www.merckmanuals.com/professional/infectious_diseases/approach_to_parasitic_infections/approach_to_parasitic_infections.html (accessed October 29, 2012).

World Health Organization. "Initiative for Vaccine Research: Parasitic Diseases." http://www.who.int/vaccine_research/diseases/soa_parasitic/en/index.html (accessed October 29, 2012).

ORGANIZATIONS

Centers for Disease Control and Prevention (CDC), 1600 Clifton Rd., Atlanta, GA 30333, (404) 639-3534, (800) CDC-INFO (800-232-4636); TTY: (888) 232-6348, inquiry@cdc.gov, http://www.cdc.gov.

National Institute of Allergy and Infectious Diseases Office of Communications and Government Relations, 6610 Rockledge Dr., MSC 6612, Bethesda, MD 20892-6612, (301) 496-5717, (866) 284-4107 or TDD: (800)877-8339, Fax: (301) 402-3573, ocpostoffice@niaid.nih.gov, http://www.niaid.nih.gov.

World Health Organization, Avenue Appia 20, 1211 Geneva 27, Switzerland, 2241 791 21 11, Fax: 2241 791 31 11, info@who.int, http://www.who.int.

Rhonda Cloos, RN
Tish Davidson, AM

Patch testing

Definition

A patch test is a method used to check for the cause or causes of irritant or allergic contact dermatitis, also known as an allergic reaction of the skin.

Description

Patch testing is a recognized and well-accepted way for dermatologists to determine which allergen or allergens are causing contact dermatitis. The test is not invasive and is extremely safe, making it a popular allergen-testing method.

Origins

Josef Jadassohn, known as the father of patch testing, discovered the possibilities of contact testing in 1895. At this time, Jadassohn was a professor of dermatology in Breslau (currently Wroclaw, Poland). He observed that one of his patients developed a skin rash to **mercury** bandages. Jadassohn realized looking at the skin's reaction to chemicals applied to it as a potential diagnostic tool.

The work of Jadassohn was expanded by Bruno Bloch, a professor in Switzerland. He wrote papers and textbooks on the clinical and experimental work he did in the field of contact testing. The field grew, and patch testing was officially brought to the United States in 1932 by Sulzberger and Wise.

The use of patch testing was slow to develop. Between its discovery and the 1960s, patch testing was heavily used by some European clinics and not at all by others. During this time, results often varied due to testing methods. The concentration of substances used and how the substances were delivered often changed depending on with who did the test and where it took place. Reading of results was not always done correctly, and at first there was little understanding of the difference between irritant and allergic contact dermatitis. As a result, the Scandinavian Committee for Standardization of Routine Patch Testing was formed in 1952, bringing standardization to patch testing. Shortly after, the North American Contact Dermatitis Group (NACDG) was also formed.

The work done by the NACDG was often informal, and in the 1980s, the Federal Drug Administration (FDA) banned the production and sale of patch test allergens in the United States. This decision forced the NACDG to do serious research on patch testing with the goal of getting the Hermal/Trolab's twenty-allergen patch test kit approved. Through the work of the NACDG and the foundation of other groups, such as the American Contact Dermatitis Society, research and funding for education about patch testing accelerated. As of 2012, patch testing is considered the gold standard for diagnosing contact dermatitis and is a common part of the curriculum in dermatology residency programs.

Purpose

The purpose of a patch test is to determine what allergen is causing contact dermatitis. There are two types of contact dermatitis. Irritant contact dermatitis is the most common type and occurs when the skin is repeatedly exposed over time to acids or alkaline materials that irritate the skin. Common irritants include soap, rubber gloves, and detergent. People with irritant contact dermatitis may experience red rashes that look like burns, dry skin, cuts on the hands, and pain.

Allergic contact dermatitis occurs when the skin comes in contact with a substance that it is extra sensitive or allergic to. Fabrics, adhesives, fragrances, hair dye, and material found in jewelry, such as nickel,

KEY TERMS

Allergen—A foreign substance that causes an allergic reaction in some sensitive people but not in most others.

Antihistamine—A medication used most commonly to treat allergic reactions and to block the effects of histamines, which can cause swelling and inflammation.

Dermatologist—A doctor who specializes in diseases and disorders of the skin.

and certain plants (e.g., poison ivy) are common allergens. Allergic contact dermatitis may also be caused by airborne allergies, such as insecticide, but this is much less common than direct contact. Red and patchy rashes are the common allergic reactions to these allergens. These rashes may have red bumps and blisters, feel warm and tender, or become thick and scaly. Often times, a reaction will not take place immediately, but instead appear 24–48 hours after exposure.

Limitations

Although patch testing is considered the gold standard in contact dermatitis testing, it does have some limitations. Patch testing uses only the most common allergens. Therefore, less common allergies will not be detected through patch testing. Additionally, patch testing can only be used for allergens that cause a reaction due to direct skin contact; it cannot detect allergies due to diet or inhaled substances. Patch testing should not be performed on women who are pregnant and nursing, and although it has been found to be safe, patch testing is not typically performed on children.

Patch testing results can be influenced by the use of creams, lotions, or antihistamines within 48 hours of testing. Sunbathing within four weeks before testing takes place also can influence results. It is important that tested areas remain dry during the test period, because patches that become wet or are removed too early cannot be read for correct results. Additionally, it is possible for false positives and negatives to occur.

Procedure

Patch testing is a relatively simple but time-consuming procedure. It requires three visits to the dermatologist within one week. Before having a patch test, patients should tell their physician of any medication they are taking and refrain from taking any antihistamines at least 48 hours before the first visit. Creams and lotions should also not be applied to the area where the patch test will take place for at least 48 hours before the procedure, and sunbathing should be avoided the four weeks before the test.

During the first visit, small patches are taped to the skin using hypoallergenic tape. Patches are almost always attached to a person's back because this is a large, flat, and out of the way area. Each patch contains a different substance that is a possible allergen. Depending on the number of patches being applied, this process can take 20 minutes or longer. Typically, anywhere from 30 to 160 patches may be used. Once the patches are taped, the position of each patch is marked with a special pen. The patient must keep the area with the patches dry until the final appointment. This means avoiding showering, bathing, or excessive exercise that will cause the person to sweat. Excessive bending and stretching should also be avoided in order to make sure the patches stay in place.

After the patches have been on for 48 hours, the patient must return to the dermatologist's office to have the patches removed. During this visit, the location of each patch may be once again marked as the tape and patches are taken off. The dermatologist will make a first reading of the area; however, no conclusions can be drawn at that time.

The patient must return to the dermatologist a third time to have the area read a second time and to receive results. This third visit typically takes place 48 hours after the patches have been removed (or 72–96 hours after the initial visit). During this visit, the dermatologist will be able to make conclusions about the test results.

Results

The dermatologist will read the area where the patches were located during the second and third visits. There are three possible results for each test site. A negative reaction has taken place when the skin does not show any irritation to the substance on the patch. A positive reaction occurs when there is an irritation. This reaction may range from weak to extreme. An uncertain reaction occurs when the dermatologist is not able to read the site for any clear positive or negative reaction.

A positive reaction signifies that a person is allergic to the substance on the patch. With this knowledge, a person should avoid further contact with this substance and wash away any trace of the irritant that

> **QUESTIONS TO ASK YOUR DOCTOR**
>
> - What should I do if one of my patches falls off before my second appointment?
> - Is patch testing safe for children?
> - How long will it take the irritation from a positive result to go away?

may be left behind. It is possible, but uncommon, for a person to be allergic to a substance that gave a negative result, or for a false positive takes place.

Side effects

The most common side effect of a patch test is irritation of the area where a positive reading was made. This can range from a small rash to blistering, scarring, or pigmentation of the skin in this area. Water should be used to wash away any trace of the irritant and moisturizers or anti-itch lotions may soothe the irritated area. Most often, the passing of time and the avoidance of the irritant is the best treatment. The irritation should go away on its own within two to three weeks. In extreme cases, a person may be prescribed corticosteroid pills. These pills are started with a high dose, which is then tapered off over 12 days.

Bacterial skin infections are a possible, but extremely rare, complication of patch tests. These infections are typically treated by a dermatologist or family physician.

Resources

BOOKS

Lachapelle, Jean Marie and Howard I. Maibach. *Patch Testing and Prick Testing*. New York: Springer, 2012.

WEBSITES

Cambridge University Hospitals. "What Does Patch Testing Involve?" http://www.cuh.org.uk/resources/pdf/patient_information_leaflets/PIN1300_patch_testing.pdf (accessed October 12, 2012).

MedlinePlus. "Allegery Testing—Skin." http://www.nlm.nih.gov/medlineplus/ency/article/003519.htm (accessed October 12, 2012).

MedlinePlus. "Contact Dermatitis." http://www.nlm.nih.gov/medlineplus/ency/article/000869.htm (accessed October 12, 2012).

ORGANIZATIONS

American Academy of Allergy, Asthma, and Immunology (AAAAI), 555 East Wells Street, Suite 1100, Milwaukee, WI 53202-3823, (414) 272-6071, info@aaaai.org, http://www.aaaai.org.

American Academy of Dermatology, P. O. Box 4014, Schaumburg, IL 60168, (847) 240-1859, (866) 503-7546, Fax: (847) 240-1859, MRC@aad.org, http://www.aad.org.

American Contact Dermatitis Society, 2323 North State Street #30, Bunnell, FL 32110, (386) 437-4405, Fax: (386) 437-4427, info@contactderm.org, http://www.contactderm.org.

Tish Davidson, AM

Pertussis *see* **Whooping cough**

Pesticide poisoning *see* **Insecticide poisoning**

Plague

Definition

Plague is a serious, potentially life-threatening infectious disease that is usually transmitted to humans by the bites of rodent fleas. There are three major forms of the disease: bubonic, septicemic, and pneumonic.

Description

Plague was one of the scourges of early human history. It has been responsible for three great world pandemics, which caused millions of deaths and significantly altered the course of history. A **pandemic** is a disease occurring in epidemic form throughout the entire population of a country, a people, or the world. Although the cause of the plague was not identified until the third pandemic in 1894, scientists are virtually certain that the first two pandemics were plague because a number of the survivors wrote about their experiences and described the symptoms.

The first great pandemic appeared in AD 542 and lasted for 60 years. It killed millions of citizens, particularly people living along the Mediterranean Sea. This sea was the busiest coastal trade route at that time and connected what is now southern Europe, northern Africa, and parts of coastal Asia. This pandemic is sometimes referred to as the Plague of Justinian, named for the great emperor of Byzantium who was ruling at the beginning of the outbreak. According to the historian Procopius, this outbreak of plague killed 10,000 people per day at its height just within the city of Constantinople.

The second pandemic occurred during the fourteenth century, and was called the Black Death because its main symptom was the appearance of black patches (caused by bleeding) on the skin. It was also a subject found in many European paintings, drawings, plays, and writings of that time. The connections between large active trading ports, rats coming off the ships, and the severe outbreaks of the plague were understood by people at the time. This was the most severe of the three, beginning in the mid–1300s with an origin in central Asia and lasting for 400 years. Between a fourth and a third of the entire European population died within a few years after plague was first introduced. Some smaller villages and towns were completely wiped out.

The final pandemic began in northern China, reaching Canton and Hong Kong by 1894. From there, it spread to all continents, killing millions.

The great pandemics of the past occurred when wild **rodents** spread the disease to rats in cities, and then to humans when the rats died. Another route for infection came from rats coming off ships that had traveled from heavily infected areas. Generally, these were busy coastal or inland trade routes. Plague was introduced into the United States during this pandemic and it spread from the West towards the Midwest and became **endemic** in the Southwest of the United States.

Risk factors

Plague occurs in areas where the bacteria are present in wild rodent populations. The risks are generally highest in rural areas, including homes that provide food and shelter for various rodents, such as ground squirrels, chipmunks and wood rats.

While plague is found in several countries, there is little risk to United States travelers within endemic areas (regions where a disease is known to be present) if they travel to urban areas with modern hotel facilities.

Demographics

According to the Centers for Disease Control (CDC), between 1900 and 2010, 999 confirmed or probable human plague cases occurred in the United States. Over 80% of cases have been the bubonic form. In recent decades, an average of 7 human plague cases are reported each year. Plague has occurred in people of all ages (infants up to age 96), though 50% of cases occur in people ages 12–45. Plague is most common in the southwestern states, particularly New Mexico, Arizona, and Colorado. Most cases in the United States are acquired from late spring to early fall. Around the world, there are between 1,000 and 2,000 cases of plague each year. Recent outbreaks in humans occurred in Africa, South America, and Southeast Asia.

Causes and symptoms

Fleas carry the bacterium *Yersinia pestis*, formerly known as *Pasteurella pestis*. The plague bacillus can be stained with Giemsa stain and typically looks like a safety pin under the microscope. When a flea bites an infected rodent, it swallows the plague bacteria. The bacteria are passed on when the fleas, in turn, bite a human. Interestingly, the plague bacterium grows in the gullet of the flea, obstructing it and not allowing the flea to eat. Transmission occurs during abortive feeding with regurgitation of bacteria into the feeding site. Humans also may become infected if they have a break or cut in the skin and come in direct contact with body fluids or tissues of infected animals.

More than 100 species of fleas have been reported to be naturally infected with plague; in the western United States, the most common source of plague is the golden-manteled ground squirrel flea. Chipmunks and prairie dogs have also been identified as hosts of infected fleas.

Since 1924, there have been no documented cases in the United States of human-to-human spread of plague from droplets. All but one of the few pneumonic cases have been associated with handling infected cats. While dogs and cats can become infected, dogs rarely show signs of illness and are not believed to spread disease to humans. However, plague has been spread from infected coyotes (wild dogs) to humans. In parts of central Asia, gerbils have been identified as the source of cases of bubonic plague in humans.

Bubonic plague

Two to five days after infection, patients experience a sudden fever, chills, seizures, and severe headaches, followed by the appearance of swellings or "buboes" in armpits, groin, and neck. The most commonly affected sites are the lymph glands near the site of the first infection. As the bacteria multiply in the glands, the lymph node becomes swollen. As the nodes collect fluid, they become extremely tender. Occasionally, the bacteria will cause an ulcer at the point of the first infection.

Septicemic plague

Bacteria that invade the bloodstream directly (without involving the lymph nodes) cause septicemic plague. (Bubonic plague also can progress to septicemic plague if not treated appropriately.) Septicemic plague that does not involve the lymph glands is particularly dangerous because it can be hard to diagnose the disease. The bacteria usually spread to other sites, including the liver, kidneys, spleen, lungs, and sometimes the eyes, or the lining of the brain. Symptoms include fever, chills, prostration, abdominal pain, shock, and bleeding into the skin and organs.

Pneumonic plague

Pneumonic plague may occur as a direct infection (primary) or as a result of untreated bubonic or septicemic plague (secondary). Primary pneumonic plague is caused by inhaling infective drops from another person or animal with pneumonic plague. Symptoms, which appear within one to three days after infection, include a severe, overwhelming pneumonia, with shortness of breath, high fever, and blood in the phlegm. If untreated, half the patients will die; if blood poisoning occurs as an early complication, patients may die even before the buboes appear.

Life-threatening complications of plague include shock, high fever, problems with blood clotting, and convulsions.

Diagnosis

Plague should be suspected if there are painful buboes, fever, exhaustion, and a history of possible exposure to rodents, rabbits, or fleas in the West or Southwest. The patient should be isolated. Chest

> **KEY TERMS**
>
> **Bioterrorism**—The use of disease agents to terrorize or intimidate a civilian population.
>
> **Buboes**—Smooth, oval, reddened, and very painful swellings in the armpits, groin, or neck that occur as a result of infection with the plague.
>
> **Endemic**—A disease that occurs naturally in a geographic area or population group.
>
> **Epidemic**—A disease that occurs throughout part of the population of a country.
>
> **Pandemic**—A disease that occurs throughout a regional group, the population of a country, or the world.
>
> **Septicemia**—The medical term for blood poisoning, in which bacteria have invaded the bloodstream and circulates throughout the body.

x rays are taken, as well as blood cultures, antigen testing, and examination of lymph node specimens. Blood cultures should be taken 30 minutes apart, before treatment.

A group of German researchers reported in 2004 on a standardized enzyme-linked immunosorbent assay (ELISA) kit for the rapid diagnosis of plague. The test kit was developed by the German military and has a high degree of accuracy as well as speed in identifying the plague bacillus. The kit could be useful in the event of a bioterrorist attack as well as in countries without advanced microbiology laboratories.

Treatment

As soon as plague is suspected, the patient should be isolated, and local and state departments notified. Drug treatment reduces the risk of death to less than 5%. The preferred treatment is streptomycin administered as soon as possible. Alternatives include gentamicin, chloramphenicol, tetracycline, or trimethoprim/sulfamethoxazole.

Public health role and response

Plague is one of three diseases still subject to international health regulations. These rules require that all confirmed cases be reported to the **World Health Organization** (WHO) within 24 hours of diagnosis. According to the regulations, passengers on an international voyage who have been to an area where there is an epidemic of pneumonic plague must be placed in isolation for six days before being allowed to leave.

Over the past few years, this infection primarily of antiquity has become a modern issue. This change has occurred because of the concerns about the use of plague as a weapon of biological warfare or terrorism (**bioterrorism**). Along with **anthrax** and **smallpox**, plague is considered to be a significant risk. In this scenario, the primary manifestation is likely to be pneumonic plague transmitted by clandestine aerosols. It has been reported that during World War II the Japanese dropped "bombs" containing plague-infected fleas in China as a form of biowarfare.

Prognosis

Plague can be treated successfully if it is caught early; the mortality rate for treated disease is 1–15% but 40–60% in untreated cases. Untreated pneumonic plague is almost always fatal, however, and the chances of survival are very low unless specific antibiotic treatment is started within 15–18 hours after symptoms appear. The presence of plague bacteria in a blood smear is a grave sign and indicates septicemic plague. Septicemic plague has a mortality rate of 40% in treated cases and 100% in untreated cases.

QUESTIONS TO ASK YOUR DOCTOR

- What is plague?
- How is it transmitted?
- What are the different forms of plague?
- What is the best course of treatment?
- What are the best prevention measures?

Prevention

Anyone who has come in contact with a plague pneumonia victim should be given antibiotics, since untreated pneumonic plague patients can pass on their illness to close contacts throughout the course of the illness. All plague patients should be isolated for 48 hours after antibiotic treatment begins. Pneumonic plague patients should be completely isolated until sputum cultures show no sign of infection.

Residents of areas where plague is found should keep rodents out of their homes. Anyone working in a rodent-infested area should wear insect repellent on skin and clothing. Pets can be treated with insecticidal dust and kept indoors. Handling sick or dead animals (especially rodents and cats) should be avoided.

Plague vaccines have been used with varying effectiveness since the late nineteenth century. Experts believe that **vaccination** lowers the chance of infection and the severity of the disease. However, the effectiveness of the vaccine against pneumonic plague is not clearly known.

Vaccinations against plague are not required to enter any country. Because immunization requires multiple doses over a 6–10 month period, plague vaccine is not recommended for quick protection during outbreaks. Moreover, its unpleasant side effects make it a poor choice unless there is a substantial long-term risk of infection. The safety of the vaccine for those under age 18 has not been established. Pregnant women should not be vaccinated unless the need for protection is greater than the risk to the unborn child. Even those who receive the vaccine may not be completely protected. The inadequacy of the vaccines available as of the early 2000s explains why it is important to protect against rodents, fleas, and people with plague. A team of researchers in the United Kingdom reported in the summer of 2004 that an injected sub-unit vaccine is likely to offer the best protection against both bubonic and pneumonic forms of plague.

Resources

BOOKS

Aberth, John. *Plagues in World History*. Lanham, MD: Rowman & Littlefield Publishers, 2011.

Beers, Mark H., Robert S. Porter, and Thomas V. Jones, eds. *The Merck Manual of Diagnosis and Therapy*. 18th ed. Whitehouse Station, NJ: Merck Research Laboratories, 2006.

Slack, Paul. *Plague: A Very Short Introduction*. New York, NY: Oxford University Press, 2012.

PERIODICALS

Bitam, Idir, et al. "Fleas and flea–borne diseases." *International Journal of Infectious Diseases* (August 2010): 667–676.

Chouikha, I., and B. J. Hinnebusch. "Yersinia—flea interactions and the evolution of the arthropod–borne transmission route of plague." *Current Opinion in Microbiology* 15, no. 3 (June 2012): 239–246.

Gage, K. L. "Factors affecting the spread and maintenance of plague." *Advances in Experimental Medicine and Biology* 953 (2012): 79–94.

Oyston, P. C., and E. D. Williamson. "Modern Advances against Plague." *Human Pathology* 81 (2012): 209–241.

WEBSITES

Plague. Centers for Disease Control. http://www.cdc.gov/plague/ (accessed June 13, 2012).

Plague. Medline Plus. http://www.nlm.nih.gov/medlineplus/plague.html (accessed June 6, 2012).

Plague. NIAID. http://www.niaid.nih.gov/topics/plague/pages/default.aspx (accessed October 13, 2012).

ORGANIZATIONS

Centers for Disease Control and Prevention (CDC), 1600 Clifton Road, Atlanta, GA 30333, (800) 232-4636, cdcinfo@cdc.gov, http://www.cdc.gov.

National Institute of Allergies and Infectious Diseases, 6610 Rockledge Drive, MSC 6612, Bethesda, MD 208926612, ((301)) 496-5717, Fax: ((301)) 402-3573, ((866)) 284-4107, ocpostoffice@niaid.nih.gov, http://www.niaid.nih.gov.

World Health Organization (WHO), Avenue Appia 201211, Geneva, Switzerland 27, 41 22 791-2111, info@who.int, http://www.who.int.

Arnold Cua, MD
Rebecca J. Frey, PhD

Pneumoconioses *see* **Silicosis**

Polio

Definition

Poliomyelitis, or polio, is an infectious disease caused by a virus that normally lives in the human digestive tract. About 90% of persons infected by the virus have no symptoms at all. In the other 10%, the polio virus causes an infection with symptoms ranging from a mild flu-like illness to paralysis of the lower limbs or death from paralysis of the muscles that control breathing.

Description

The term poliomyelitis comes from the Greek words *polio*, meaning gray, and *myelon*, referring to the spinal cord. The term is accurate, as an important consequence of the disease is the involvement of the spinal cord.

Polio was widespread in the developed countries of Europe and North America in the first part of the twentieth century. The epidemics not only became more severe, but also affected adolescents and adults rather than mostly children. The older average age of patients was also marked by increased severity of symptoms. Since the introduction of effective vaccines, paralytic polio is almost unknown in the United States except for a few cases among recent immigrants and travelers who have contracted the disease outside the United States; the last case of wild polio occurred in the United States in 1979. In 1988, the **World Health Organization** (WHO) began the Global Polio Eradication Initiative with the goal of wiping out **endemic** polio by 2006.

There are three known types of polioviruses (called 1, 2, and 3), each causing a different strain of the disease. All are members of the viral family of enteroviruses, which are **viruses** that infect the gastrointestinal tract. Type 1 is the cause of epidemics and about 85% of cases of paralysis, which is the most severe manifestation of the infection.

When the poliovirus reaches the central nervous system, inflammation and destruction of the spinal cord motor cells (anterior horn cells) occurs, which prevents them from sending out impulses to muscles. Loss of impulse transmission causes the muscles to become limp or soft and they cannot contract. This condition is referred to as flaccid paralysis. The extent of the paralysis depends on where the virus strikes and the number of cells that it destroys. Usually, some of the limb muscles are paralyzed; the abdominal muscles or muscles of the back may be paralyzed, affecting the

JONAS E. SALK (1914–1995)

Jonas Salk was born in New York, New York, on October 28, 1914. He received his medical degree from New York University in 1939. In 1942, Salk began working for a former teacher, Thomas Francis, Jr., to produce influenza vaccines, a project that continued until 1949. That year, as a research professor, Salk began a three-year project sponsored by the National Foundation for Infantile Paralysis, also known as the March of Dimes. Caused by the poliomyelitis virus, polio was also known as infantile paralysis. Periodic outbreaks of the disease, which attacks the nervous system, caused death or a lifetime of paralysis, especially in children. It was a difficult disease to study because sufficient viruses could not be obtained. Unlike bacteria that can be grown in cultures, viruses need living tissue on which to grow. Once a method for preparing viruses was discovered and improved, sufficient viruses became available for research.

Salk first set out to confirm that there were three virus types responsible for polio and then began to experiment with ways to kill the virus and yet retain its ability to produce an immune response. By 1952, he had produced a dead virus vaccine that worked against the three virus types. He began testing. First the vaccine was tested on monkeys, then on children who had recovered from the disease, and finally on Salk's family and children, none of whom had ever had the disease. Following large-scale trials in 1954, the vaccine was finally released for public use in 1955. The Salk vaccine was not the first vaccine against polio, but it was the first to be found safe and effective. By 1961, there was a 96% reduction in polio cases in the United States.

---

person's posture. The neck muscles may become too weak for the head to be lifted. Paralysis of the face muscles may cause the mouth to twist or the eyelids to droop. According to WHO, one of every 200 infections leads to paralysis. Of those, between 5% and 10% die because their breathing muscles become paralyzed.

Risk factors

Humans are the only natural host of polioviruses; these viruses are not transmitted by animals. Some people are more likely than others to develop the paralytic form of the disease if they do become infected. These include:

- young children
- elderly adults
- people who engage in hard physical labor or strenuous exercise
- people who have recently had a tonsillectomy or dental surgery
- pregnant women
- people who travel frequently to areas where polio is still endemic
- people with an immune system weakened by HIV/AIDS or certain types of cancer treatment

Demographics

According to the Centers for Disease Prevention and Control (CDC), the incidence rate has been less than 0.01 cases per 100,000 people in the United States since 1965.

Worldwide, polio has come close to being eradicated. In 1988, polio was endemic in 125 countries. By mid-2012, it was endemic in only 3—Afghanistan, Pakistan, and Nigeria. However, in June 2012, the Taliban, a fundamentalist insurgent group in Afghanistan and Pakistan, forced stoppage of the polio **vaccination** program in Pakistan for fear that doctors with the program were working as spies for the United States. A similar boycott of the polio vaccination program occurred in Nigeria in 2003 when rumors were spread that the vaccine contained anti-fertility drugs to prevent Muslim men from fathering children. Although the vaccination program resumed 12 months later, The disease had returned to large areas of Nigeria and as of 2012 had not yet been eradicated.

Causes and symptoms

Polio is caused by a virus that enters the mouth through food or water that has been contaminated by fecal matter. It is an extremely contagious illness; anyone living with a recently infected person is likely to become infected too. Although people carrying the poliovirus are most contagious for 7–10 days before and after symptoms (if any) appear, they can spread the virus for weeks in their bowel movements.

Once inside the body, the polio virus takes between 6 and 20 days to incubate. It finds its way to the tissues lining the throat and the intestinal tract, where it multiplies rapidly. After about a week in the intestines, the virus travels to the tonsils and the lymph nodes, where it multiplies further and then enters the bloodstream. It can remain within the blood and lymphatic system for as long as 17 weeks. In a minority of cases, the virus enters the central nervous system from the blood and lymph. It then multiplies in and destroys the nerve cells (motor neurons) in the brain and spinal cord that control the movements of the muscles. The location and severity of the paralytic polio that results when the motor neurons are damaged varies with the part of the central nervous system that is affected.

Minor forms of acute polio infection

Between 4 and 8% of acute polio infections are characterized by influenza-like symptoms. This type of infection is called abortive poliomyelitis. People with this form of polio infection experience sore throat and fever, nausea, vomiting, abdominal pain, constipation, or diarrhea. Abortive polio is difficult to distinguish from influenza or other viral infections. Patients recover completely in about a week.

About 10% of people infected with poliovirus develop severe headache and pain and stiffness of the neck and back. These symptoms are due to an inflammation of the meninges (tissues that cover the spinal cord and brain). This syndrome is called nonparalytic or aseptic **meningitis**. The term "aseptic" is used to differentiate this type of meningitis from those caused by bacteria. Patients with nonparalytic meningitis may experience a brief period of general illness followed by stiffness in the neck, back, or legs. They may also experience other abnormal sensations for a period of 2–10 days. As with abortive polio, patients with nonparalytic meningitis recover completely.

Paralytic polio

Between 1 and 2% of people infected with poliovirus develop the most severe form, paralytic polio. Some of these individuals may have 2–3 symptom-free days between the minor illness and the major illness, but often the symptoms appear without any previous minor illness. Symptoms again include headache and back and neck pain. The major symptoms, however, are due to invasion of the motor nerves, which are responsible for movement of the muscles.

Paralytic polio is usually divided into three types, depending on whether the paralysis affects the arms and legs (spinal polio; accounts for 79% of cases of paralytic polio); breathing, speaking, and swallowing (bulbar polio; 2% of cases); or the limbs as well as breathing and other functions (bulbospinal polio; 19% of cases). Bulbar polio is particularly likely to lead to death if the patient is not placed on a respirator because the virus affects the brain stem—the part of the brain that controls heartbeat as well as breathing and other vital functions.

The maximum state of paralysis in paralytic polio is usually reached within a few days of the onset of symptoms. The remaining unaffected nerves then begin the process of attempting to grow branches to compensate for the destroyed nerves. Often, the nerve cells are not completely destroyed. By the end of a month, the nerve impulses start to return to the apparently paralyzed muscle and by the end of six months, recovery is almost complete. In cases where the nerve cells are completely destroyed, however, paralysis is permanent.

Diagnosis

The diagnosis of polio is based on a combination of the patient's history and the type and location of symptoms—particularly such symptoms as a stiff neck, difficulty breathing, or abnormal reflexes. Fever and asymmetric flaccid paralysis without sensory loss in a child or young adult almost always indicate poliomyelitis. Nonparalytic poliomyelitis cannot be distinguished clinically from aseptic meningitis due to other agents. Virus isolated from a throat swab and/or feces or blood tests that demonstrate the rise in a specific antibody are required to confirm the diagnosis.

Examination

TESTS. To confirm the diagnosis, samples of the patient's stool, spinal fluid, or throat mucus may be collected and sent to a laboratory for analysis to see whether the sample contains the virus itself. A blood sample early in the infection may also be analyzed for evidence of antibodies to the poliovirus.

PROCEDURES. A lumbar puncture is the procedure performed in order to obtain a sample of the patient's spinal fluid. A long, thin needle is inserted into the lower back between the vertebrae to withdraw spinal fluid. This test can be used to reveal an increased number of white blood cells and no bacteria (aseptic meningitis).

Treatment

There is no drug that can cure polio as of 2012. Antibiotics are ineffective against any viral infection, including polio. Patients with abortive polio or nonparalytic meningitis do not usually need treatment other than resting at home.

Patients with paralytic polio may be placed on a respirator to help them breathe, particularly if they are diagnosed with bulbar polio. Other treatments include painkillers and hot packs for muscle aches, physical therapy to restore muscle strength, and occupational or speech therapy as needed. Physical therapy is the most important part of management of paralytic polio during recovery. Braces or special shoes may be recommended for some patients. A few patients may undergo surgery to restore limb function.

Prognosis

The overall prognosis for recovery from an acute attack of paralytic polio is generally good. Mortality is about 5–10%, mostly in elderly and very young patients; however, the death rate can reach 20–60% in cases of bulbar involvement. Half the patients with spinal polio recover fully; 25% have mild disabilities; and the remaining 25% are left with severe disabilities. Most patients recover from breathing problems, and only a small percentage of patients need long-term treatment on a respirator. Patients with muscle paralysis typically recover about 60% of their strength in the first 3–4 months of treatment.

About a quarter of patients who have recovered from paralytic polio develop a disorder called post-polio syndrome (PPS) between 10 and 40 years after the initial infection. PPS is not a re-infection although its cause is not completely understood as of 2009. PPS is marked by:

- muscular weakness
- fatigue
- being easily exhausted after even small amounts of activity
- joint pain
- sleep disorders
- difficulty breathing or swallowing
- inability to tolerate cold temperatures

PPS is treated with rest and such supportive measures as powered wheelchairs, pain relievers, and medications to help the patient sleep. Patients are also encouraged to simplify their work habits and take frequent rest breaks.

Public health role and response

The World Health Organization has sponsored the initiative to eradicate polio. They work in conjunction with public health agencies and non-governmental organizations around the world, with their effort concentrated in countries where polio is still present.

KEY TERMS

Aseptic—Sterile; containing no microorganisms, especially no bacteria.

Asymptomatic—Having no symptoms of a disease even though the person may be infected by the organism that causes the disease.

Brainstem—The stalk of the brain that connects the two cerebral hemispheres to the spinal cord.

Endemic—A term applied to a disease that maintains itself in a particular area without reinforcement from outside sources of infection.

Flaccid—Weak, soft, or floppy.

Gastrointestinal—Pertaining to the stomach and intestines.

Lymph/lymphatic—One of the three body fluids that is transparent and a slightly yellow liquid that is collected from the capillary walls into the tissues and circulates back to the blood supply.

Meningitis—Inflammation of the membranes that cover the brain and spinal cord.

Motor neuron—A type of cell in the central nervous system that controls the movement of muscles either directly or indirectly.

Neurologic—Pertaining to the nervous system.

Paralysis—The inability to voluntarily move.

Because humans are the only host to the polio virus, it is possible that the virus can, like the **smallpox** virus, be completely eliminated by properly supported and coordinated vaccination efforts.

Prevention

Polio can easily be prevented by administration of either the Salk vaccine, which contains an inactivated poliovirus, or the Sabin oral vaccine, which contains a weakened live virus. The Salk vaccine (also called the inactivated polio vaccine or IPV) is given as a series of four shots administered at 2 months, 4 months, between 6 and 18 months and a booster given between 4 and 6 years. This immunization contains no live virus, just the components of the virus that provoke the recipient's immune system to react as if the recipient were actually infected with the poliovirus without causing polio symptoms. The recipient thus becomes immune to infection with the poliovirus in the future. The United States switched exclusively to using IPV rather than oral polio vaccine in 1999. It is the only

> **QUESTIONS TO ASK YOUR DOCTOR**
>
> - Why is it necessary for my baby to be immunized against polio when the disease is no longer found in my country?
> - I have read a lot about the side effects of various vaccines. What are the risks associated with administration of the polio vaccine to infants?
> - I am going to travel to a country where polio is still found. I was vaccinated against the disease as a child. Should I be re-vaccinated?
> - If I travel to a place where polio exists, what other precautions besides vaccination should I take?

polio vaccine that can safely be given to people with weakened immune systems.

The Sabin vaccine (also called the oral polio vaccine or OPV) is given to infants and adults by mouth in several doses. OPV contains the live, but weakened, poliovirus, which make the recipient immune to future infections with poliovirus. OPV is less expensive to administer than IPV. It requires no injections, thus no sterile needles, and is easily administered to both children and adults. For these reason, it is often used in the developing world. It is not routinely given to people with weakened immune systems because it contains a live virus and can very rarely cause polio.

Resources

BOOKS

Closser, Svea. *Chasing Polio in Pakistan: Why the World's Largest Public Health Initiative May Fail.* Nashville, TN: Vanderbilt University Press, 2010.

Hecht, Alan. *Polio.* New York: Chelsea House, 2009.

Krasner, Robert I. *Twentieth-century Microbe Hunters: Their Lives, Accomplishments, and Legacies.* Sudbury, MA: Jones and Bartlett Publishers, 2008.

Presley, Gary. *Seven Wheelchairs: A Life beyond Polio.* Iowa City: University of Iowa Press, 2008.

WEBSITES

Polio and Post-Polio Syndrome. MedlinePlus March 6, 2012 [accessed June 25, 2012]. http://www.nlm.nih.gov/medlineplus/polioandpostpoliosyndrome.html

Polio Vaccination. Centers for Disease Control and Prevention. January 3, 2012 [accessed June 25, 2012]. http://www.cdc.gov/vaccines/vpd-vac/polio/default.htm

Weiler, Christine. Acute Poliomyelitis. Medscape.com January 18, 2012 [accessed June 25, 2012]. http://emedicine.medscape.com/article/306440-overview

World Health Organization (WHO). Poliomyelitis 2012 [accessed June 25, 2012]. http://www.who.int/topics/poliomyelitis/en

ORGANIZATIONS

American Physical Therapy Association, 1111 North Fairfax Street, Alexandria, VA 22314-1488, (703) 684-APTA (2782). TDD: (703) 683-6748, (800) 999-APTA (2782, Fax: (703) 683-6748, http://www.apta.org.

March of Dimes Foundation, 1275 Mamaroneck Avenue, White Plains, NY 10605, (914)997-4488, askus@marchofdimes.com, http://www.marchofdimes.com.

National Institute of Allergy and Infectious Diseases Office of Communications and Government Relations, 6610 Rockledge Drive, MSC 6612, Bethesda, MD 20892-6612, (301) 496-5717, (866) 284-4107 or TDD: (800)877-8339 (for hearing impaired), Fax: (301) 402-3573, http://www3.niaid.nih.gov.

United States Centers for Disease Control and Prevention (CDC), 1600 Clifton Road, Atlanta, GA 30333, (404) 639-3534, 800-CDC-INFO (800-232-4636). TTY: (888) 232-6348, inquiry@cdc.gov, http://www.cdc.gov.

World Health Organization, Avenue Appia 20, 1211 Geneva 27, Switzerland, +22 41 791 21 11, Fax: +22 41 791 31 11, info@who.int, http://www.who.int.

Linda K. Bennington, CNS
Rebecca J. Frey, PhD
Tish Davidson, AM

Pollution *see* **Air pollution, Noise pollution, Water pollution**

Population and disease

Definition

The study of the relationship between population and disease generally falls under the discipline of **epidemiology**, although it may also be studied under the relatively new field of disease ecology.

Description

Epidemiology is defined by the **World Health Organization** (WHO) as "the study of the distribution and determinants of health-related states (including disease), and the application of this study to the control of diseases and other health problems." This means is that epidemiologists look at where specific health problems are found and how they spread among the population as a whole and among certain subgroups of the population (i.e., distribution) and the factors and causes (i.e., determinants) of these diseases and disorders. They then use this information to help prevent and control diseases and disorders and improve public health. Epidemiologists differ from clinical physicians because they work to understand the steps needed to prevent or cure disease in whole populations or subpopulations, while clinical physicians generally are focused on preventing or curing disease in individual patients.

Origins

The word epidemiology comes from three Greek words. *Epi* means "among", *demos* refers to "people", and *ology* means "study". Thus, epidemiology means the study of what (health issues) are among the people.

From the earliest times, physicians have sought to understand the causes of disease, but a systematic study of the causes and spread of disease in entire populations did not take off until the mid-1800s. A massive **cholera** outbreak occurred in London in late August 1854. Within three days 127 people died. The death rate of those who became ill was about 12%. Before the outbreak was over, more than 600 people died. John Snow (1813–1858), a physician, essentially established the science of epidemiology when he had the idea of mapping the locations where cholera cases occurred. Snow's map showed that most cholera cases clustered around certain city water pumps, while very few cases of cholera occurred in buildings with private wells.

Snow convinced the municipal authorities to disable a public pump in the Soho area of London where the number of cholera cases was highest. Almost immediately, the cholera outbreak subsided in that area. From this, Snow as able to deduce that cholera was caused by contamination of the water. Snow's discovery was the beginning of the science that became epidemiology. His findings were a major event in public health and helped shift the focus of water treatment from taste and clarity to controlling waterborne pathogens.

The history of epidemiology is closely connected to the history of public health. Until the 1940s, epidemiologists were primarily concerned with learning how **communicable diseases** were cause and how they spread. It was well known that when people were crowded together, disease was common and spread quickly and easily. In studying diseases such as **tuberculosis**, epidemiologists came to understand that population density alone was not responsible for disease distribution. Socioeconomic factors were also at work.

KEY TERMS

Cholera—An infection of the small intestine caused by a type of bacterium. The disease is spread by drinking water or eating seafood or other foods that have been contaminated with the feces of infected people. It occurs in parts of Asia, Africa, Latin America, India, and the Middle East. Symptoms include watery diarrhea and exhaustion. It is often fatal to young children and the elderly.

Pathogen—Any disease-causing microorganism.

Severe acute respiratory syndrome (SARS)—A potentially fatal viral respiratory illness that emerged from Asia in 2003.

Tuberculosis—A highly contagious, often fatal, bacterial infection of the lungs.

People who lived in crowded conditions generally were less well nourished, had limited access to health care, were less well educated about disease, often shared living space with disease-carrying animals (rats, insects), and tended to have more physically stressful lives than people who lived in less crowded conditions. Understanding the connection between socioeconomic factors and disease informed public health policy throughout the first half of the twentieth century.

Populations and environmental disease

Beginning in the middle of the twentieth century, epidemiologists began to look beyond the distribution and determinants of infectious disease to study the effect of behavior and environmental conditions on noncommunicable diseases. The relationship between tobacco use and lung cancer was one of the earliest studies of this nature. By 1964, this relationship was soundly established. The tobacco-health connection and resulted in legal changes in the way cigarettes were advertised and label, along with a major push by public health organizations to develop **smoking** cessation programs.

The publication of Rachel Carson's book *Silent Spring* in 1962 increased awareness of chemicals and toxins in the environment and started the environmental movement. Epidemiology expanded into studying the relationship between environmental toxins other noncommunicable diseases. Examples include the relationship between **asthma** and **air** pollution, **asbestos** exposure and mesothelioma, and ultraviolet light and malignant **melanoma**. Legal changes in allowable exposure to toxins, banning of certain chemicals, and better product labeling have occurred and will continue to occur because of this research.

Other branches of epidemiology still focus on tracking emergent communicable diseases such as avian influenza and **SARS**, while still others concentrate on the relationship between social habits, living environments, and disease in various subpopulations. As more and more is learned about the connection between changes in genes and the development of specific diseases, epidemiologists will likely expand their study of the role environmental toxins play as triggers for genetic changes in specific subpopulations.

Resources

BOOKS

Merril, Ray M. *Introduction to Epidemiology.*. Burlington, MA: Jones & Bartlett Learning, 2013.

Sinha, B. R. K. *Population, Environment and Development.*. New Delhi, India: New Century Publications, 2009.

PERIODICALS

Dobson, Andrew P. and E. Robin Carper. "Infectious Diseases and Human Population History." *BioScience*. 46 no.2 (February 1996):115–126.

McMichael, Anthony J. "Population, Environment, Disease, and Survival: Past Patterns, Uncertain Futures." *Lancet*. 359 no. 9312 (March 2002): 1145–1148.

WEBSITES

Saracci, Rudolph. "Introducing the History of Epidemiology." http://fds.oup.com/www.oup.com/pdf/13/9780192630667.pdf (accessed October 24, 2012).

"The WWW Virtual Health Library: Medicine and Health: Epidemiology;." University of California San Francisco Department of Epidemiology and Biostatistics. http://www.epibiostat.ucsf.edu/epidem/epidem.html (accessed October 23, 2012).

ORGANIZATIONS

National Institute of Environmental Health Science, P.O. Box 12233, MD K3-16, Research Triangle Park, NC 27709, (919) 541-1919, Fax: (919) 541-4395, http://www.niehs.nih.gov.

United States Centers for Disease Control and Prevention (CDC), 1600 Clifton Road, Atlanta, GA 30333, (404) 639-3534, (800) CDC-INFO (800-232-4636); TTY: (888) 232-6348, inquiry@cdc.gov, http://www.cdc.gov.

World Health Organization, Avenue Appia 20, 1211 Geneva 27, Switzerland, +2241 791 21 11, Fax: +2241 791 31 11, info@who.int, http://www.who.int.

Tish Davidson, AM

Population pyramid

Definition

A populations pyramid, or age picture diagram, is a sociological tool used to illustrate age distribution within age groups in a population (as of a country or region).

Description

The graphical representation is designed as a back-to-back bar graph with an X and Y axis, one side for males, one side for females within an age group, typically 5- or 10-year increments. Bars are drawn starting from the central Y-axis as a percentage of the population with the total amount on both sides of the Y-axis equal 100% of the population. The model is called a population pyramid because of the frequent pyramidal formation that age distribution takes in a society, with more young persons than elderly.

Origins

The originator of the population pyramid is unknown. Population pyramid data come from primary sources, including the **World Health Organization** (WHO), World Bank, UNESCO, CIA, and individual country databases for global health and causes of death. In the United States, the National Institutes for Health (NIH) and census data completed at the federal level are used. In areas without central government population, information can be gathered through privately organized and operated surveying, usually done through academic research groups.

Stages of demographic transition

- Stable pyramid: A population pyramid with practically straight lines indicating equal numbers of individuals in all age ranges shows an unchanging pattern of fertility and mortality has steady population, with no populations growth rate.
- Stationary pyramid: This low fertility, high mortality rate pyramid shows a country where population growth is at a low percentage.
- Expansive pyramid: A population pyramid that shows a high proportion of youth, with rapid rate of population growth, and a low proportion of older people indicates a booming population, possibly as a result of poor family planning. A steady narrowing as the age increases indicates increased death rates at each age range. A high birth rate, a high death rate, and a short life expectancy can be the typical pattern of a less economically developed country.

- Constrictive or contracting pyramid: Population pyramids that have lower numbers of youth and a larger elderly population indicate longer life spans and a low death rate due to better medical care, access to birth control, and other population control measures as for very developed countries, where high levels of education lead to better medicine and family planning.

Results

Population pyramids can tell sociologists more than just the fertility and morality rates of a country. These graphical depictions also tell a story of the equality a population has between the sexes. For example, the population pyramid for China would show a significant number of male youths because after the one child policy went into effect, parents chose to keep male children over female children. Similarly, male dominated societies and countries that devalue females would have a male-skewed pyramid.

Economists and corporations can also use population pyramids, among other tools, for applications such as choosing the best markets for certain goods and services. They also show how a population is growing, allowing for infrastructure planning, and other such population-based decision making.

Furthermore, some demographers claim that historical and future periods of social unrest can be predicted by identifying a so-called youth bulge. A youth bulge occurs when a country has a large unemployed youth population, as in the case of the modern-day Middle East.

Resources

BOOKS

Fuller, Gary. "The Demographic Backdrop to Ethnic Conflict: A Geographic Overview." Washington, DC: CIA.

WEBSITES

Population Action. "The Shape of Things to Come." http://populationaction.org/Publications2/Data_and_Maps/Shape_of_Things_to_Come/Summary.php (accessed October 12, 2012).

World Life Expectancy. "World Population Pyramid." http://www.worldlifeexpectancy.com/world-population-pyramid (accessed October 12, 2012).

ORGANIZATIONS

National Institutes of Health, 9000 Rockville Pike, Bethesda, MD 20892, (301) 496-4000, NIHinfo@od.nih.gov, nih.gov.

World Health Organization, Avenue Appia 20, 1211 Geneva 27, Switzerland, 2241 791 21 11, Fax: 2241 791 31 11, info@who.int, http://www.who.int.

Alyson C. Heimer, MA

Post-traumatic stress disorder

Definition

Post-traumatic stress disorder (PTSD) is a complex psychiatric condition that specifically involves anxiety. It may also be written as posttraumatic stress disorder. People develop PTSD after they experience or witness an event that is perceived to be a threat or considered to be life-threatening and in which they experience fear, terror, or helplessness.

Description

PTSD is sometimes summarized as "a normal reaction to abnormal events." It was first defined as a distinctive disorder in 1980. Originally diagnosed in veterans of the Vietnam War (1955–1975), it is now recognized in civilian survivors of rape or other criminal assaults; natural disasters; aircraft crashes, train collisions, serious accidents, or industrial explosions; acts of terrorism; child abuse; or military combat. Most people who have experienced such trauma return to a normal life. However, some people continue to experience the stress of reliving such trauma, often in the form of nightmares, flashbacks, sleep problems, and other such symptoms that impair daily life. These persons may develop PTSD.

Soldiers in the early nineteenth century were diagnosed by medical doctors with exhaustion after experiencing the trauma and stress of war. Often these soldiers displayed degraded mental facilities that sometimes included physical symptoms, which forced them into treatment until their symptoms subsided and they could return to combat. Although these soldiers were diagnosed with such terms as battle fatigue, shell shock, and stress syndrome, the medical community did not recognize PTSD until the 1970s, during the Vietnam War.

The experience of PTSD has sometimes been described as being in a horror film that keeps replaying and cannot be shut off. It is common for people with PTSD to feel intense fear and helplessness, and to relive the frightening event in nightmares or in their waking hours. Sometimes the memory is triggered by a sound, smell, or image that reminds the individual of the traumatic event. These re-experiences of the event are called flashbacks. Persons with PTSD are likely to be jumpy and easily startled or to go numb emotionally and lose interest in activities they used to enjoy. They may have problems with memory and with getting enough sleep. In some cases, they may feel disconnected from the real world or have moments in which their own bodies seem unreal. These symptoms are indications of dissociation, a process in which the mind splits off certain memories or thoughts from conscious awareness. Many people with PTSD turn to alcohol or drugs in order to escape the flashbacks and other symptoms of the disorder, even if only for a few minutes.

Risk factors

Factors that influence the likelihood of a person developing PTSD include:

- The nature, intensity, and duration of the traumatic experience: For example, someone who just barely escaped from the World Trade Center in New York City before the towers collapsed on September 11, 2001, is at greater risk of PTSD than someone who saw the collapse from a distance or on television.
- A person's previous history: People who were abused as children, who were separated from their parents at an early age, or who have a previous history of anxiety or depression are at increased risk of PTSD.
- Genetic factors: Vulnerability to PTSD is known to run in families.
- The availability of social support after the event: People who have no family or friends are more likely to develop PTSD than those who do.

HIGH-RISK POPULATIONS. About 8% of Americans experience PTSD at some point in their lives; however, women (10.4%) are just over twice as likely as men (5%) to develop PTSD. Around 3.5% of adults in the United States from the age of 18 to 54 years have PTSD during any given year. Some subpopulations in the United States are at greater risk of developing PTSD. The lifetime prevalence of PTSD among persons living in depressed urban areas or on Native American reservations is estimated at 23%. For victims of violent crimes, the estimated rate is 58%.

PTSD also appears to be more common in seniors than in younger people. Thirteen percent of the members of a senior population report they are affected by PTSD in comparison to 7–10% of the entire population. Reports of elder abuse crimes have increased 200% since 1986. In addition, the incidence of PTSD is known to be higher in Holocaust survivors, war veterans, and cancer or heart surgery survivors, which account for a significant portion of older Americans. Of those seniors who are military veterans, there is an increasing number who are isolated and/or in poor health as a result of PTSD.

Children are also susceptible to PTSD and their risk is increased exponentially as their exposure to the event increases. Children experiencing abuse, the death of a parent, or those located in a community experiencing a traumatic event can develop PTSD. Two years after the Oklahoma City (Oklahoma) bombing of 1995, 16% of children within a 100-mi. (160-km) radius of Oklahoma City with no direct exposure to the bombing had increased symptoms of PTSD. Weak parental response to the event, having a parent with PTSD symptoms, and intensified exposure to the event via the media all increase the possibility of a child developing PTSD symptoms. In addition, a developmentally inappropriate sexual experience for a child may be considered a traumatic event, even though it may not have actually involved violence or physical injury.

MILITARY VETERANS. Studies conducted between 2004 and 2006 with veteran participants from Operation Iraqi Freedom and Operation Enduring Freedom (Afghanistan) found a strong correlation between duration of combat exposure and PTSD. Veterans of combat in Iraq reported a higher rate of PTSD than those deployed to Afghanistan because of longer exposure to warfare.

Information about PTSD in veterans of the Vietnam era is derived from the National Vietnam Veterans Readjustment Survey (NVVRS), conducted between 1986 and 1988. The estimated lifetime prevalence of PTSD among American veterans of this war is 31% for men and 27% for women. An additional 22.5% of the men and 21% of the women have been diagnosed with partial PTSD at some point in their lives. The lifetime prevalence of PTSD among veterans of World War II (1939–1945) and the Korean War (1950–1953) is estimated at 20%.

Generally, military personnel, whether men or women, who have spent time in war zones experience PTSD about 30% of the time. Another 20–25% of these veterans are diagnosed with partial PTSD at some time after their military experiences. In the 2010s, estimates of PTSD in U.S. military personnel who served in Iraq vary from 12% to 20%.

CROSS-CULTURAL ISSUES. Further research needs to be done on the effects of ethnicity and culture on post-traumatic symptoms. As of the early 2010s, Western clinicians working with patients from a similar background have done most PTSD research. Researchers do not yet know whether persons from non-Western societies have the same psychological reactions to specific traumas or whether they develop the same symptom patterns.

Demographics

PTSD can develop in almost anyone in any age group exposed to a sufficiently terrifying event or chain of events. The National Institute of Mental Health (NIMH) states, "Anyone can get PTSD at any age. This includes war veterans and survivors of physical and sexual assault, abuse, accidents, disasters, and many other serious events. Not everyone with PTSD has been through a dangerous event. Some people get PTSD after a friend or family member experiences danger or is harmed. The sudden, unexpected death of a loved one can also cause PTSD."

The NIMH estimated in 2007, the last year in which it was reported, that about 7.7 million adults in the United States have PTSD. One study found that 3.7% of a sample of teenage boys and 6.3% of adolescent girls had PTSD. It is estimated that a person's risk of developing PTSD over the course of their life is between 8% and 10%. On average, 30% of soldiers who have been in a war zone develop PTSD. Women are at greater risk of PTSD following sexual assault or domestic violence, while men are at greater risk of developing PTSD following military combat.

Traumatic experiences are surprisingly common in the general North American population. More than 10% of the men and 6% of the women in one survey reported experiencing four or more types of trauma in their lives. The most frequently mentioned traumas are:

- witnessing someone being badly hurt or killed
- involvement in a fire, flood, earthquake, severe hurricane, or other natural disaster
- involvement in a life-threatening accident (workplace explosion or transportation accident)
- military combat

PTSD is more likely to develop in response to an intentional human act of violence or cruelty such as a rape or mugging than as a reaction to an impersonal catastrophe like a flood or hurricane. It is not surprising that the traumatic events most frequently mentioned by men diagnosed with PTSD are rape, combat exposure, childhood neglect, and childhood physical abuse. For women diagnosed with PTSD, the most common traumas are rape, sexual molestation, physical attack, being threatened with a weapon, and childhood physical abuse.

PTSD can also develop in therapists, rescue workers, or witnesses of a frightening event as well as in those who were directly involved. This process is called vicarious traumatization.

Causes and symptoms

The causes of PTSD are not completely understood. One major question that has not been answered, is why some people involved in a major disaster develop PTSD and other survivors of the same event do not. For example, a survey of 988 adults living close to the World Trade Center conducted in November 2001 found that only 7% had been diagnosed with PTSD following the events of September 11th; the other 93% were anxious and upset, but they did not develop PTSD. Research into this question is ongoing in the 2010s.

Causes

When PTSD was first suggested as a diagnostic category for *DSM-III* (*Diagnostic and Statistical Manual of Mental Disorders 3*) in 1980, it was controversial precisely because of the central role of outside stressors as causes of the disorder. Psychiatry has generally emphasized the internal abnormalities of individuals as the source of mental disorders; prior to the 1970s, war veterans, rape victims, and other trauma survivors were often blamed for their symptoms and they were regarded as cowards, moral weaklings, or masochists. The high rate of psychiatric casualties among Vietnam veterans, however, led to studies conducted by the Veterans Administration. These studies helped to establish PTSD as a legitimate diagnostic entity with a complex set of causes.

BIOCHEMICAL/PHYSIOLOGICAL CAUSES. Present neurobiological research indicates that traumatic events cause lasting changes in the human nervous system, including abnormal levels of secretion of stress hormones. In addition, in PTSD patients, researchers have found changes in the amygdala and the hippocampus—the parts of the brain that form links between fear and memory. Experiments with ketamine, a drug that inactivates one of the neurotransmitters in the central nervous system, suggest that trauma works in a similar way to damage associative pathways in the brain. Positron emission tomography (PET) scans of PTSD patients suggest that trauma affects the parts of the brain that govern speech and language.

SOCIOCULTURAL CAUSES. Studies of specific populations of PTSD patients (such as combat veterans, survivors of rape or genocide, and former political hostages or prisoners) have shed light on the social and cultural causes of PTSD. In general, societies that are highly authoritarian, glorify violence, or sexualize violence have high rates of PTSD even among civilians.

OCCUPATIONAL FACTORS. Persons whose work exposes them to traumatic events or who treat trauma survivors may develop secondary PTSD (also known as compassion fatigue or burnout). These occupations include specialists in emergency medicine, police officers, firefighters, search-and-rescue personnel, psychotherapists, and disaster investigators. The degree of risk for PTSD is related to three factors: (1) the amount and intensity of exposure to the suffering of trauma victims, (2) the worker's degree of empathy and sensitivity, and (3) unresolved issues from the worker's personal history.

PERSONAL VARIABLES. Although the most important causal factor in PTSD is the traumatic event itself, individuals differ in the intensity of their cognitive and emotional responses to trauma; some persons appear to be more vulnerable than others. In some cases, this greater vulnerability is related to temperament or natural disposition, with shy or introverted people being at greater risk. In other cases, the person's vulnerability results from chronic illness, a physical disability, or previous traumatization—particularly abuse in childhood. As of 2012, researchers have not found any correlation between race or ethnicity and biological vulnerability to PTSD. The NIMH states, "Researchers are studying the importance of various risk and resilience factors. With more study, it may be possible someday to predict who is likely to get PTSD and prevent it."

Symptoms

DSM-IV-TR (published in 2000; with version 5 expected to be published in May 2013) specifies six diagnostic criteria for PTSD:

- Traumatic stressor: The patient has been exposed to a catastrophic event involving actual or threatened death or injury, or a threat to the physical integrity of the self or others. During exposure to the trauma, the person's emotional response was marked by intense fear, feelings of helplessness, or horror. In general, stressors caused intentionally by human beings (genocide, rape, torture, abuse, etc.) are experienced as more traumatic than accidents, natural disasters, or "acts of God."
- Intrusive symptoms: The patient experiences flashbacks, traumatic daydreams, or nightmares, in which he or she relives the trauma as if it were recurring in the present. Intrusive symptoms result from an abnormal process of memory formation. Traumatic memories have two distinctive characteristics: (1) they can be triggered by stimuli that remind the patient of the traumatic event; (2) they have a "frozen" or wordless quality, consisting of images and sensations rather than verbal descriptions.
- Avoidant symptoms: The patient attempts to reduce the possibility of exposure to anything that might trigger memories of the trauma, and to minimize his or her reactions to such memories. This cluster of symptoms includes feeling disconnected from other people, psychic numbing, and avoidance of places, persons, or things associated with the trauma. Patients with PTSD are at increased risk of substance abuse as a form of self-medication to numb painful memories.
- Hyperarousal: Hyperarousal is a condition in which the patient's nervous system is always on "red alert" for the return of danger. This symptom cluster includes hypervigilance, insomnia, difficulty concentrating, general irritability, and an extreme startle response. Some clinicians think that this abnormally intense startle response may be the most characteristic symptom of PTSD.
- Duration of symptoms: The symptoms must persist for at least one month.
- Significance: The patient has significant social, interpersonal, or work-related problems as a result of the PTSD symptoms. A common social symptom of PTSD is a feeling of disconnection from other people (including loved ones), from the larger society, and from spiritual, religious, or other significant sources of meaning.

Diagnosis

The diagnosis of PTSD is based on the patient's history, including the timing of the traumatic event and the duration of the patient's symptoms.

Examination

Consultation with a mental health professional for diagnosis and a plan of treatment is always advised. Many of the responses to trauma, such as shock, terror, irritability, blame, guilt, grief, sadness, emotional numbing, and feelings of helplessness, are natural reactions. For most people, resilience is an overriding factor and trauma effects diminish within 6 to 16 months. It is when these responses continue or become debilitating that PTSD is often diagnosed.

As outlined in DSM-IV, exposure to a traumatic stressor means that an individual experienced, witnessed or was confronted by an event or events involving death or threat of death, serious injury or the threat of bodily harm to oneself or others. The individual's response must involve intense fear, helplessness, or horror. A two-pronged approach to evaluation is considered the best way to make a valid diagnosis because it can gauge under-reporting or over-reporting of symptoms. The two primary forms are structured interviews and self-report questionnaires. Spouses, partners, and other family members may also be interviewed. Because the evaluation may involve subtle reminders of the trauma in order to gauge a patient's reactions, individuals should ask for a full description of the evaluation process beforehand. Asking what results can be expected from the evaluation is also advised.

A number of structured interview forms have been devised to facilitate the diagnosis of PTSD:

- The Clinician Administered PTSD Scale (CAPS) developed by the National Center for PTSD
- The Structured Clinical Interview for DSM (SCID)
- Anxiety Disorders Interview Schedule-Revised (ADIS)
- PTSD-Interview
- Structured Interview for PTSD (SI-PTSD)
- PTSD Symptom Scale Interview (PSS-I)

Self-reporting checklists provide scores to represent the level of stress experienced. Some of the most commonly used checklists are:

- The PTSD Checklist (PCL), which has one list for civilians and one for military personnel and veterans
- Impact of Event Scale-Revised (IES-R)
- Keane PTSD Scale of the MMPI-2
- The Mississippi Scale for Combat Related PTSD and the Mississippi Scale for Civilians
- The Post Traumatic Diagnostic Scale (PDS)
- The Penn Inventory for Post-Traumatic Stress
- Los Angeles Symptom Checklist (LASC)

Tests

There are no laboratory or imaging tests that can detect PTSD, although the doctor may order imaging studies of the brain to rule out head injuries or other physical causes of the patient's symptoms.

Treatment

Treatment for post-traumatic stress disorder includes both traditional and alternative methods.

Treatment for PTSD usually involves a combination of medications and psychotherapy. If patients have started to abuse alcohol or drugs, they must be treated for the substance abuse before being treated for PTSD. If the patient is diagnosed with coexisting depression, treatment should focus on the PTSD because its course, biology, and treatment response are different from those associated with major depression. Patients with the disorder are usually treated as outpatients; they are not hospitalized unless they are threatening to commit suicide or harm other people.

Mainstream forms of psychotherapy used to treat patients who have already developed PTSD include:

- Cognitive-behavioral therapy: There are three treatment approaches to PTSD included under this heading: (1) exposure therapy, which seeks to desensitize the patient to reminders of the trauma; (2) cognitive restructuring, which helps people to better understand their bad feelings and memories and to look at the experience in a more realistic way; and (3) stress inoculation training (sometimes called anxiety management training), which reduces the symptoms of PTSD by showing the patient how to reduce anxiety. These strategies may include relaxation training, biofeedback, social skills training, or distraction techniques.
- Psychodynamic psychotherapy: This approach helps the patient recover a sense of self and learn new coping strategies and ways to deal with intense emotions related to the trauma. Typically, it consists of three phases: (1) establishing a sense of safety for the patient; (2) exploring the trauma itself in depth; (3) helping the patient re-establish connections with family, friends, the wider society, and other sources of meaning.
- Discussion groups or peer-counseling groups: These groups are usually formed for survivors of specific traumas, such as combat, rape/incest, and natural or transportation disasters. They help patients to recognize that other survivors of the shared experience have had the same emotions and reacted to the trauma in similar ways. They appear to be especially beneficial for patients with guilt issues about their behavior during the trauma (e.g., submitting to rape to save one's life, or surviving the event when others did not).
- Family therapy: This form of treatment is recommended for PTSD patients whose family life has been affected by the PTSD symptoms.

Drugs

Medications are used most often in patients with severe PTSD to treat the intrusive symptoms of the disorder as well as feelings of anxiety and depression. These drugs are usually given as one part of a treatment plan that includes psychotherapy or group therapy. As of 2012, there is no single medication used to treat PTSD. The selective serotonin reuptake inhibitors (SSRIs), which are a class of compounds often used as antidepressants, appear to help the core symptoms when given in higher doses for five to eight weeks, while the tricyclic antidepressants (TCAs) or the monoamine oxidase inhibitors (MAOIs) are most useful in treating anxiety and depression.

Sleep problems can be lessened with brief treatment with an anti-anxiety drug, such as a benzodiazepine like alprazolam (Xanax), but long-term usage can lead to disturbing side effects, such as increased anger, drug tolerance, dependency, and abuse. Benzodiazepines are also not given to PTSD patients diagnosed with coexisting drug or alcohol abuse.

Alternative treatment

Relaxation training, which is sometimes called anxiety management training, includes breathing exercises and similar techniques intended to help the patient prevent hyperventilation and relieve the muscle tension associated with the fight-or-flight reaction of anxiety. Yoga, aikido, t'ai chi, and dance therapy help patients work with the physical as well as the emotional tensions that either promote anxiety or are created by the anxiety.

Other alternative or complementary therapies are based on physiological and/or energetic understanding of how the trauma is imprinted in the body. These therapies affect a release of stored emotions and resolution of them by working with the body rather than merely talking through the experience. One example of such a therapy is Somatic Experiencing (SE), developed by American therapist Peter Levine (1942–). SE is a short-term, biological, body-oriented approach to PTSD or other trauma. This approach heals by emphasizing physiological and emotional responses, without re-traumatizing the person, without placing the person on medication, and without the long hours of conventional therapy.

When used in conjunction with therapies that address the underlying cause of PTSD, such relaxation therapies as hydrotherapy, massage therapy, and aromatherapy are useful to some patients in easing PTSD symptoms. Essential oils of lavender, chamomile, neroli, sweet marjoram, and ylang-ylang are commonly recommended by aromatherapists for stress relief and anxiety reduction.

Some patients benefit from spiritual or religious counseling. Because traumatic experiences often affect patients' spiritual views and beliefs, counseling with a trusted religious or spiritual advisor may be part of a treatment plan. A growing number of pastoral counselors in the major Christian and Jewish bodies in North America have advanced credentials in trauma therapy. Native Americans are often helped to recover from PTSD by participating in traditional tribal rituals for cleansing memories of war and other traumatic events. These rituals may include sweat lodges, prayers and chants, or consultation with a shaman or tribal healer.

Several controversial methods of treatment for PTSD have been introduced since the mid-1980s. Mainstream medical researchers have developed some methods, while others are derived from various forms of alternative medicine. These methods are controversial because they do not offer any scientifically validated explanations for their effectiveness. They include:

- Eye Movement Desensitization and Reprocessing (EMDR): This is a technique in which the patient reimagines the trauma while focusing visually on movements of the therapist's finger. It is claimed that the movements of the patient's eyes reprogram the brain and allow emotional healing.

> **KEY TERMS**
>
> **Benzodiazepines**—A class of drugs that have a hypnotic and sedative action, used mainly as tranquilizers to control symptoms of anxiety.
>
> **Cognitive-behavioral therapy**—A type of psychotherapy used to treat anxiety disorders (including PTSD) that emphasizes behavioral change as well as alteration of negative thought patterns.
>
> **Cortisol**—A hormone produced by the adrenal glands near the kidneys in response to stress.
>
> **Dissociation**—The splitting off of certain mental processes from conscious awareness. Many PTSD patients have dissociative symptoms.
>
> **Flashback**—A temporary reliving of a traumatic event.
>
> **Hyperarousal**—A state of increased emotional tension and anxiety, often including jitteriness and being easily startled.
>
> **Hypervigilance**—A condition of abnormally intense watchfulness or wariness. It is one of the most common symptoms of PTSD.
>
> **Prevalence**—The percentage of a population that is affected by a specific disease at a given time.
>
> **Selective serotonin reuptake inhibitors (SSRIs)**—A class of antidepressants that work by blocking the reabsorption of serotonin in the brain, raising the levels of serotonin. Examples include Prozac, Zoloft, and Paxil.
>
> **Trauma**—A severe injury or shock to a person's body or mind.

- Tapas Acupressure Technique (TAT): TAT was developed in 1993 by a licensed acupuncturist named Tapas Fleming. It is derived from traditional Chinese medicine (TCM), and its practitioners maintain that a large number of acupuncture meridians enter the brain at certain points on the face, especially around the eyes. Pressure on these points is thought to release traumatic stress.
- Thought Field Therapy: This therapy combines the acupuncture meridians of TCM with analysis of the patient's voice over the telephone. The therapist then provides an individualized treatment for the patient.
- Traumatic Incident Reduction: This is a technique in which the patient treats the trauma like a video and "runs through" it repeatedly with the therapist until all negative emotions have been discharged.
- Emotional Freedom Techniques (EFT): EFT is similar to TAT in that it uses the body's acupuncture meridians, but it emphasizes the body's entire energy field rather than just the face.
- Counting Technique: Developed by a physician, this treatment consists of a preparation phase, a counting phase in which the therapist counts from 1 to 100 while the patient reimagines the trauma, and a review phase. Like Traumatic Incident Reduction, it is intended to reduce the patient's hyperarousal.

Public health role and response

The United States offers help with PTSD through its National Center for PTSD—headquartered in Washington, D.C.—which is a part of the Department of Veterans Affairs (VA). Its website (http://www.ptsd.va.gov/) states, "We are the center of excellence for research and education on the prevention, understanding, and treatment of PTSD. Our Center has seven divisions across the country. Although we provide no direct clinical care, our purpose is to improve the well-being and understanding of American Veterans. We conduct cutting edge research and apply resultant findings to: 'Advance the Science and Promote Understanding of Traumatic Stress.'" These seven divisions are:

- Executive Division: White River Junction, Vermont
- Clinical Neurosciences Division: West Haven, Connecticut
- Evaluation Division: West Haven, Connecticut
- Behavioral Sciences Division: Boston, Massachusetts
- Women's Health Sciences Division: Boston, Massachusetts
- Dissemination and Training Division: Palo Alto, California
- Pacific Islands Division: Honolulu, Hawaii

QUESTIONS TO ASK YOUR DOCTOR

- Where can I go for help? Should I see a mental health specialist?
- How can I help myself? Do you recommend any changes at home, work, or school to help my recovery?
- What should I do if I have a friend or relative with PTSD?
- Will I completely recover from PTSD?
- Why did I get PTSD when other fellow veterans did not?
- What do you believe is causing my symptoms?
- How will you determine my diagnosis?
- Do you recommend treatment? If yes, with what types of therapy?
- How soon do you expect my symptoms to improve?
- Where can I learn more about PTSD?

Prognosis

The prognosis of PTSD is difficult to determine because patients' personalities and the experiences they undergo vary widely. A majority of patients get better, including some who do not receive treatment. One study reported that the average length of PTSD symptoms in patients who get treatment is 32 months, compared to 64 months in patients who are not treated.

Factors that improve a patient's chances for full recovery include prompt treatment, early and ongoing support from family and friends, a high level of functioning before the frightening event, and an absence of alcohol or substance abuse.

About 30% of people with PTSD never recover completely. A few commit suicide because their symptoms get worse rather than improving.

Prevention

PTSD is impossible to prevent completely because natural disasters and human acts of violence will continue to occur. In addition, it is not possible to tell beforehand how any given individual will react to a specific type of trauma. Prompt treatment after a traumatic event may lower the survivor's risk of developing severe symptoms.

Resources

BOOKS

American Psychiatric Association. *Diagnostic and Statistical Manual of Mental Disorders.* 4th ed., text rev. Washington, D.C.: American Psychiatric Association, 2000.

Antony, Martin M., and Murray B. Stein, eds. *Oxford Handbook of Anxiety and Related Disorders.* New York: Oxford University Press, 2009.

Beck, J. Gayle, and Denise M. Sloan, eds. *The Oxford Handbook of Traumatic Stress Disorders.* Oxford: Oxford University Press, 2012.

Chu, James. *Rebuilding Shattered Lives: Treating Complex PTSD and Dissociative Disorders.* Hoboken, NJ: John Wiley & Sons, 2011.

Grey, Nick, ed. *A Casebook of Cognitive Therapy for Traumatic Stress Reactions.* New York: Routledge, 2009.

Ringel, Shoshana, and Jerrold R. Brandell, eds. *Trauma: Contemporary Directions in Theory, Practice, and Research.* Thousand Oaks, CA: SAGE, 2012.

Slone, Laurie B., and Matthew J. Friedman. *After the War Zone: A Practical Guide for Returning Troops and Their Families.* Cambridge, MA: Da Capo Lifelong, 2008.

PERIODICALS

Cohen, J. A., and M. S. Scheeringa. "Post-traumatic Stress Disorder Diagnosis in Children: Challenges and Promises." *Dialogues in Clinical Neuroscience* 11 (2009): 91–99.

Evans, S., et al. "Disability and Posttraumatic Stress Disorder in Disaster Relief Workers Responding to September 11, 2001 World Trade Center Disaster." *Journal of Clinical Psychology* 65 (April 22, 2009): 684–94.

Hamblen, J. L., et al. "Cognitive Behavioral Therapy for Postdisaster Distress: A Community-Based Treatment Program for Survivors of Hurricane Katrina." *Administration and Policy in Mental Health* 36 (May 2009): 206–14.

Smith, T. C., et al. "PTSD Prevalence, Associated Exposures, and Functional Health Outcomes in a Large, Population-Based Military Cohort." *Public Health Reports* 124 (January-February 2009): 90–102.

WEBSITES

Helping Children Cope with Violence and Disasters: What Parents Can Do. National Institute of Mental Health. 2008. http://www.nimh.nih.gov/health/publications/helping-children-and-adolescents-cope-with-violence-and-disasters-parents/complete-index.shtml (accessed October 13, 2012).

National Center for Posttraumatic Stress Disorder. U.S. Department of Veterans Affairs. http://www.ptsd.va.gov/ (accessed October 13, 2012).

Post-Traumatic Stress Disorder. National Alliance on Mental Illness. http://www.nami.org/Template.cfm?Section=Posttraumatic_Stress_Disorder (accessed October 13, 2012).

Post-traumatic Stress Disorder (PTSD). Mayo Clinic. April 1, 2011. http://www.mayoclinic.com/health/post-traumatic-stress-disorder/DS00246/DSECTION=preparing-for-your-appointment (accessed October 13, 2012).

Post Traumatic Stress Disorder (PTSD). National Institute of Mental Health. http://www.nimh.nih.gov/health/publications/post-traumatic-stress-disorder-ptsd/index.shtml (accessed October 13, 2012).

What Is PTSD? National Center for Posttraumatic Stress Disorder, U.S. Department of Veterans Affairs. May 29, 2012. http://www.ptsd.va.gov/public/pages/what-is-ptsd.asp (accessed October 13, 2012).

ORGANIZATIONS

American Psychiatric Association, 1000 Wilson Blvd, Ste. 1825, Arlington, VA 22209-3901, (703) 907-7300, (888) 357-7924, apa@psych.org, http://www.psych.org.

Anxiety Disorders Association of America, 8701 Georgia Ave., Ste. 412, Silver Spring, MD 20910, (240) 485-1001, http://www.adaa.org.

International Society for Traumatic Stress Studies, 111 Deer Lake Rd., Ste. 100, Deerfield, IL 60015, (847) 480-9028, Fax: (847) 480-9282, http://www.istss.org.

National Alliance on Mental Illness, 3803 N. Fairfax Dr., Ste. 100, Arlington, VA 22203, (703) 524-7600, Fax: (703) 524-9094, (800) 950-6264, http://www.nami.org.

National Center for Posttraumatic Stress Disorder, 810 Vermont Ave. NW, Washington, DC 20420, http://www.ptsd.va.gov.

National Institute of Mental Health, 6001 Executive Bvld, Rm. 8184, MSC 9663, Bethesda, MD 20892-9663, (301) 443-4513, Fax: (301) 443-4279, (866) 615-6464, nimhinfo@nih.gov, http://www.nimh.nih.gov.

Rebecca J. Frey, PhD
William A. Atkins, BB, BS, MBA

Protein-calorie malnutrition *see* **Protein-energy malnutrition**

Protein-energy malnutrition

Definition

Protein-energy malnutrition (PEM), also referred to as protein-calorie malnutrition, is a potentially fatal body-depletion disorder. It is a leading cause of death in children in developing countries.

Demographics

Although PEM is not prevalent among the general population of the United States, one governmental study estimated that up to half of elderly patients in nursing home are suffering from PEM. Additionally, PEM seen in children in the United States is often a sign of child abuse or severe neglect. Other groups who may suffer from PEM in industrialized nations such as the United States are cancer patients, those with anorexia nervosa, and patients who have had gastric bypass surgery in order to control obesity.

Outside industrialized nations, PEM is common in areas with high rates of impoverishment, especially in Africa. It is also prevalent after large natural disasters, such as **drought**, or during political unrest, which leads to a shortage of food in an area.

Description

PEM develops in children and adults whose consumption of protein and energy (measured by calories) is insufficient to satisfy the body's nutritional needs. Whereas pure protein deficiency can occur when a person's diet provides enough energy but lacks the protein minimum, in most cases the deficiency will be dual. PEM may also occur in persons who are unable to absorb vital nutrients or convert them to energy essential for healthy tissue formation and organ function.

Types of PEM

Primary PEM results from a diet that lacks sufficient sources of protein and/or energy. Secondary PEM is more common in the United States, where it usually occurs as a complication of **AIDS**, cancer, chronic kidney failure, inflammatory bowel disease, or other illnesses that impair the body's ability to absorb or use nutrients or to compensate for nutrient losses. PEM can develop gradually in a patient who has a chronic illness or who experiences chronic semi-starvation. It may appear suddenly in a patient who has an acute illness.

Kwashiorkor

Kwashiorkor, also called wet protein-energy malnutrition, is a form of PEM characterized primarily by protein deficiency. This condition usually appears at the age of about 12 months when breastfeeding is discontinued, but it can develop at any time during a child's formative years. It causes fluid retention (edema); dry, peeling skin; and hair discoloration.

Marasmus

Primarily caused by energy deficiency, marasmus is characterized by stunted growth and wasting of muscle and tissue. Marasmus usually develops between the ages of six months and one year in children who have been weaned from breast milk or who suffer from weakening conditions such as chronic diarrhea.

Causes and symptoms

Secondary PEM symptoms range from mild to severe and can alter the form or function of almost every organ in the body. The type and intensity of symptoms depend on the patient's prior nutritional status, the nature of the underlying disease, and the speed at which it is progressing.

Mild, moderate, and severe classifications have not been precisely defined, but patients who lose 10–20% of their body weight without trying are usually said to have moderate PEM. This condition is also characterized by a weakened grip and inability to perform high-energy tasks.

Losing 20% of body weight or more is generally classified as severe PEM. People with this condition cannot eat normal-sized meals. They have slow heart rates and low blood pressure and body temperatures. Other symptoms of severe secondary PEM are baggy, wrinkled skin; constipation; dry, thin, brittle hair; lethargy; and pressure sores or other skin lesions.

Kwashiorkor

People who have kwashiorkor often have extremely thin arms and legs, but liver enlargement and ascites (abnormal accumulation of fluid) can distend the abdomen and disguise weight loss. Hair may turn red or yellow. Anemia, diarrhea, and fluid and electrolyte disorders are common. The body's immune system is often weakened, behavioral development is slow, and mental retardation may occur. Children may grow to normal height but are abnormally thin.

Kwashiorkor-like secondary PEM usually develops in patients who have been severely burned, suffered trauma, or had sepsis (tissue-destroying infection) or another life-threatening illness. The condition's onset is so sudden that body fat and muscle mass of normal-weight people may not change. Some obese patients even gain weight.

Marasmus

Profound weakness accompanies severe marasmus. Since the body breaks down its own tissue to use as calories, people with this condition lose all their body fat and muscle strength, and acquire a skeletal appearance most noticeable in the hands and in the temporal muscle in front of and above each ear. Children with marasmus are small for their age. Since their immune systems are weakened, they experience frequent infections. Other symptoms include loss of appetite, diarrhea, skin that is dry and baggy, sparse hair that is dull brown or reddish yellow, mental retardation, behavioral retardation, low body temperature (hypothermia), and slow pulse and breathing rates.

The absence of edema distinguishes marasmus-like secondary PEM, a gradual wasting process that begins with weight loss and progresses to mild, moderate, or severe malnutrition (cachexia). It is usually associated with cancer, chronic obstructive pulmonary disease (COPD), or another chronic disease that is inactive or progressing very slowly.

Some individuals have kwashiorkor and marasmus at the same time. This situation most often occurs when a person who has a chronic, inactive condition develops symptoms of an acute illness.

Hospitalized patients

Difficulty chewing, swallowing, and digesting food, as well as pain, nausea, and lack of appetite are among the most common reasons that many hospital patients do not consume enough nutrients. Nutrient loss can be accelerated by bleeding, diarrhea, abnormally high sugar levels (glycosuria), kidney disease, malabsorption disorders, and other factors. Fever, infection, surgery, and benign or malignant tumors increase the amount of nutrients hospitalized patients need. So do trauma, burns, and some medications.

Diagnosis

A thorough physical examination and a health history that probes eating habits and weight changes, checks body-fat composition and muscle strength, and assesses gastrointestinal symptoms, underlying illness, and nutritional status is often as accurate as blood tests and urinalyses used to detect and document abnormalities.

Some doctors further quantify a patient's nutritional status by the following:

- comparing height and weight to standardized norms
- calculating body mass index (BMI)
- measuring skinfold thickness or the circumference of the upper arm

Treatment

Treatment is designed to provide adequate nutrition, restore normal body composition, and cure the condition that caused the deficiency. Tube feeding or intravenous feeding is used to supply nutrients to patients who cannot or will not eat protein-rich foods.

> **KEY TERMS**
>
> **Ascites**—Abnormal accumulation of fluid in the abdomen, making the abdomen appear distended.
>
> **Cachexia**—Severe malnutrition involving muscle wasting and organ damage.
>
> **Edema**—Fluid retention, generally seen in the limbs.
>
> **Hypothermia**—Low body temperature.

In patients with severe PEM, the first stage of treatment consists of correcting fluid and electrolyte imbalances, treating infection with antibiotics that do not affect protein synthesis, and addressing related medical problems. The second phase involves replenishing essential nutrients slowly to prevent taxing the patient's weakened system with more food than it can handle. Physical therapy may be beneficial to patients whose muscles have deteriorated significantly.

Prognosis

Most people can lose up to 10% of their body weight without side effects, but losing more than 40% is almost always fatal. Death usually results from heart failure, an electrolyte imbalance, or low body temperature. Patients with certain symptoms, including semi-consciousness, persistent diarrhea, jaundice, and low blood sodium levels, have a poorer prognosis than other patients. Recovery from marasmus usually takes longer than recovery from kwashiorkor. The long-term effects of childhood malnutrition are uncertain. Some children recover completely, whereas others may have a variety of lifelong impairments, including an inability to properly absorb nutrients in the intestines and mental retardation. The outcome appears to be related to the length and severity of the malnutrition, as well as to the age of the child when the malnutrition occurred.

Prevention

Breastfeeding a baby for at least six months is considered the best way to prevent early childhood malnutrition. Preventing malnutrition in developing countries is a complicated and challenging problem. Providing food directly during **famine** can help in the short term, but more long-term solutions are needed, including agricultural development, public health programs (especially programs that monitor growth and development, as well as programs that provide nutritional information and supplements), and improved food distribution systems.

> **QUESTIONS TO ASK YOUR DOCTOR**
>
> - If I am unable to breastfeed, what precautions can I take against my baby developing PEM?
> - How much weight loss is abnormal?
> - What type of foods should my elderly parents be eating to reduce their chances of PEM?

Programs that distribute infant formula and discourage breastfeeding are believed to hurt the reduction of PEM cases, and many believe these programs should be discontinued, except in areas where many mothers are infected with HIV.

Every patient being admitted to a hospital should be screened for the presence of illnesses and conditions that could lead to PEM. The nutritional status of patients at higher-than-average risk should be more thoroughly assessed and periodically reevaluated during extended hospital stays or nursing home residence.

Resources

BOOKS

Shalin, Judith, and Sari Edelstein. *Essentials of Life Cycle Nutrition*. New York: Jones & Bartlett, 2010.

PERIODICALS

Zubin, Grover, and C. Looi. "Protein Energy Malnutrition." *Pediatric Clinics of North America*. 56, no. 5 (2009): 1055–68. http://xa.yimg.com/kq/groups/23515872/1742863024/name/Pediatric#page=27 (accessed September 25, 2012).

WEBSITES

A.D.A.M. Medical Encyclopedia. "Kwashiorkor." http://www.ncbi.nlm.nih.gov/pubmedhealth/PMH0002571 (accessed September 25, 2012).

MedlinePlus. "Kwashiorkor." http://www.nlm.nih.gov/medlineplus/ency/article/001604.htm (accessed September 25, 2012).

Scheinfeld, Noah S., et al. "Protein-Energy Malnutrition." http://emedicine.medscape.com/article/1104623-overview (accessed September 26, 2012).

ORGANIZATIONS

American Academy of Pediatrics (AAP), 141 Northwest Point Blvd., Elk Grove, IL 60007-1098, (847) 434-8000, http://www.aap.org.

American College of Nutrition, 300 S. Duncan Ave., Ste. 225, Clearwater, FL 33755, (727) 446-6086, Fax: (727) 446-6202, office@AmericanCollegeofNutrition.org, http://www.americancollegeofnutrition.org.

American Society for Nutrition, 9650 Rockville Pike, Bethesda, MD 20814, (301) 634-7050, Fax: (301) 634-7894, http://www.nutrition.org.

National Institute of Child Health and Human Development (NICHD), PO Box 3006, Rockville, MD 20847, (800) 370-2943, Fax: (866) 760-5947, NICHDInformationResourceCenter@mail.nih.gov, http://www.nichd.nih.gov.

World Health Organization, Avenue Appia 20, 1211 Geneva 27, Switzerland, +2241 791 21 11, Fax: +2241 791 31 11, info@who.int, http://www.who.int.

Maureen Haggerty
Tish Davidson, AM

Public Health Service

Description

The United States Public Health Service is the health component of the **U.S. Department of Health and Human Services**. It originated in 1798 with the organization of the Marine Hospital Service, out of concern for the health of the nation's seafarers who brought diseases back to this country. As immigrants came to America, they brought with them **cholera**, **smallpox**, and **yellow fever**; the Public Health Service was charged with protecting the nation from infectious diseases.

Today the Service helps city and state health departments with health problems. Its responsibilities include controlling infectious diseases, immunizing children, controlling sexually transmitted diseases, preventing the spread of **tuberculosis**, and operating a quarantine program.

The Centers for Disease Control in Atlanta, Georgia, is the Public Health Service agency responsible for disease identification, research, and prevention.

Pulmonary dust disorders *see* **Talcosis**

R

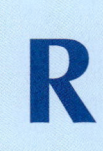

Rachel Carson Council

Definition

The Rachel Carson Council is a nonprofit organization that focuses on the dangers of pesticides and other toxic chemicals and their impact on human health, wildlife, and the environment.

Purpose

The purpose of the Rachel Carson Council is to work for conservation of natural resources, to increase knowledge about threats to the environment, and to serve as a clearinghouse of information for scientists, government officials, environmentalists, journalists, and the public.

Description

The Rachel Carson Council is a nonprofit organization that promotes the use of alternative and benign pest management. The organization maintains that using these methods can lead to healthier and more sustainable living. The council's board of directors includes experts and leaders in the fields of environmental science, medicine, education, law, and consumer interest, and a board of consulting experts with scientists from many fields.

Origins

Rachel Carson's *Silent Spring*, her 1962 book on pesticides, generated enormous interest in the subject of pesticides. People asked for information and advice. Shortly after Carson died in April 1964, her colleagues and friends established an organization to keep the public informed on new developments in the field of chemical contamination. Originally called the Rachel Carson Trust for the Living Environment, the organization was incorporated in 1965, and in 1980, it became known as the Rachel Carson Council.

Research and general acceptance

The Council has long warned that many pesticides, regulated by the U.S. **Environmental Protection Agency (EPA)** and widely used by homeowners, farmers, and industry, are extremely harmful. Many of these chemicals can cause cancer, miscarriages, birth defects, genetic damage, and harm to the central nervous system in humans, as well as destroy wildlife and poison the environment and food chain/web for years to come.

Other, less acutely toxic chemicals that are commonly used, the organization points out, can cause delayed neurotoxicity, a milder form of nerve damage that can show up in subtle behavior changes such as memory loss, fatigue, irritability, sleep disturbance, and altered brain wave patterns. Concerning termiticides used in schools, "children are especially vulnerable to this kind of poisoning," the Council observes, "and the implications for disturbing their ability to learn are especially serious."

Through its studies, publications, and information distribution, the Council has provided data strongly indicating that many pesticides now in widespread use should be banned or carefully restricted. The group has urged and petitioned the **EPA** to take such action on a variety of chemicals that represent serious potential dangers to the health and lives of millions of Americans and to future generations.

The Council has also expressed strong concern about and sponsored extensive research on the link between exposure to toxic chemicals and the dramatic increase in cancer incidence and death rates. The group's publications and officials have warned that the presence of dozens of cancer-causing chemicals in food, air, and water is constantly exposing Americans to deadly carcinogens and is contributing to the mounting incidence of cancer, which eventually strikes almost one American in three, and kills more than 500,000 Americans every year.

The Council publishes numerous books, booklets, and brochures on pesticides, toxic chemicals, and alternatives to their use. Other publications discuss the least

RACHEL CARSON (1907–1964)

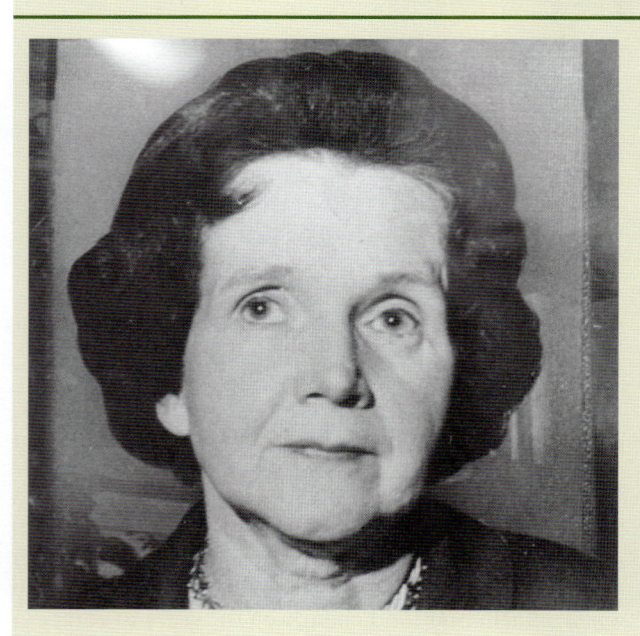

Rachel Carson initially pursued an English degree, but eventually changed her college major to zoology. She was able to pair her two passions, biology and writing, into a successful career as a biologist and a writer for the Bureau of Fisheries. Upon leaving the Bureau, she was a biologist and chief editor for the United States Fish and Wildlife Service.

Eventually, Carson devoted all of her time to her writing—creating best-selling environmental literature classics. One of these classics, Silent Spring, is considered required reading for those interested in the environment. The bulk of the book details the effects of pesticides on living things.

The book quickly gained mass market appeal and appeared on the New York Times best-seller list. People became aware and concerned about their role in the environment's future. Silent Spring is credited with the United States' 1972 ban of DDT as well as the creation of the Environmental Protection Agency (EPA).

Rachel Carson. (The Library of Congress.)

toxic methods of dealing with pests in the home, garden, and greenhouse; nontoxic gardening; ways to safely cure and prevent lawn diseases; and the dangers of poisons used to keep lawns green. The Council also highlights the increased use of spot-on flea control treatments for pets, providing pet owners with a guide for safe usage of the pesticides and pushing for manufacturers to more accurately list the products' ingredients and possible side effects. Additionally, the Council provides information to veterinarians and pet owners on the effects of common household and yard pesticides on pets, including advising New York City animal shelters in 2012 on the least-harmful pet care products.

Criticism has been aimed at Rachel Carson, her book, and the Rachel Carson Council. An uproar developed over dichlorodiphenyltrichloroethane (DDT) in the 2000s. Critics of Carson said that she had called for the ban of DDT in her book, which led to millions of people dying worldwide from **malaria** that could have been easily prevented using DDT. The Rachel Carson Council released a statement that Rachel Carson never called for banning of DDT completely, and that a year after the publication of Silent Spring, an independent body, the President's Science Advisory Commission, recommended a ban on DDT. Many critics continue to publicly criticize Rachel Carson and have put a special emphasis on their arguments during the celebration of the fiftieth anniversary of her book in September 2012.

Resources

BOOKS

Carson, Rachel. Silent Spring. Boston: Houghton Mifflin, 1962.

WEBSITES

Griswold, Eliza. "How Silent Spring Ignited the Environmental Movement." http://www.nytimes.com/2012/09/23/magazine/how-silent-spring-ignited-the-environmental-movement.html?pagewanted=all (accessed October 29, 2012).

Mahoney, Linda. "Rachel Carson (1907–1964)." http://www.nwhm.org/education-resources/biography/biographies/rachel-carson (accessed October 29, 2012).

Rachel Carson Council. "Tips for Researching a Pesticide Product." http://www.rachelcarsoncouncil.org/index.php?page=pesticides (accessed October 29, 2012).

U.S. Environmental Protection Agency. "DDT: A Brief History and Status." http://www.epa.gov/pesticides/factsheets/chemicals/ddt-brief-history-status.htm (accessed October 29, 2012).

ORGANIZATIONS

Rachel Carson Council, PO Box 10779, Silver Spring, MD 20914, (301) 593-7507, rccouncil@aol.com, http://www.rachelcarsoncouncil.org.

> **KEY TERMS**
>
> **Benign**—Harmless, not disease causing. Most often, benign is used to mean not malignant or noncancerous.
>
> **Carcinogen**—Any substance capable of causing cancer.
>
> **Dichlorodiphenyltrichloroethane (DDT)**—A synthetic organic compound first developed in 1874 and made popular in the 1940s for its use as an insecticide. DDT was banned by most developed countries in the 1970s, including by the United States in 1972. In 2006, the World Health Organization promoted the use of DDT indoors as a vector control in African countries.
>
> **Malaria**—Disease caused by the presence of sporozoan parasites of the genus Plasmodium in the red blood cells, transmitted by the bite of anopheline mosquitoes and characterized by severe and recurring attacks of chills and fever.
>
> **Termiticide**—An insecticide used against termites.

U.S. Environmental Protection Agency (EPA), Ariel Rios Bldg.,1200 Pennsylvania Avenue NW, Washington, DC 20460, (202) 272-0167; TTY (202) 272-0165, http://www.epa.gov.

Lewis G. Regenstein
Tish Davidson, AM

Radiation

Definition

Radiation and radioisotopes are extensively used medications to allow physicians and other medical professionals to image internal structures and processes *in vivo* (in the living body) with a minimum of invasion to the patient. Higher doses of radiation are also used as means to kill cancerous cells.

Radiation is actually a term that includes a variety of different physical phenomena. However, in essence, all these phenomena can be divided in two classes: phenomena connected with nuclear radioactive processes are one class, the so-called radioactive radiation (RR); electromagnetic radiation (EMR) may be considered as the second class.

Both classes of radiation are used in diagnoses and treatment of neurological disorders.

Demographics

Devices such as x-ray machines and computed tomography (CT) medical imaging instruments are used commonly in the medical community. Any patient of a physician or other such medical professional in need of such devices for diagnosis and/or treatment would be subjected to various amounts of radiation or radioisotopes.

Description

There are three kinds of radiation useful to medical personnel: alpha, beta, and gamma radiation. Alpha radiation is a flow of alpha particles that have been emitted by an atomic nucleus; beta radiation is a flow of electrons (or positrons) emitted by radioactive nuclei such as strontium-90; and gamma radiation is electromagnetic radiation of very high frequency (very short wavelength), otherwise called gamma rays.

Radioisotopes for medical use, containing unstable combinations of protons and neutrons, are made by neutron activation. This process involves the capture of a neutron by the nucleus of an atom, resulting in an excess of neutrons (neutron rich). Proton-rich radioisotopes are manufactured in cyclotrons. During radioactive decay, the nucleus of a radioisotope seeks energetic stability by emitting particles (alpha, beta, or positron) and photons (including gamma rays).

Radiation produced by radioisotopes allows accurate imaging of internal organs and structures. Radioactive tracers are formed from the bonding of short-lived radioisotopes with chemical compounds that, when in the body, allow the targeting of specific body regions or physiologic processes. Emitted gamma rays (photons) can be detected by gamma cameras and computer enhancement of the resulting images and allows quick and relatively noninvasive (compared to surgery) assessments of trauma or physiological impairments.

Causes and symptoms

Radiation can damage any and all tissues in the body. The particular manifestation will depend upon the amount of radiation, the time during which it is absorbed, and the susceptibility of the particular type of tissue. However, in small doses, radiation can be helpful in the diagnosis and treatment of medical conditions. Some symptoms may occur when radiation is used on humans.

These symptoms depend on the amount of dosage used and the region of the body in which the radiation is applied. Commonly felt symptoms include skin reactions (such as redness or itchiness), tiredness, and loss of appetite. Inflammation of the tissues in and around the affected area can also occur. Such tissue inflammation depends on the particular organs affected. For instance, radiation of the colon may cause diarrhea, whereas radiation to the lungs may cause radiation pneumonitis (or inflammation of lung tissue caused by radiation), with symptoms that include difficulty breathing, chest pain, and coughing. Other signs of **radiation exposure** are bruising, skin burns, vomiting of blood, hair loss, mouth ulcers, and open sores. Even though undesirable and temporary symptoms often occur, they can be minimized with the use of caution and expertise by medical professionals.

Diagnosis

The use of radiation for the diagnosis of disease or damage to the body can greatly benefit patients, but the benefit must outweigh its risk when recommending such procedures. In almost all cases the amount of radiation given in such diagnoses is generally low. For instance, a single diagnostic radiology examination of the (lateral) chest provides about 4 millirem (mrem), or 0.04 milli-Sievert (mSv), of radiation to the patient, while an exam to the abdomen gives approximately 53 mrem (0.53 mSv). As a comparison, the amount of natural **background radiation** that the average American receives each year is approximately 300 mrem (3 mSv). Consequently, the benefits typically outweigh the risks. Research has consistently shown that such low doses of radiation, used for diagnostic radiological examinations, do not cause any serious harm to the human body. However, the increasing use of medical radiation is a growing concern to the medical profession. In fact, a 2010 article in *The Wall Street Journal* stated that "Americans get the most medical radiation in the world—even more than folks in other rich countries—and the average American's dose has grown six-fold over the last couple of decades."

Nuclear radiation

The diagnosis of certain medical conditions is commonly performed with the use of nuclear radiation. Some of these methods include the use of x rays and tomography.

X RAYS. The use of x rays for examining people and animals is called diagnostic radiology. Because the density of tissues is unequal, x rays (a high frequency and energetic form of electromagnetic radiation) pass through tissues in an unequal manner. The beam passed through the body layer is recorded on special film to produce an image of internal structures. However, conventional x rays produce only a two-dimensional (2D) picture of the body structure under investigation.

TOMOGRAPHY. Tomography (from the Greek *tomos*, meaning "to slice") is a method developed to allow the detailed construction of images of the target object. Initially using the x rays to scan layers of the area in question, with computer assisted tomography, a computer then analyzes data of all layers to construct a three-dimensional (3D) image of the object.

Computed tomography (also known as CT, CT scan) and computerized axial tomography (CAT) scans use x rays to produce images of anatomical structures.

Single proton (or photon) emission computed tomography (SPECT) produces three-dimensional images of an organ or body system. SPECT detects the presence and course of a radioactive substance that is injected, ingested, or inhaled. In neurology, a SPECT scan can allow physicians to examine and observe the cerebral circulation. SPECT produces images of the target region by detecting the presence and location of a radioactive isotope. The photon emissions of the radioactive compound containing the isotope can be detected in a manner that is similar to the detection of x rays in computed tomography (CT). At the end of the SPECT scan, the stored information can be integrated to produce a computer-generated composite image.

Positron emission tomography (PET) scans use isotopes produced in a cyclotron. Positron-emitting radionuclides are injected and allowed to accumulate in the target tissue or organ. As the radionuclide decays, it emits a positron that collides with nearby electrons to result in the emission of two identifiable gamma photons. PET scans use rings of detectors that surround the patient to track the movements and concentrations of radioactive tracers. PET scans have attracted the interest of physicians because of their potential use in research into metabolic changes associated with mental diseases such as schizophrenia and depression. PET scans are used in the diagnosis and characterizations of certain cancers and heart disease, as well as clinical studies of the brain. PET uses radiolabeled tracers, including deoxyglucose, which is chemically similar to glucose and is used to assess metabolic rate in tissues and to image tumors, and dopa (3,4-dihydroxyphenylalanine), within the brain.

Another type of CT scan device was first tested in 2007. Using what is called super x rays, the device has the capability of directing a much more concentrated beam of x rays than any older type of technology. The new super x-ray device is called 64-slice CT because it uses 64 detectors to produce the images. It is faster and less expensive at diagnosing heart disease. One day, such advanced technology may eliminate the need for millions of cardiac catheterizations (procedures to unblock clogged arteries) performed annually in the United States. However, a much larger amount of radiation is directed into the patient, which raises considerable controversy in the medical profession. The risk for cancer when such procedures are performed is a major concern of doctors and patients alike.

Electromagnetic radiation

In contrast to imaging produced through the emission and collection of nuclear radiation (e.g., x rays, CT scans), magnetic resonance imaging (MRI) scanners rely on the emission and detection of electromagnetic radiation.

MAGNETIC RESONANCE IMAGING. Electromagnetic radiation consists of oscillations of components of electric and magnetic fields. In the simplest cases, these oscillations occur with definite frequency; the unit of frequency measurement is 1 hertz (Hz), which is one oscillation per second. Arising in some point (under the action of the radiation source), electromagnetic radiation travels with velocity that is equal to the velocity of the light, and this velocity is equal for all frequencies. Another quantity, wavelength, is often used for the description of electromagnetic radiation (this quantity is similar to the distance between two neighboring crests of waves spreading on a water surface, which appeared after dropping a stone on the surface). Because the product of the wavelength and frequency must equal the velocity of light, the greater the wave frequency, the less its wavelength.

MRI scanners rely on the principles of atomic nuclear-spin resonance. Using strong magnetic fields and radio waves, MRIs collect and correlate deflections caused by atoms into images. MRIs allow physicians to see internal structures with great detail and also allow earlier and more accurate diagnosis of disorders.

MRI technology was developed from nuclear magnetic resonance (NMR) technology. Groups of nuclei brought into resonance, that is, nuclei absorbing and emitting photons of similar electromagnetic radiation such as radio waves, make subtle yet distinguishable changes when the resonance is forced to change by altering the energy of impacting photons. The speed and extent of the resonance changes permit a nondestructive (because of the use of low-energy photons) determination of anatomical structures.

MRI images do not utilize potentially harmful ionizing radiation generated by three-dimensional x-ray

---

KEY TERMS

Computed tomography—Abbreviated CT, a medical imaging method that uses tomography along with computer processing to generate three-dimensional images from a series of two-dimensional x-ray images.

Electromagnetic radiation—Abbreviated EMR or EM radiation, a form of energy that contains components of both an electric field and a magnetic field.

Radioactive radiation—Radiation produced from radioactive substances.

Radioisotope—An unstable isotope that emits radiation when it decays or returns to a stable state.

Radiotherapy—The use of x rays or radioactive substances to treat disease.

Rem—Short for roentgen equivalent in man, it is a dose equivalent radiation. One rem is equal to 0.01 Sievert (Sv).

Sievert—Abbreviated Sv, it is a unit of dose equivalent radiation in the International System of Units (SI). One Sv is equal to 100 rem, or 100,000 millirem (mrem).

Tomography—Any of a number of medical imaging procedures that image sections of a body with the use of various types of penetrating waves, such as x rays.

CT scans; rather, they rely on the atomic properties (nuclear resonance) of protons in tissues when they are scanned with radio frequency radiation. The protons in the tissues, which resonate at slightly different frequencies, produce a signal that a computer uses to tell one tissue from another. MRI provides detailed three-dimensional soft tissue images.

Treatment

These methods are used successfully for the treatment of medical conditions. Because higher doses of radiation are used, when compared to diagnosis procedures, the risks are much greater. Consequently, physicians seriously consider the risks and benefits of the treatments for the patient.

Radiation therapy (radiotherapy)

When radiation beams are used for the treatment of patients, the procedure is called radiotherapy. As such, radiotherapy requires the use of radioisotopes and higher doses of radiation that are used diagnostically

> **QUESTIONS TO ASK YOUR DOCTOR**
>
> - How does radiation therapy work?
> - How much does radiation therapy cost? Will my health insurance cover it?
> - What should I expect as side effects of radiation? Are there any long-term effects that I should consider?
> - Can you help me assess the benefits compared to the risks?

to treat some cancers (including brain cancer) and other medical conditions that require destruction of harmful cells.

Radiation therapy is delivered via external radiation or via internal radiation therapy (the implantation/injection of radioactive substances).

Cancer, tumors, and other rapidly dividing cells are usually sensitive to damage by radiation. The goal of radiation therapy is to deliver the minimally sufficient dosage to kill cancerous cells or to keep them from dividing. Cancer cells divide and grow at rates more rapid than normal cells and so are particularly susceptible to radiation. Accordingly, radioisotope irradiation can restrict or eliminate some cancerous growths. The most common forms of external radiation therapy use gamma rays and x rays. During the last half of the twentieth century, the radioisotope cobalt-60 was the frequently used source of radiation used in such treatments. Subsequent methods of irradiation included the production of x rays from linear accelerators.

Iodine-131 and phosphorus-32 are commonly used in radiotherapy. The use of boron-10 to specifically attack tumor cells is one of several more radical uses of radioisotopes. Boron-10 concentrates in tumor cells and is then subjected to neutron beams that result in highly energetic alpha particles that are lethal to the tumor tissue.

Precautions

Radiation therapy is not without risk to healthy tissue and to persons on the healthcare team, and precautions (shielding and limiting exposure) are taken to minimize exposure to other areas of the patient's body and to personnel on the treatment team.

Therapeutic radiologists, radiation oncologists, and a number of technical specialists use radiation and other methods to treat patients who have cancer or other tumors.

Care is taken in the selection of the appropriate radioactive isotope. Ideally, when the radioactive compound is used it loses its radioactive potency rapidly (this is expressed as the half-life of a compound). For example, gamma-emitting compounds used in SPECT scans can have a half-life of just a few hours. This is beneficial for the patients, as it limits the contact time with the potentially damaging radioisotope.

The selection of radioisotopes for medical use is governed by several important considerations involving dosage and half-life. Radioisotopes must be administered in sufficient dosages so that emitted radiation is present in sufficient quantity to be measured. Ideally the radioisotope has a short enough half-life that, at the delivered dosage, there is insignificant residual radiation following the desired length of exposure.

Prognosis

The use of radiation for therapy widely varies due primarily to the type of cancer being treated, the location of the cancer, the degree that the cancer has spread in the body, and the type of radiation therapy being administered to the patient. In some cases, radiation can cure the cancer, such as in the treatment for skin tumors, laryngeal cancer (of the vocal cords), and early-stage breast cancer (after a lumpectomy has been performed). In other cases, radiation does not cure the cancer but prevents the cancer from spreading and improves the patient's quality of life.

Prevention

New areas of radiation therapy that may prove more effective in treating brain tumors (and other forms of cancers) include three-dimensional conformal radiation therapy (a process where multiple beams are shaped to match the contour of the tumor) and stereotactic radiosurgery (used to irradiate certain brain tumors and obstructions of the cerebral circulation). Gamma knives use focused beams (with the patient often wearing a special helmet to help focus the beams), while cyberknifes use hundreds of precise pinpoint beams emanating from a source of irradiation that moves around the patient's head.

Resources

BOOKS

Adler, Arlene M, and Richard R. Carlton, eds. *Introduction to Radiologic Sciences and Patient Care*. St. Louis: Elsevier Saunders, 2012.

Khalil, Magdy M. *Basic Sciences of Nuclear Medicine*. Berlin: Springer, 2011.

Saha, Gopal B. *Fundamentals of Nuclear Pharmacy*. New York: Springer, 2010.

Yarbro, Connie Henke, Debra Wujcik, and Barbara Holmes Gobel, eds. *Cancer Nursing: Principles and Practice.* Sudbury, MA: Jones and Bartlett, 2011.

WEBSITES

"Medical Radiation Is a Growing Concern." The Wall Street Journal, June 15, 2010. http://online.wsj.com/article/SB10001424052748704324304575306940440759082.html (accessed March 23, 2011).

"Radiation, People, and the Environment." International Atomic Energy Agency. http://www.iaea.org/Publications/Booklets/RadPeopleEnv/index.html (accessed March 21, 2011).

Stabin, Michael G. "Doses from Medical Radiation Sources." Health Physics Society. http://www.hps.org/hpspublications/articles/dosesfrommedicalradiation.html (accessed March 21, 2011).

"'Super X-rays' Spot Heart Ills, Spark Debate." MSNBC. http://www.msnbc.msn.com/id/21642624/ns/health-heart_health/ (accessed March 21, 2011).

"What Is Nuclear Medicine?" Society of Nuclear Medicine. http://www.snm.org/index.cfm?PageID=3106&RPID (accessed March 21, 2011).

ORGANIZATIONS

Environmental Protection Agency, 1200 Pennsylvania Ave. NW, Washington, DC 20460, (202) 272-0167, http://water.epa.gov.

National Cancer Institute, 6116 Executive Blvd., Rm. 3036A, Bethesda, MD 20892-8322, (800) 422-6237, cancergovstaff@mail.nih.gov, http://www.cancer.gov.

Alexander Ioffe

Radiation exposure

Definition

Radiation is the emission of energy from an atom in the form of a wave or particle.

Description

Radiation is emitted when an atomic nucleus undergoes decay (change), which is associated with

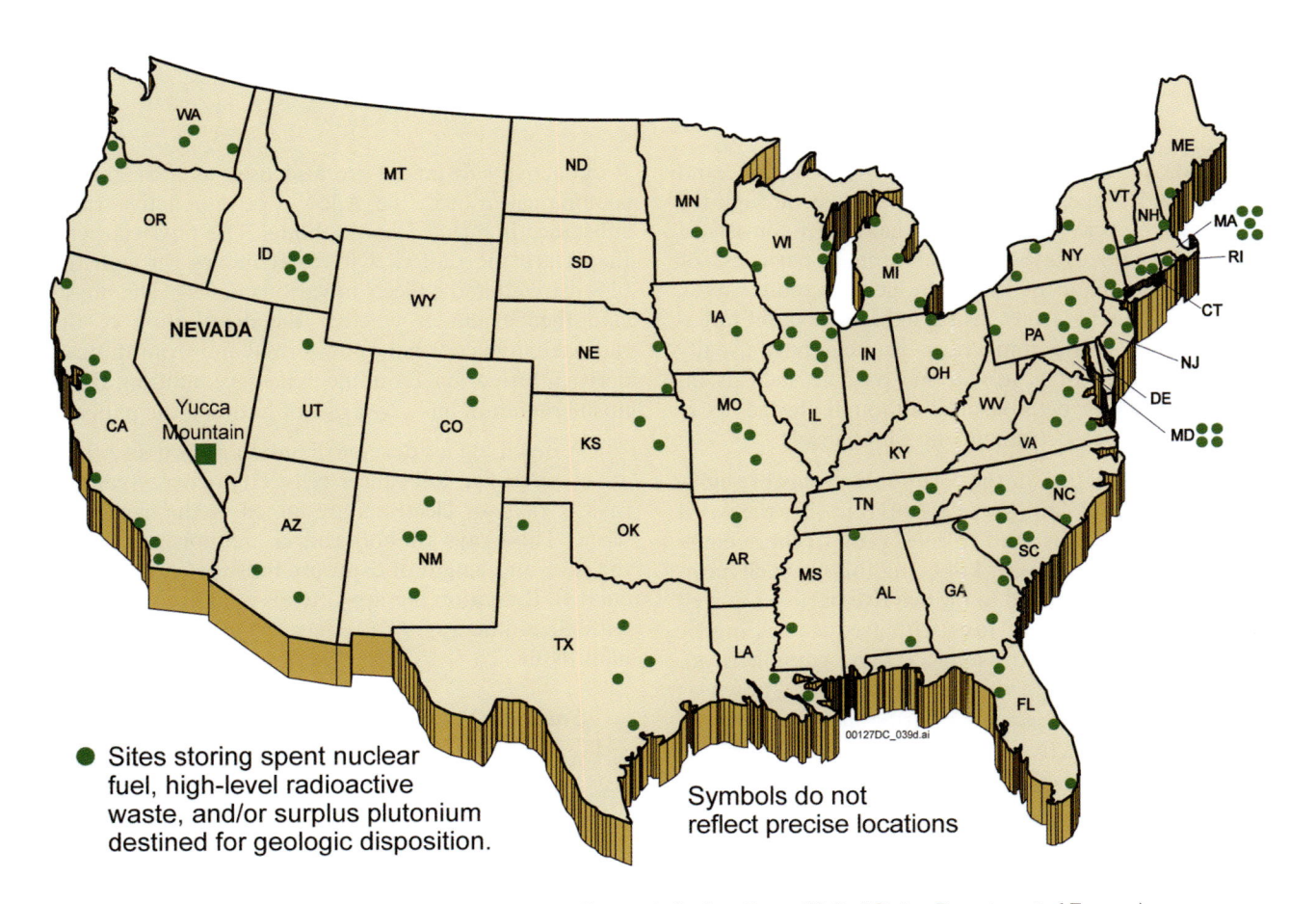

A map of the United States showing radioactive waste disposal site locations *(United States Department of Energy.)*

HIROSHIMA AND NAGASAKI (1945)

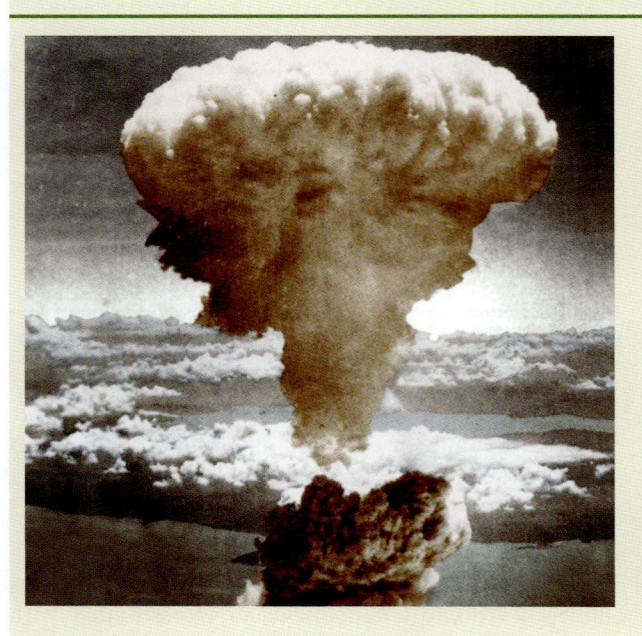

The American military's atomic bombings of Hiroshima and Nagasaki directly influenced Japan's unconditional surrender in World War II. In August of 1945, the first atomic bomb was dropped by the *Enola Gay*, an American B-29 bomber. The atomic bomb, known as "Little Boy", hit the Japanese city of Hiroshima, killing approximately 80,000 people and wiping out most of the town.

Three days later, a second atomic bomb was dropped on the major Japanese shipbuilding port of Nagasaki, killing approximately 40,000. With his country reeling from the devastating power of nuclear warfare, the Japanese emperor surrendered on August 15.

Survivors of the nuclear attacks have an increased health threat of radiation-induced cancer. The Radiation Effects Research Foundation (RERF), a Japanese/United States joint commission, monitors these atomic bomb survivors and studies the long-term health effects of radiation exposure.

The mushroom cloud of the first atomic bomb over Nagasaki, Japan, 9 August 1945. *(Photo by Apic/Getty Images.)*

---

the radioactivity of certain naturally occurring and manmade isotopes. The radiation emitted through the radioactive decay of certain atomic nuclei consists of electromagnetic waves, or sub-atomic particles, or both. Electromagnetic radiation includes radio waves, infrared waves (or heat), visible light, **ultraviolet radiation**, x-rays, and gamma rays. Radioactivity usually takes the form of a sub-atomic particle such as an alpha particle or beta particle, although atomic decay can also release electromagnetic gamma rays.

While radiation in the form of heat, visible light, and even ultraviolet light is essential to life, the word "radiation" often is used to refer only to those emissions that can damage or kill living things. Such harm is specifically attributed to radioactive particles as well as the electromagnetic rays with frequencies higher than visible light (ultraviolet, x rays, gamma rays). Harmful electromagnetic radiation is also known as ionizing radiation because it strips atoms of one or more of their electrons, leaving highly reactive ions called free radicals that can damage tissue or genetic material (DNA).

Radiation is used safely in medical settings as both a diagnostic tool and a therapeutic agent. X rays are the most common diagnostic tool that uses radiation.

Radioactive substances are also used as a diagnostic tool in nuclear medicine. A low-dose radioactive tracer substance is injected in the body. The physician can then trace the radioactivity as it moves through the bloodstream and collects in various tissues. The physician then evaluates whether the distribution of the radioactivity is normal or abnormal and from this can derive information about the patient's condition. Diagnostic radiation has a low risk of harming the patient.

A much higher dose of radiation is used as a therapeutic agent to kill cancer cells. High-energy gamma rays, x rays, or electrons are aimed at the cancerous tissue. These rays kill both cancer and normal cells, so the dose and length of exposure must be carefully calculated. Radiation therapy often is used in conjunction with chemotherapy or after surgery to remove malignant tissue.

Sources of radiation

About 82% of the average American's radiation exposure comes from natural sources. These sources include radon gas emissions from underground, cosmic rays from space, naturally occurring radioactive elements within our own bodies, and radioactive particles emitted from soil and rocks.

Manmade radiation, the other 18%, comes primarily from medical x rays and nuclear medicine, but it is also emitted from some other sources (e.g., smoke detectors; airport body scanners; blue topaz jewelry), or originates in the production and testing of nuclear weapons and the manufacture of nuclear fuels.

Although artificial sources of radiation contribute only a small fraction to overall radiation exposure, they remain a strong concern for two reasons. First, they are preventable or avoidable, unlike cosmic radiation, for example. Second, while the average individual may not receive a significant dose of radiation from artificial sources, geographic and occupational factors may mean exposure to dramatically higher doses of radiation for large numbers of people. For instance, many Americans have been exposed to radiation from nearly 600 nuclear tests conducted at the Nevada Test Site. From the early 1950s to the early 1960s, atmospheric blasts caused a lingering increase in radiation-related sickness downwind of the site and increased the overall dose of radiation received by Americans by as much as 7%. Once the tests were moved underground, that figure fell to less than 1%.

A February 1990 study of the Windscale plutonium processing plant in Britain clearly demonstrated the importance of the indirect effects of radiation exposure. The study correlated an abnormally high rate of **leukemia** among children in the area with male workers at the plant, who evidently passed a tendency to leukemia to their children even though they had been receiving radiation doses that were considered "acceptable."

Environmental scientists believe that radon, a radioactive gas, accounts for most of the radiation dose Americans receive. Released by the decay of uranium in the earth, radon can infiltrate a house through pores in block walls, cracks in basement walls or floors, or around pipes. In 2010, the **Environmental Protection Agency (EPA)** estimated that roughly one in every fifteen homes in the United States had elevated levels of radon. The **EPA** called radon "the largest environmental radiation health problem affecting Americans." Inhaled radon may contribute to as many as 21,000 lung cancer deaths each year in the United States. The EPA now recommends that homeowners test their houses for radon gas and install a specialized ventilation system if excessive levels of gas are detected. Some states require radon testing whenever an existing house changes ownership.

The 2008–2009 report from the *President's Cancer Panel* recognized the health danger and ubiquitous nature of radon gas in the United States. The Panel offered a number of recommendations, such as a requirement of radon-resistant features as part of all new home construction; improvements in the reliability and accuracy of testing methods to uncover radon in buildings; as well as calling for mandatory testing of radon exposure levels in the workplace, at school, and in daycare facilities.

> ## KEY TERMS
>
> **Alpha particle**—A positively charged particle emitted during radioactive decay. It contains two protons and two neutrons and is the same as the nucleus of the helium atom.
>
> **Beta particle**—High-energy electrons (negatively charged) or positrons (positively charged) emitted during radioactive decay. They are a form of ionizing radiation.
>
> **Free radical**—A molecule with an unpaired electron that has a strong tendency to react with other molecules in DNA (genetic material), proteins, and lipids (fats), resulting in damage to cells.
>
> **Hemorrhage**—Heavy bleeding.
>
> **White blood cells**—A group of several cell types that occur in the bloodstream and are essential for a properly functioning immune system.

Causes and symptoms

The effects of radiation depend upon the type of radiation absorbed, the amount or dose received, and the part of the body irradiated. Alpha and beta particles have limited power to penetrate the body; gamma rays and x rays are far more potent. The damage potential of a radiation dose is expressed in *rems*, a quantity equal to the actual dose in *rads* (units per kg) multiplied by a quality factor, called Q, representing the potency of the radiation in living tissue.

Over a lifetime, a person typically receives 7–14 rems from natural sources. Exposure to 5–75 rems causes few observable symptoms. Exposure to 75–200 rems leads to vomiting, fatigue, and loss of appetite. Exposure to 300 rems or more leads to severe changes in blood cells accompanied by hemorrhage. Such a dosage delivered to the whole body is lethal 50% of the time. An exposure of more than 600 rems causes loss of hair, loss of the body's ability to fight infection, and results in death. A dose of 10,000 rem will kill quickly through damage to the central nervous system.

The symptoms that follow exposure to a harmful dose of radiation are often termed radiation sickness or radiation burn. Bone marrow and lymphoid tissue cells, testes and ovaries, and embryonic tissue are most sensitive to radiation exposure. Since the lymphatic tissue manufactures white blood cells (WBCs), radiation sickness usually is accompanied by a reduction in WBC production within seventy-two hours, and recovery from a radiation dose is first indicated by an increase in WBC production.

Any exposure to radiation increases the risk of cancer, birth defects, and genetic damage, as well as accelerating the aging process, and causing other health problems including impaired immunity. Various cancers, stroke, diabetes, hypertension, and cardiovascular and renal disease are among the chronic diseases often experienced by those exposed to excessive radiation.

Treatment

Treatment of radiation exposure or contamination is complicated by the need to prevent contamination or exposure of the attending healthcare professionals. Exposure occurs when the individual has been exposed to a radioactive source, but does not carry radioactive material in or on his or her body or clothing. Contamination occurs when the body or clothing of the individual contains radioactive material. Contamination can be external (clothing or skin) or internal (airways, lungs). Internal contamination is much less common than external contamination, but is also much more difficult to remedy.

Basic treatment steps include protecting the attending healthcare professionals and preventing contamination of the treatment area. When contamination is suspected, a probe attached to a survey Geiger counter is used to identify the location and extent of external contamination. In addition, samples of urine, feces, swabs of the airways, open wounds, and stomach contents may be monitored for radioactivity.

Clothing is removed and quarantined. The body is then decontaminated by washing skin and hair with water and a mild soap until the level of radioactivity is reduced. The used wash water will contain radioactivity and must also be quarantined. Much of the difficulty in treating radiation contamination comes from the need to protect those providing the treatment and to prevent radiation, which can be neither seen nor smelled, from spreading and contaminating new areas.

After the body is free of radiation, care is supportive and depends on symptoms. Long-term follow-up and monitoring for the development of cancers and other health problems is essential

Prevention

Protection basics for people working in environments where radiation is present consist of shielding

> **QUESTIONS TO ASK YOUR DOCTOR**
>
> - Do the diagnostic tests you have ordered expose me to radiation? If so, what are the short-term and long term risks?
> - I fly frequently. Should I be worried about the amount of radiation I am exposed to when I pass through body scanners at the airport?
> - How can I protect my children from unnecessary radiation exposure?
> - I have been told there is a low level of radon in my basement. Is it safe for my children to play there?

and monitoring. Shielding creates a barrier to radiation. The degree of shielding necessary to keep workers safe depends on the type of radiation present and how close they must work to the radiaation source. High-energy radiation has more penetrating power than low-energy radiation and thus greater shielding is necessary. All workers should wear monitoring badges that record their level of radiation exposure so that it does not exceed allowable levels.

The benefits of radiation exposure when used for diagnostic and therapeutic purposes generally outweighs the risks. However, patients should avoid unnecessary diagnostic tests such as x rays and should speak to their physicians and technicians about any concerns they may have about safety.

Resources

WEBSITES

Centers for Disease Control and Prevention (CDC). "Radiation Emergencies." http://emergency.cdc.gov/radiation (accessed October 23, 2012).

Environmental Protection Agency. "Radiation Protection: Health Effects." http://www.epa.gov/radiation/understand/health_effects.html (accessed October 23, 2012).

International Atomic Energy Agency. "Radiation, People and the Environment." http://www.iaea.org/Publications/Booklets/RadPeopleEnv/intro.html (accessed October 23, 2012).

Mayo Clinic. "Radiation sickness." http://www.mayoclinic.com/health/radiation-sickness/DS00432 (accessed October 23, 3012).

MedlinePlus. "Radiation Exposure." October 18, 2012 http://www.nlm.nih.gov/medlineplus/radiationexposure.html (accessed October 23, 2012).

Pae, Jeanne S. "Radiation Emergencies" Medscape Reference September 26, 2011. http://emedicine.medscape.com/article/834015-overview (accessed October 23, 2012).

United States Department of Energy. "Understanding Radiation." http://www.ne.doe.gov/pdfFiles/UNDERRAD.PDF (accessed October 23, 2012).

ORGANIZATIONS

International Atomic Energy Agency (IAEA), Vienna International Center, PO Box 100, Vienna, Austria A-1400, +4312600-0, Fax: +4312600-7, Official.Mail@iaea.org, http://www.iaea.org.

United States Centers for Disease Control and Prevention (CDC), 1600 Clifton Road, Atlanta, GA 30333, (404) 639-3534, (800) CDC-INFO (800-232-4636); TTY: (888) 232-6348, inquiry@cdc.gov, http://www.cdc.gov.

United States Environmental Protection Agency (EPA), Ariel Rios Building, 1200 Pennsylvania Avenue, N.W., Washington, DC 20460, (202) 272-0167; TTY (202) 272-0165, http://www.epa.gov.

Jeffrey Muhr
Tish Davidson, AM

Radiation injuries

Definition

Radiation injuries are caused by ionizing radiation emitted by sources such as the sun, x-ray and other diagnostic machines, tanning beds, and radioactive elements released in nuclear power plant accidents and detonation of nuclear weapons during war and as part of terrorist acts.

Demographics

Anyone has the potential for being injured by radiation, whether it is naturally, such as from a severe sunburn, or artificially, such as from radiation leaked from a nuclear power plant or expelled through a nuclear weapon.

Description

Ionizing radiation derives from unstable atoms that contain an excess amount of energy. In an attempt to stabilize, the atoms emit the excess energy creating radiation. Radiation can either be electromagnetic (in the form of a wave) or as particles.

The energy of electromagnetic radiation is a direct function of its frequency. The high-energy, high-frequency waves that can penetrate solids to various depths cause damage by separating molecules into electrically charged pieces, a process known as ionization. X rays are a type of electromagnetic radiation. Sub-atomic particles come from radioactive isotopes as they decay to stable elements. Electrons traveling at high velocity form beta radiate. Alpha particles are the nuclei of helium atoms—two protons and two neutrons—without the surrounding electrons. Alpha particles interact so strongly with matter that they cannot penetrate a piece of paper unless greatly accelerated in electric and magnetic fields. Both beta and alpha particles are typical of ionizing particulate radiation. Exposure to ionizing radiation can lead to chromosomal damage in deoxyribonucleic acid (DNA), although DNA is very good at repairing itself; both strands of the double helix must be broken to produce genetic damage.

Because radiation is energy, it can be measured. There are a number of units used to quantify radiation energy. Some refer to effects on air, others to effects on living tissue. The roentgen, named after German physicist Wilhelm Conrad Röentgen (1845–1923), sometimes spelled Roentgen, who discovered x rays in 1895, measures ionizing energy in air. A rad expresses the energy transferred to tissue. The rem measures tissue response. A roentgen generates about a rad of effect and produces about a rem of response. The gray and the sievert are international units equivalent to 100 rads and rems, respectively. A curie, named after French physicists Marie Curie (1867–1934) and Pierre Curie (1859–1906) who experimented with radiation, is a measure of actual radioactivity given off by a radioactive element, not a measure of its effect. The average annual human exposure to natural **background radiation** is roughly 3 milliSieverts (mSv). The gray, Becquerel, and sievert have increasingly replaced the curie, rad, rem and roentgen.

Any amount of ionizing radiation will produce some damage; however, radiation is everywhere, from the sun (cosmic rays) and from traces of radioactive elements in the air (radon) and the ground (uranium, radium, carbon-14, potassium-40 and many others). Earth's atmosphere protects humans and other living beings from most of the sun's radiation. However, living at 5,000 feet (1,500 m) altitude in Denver, Colorado, approximately doubles exposure to radiation. Further, a flight in a commercial airliner increases it by about 24 times more when lifting humans above 80% of the atmosphere, or at about 32,800 feet (10,000 m) in altitude. Because no amount of radiation is perfectly safe and because radiation is ever present, arbitrary limits have been established to provide some measure of safety for those humans exposed to unusual amounts. Less than 1% of them reach the current annual permissible maximum of 2,000 mrem (20 mSv).

A 2001 ruling by the Federal Court of Australia indicated that two soldiers died from cancer caused by exposure to radiation while occupying Hiroshima in 1945. The soldiers were exposed to less than 500 rem (5 Sv) of radiation. The international recommendation for workers, as of 2010 and after over a century of scientific study, is a safety level of up to 2,000 mrem (20 mSv). Further, according to the U.S. Nuclear Regulatory Commission, the average U.S. nuclear worker receives about 120 mrem (1.2 mSv) per year, whereas a typical x-ray scan produces about 10 mrem (0.1 mSv).

Many international agencies, such as the International Agency for Research on Cancer (IARC), part of the **World Health Organization** (WHO), suggests that even extremely low doses of radiation can be potentially harmful. For the most part, such doses are generally safe for nuclear workers, but the potential for harm remains, as based on internationally recognized scientific studies. Specifically, the IARC conducted an international study of nearly half a million nuclear workers in 15 countries. Their exposure to low levels of radiation was found to be "statistically compatible with the current bases for radiation protection standards."

Ultraviolet (UV) radiation exposure

UV radiation from the sun (naturally produced by the closest star to Earth) and tanning beds and lamps (artificially produced by humans) can cause skin damage, premature aging, and skin cancers. Malignant **melanoma** is the most dangerous of skin cancers. Thus, a definite link exists between type UVA exposure used in tanning beds and its occurrence. UVB type UV radiation is associated with sunburn, and while not as penetrating as UVA, it still damages the skin during high exposures. Skin damage accumulates over time, and effects do not often manifest until individuals reach middle age. Light-skinned people who most often burn rather than tan are at a greater risk of skin damage than darker-skinned individuals who rarely burn. The U.S. **Food and Drug Administration** (FDA) and the **Centers for Disease Control and Prevention** (CDC) discourage the use of tanning beds and sun lamps and encourage all people to use sunscreen with a sun protection factor (SPF) of 15 or greater. In 2009, the International Agency for Research on Cancer classified tanning beds as "carcinogenic to humans", with carcinogenic meaning that they cause cancer. This classification by the IARC is its highest cancer risk category. In fact, IARC studies that prompted the cancer classification found that UVA, UVB, and UVC radiation all cause cancer in laboratory animals.

Over exposure during medical procedures

Ionizing radiation has many uses in medicine, both in diagnosis and in treatment. X rays, CT (computed tomography) scanners, and fluoroscopes use it to form images of the body's insides. Nuclear medicine uses radioactive isotopes to diagnose and to treat medical conditions. In the body, radioactive elements localize to specific tissues and give off tiny amounts of radiation. Detecting that radiation provides information on both anatomy and function. Between 1995 and 2010, skin injuries caused by too much exposure during medical procedures were documented. In 1995, the FDA issued a recommendation to physicians and medical institutions to record and monitor the dosage of radiation used during medical procedures on patients in order to minimize the amount of skin injuries. The FDA suggested doses of radiation not exceed 1 Grey (Gy). (A Grey is roughly equivalent to a sievert.)

As of 2001, the FDA was preparing further guidelines for fluoroscopy, the procedure most often associated with medical-related radiation skin injuries such as rashes and more serious burns and tissue death. Injuries occurred most often during angioplasty procedures using fluoroscopy. As of late 2010, the FDA was still in the process of issuing updated guidelines for radiation safety performance standards for diagnostic x-ray systems, such as flurorscopic x-ray systems. These updated standards were expected to parallel developments in technology and product usage, along with being more similar to international standards.

CT scans of children have also been problematic. Oftentimes the dosage of radiation used for an adult is not decreased for a child, leading to radiation over exposure. Children are more sensitive to radiation and a February 2001 study indicated 1,500 out of 1.6 million children under 15 years of age receiving CT scans annually were expected to develop cancer. Studies showed that decreasing the radiation by half for CT scans of children would effectively decrease the possibility of over exposure while still providing an effective diagnostic image. The benefits to receiving the medical treatment utilizing radiation is still greater than the risks involved; however, more stringent control over the amount of radiation used during the procedures was expected to go far in minimizing the risk of radiation injury to the patient.

Minimizing the risk of medical **radiation exposure** in children can be accomplished by doing the following:

- only image when there is a definite medical benefit
- use the minimum amount of radiation for adequate imaging based on size of the child
- image only the indicated area
- avoid multiple scans

- use alternative diagnostic studies (such as ultrasound or MRI [magnetic resonance imaging]) when possible

Radiation exposure from nuclear accidents and weaponry

Between 1945 and 1987, there were 285 nuclear reactor accidents, injuring more than 1,550 people and killing 64. The most striking example was the meltdown of the graphite core nuclear reactor at Chernobyl (in Ukraine, part of the former Soviet Union) in 1986, which spread a cloud of radioactive particles across the entire continent of Europe. Over the following decades, information about radiation effects continued to be gathered from that disaster, but 31 people were killed in the immediate accident, and at least 1,800 children were subsequently diagnosed with thyroid cancer. In a study published in May 2001 by the British Royal Society, children born to individuals involved in the cleanup of Chernobyl and born after the accident are six times more likely to have genetic mutations than children born before the accident.

After the terrorist attacks on the World Trade Center and the Pentagon on September 11, 2001, the possibility of terrorist-caused nuclear accidents became a concern. As of 2008, All 104 active nuclear power plants in the United States were on full alert, but they were still vulnerable to sabotage such as bombing or attack from the air. The Federal Aviation Administration (FAA) established a no-fly zone of 12 miles (19 km), at an altitude of below 18,000 feet (5,500 m), around nuclear power plants. There was also growing concern over the security of spent nuclear fuel: More than 40,000 tons of spent fuel is housed in buildings at closed plants around the country. Unlike the active nuclear reactors that are enclosed in concrete-reinforced buildings, the spent fuel is stored in nonreinforced buildings. Housed in cooling pools, the spent fuel could emit dangerous levels of radioactive material if exploded or used in makeshift weaponry. Radioactive medical and industrial waste could also be used to make so-called dirty bombs. After 1993, the Nuclear Regulatory Commission (NRC) reported 376 cases of stolen radioactive materials.

On March 15, 2011, the Japanese government imposed a 18-mile (30-km) no-fly zone around the Fukushima Daiichi Nuclear Power Plant after it was damaged from a 9.0-magnitude earthquake (commonly called the 2011 Tōhoku earthquake) that hit on March 11, 2011, off the coast of northeastern Japan. At least three nuclear reactors sustained damage from the tsunamis that followed this major earthquake. Explosions arose from a build-up of gas within their containment walls. On March 18, 2011, the International Atomic Energy Agency (IAEA) described the situation as extremely serious.

Causes and symptoms

Radiation can damage every tissue in the body. The particular manifestation will depend upon the amount of radiation, the time over which it is absorbed, and the susceptibility of the tissue. The fastest growing tissues are the most vulnerable because radiation as much as triples its effects during the growth phase. Bone marrow cells that make blood are the fastest growing cells in the body. A fetus is equally sensitive. The germinal cells in the testes and ovaries are only slightly less sensitive. Both can be rendered useless with very small doses of radiation. More resistant are the lining cells of the body, the skin and intestines. Most resistant are the brain cells, because they grow the slowest.

Many signs and symptoms can occur after a person has been exposed to a large amount of radiation. Some of these signs and symptoms from radiation sickness (radiation poisoning) are:

- bleeding of the mouth, gums, nose, and rectum
- bloody stool
- bruising of the body
- burning of the skin
- dehydration
- diarrhea
- fainting and dizziness
- fatigue, tiredness, and weakness
- hair loss
- inflammation of body areas (that were not covered at the time of exposure)
- mouth ulcers
- open sores on skin, especially those uncovered at the time of radiation exposure
- vomiting and nausea
- ulcers of the esophagus, intestines, and stomach
- ulcers of the mouth

The length of exposure makes a big difference in what happens afterward. Over time the accumulating damage, if not enough to kill cells outright, distorts their growth and causes scarring and/or cancers. In addition to leukemias and cancers of the thyroid, brain, bone, breast, skin, stomach, and lung, all may arise after radiation. Damage depends, too, on the ability of the tissue to repair itself. Some tissues and some types of damage produce much greater consequences than others.

There are three types of radiation injuries.

KEY TERMS

Computed tomography (CT)—A medical imaging method that uses tomography along with computer processing to generate three-dimensional images from a series of two-dimensional x-ray images.

Deoxyribonucleic acid (DNA)—The chemical of chromosomes and hence the vehicle of heredity.

Dirty bomb—A radiological weapon that combines radioactive material and conventional explosives; in other words, a conventional bomb could be exploded near radioactive material causing the area to become contaminated with radioactive material.

Gray—Abbreviated Gy, a unit within the International System of Units (SI) that refers to absorbed radiation dose of ionizing radiation. One Gray is defined as the absorption of one joule of ionizing radiation by one kilogram of matter.

Isotope—An unstable form of an element that gives off radiation to become stable. Elements are characterized by the number of electrons around each atom. One electron's negative charge balances the positive charge of each proton in the nucleus. To keep all those positive charges in the nucleus from repelling each other (like the same poles of magnets), neutrons are added. Only certain numbers of neutrons work. Other numbers cannot hold the nucleus together, so it splits apart, giving off ionizing radiation. Sometimes one of the split products is not stable either, so another split takes place. The process is called radioactivity.

Rem—short for roentgen equivalent in man, rem is a dose equivalent radiation. One rem is equal to 0.01 Sievert (Sv).

Sievert—Abbreviated Sv, it is a unit of dose equivalent radiation in the International System of Units (SI). One Sv is equal to 100 rem, or 100,000 millirem (mrem).

Tomography—Any of a number of medical imaging procedures that image sections of a body with the use of various types of penetrating waves, such as x rays.

UVA—Ultraviolet A, a long wave of ultraviolet radiation, with a wavelength of 400 to 315 nanometers and an energy level of 3.10 to 3.94 electron volts.

UVB—Ultraviolet B, a medium wave of ultraviolet radiation, with a wavelength of 315 to 280 nanometers and an energy level of 3.94 to 4.43 electron volts.

UVC—Ultraviolet C, a short wave of ultraviolet radiation, with a wavelength of 280 to 1000 nanometers and an energy level of 4.43 to 12.4 electron volts.

- External irradiation: As with x-ray exposure, all or part of the body is exposed to radiation that either is absorbed or passes through the body.
- Contamination: As with a nuclear accident, the environment and its inhabitants are exposed to radiation. People are affected internally, externally, or with both internal and external exposure.
- Incorporation: Dependent on contamination, the bodies of individuals affected incorporate the radiation chemicals within cells, organs, and tissues and the radiation is dispersed throughout the body.

Immediately after sudden irradiation, the fate of those affected depends mostly on the total dose absorbed. This information comes mostly from survivors of the two atomic bombs the United States dropped over two cities in Japan in 1945.

- Massive doses incinerate immediately and are not distinguishable from the heat of the source.
- A sudden whole body dose over 50 Sv (5,000 rem, or 5 mrem) produces such profound neurological, heart, and circulatory damage that patients die within the first two days (100% chance of fatalities).
- Doses around 10 to 20 Sv (1,000 to 2,000rem, or 1 to 2 mrem) range affect the intestines, stripping their lining and leading to death within three months from vomiting, diarrhea, starvation, and infection.
- Victims receiving around 6 to 10 Sv (600 to 1,000 rem, or 0.6 to 1.0 mrem) instantaneously usually escape an intestinal death, facing instead bone marrow failure and death within two months from loss of blood coagulation factors and the protection against infection provided by white blood cells.
- A dose of from 2 to 6 Sv (200 to 600 rem, or 1 to 2 mrem) gives some chance for survival if victims are supported with blood transfusions and antibiotics (generally no fatalities occur if proper medical procedures are followed).
- People suffering from 1 to 2 Sv (100 to 200 rem, or 0.5 to 1.0 mrem) will have a brief, nonlethal sickness with

vomiting, loss of appetite, and generalized discomfort. At this level, victims still receive several thousand times more than an average person does in normal exposure over one year.

Diagnosis

A person who has been exposed to a high dose of radiation should seek out immediate assistance from medical personnel. When a known major incident has occurred, medical personnel will be at the site within a short period. In any case, medical personnel will take the necessary steps to measure the amount of radiation absorbed into the body of these victims. The amount of radiation absorbed into the human victims will dictate which treatments will be used and how likely the person will survive over the next few days, weeks, and months.

Critical information is acquired in order to provide the best diagnosis and, thus, treatment, for these victims. This vital information is:

- Symptoms: Onset of vomiting and other signs and symptoms with respect to the time of initial exposure (generally, the shorter [longer] the time of vomiting from initial exposure, the higher [lower] the radiation dose received).
- Distance from source: Distance the victim was from the radiation source, along with the duration of the exposure (generally, the further away from the radiation source, the less radiation exposure).
- Blood tests: Taken over several days to determine white blood cell counts and any changes in the DNA of blood cells, which help to verify the amount of bone marrow damage and, thus, the amount of radioactive material in the body.
- Dosimeter: If such a device was exposed to the same radiation event, it can be effectively used to compare the amount absorbed by people.
- Geiger counter: A survey-meter device can be scanned across the body to determine the amount of radioactive particles on the victim.
- Radiation type: A determination as to the type of radiation people have been exposed to can help to treat victims in a more effective manner.

Treatment

It is clearly important to have some idea of the dose received as early as possible, so that attention can be directed to those victims in the 2–10 Sv range who might survive with treatment. Blood transfusions, protection from infection in damaged organs, and

> ### QUESTIONS TO ASK YOUR DOCTOR
>
> - What should I do if I begin to show signs and symptoms from radiation exposure?
> - What should I expect from the side effects of radiation? Are there any long-term effects that I should be concerned about?
> - How much radiation have I been exposed to?
> - What is my prognosis for recovery? What are my chances of surviving?
> - Are there special medical facilities that treat people with radiation exposure? If so, how do I contact them?

possibly the use of newer stimulants to blood formation can save many victims in this category.

Local radiation exposures usually damage the skin and require careful wound care, removal of dead tissue, and skin grafting if the area is large. Again infection control is imperative.

One of the best known, and perhaps even mainstream, treatments of radiation injury is the use of *Aloe vera* preparations on damaged areas of skin. It has demonstrated remarkable healing properties even for chronic ulcerations resulting from radiation exposure.

Alternative treatment

There is considerable interest in benevolent chemicals called free radical scavengers. How well they work is yet to be determined, but population studies strongly suggest that certain diets are better than others and that those better diets are full of free radical scavengers, otherwise known as antioxidants. The recommended ingredients are beta-carotene, vitamins E and C, and selenium, all available as commercial preparations. Beta-carotene is yellow-orange and is present in yellow and orange fruits and vegetables. Vitamin C can be found naturally in citrus fruits. Traditional Chinese medicine (TCM) and acupuncture, botanical medicine, and homeopathy all have contributions to make to recovery from the damage of radiation injuries. The level of recovery will depend on the exposure.

Prognosis

The degree to which one has been exposed to radiation and the length of time of that exposure will determine the prognosis of individual cases. If people survive ten to fifteen years after the radiation exposure, most illnesses associated with the exposure will have presented themselves. Illnesses involving the endocrine glands, thyroid, nervous system, digestive organs, and sensory organs seem to be especially prevalent in such people.

Prevention

Injuries caused by radiation exposure can be avoided by not working or living around known sources of radiation. If such sites cannot be avoided, then workers should wear badges that consistently measure exposure levels. When being diagnosed or treated with radiation, individuals ought to make sure protective shields are used over the part of their body not be diagnosed or treated. In addition, they should discuss with their family doctor or other medical professionals whenever radiation devices are used to make sure they are essentially needed.

Resources

BOOKS

Adler, Arlene M., and Richard R. Carlton, eds. *Introduction to Radiologic Sciences and Patient Care*. St. Louis: Elsevier Saunders, 2012.

Khalil, Magdy M. *Basic Sciences of Nuclear Medicine*. Berlin: Springer, 2011.

Saha, Gopal B. *Fundamentals of Nuclear Pharmacy*. New York: Springer, 2010.

Yarbro, Connie Henke, Debra Wujcik, and Barbara Holmes Gobel, eds. *Cancer Nursing: Principles and Practice*. Sudbury, MA: Jones and Bartlett, 2011.

WEBSITES

"How Radioactivity Can Affect You." Oasis LLC. http://www.oasisllc.com/abgx/effects.htm (accessed March 22, 2011).

"Japan Imposes No-Fly Zone Above Crippled Nuclear Plant." NYC Aviation News, March 15, 2011. http://nycaviation.com/2011/03/japan-imposes-no-fly-zone-above-crippled-nuclear-plant/ (accessed March 22, 2011).

"Japan's Crisis Extremely Serious: IAEA Chief." Hindustan Times, March 18, 2011. http://www.hindustantimes.com/News-Feed/restofasia/IAEA-chief-says-Japan-s-crisis-extremely-serious/Article1-674806.aspx (accessed March 22, 2011).

"Radiation-Emitting Products: Medical Imaging." U.S. Food and Drug Administration, October 3, 2010. http://www.fda.gov/Radiation-EmittingProducts/RadiationEmittingProductsandProcedures/MedicalImaging/MedicalX-Rays/ucm135572.htm (accessed March 22, 2011).

"Radiation Sickness." Mayo Clinic. http://www.mayoclinic.com/health/radiation-sickness/DS00432 (accessed March 22, 2011).

"Radiation Sickness." MedlinePlus, U.S. National Library of Medicine and National Institutes of Health. http://www.nlm.nih.gov/medlineplus/ency/article/000026.htm (accessed March 22, 2011).

"Radiation Standards and Organizations Provide Safety for Public and Workers." Nuclear Energy Institute. http://www.nei.org/resourcesandstats/documentlibrary/safetyandsecurity/factsheet/radiationstandards/ (accessed March 22, 2011).

"WHO: Tanning Beds Cause Cancer." World Health Organization. http://www.webmd.com/skin-problems-and-treatments/news/20090728/who-tanning-beds-cause-cancer (accessed March 22, 2011).

ORGANIZATIONS

International Agency for Research on Cancer, 150 Cours Albert Thomas, CEDEX 08, LyonsRhône-Alpes, France 69372, 33 0 4 72 73 8485, Fax: 33 0 4 72 73 8575, http://www.iarc.fr.

Jacqueline L. Longe

Ragpicker's disease *see* **Anthrax**

Red Cross

Definition

The Red Cross is the common name given to the International Federation of Red Cross and Red Crescent Societies, the International Committee of the Red Cross, and the 191 national member organizations. Together, these organizations make up the largest humanitarian organization in the world.

Purpose

The International Federation of Red Cross and Red Crescent Societies (IFRC) encourages, facilitates, and promotes assistance and other humanitarian activities to those in need without discrimination. The IFRC's vision also includes the goal of preventing and alleviating human suffering around the world and to contribute to the maintenance and promotion of human dignity and peace. The IFRC focuses on **disaster preparedness** and response and health and community care. Each individual National Red Cross Society may have a deeper focus on one area than the others, but all of the organizations follow the same seven fundamental principles that were developed in 1965. These principles include:

- humanity. Protect human health and promote cooperation, friendship, mutual understanding, and lasting peace amongst all people.

- impartiality. Relieve suffering based on needs by giving priority to the most urgent cases of distress. Do not discriminate in terms of class, nationality, political opinion, race, or religious belief.
- independence. Remain independent from government or other organizations in order to always be able to live the principles of the IFRC.
- voluntary service. Remain a voluntary relief movement not motivated by gain.
- neutrality. Do not take sides in hostilities or engage in conversations about ideology, politics, race, or religion.
- unity. There may only be one Red Cross or Red Crescent Society (or the country's equivalent) in each country. The group must be open to all and do humanitarian work throughout its territory.
- universality. All societies within the IFRC have equal status and share equal responsibility in helping each other.

The International Committee of the Red Cross (ICRC) is an independent neutral organization that bases its purpose on the Geneva Conventions and the fundamental principles and goals of the IFRC. The ICRC is focused on humanitarian protection and assistance for victims affected by war and armed violence. The organization responds to emergencies and promotes the respect of international humanitarian law.

Demographics

The International Federation of Red Cross and Red Crescent Societies is made up of 191 member organizations represented by almost 100 million members, volunteers, and supporters. About 50% of Red Cross volunteers are women, and societies represent nearly every country. The American Red Cross alone has more than 1.33 million volunteers and almost 30,000 paid staff. As of 2012, the ICRC had more than 1,400 delegates and specialized staff on field missions around the world. The organization also has 800 staff members based at its headquarters in Geneva and works with almost 11,000 local employees in field mission locations.

Description

The Red Cross is made up of many organizations throughout the world that together follow the same principals and have similar goals. Each organization and chapter is both independent and interrelated at the same time.

The ICRC is a private, independent group made up of an assembly of 25 Swiss citizens. Beyond these 25 people, the ICRC has both headquarter staff (around 800 people) located in Geneva and specialized staff that go on field missions around the world (around 1,400 people). The ICRC acts during times of war when a neutral body is necessary. For example, the ICRC may send in someone to supervise repatriation, go into prisoner of war camps, or supply relief. The ICRC is considered a guardian of the Geneva Conventions and basis its own principles off of the Geneva Conventions and the fundamental principles and goals of the IFRC. The ICRC has won three Nobel Peace Prizes. The first in 1917 and second in 1944, were awarded solely to the ICRC. The third, won in 1963, was won jointly with the League of Red Cross Societies (now called the International Federation of Red Cross and Red Crescent Societies).

The International Federation of Red Cross and Red Crescent Societies was created in 1919 under the name the League of Red Cross Societies. The IFRC was developed in order to coordinate efforts by the various National Red Cross Societies. The organization is a clearinghouse for information, maintains contact between individual societies, assists individual societies in expanding and improving old programs and in setting up new ones, and helps coordinate international disaster relief. The IFRC has its own executive committee and each national society is represented on the board of governors.

As of 2012, there were 191 individual National Red Cross Societies. These societies must be approved by the IFRC and follow the IFRC principals. There may only be one national society per country, however, there may be numerous chapters within one country. For example, as of 2012, the American Red Cross had more than 1,300 chapters, 38 Blood Services regions, 18 Tissue Services centers, and hundreds of additional centers on U.S. military basis around the globe. Each National Red Cross Society must focus on **humanitarian aid** within their country, and some societies may choose to focus on additional projects. The American Red Cross chooses to separate disaster relief Red Cross chapters and Blood Services chapters. National Societies may also provide humanitarian aid to places of need outside of their country.

The International Red Cross Conference is the highest Red Cross legislative body. It is made up of representatives from the National Red Cross Societies, the IFRC, and the governments that have signed the Geneva Conventions. The body meets every four to six years. The 31st International Conference took

CLARA BARTON (1821–1912)

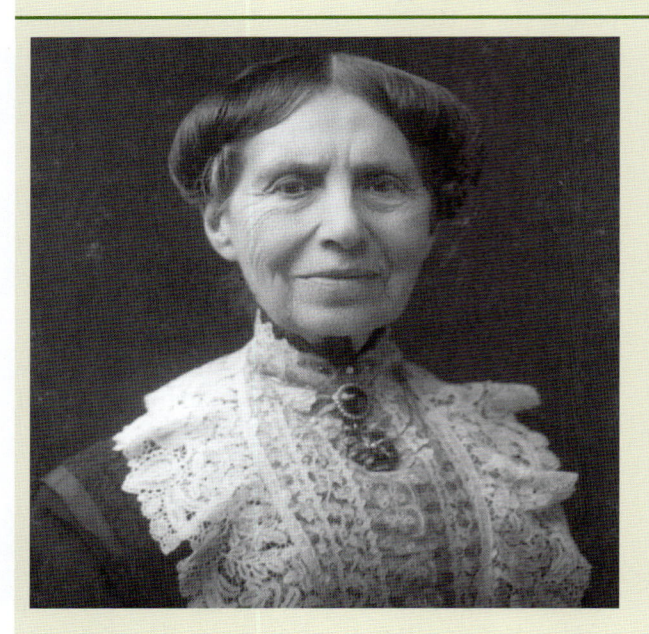

Clara Barton was interested in the medical profession from an early age. During the Civil War, she was omnipresent on the front line, providing necessary aid and supplies to soldiers. She also provided emotional support, praying with them and listening to them. After the Civil War, Barton went to Europe and was introduced to the Red Cross Organization. She realized a need for a disaster relief organization in the United States.

In 1881, Barton led a group in the creation of the American Red Cross. In that same year, the organization was utilized when Michigan experienced tragic forest fires. Barton organized relief efforts, sending clothes and food to the victims of the fires. The American Red Cross also helped those in need outside of the United States.

The American Red Cross is still very involved in disaster assistance, helping people with emergency preparedness and those that have suffered devastation.

(Courtesy of the Library of Congress, Copyright 1904 by J.E. Purdy, Boston.)

---

place from November 28 to December 1, 2011. The body meets to discuss Red Cross activities and to review any suggested or newly adopted revisions of the Convention. Between meetings, the Standing Commission of the International Red Cross coordinates work between the International Red Cross Conference and the IFRC.

Origins

The Red Cross has a long history of humanitarian aid around the world that is said to have been founded on the words of one individual. Henry Dunant, a Swiss businessman, wrote the book, *A Memory of Solferino*, after seeing a battlefield in Solferino, Italy in 1859. During this battle, more than 40,000 troops were killed or wounded and left without any aid. In his book, Dunant described the battle and his concerns about protecting the sick and wounded, including making two proposals for the future. First, Dunant proposed that during peacetime, volunteer groups in every country should be created to take care of the causalities in wartime. Secondly, he proposed to get countries to agree to protect the wounded on the battlefield and the first aid volunteers who help them. Dunant's book and his proposals led to the founding of the Red Cross.

The basic foundation of the Red Cross began in February 1863, when the Geneva Public Welfare Society developed a committee of five Swiss citizens to look into the ideas put forth in Henry Dunant's book. This committee was made up of Henry Dunant himself, Guillaume Henri Dufour, a general of the Swiss army, Gustave Moynier, a lawyer and president of the Public Welfare Society which sponsored the foundation of the group, and two medical doctors, Louis Appia and Theodore Maunoir.

The committee quickly got to work and held an international conference in October of 1863, only months after its foundation. Delegates from sixteen nations and fourteen philanthropic institutions attended the conference and adopted resolutions, principals, and an international emblem. The conference also discussed the creation of voluntary units to help care for the sick and wounded during war. These voluntary units later became National Red Cross Societies (all working together under the International Federation of Red Cross and Red Crescent Societies). The group of five committee members from Switzerland later became the International Committee of the Red Cross.

In 1864, the Swiss government held an international diplomatic meeting. This gathering led to the Geneva Convention of 1864, which protected the wartime sick and wounded on land and had provisions that guaranteed neutrality for medical personnel and medical equipment. It also adopted the emblem, which is now known around the world, the red cross on a white field. The ideas in Dunant's book are also credited for the other international treaties that came out of the Geneva Conventions, such as the protection of the wartime sick and wounded at sea (1906), prisoners of war (1929), and civilians (1949). These treaties not only served to protect the sick and wounded during war, but allowed the ICRC to continue its mission around the world. Henry Dunant won a Nobel Peace Prize for his work in 1901.

Before there was the IFRC, individual National Red Cross Societies were developed. For example, the American Red Cross began in 1881, and was developed for humanitarian aid and emergency services within the United States. In Paris in 1919, the League of Red Cross Societies was born. This organization was developed after World War I when members recognized that individual societies needed to cooperate closely in order to be as successful as possible. Henry Davison, president of the American Red Cross War Committee, came up with the idea to create a national federation to allow for better coordination among individual national societies. This organization changed its name to the League of Red Cross and Red Crescent Societies in 1983.

The addition of Red Crescent Societies developed from Muslim nations who did not want to be represented by the Christian cross. The red crescent was first used in 1876 during the war between Russia and Turkey, but not officially recognized until 1929 at the Diplomatic Conference. At this time, the Turkish, Persian, and Egyptian delegations requested that both the red crescent and another symbol, the red lion and sun, be recognized. The symbols were recognized, but use was limited to the countries that already used them. Over time, other countries submitted their own requests to use a different symbol, such as the red shield of David by Israel. All of these proposals were rejected. The International Conference of the Red Cross and Red Crescent developed a committee to create a new symbol that could be used by all, regardless of religious background. In 2005, the red crystal was adopted to be used, not instead of but in addition to, the red cross and red crescent. Countries then had the ability to use the red cross, the red crescent, the red crystal, or the red cross and red crescent next to each other. Iran, the only country using the red lion and sun, switched to the red crescent in 1980, but held onto the right to change back to the red lion and sun if it ever wishes to. In 2006, it was decided that Magen David Adom, Israel's equivalent to the National Red Cross, could use the red shield of David emblem inside Israel. When working outside of Israel, the society must work in requirements to the host country.

In 1991, the organization went through another name change becoming the International Federation of Red Cross and Red Crescent Societies. As of 2012, there were 191 individual National Red Cross Societies that make up the IFRC and 194 countries that had signed the Geneva Convention to protect the wounded and aid workers during times of war, fulfilling the visions of Henry Dunant.

Results

Due to the large number of individual organizations and chapters, it is difficult to estimate exactly how many people are affected by the work of Red Cross Societies each year. In 2010, the IFRC estimated that disaster relief given by volunteers of the Red Cross provided services worth over $6 billion and reached more than 30 million people. An example of work done by Red Cross Societies includes the 2010 earthquake in Haiti, when 120 National Red Cross Societies provided aid. This was one out of the over 400 disasters responded to by Red Cross Societies that year.

Research and general acceptance

Worldwide, the Red Cross is an overwhelmingly trusted name. Over the years, however, individual national societies have received criticism and bad publicity regarding employees, donations, and publications. For example, in October 2012, the Australian Red Cross came under fire for an anti-gay Facebook post, which they later apologized for as a mistake. The American Red Cross has suffered various problems, from employees stealing donations to not being properly prepared at disasters. In 2012, the organization was fined $9.6 million by the United States Federal Drug Administration for unsafe blood management practices, the second multi-million dollar penalty filed again the American Red Cross since 2010. Even with this bad publicity, the Red Cross is considered a trusted and well-watched organization that positively affects millions of people in need each year.

Resources

PERIODICALS

Ratner, Steven R. "Law Promotion Beyond Law Talk: The Red Cross, Persuasion, and the Laws of War." *European Journal of International Law* (2011) 22(2): 459–506. http://ejil.oxfordjournals.org/content/22/2/459.full (accessed October 22, 2012).

WEBSITES

Aleccia, JoNel. "FDA Fines Red Cross Nearly $9.6 Million for Blood Safety Lapses." NBC News. http://vitals.nbcnews.com/_news/2012/01/16/10168484-fda-fines-red-cross-nearly-96-million-for-blood-safety-lapses?lite (accessed October 22, 2012).

International Committee of the Red Cross. "About the International Committee of the Red Cross." http://www.icrc.org/eng/who-we-are/index.jsp (accessed October 22, 2012).

International Federation of Red Cross and Red Crescent Societies. "Our Vision and Mission." http://www.ifrc.org/en/who-we-are/vision-and-mission (accessed October 22, 2012).

International Federation of Red Cross and Red Crescent Societies. "Saving Lives Changing Minds: Strategy 2020." http://www.ifrc.org/Global/Publications/general/strategy-2020.pdf (accessed October 22, 2012).

International Federation of Red Cross and Red Crescent Societies. "Where We Work." http://www.ifrc.org/en/what-we-do/where-we-work (accessed January 14, 2013).

ORGANIZATIONS

American Red Cross, 2025 E Street, Washington, DC 20006, (202) 303 4498, (800) 733 2767, http://www.redcross.org.

International Committee of the Red Cross, 19 Avenue de la paix, Geneva, Switzerland 1202, 41 22 734 60 01, Fax: 41 22 733 20 57, webmaster@icrc.org, http://www.icrc.org.

International Federation of Red Cross and Red Crescent Societies, PO Box 372, Geneva, Switzerland 1211, 41 22 730 42 22, Fax: 41 22 733 03 95, http://www.ifrc.org.

Tish Davidson, AM

Resource Conservation and Recovery Act

Definition

The Resource Conservation and Recovery Act (RCRA), an amendment to the Solid Waste Disposal Act, was enacted in 1976 to address the problem of how to safely dispose of the huge volumes of municipal and industrial solid waste generated nationwide.

Purpose

The goals set by RCRA are: to protect human health and the environment; to reduce waste and conserve energy and natural resources; and to reduce or eliminate the generation of **hazardous waste** as expeditiously as possible.

To achieve these goals, four distinct yet interrelated programs exist under RCRA. The first program, under Subtitle D, encourages states to develop comprehensive plans to manage primarily nonhazardous solid waste, typically household waste. The second program, under Subtitle C, establishes a system for controlling hazardous waste from the time it is generated until its ultimate disposal—or from "cradle-to-grave." The third program, under Subtitle I, regulates certain underground storage tanks. It establishes performance standards for new tanks and requires leak detection, prevention, and corrective action at underground tank sites. The newest program to be established is the **medical waste** program under Subtitle J. It establishes a demonstration program to track medical waste from generation to disposal.

Description

RCRA is a law that describes the kind of waste management program that Congress wants to establish. This description is written in very broad terms. It directs the **Environmental Protection Agency (EPA)** to develop and promulgate criteria for identifying the characteristics of hazardous waste. The Act also provides the Administrator of the **EPA** (or designated representative) with the authority necessary to carry out the intent of the act, including the authority to conduct inspections.

The act includes a congressional mandate for the EPA to develop a comprehensive set of regulations. Regulations are legal mechanisms that define how a statute's broad policy directives are to be implemented. RCRA regulations have been developed by the EPA, covering a range of topics from guidelines for state solid waste plans to a framework for the hazardous waste permit program.

RCRA regulations are published according to an established process. When a regulation is proposed, it is published in the *Federal Register*. It is usually first published as a proposed regulation, allowing the public to comment on it for a period of time—typically 30–60 days. Included with the proposed regulation is a discussion of the agency's rationale for the regulatory approach and an explanation of the technical basis for the proposed regulation. Following the comment period, the EPA evaluates public comments. In addressing the comments, the EPA usually revises the proposed regulation. The final regulation is published in the *Federal Register* ("promulgated"). Regulations are compiled annually and bound in the *Code of Federal Regulations* (CFR) according to a highly structured format.

Although the relationship between an act and its regulations follows the normal legislative pattern for acts, the relationship between the 1984 amendments to RCRA, the Hazardous and Solid Waste Amendments (HSWA), and its regulations differs. HSWA is unusual in that Congress placed explicit requirements in the statute in addition to instructing the EPA in general language to develop regulations. Many of these requirements are so specific that the EPA incorporated them directly into the regulations. HSWA is all the more significant because of the ambitious schedules that Congress established to implement the act's provisions.

Another unique aspect of HSWA is that it establishes "hammer" provisions—statutory requirements that go into effect automatically as regulations if EPA fails to issue these regulations by certain dates. The EPA further clarifies its regulations through guidance documents and policy statements.

Policy statements specify operating procedures that *should* be followed. They are a mechanism used by EPA program offices to outline the manner in which pieces of the RCRA program are to be carried out. In most cases, policy statements are addressed to staff working on implementation. Many guidance and policy documents have been developed to aid in implementing the RCRA program. So that interested parties can find out what documents are available, the Office of Solid Waste's Directives System lists all RCRA-related policy guidance and memoranda and identifies where they can be obtained.

The RCRA works as follows: Subtitle D of the act encourages states to develop and implement solid waste management plans. These plans are intended to promote recycling of solid wastes and require closing or upgrading of all environmentally unsound dumps. Due to increasing volumes, solid waste management has become a key issue facing many localities and states. Recognizing this problem, Congress directed the EPA in HSWA to take an active role with the states in solving the difficult problem of solid waste management. The EPA revised standards that apply to municipal solid waste landfills. Current with the revision of these standards, the EPA formed a taskforce to analyze solid waste source reduction and recycling options. The revised solid waste standards, together with the taskforce findings, form the basis for the EPA's development of strategies to better regulate municipal solid waste management.

Subtitle C establishes a program to manage hazardous wastes from cradle-to-grave. The objective of the C program is to ensure that hazardous waste is handled in a manner that protects human health and the environment. To this end, there are Subtitle C regulations regarding the generation, transportation and treatment, storage, or disposal of hazardous wastes. In practical terms, this means regulating a large number of hazardous waste handlers.

The Subtitle C program resulted in perhaps the most comprehensive regulations the EPA ever developed. It first identified those solid wastes that are "hazardous" and then established various administrative requirements for the three categories of hazardous waste handlers: generators, transporters and owners or operators of treatment, storage, and disposal facilities (TSDFs). In addition, Subtitle C regulations set technical standards for the design and safe operation of TSDFs. These standards were designed to minimize the release of hazardous waste into the environment. Furthermore, the regulations for TSDFs served as the basis for developing and using the permits required for each facility. Issuing permits is essential to making the Subtitle C regulatory program work, since it is through the permitting process that the EPA or a state actually applies the technical standards to facilities.

Subtitle I regulates petroleum products and hazardous substances (as defined under Superfund) stored in underground tanks. The objective of Subtitle I is to prevent leakage to groundwater from tanks and to clean up past releases. Under Subtitle I, the EPA developed performance standards for new tanks and regulations for leak detection, prevention, closure, financial responsibility, and corrective action at all underground tank sites. This program may be delegated to states.

Subtitle J was added by Congress when, in the summer of 1988, medical wastes washed up on Atlantic beaches, thus highlighting the inadequacy of medical waste management practices. Subtitle J instructed the EPA to develop a two-year demonstration program to track medical waste from generation to disposal in demonstration states. The demonstration program was completed in 1991, and it was concluded that at generation, the disease-causing potential of medical waste was at its greatest and it naturally tapered off after that.

As of 2012, more than 90% of potentially infectious medical waste was incinerated. This is done to the guidelines set by the EPA in 1997 on the emissions from medical waste incinerators. The EPA is also the regulatory authority over any medical waste treatment technologies that use chemicals; however, individual states can set their own regulations on storage, packaging, transportation, and disposal.

Congress and the president set the overall national direction for RCRA programs. The EPA's Office of Solid Waste and Emergency Response translates this direction into operating programs by developing regulations, guidelines, and policy. The EPA then implements RCRA programs or delegates implementation to the states, providing them with technical and financial assistance.

Origins

Although RCRA was enacted in 1976, the problem of waste disposal has roots that go back well before that time. There was a time when the amount of waste produced in the United States was small and its impact on the environment relatively minor. However, with the industrial revolution in the latter part of the nineteenth century, the country began to grow at an unprecedented speed. New products were developed, and consumers were offered an ever-expanding array of material goods.

This growth continued through the early twentieth century and increased rapidly after World War II when the nation's industrial base, strengthened by the war, turned its energies toward domestic production. The results of this growth were not all positive. With more goods came more waste, both hazardous and nonhazardous. In the late 1940s, the United States was generating roughly 500,000 metric tons of hazardous waste a year. The EPA has estimated that in the early twenty-first century, several hundred million tons of hazardous waste are generated annually nationwide.

Waste management was slow in coming. Much of the waste produced made its way into the environment where it began to pose a serious threat to ecological systems and public health. In the mid-1970s, it became clear to both Congress and the nation that action had to be taken to ensure that solid wastes were managed properly. This realization began the process that resulted in the passage of the RCRA.

Although the RCRA created a framework for the proper management of hazardous and nonhazardous solid waste, it did not address the problems of hazardous waste encountered at inactive or abandoned sites or those resulting from spills that require emergency response. These problems are addressed by the Comprehensive Environmental Response, Compensation and Liability Act (**CERCLA**), commonly called Superfund.

The RCRA refers to the overall program resulting from the Solid Waste Disposal Act. The Solid Waste Disposal Act was enacted in 1965 for the primary purpose of improving solid waste disposal methods.

> **KEY TERMS**
>
> **Hazardous waste**—Waste that is potentially harmful to public health or the environment, for example, paints, batteries, cleaners, and oil.
>
> **Municipal**—Relating to a town or city.

It was amended in 1970 by the Resource Recovery Act and again in 1976 by RCRA. The changes embodied in the RCRA remodeled the nation's solid waste management system and added provisions pertaining to hazardous waste management.

The act continued to evolve as Congress amended it to reflect changing needs. It was amended several times since 1976, once significantly in 1984. The 1984 amendments, called the Hazardous and Solid Waste Amendments, expanded the scope and requirements of the RCRA. Provisions resulting from the 1984 amendments were significant, since they tended to deal with the waste problems resulting from more complex technology.

Results

Waste minimization or reduction is a major EPA goal. It is defined as any source reduction or recycling activity that results in either reduction of total volume of hazardous waste or reduction of toxicity of hazardous waste, or both, as long as that reduction is consistent with the general goal of minimizing present and future threats to human health and the environment. The EPA continues to work to reduce or minimize waste, but the United States has progressed steadily under the RCRA. When the act became law, the United States produced almost 300 million tons of hazardous waste each year. This was reduced to 214 million tons by 1995 (the twenty-fifth anniversary of the RCRA). In 2009, the EPA estimated that hazardous waste had been reduced to 35 million tons, 12 million tons less than just two years earlier. Additionally, as of 2010, the national recycling rate was at 34.1%, an increase from 25% in 1995 and from the low teens when the act began. These numbers show that RCRA is working and making progress when it comes to waste management.

Resources

BOOKS

McMichael, Susan M. *RCRA Permitting Deskbook*. Washington, DC: Environmental Law Institute, 2011.

VanGuilder, Clifton. *Hazardous Waste Management*. Dulles, VA: Mercury Learning and Information, 2011.

WEBSITES

U.S. Environmental Protection Agency. "Frequent Questions." http://www.epa.gov/osw/hazard/wastemin/minimize/faqs.htm (accessed October 30, 2012).

U.S. Environmental Protection Agency. "Managing Hazardous Waste (RCRA)." http://yosemite.epa.gov/r10/owcm.nsf/7468f0692f73df9a88256500005d62e8/1a9900b8c988454b8825675f00775776?opendocument (accessed October 30, 2012).

U.S. Environmental Protection Agency. "The National Biennial RCRA Hazardous Waste Report." http://www.epa.gov/lawsregs/laws/rcra.html (accessed October 30, 2012).

U.S. Environmental Protection Agency. "Summary of the Resource Conservation and Recovery Act." http://www.epa.gov/lawsregs/laws/rcra.html (accessed October 30, 2012).

ORGANIZATIONS

International Solid Waste Association, Auerspergstrasse 15, Top 41, Vienna, Austria 1080, 43 1 (253) 6001, Fax: 43 1 (253) 6001 99, iswa@iswa.org, http://www.iswa.org.

National Solid Waste Management Association, 4301 Connecticut Ave. NW, Ste. 300, Washington, DC 20008, (202) 244-4700, (800) 424-2869, Fax: (202) 966-4824, http://www.environmentalistseveryday.org.

U.S. Environmental Protection Agency (EPA), Ariel Rios Bldg., 1200 Pennsylvania Ave., NW, Washington, DC 20460, (202) 272-0167; TTY (202) 272-0165, http://www.epa.gov.

Liane Clorfene Casten
Tish Davidson, AM

Risk assessment

Definition

Risk assessment refers to the process by which the short and long-term adverse consequences to individuals or groups in a particular area resulting from the use of specific technology, chemical substance, or natural hazard are determined.

Description

Generally, quantitative methods are used to predict the number of affected individuals, morbidity or mortality, or other outcome measures of adverse consequences. Many risk assessments have been completed over the last two decades to predict human and ecological impacts with the intent of aiding policy and regulatory decisions. Well-known examples of risk assessments include evaluating potential effects of herbicides and insecticides, nuclear power plants, incinerators, **dams** (including dam failures), automobile pollution, tobacco **smoking**, and such natural catastrophes as volcanoes, **earthquakes**, and hurricanes. Risk assessment studies often consider financial and economic factors as well.

Human health risk assessments

Human health risk assessments for chemical substances that are suspected or known to have toxic or carcinogenic effects is one critical and especially controversial subset of risk assessments. These health risk assessments study small populations that have been exposed to the chemical in question. Health effects are then extrapolated to predict health impacts in large populations or to the general public who may be exposed to lower concentrations of the same chemical.

There is a mathematical formula that determines an individual's risk from chemical exposures.

$$\text{Risk} = \eqalign{{(emissions)\times(transport)\times} \cr (loss\ \{factor)\times(exposure\ period)\times} \cr {(uptake)\times(toxicity\ factor)}}$$

For the case of a **hazardous waste** incinerator, emissions might be average smokestack emissions of gas; the transport term represents dilution in the air from the stack to the community; the loss factor might represent chemical degradation of reactive contaminants as stack gases are transported in the atmosphere; the exposure period is the number of hours that the community is downwind of the incinerator; uptake is the amount of contaminants absorbed into the lung (a function of breathing rate and other factors); and toxicity is the chemical potency. Multiplying these factors indicates the probability of a specific adverse health impact caused by contaminants from the incinerator. In typical applications, such models give the incremental lifetime risk of cancer or other health hazards in the range of one in a million (equivalent to 0.000001). Cancers currently cause about one-third of deaths, thus, a one in a million probability represents a tiny increase in the total cancer incidence. However, calculated risks can vary over a large range—0.001 to 0.00000001.

While the same equation is used for all individuals, some assumptions regarding uptake and toxicity might be modified for certain individuals such as pregnant women, children, or individuals who are routinely exposed to the chemicals. In some cases, monitoring might be used to verify exposure levels. The equation illustrates the complexity of the risk assessment process.

Risk assessment process

The risk assessment/management procedure consists of five steps: (1) *Hazard assessment* seeks to identify causative agent(s). Simply put, is the substance toxic and are people exposed to it? The hazard assessment demonstrates the link between human actions and adverse effects. Often, hazard assessment involves a chain of events. For example, the release of pesticide may cause soil and ground **water pollution**. Drinking contaminated groundwater from the site or skin contact with contaminated soils may therefore result in adverse health effects.

(2) *Dose-response relationships* describe the toxicity of a chemical using models based on human studies (including clinical and epidemiologic approaches) and animal studies. Many studies have indicated a threshold or "no-effect" level, that is, an exposure level where no adverse effects are observed in test populations. Some health impacts may be reversible once the chemical is removed. In the case of potential carcinogens, linear models are used almost exclusively. Risk or potency factors are usually set using animal data, such as experiments with mice exposed to varying levels of the chemical. With a linear dose-response model, a doubling of exposure would double the predicted risk.

(3) *Exposure assessment* identifies the exposed population, detailing the level, duration, and frequency of exposure. Exposure *pathways* of the chemical include ingestion, inhalation, and dermal contact. Human and technological defenses against exposure must be considered. For example, respirators and other protective equipment reduce workplace exposures. In the case of prospective risk assessments for facilities that are not yet constructed—for example, a proposed hazardous waste incinerator—the exposure assessment uses mathematical models to predict emissions and distribution of contaminants around the site. Probably the largest effort in the risk assessment process is in estimating exposures.

(4) *Risk characterization* determines the overall risk, preferably including quantification of uncertainty. In essence, the factors listed in the equation are multiplied for each chemical and for each affected population. To arrive at the total risk, risks from different exposure pathways and for different chemicals are added. Populations with the maximum risk are identified. To gauge their significance, results are compared to other environmental and societal risks. These four steps constitute the scientific component of risk assessment.

(5) *Risk management* is the final decision-making step. It encompasses the administrative, political, and economic actions taken to decide if and how a particular societal risk is to be reduced to a certain level and at what cost. Risk management in the United States is often an adversarial process involving complicated and often conflicting testimony by expert witnesses. In recent years, a number of disputes have been resolved by mediation.

Risk management and reduction

Options that result from the risk management step include performing no action, product labeling, and placing regulations and bans. Examples of product labeling include warning labels for consumer products, such as those on tobacco products and cigarette advertising, and Material Safety Data Sheets (MSDS) for chemicals in the workplace. Regulations might be used to set maximum permissible levels of chemicals in the air and water (e.g., air and **water quality** criteria is set by the U.S. **Environmental Protection Agency**). In the workplace, maximum exposures known as Threshold Limit Values (TLVs) have been set by the U.S. **Occupational Safety and Health Administration**. Such regulations have been established for hundreds of chemicals. Governments have banned the production of a few materials, including DDT and PCBs, and product liability concerns have largely eliminated sales of some pesticides and most uses of **asbestos**. An international agreement in 2001 known as the Stockholm Convention on Persistent Organic Pollutants (POPs) banned nine chemicals including pesticides, PCBs, and dioxin from production or use. Persistent organic pollutants accumulate in the tissues of humans and other animals, and are linked to cancer and reproductive problems. POPs are also spread across worldwide by weather patterns, currents, and migrating animals. Later, the banned list increased a "dirty dozen," and in 2010, nine more chemicals were either banned or restricted by the agreement. More than 170 nations have become party to the Stockholm Convention; the United States is not a party.

A variety of social and political factors influence the outcome of the risk assessment/management process. Options to reduce risk, like banning a particular pesticide that is a suspected carcinogen, may decrease productivity, profits, and jobs. Furthermore, agricultural losses due to insects or other pests if pesticide is banned might increase malnutrition and death in subsistence economies. In general, risk assessments are most useful when used in a relative or comparative fashion, weighing the benefits of alternative chemicals or agricultural practices to another. Risk management decisions must consider what degree of risk is acceptable, whether it is a voluntary or involuntary risk, and the public's perception of the risk. A risk level of one in a million is generally considered an acceptable lifetime risk by many federal and state regulatory agencies. This risk level is mathematically equivalent to a decreased life expectancy of forty minutes for an individual with an average expected lifetime of seventy-four years. By comparison, the 40,000 traffic fatalities annually in the United States represent over a 1 percent lifetime chance of dying in a wreck—10,000 times higher than acceptable for a chemical hazard. The discrepancy between what an individual accepts for a chemical hazard in comparison to risks associated with personal choices like driving or smoking might indicate a need for more effective communication about risk management.

Risk assessments are often controversial. Scientific studies and conclusions about risk factors have been questioned. For example, animals are often used to determine dose-response and exposure relationships. Results from these studies are then applied to humans, sometimes without accounting for physiological differences. The scientific ability to accurately predict absolute risks is also poor. The accuracy of predictions might be no better than a factor of 10, thus 10 to 1,000 cancers or other health hazard might be experienced. The uncertainty might be even higher, a factor of 100, for example. Risks due to multiple factors are considered independent and additive. For instance, smoking and asbestos exposure together have been shown to greatly increase health risks than exposure to one factor alone. Conversely, multiple chemicals might inhibit or cancel risks. In nearly all cases, these factors cannot be modeled with our present knowledge. Finally, assessments often use a worst-case scenario, for example, the complete failure of a pollution control system, rather than a more modest but common failure like operator error.

Resources

BOOKS

Bennett, Peter. *Risk Communication and Public Health.* Oxford: Oxford University Press, 2010.

Campbell-Lendrum, Diarmid, Rosalie Woodruff, Annette Prüss-Üstün, and C. Corvalán. *Climate Change: Quantifying the Health Impact at National and Local Levels.* Geneva: World Health Organization, 2007.

Robson, Mark, and William Toscano. *Risk Assessment for Environmental Health.* San Francisco: Jossey-Bass, 2007.

WEBSITES

United States Environmental Protection Agency (EPA). "Air: Air Pollution Effects: Risk Assessment." http://www.epa.gov/ebtpages/airairporiskassessment.html (accessed November 6, 2010).

United States Environmental Protection Agency (EPA). "Environmental Management: Risk Assessment." http://www.epa.gov/ebtpages/enviriskassessment.html (accessed November 6, 2010).

United States Environmental Protection Agency (EPA). "Environmental Management: Risk Assessment: Human Health Risk Assessment." http://www.epa.gov/ebtpages/enviriskassessmenthumanhealthriskassessment.html (accessed November 6, 2010).

United States Environmental Protection Agency (EPA). "Pesticides: Pesticide Effects: Risk Assessment." http://www.epa.gov/ebtpages/pestpesticideeffecriskassessment.html (accessed November 6, 2010).

World Health Organization (WHO). "Risk assessment." http://www.who.int/topics/risk_assessment/en (accessed November 6, 2010).

Stuart Batterman

River blindness

Definition

River blindness, also known as onchocerciasis, is a disease caused by a parasitic worm. It is the second most common infectious cause of blindness in the world.

Description

River blindness is a disease responsible for a high incidence of partial or total blindness. The **World Health Organization** (WHO) estimates that between 18 and 37 million people are infected with the parasite that causes river blindness and that about 750,000 people have visual impairment or are blind as a result of the disease.

Risk factors

River blindness is found in tropical climates and is most common in sub-Saharan Africa. *Onchocerca volvulus*, the parasite that causes river blindness, is also found in parts of Yemen and Central and South America; however, the number of reported cases in these areas is quite low. In total, WHO estimates that over 90 million people are at risk for becoming infected with *O. volvulus*.

In the areas where river blindness is found, people who live near fast-running streams and rivers are most susceptible to being infected. The *Simulium* blackfly found in rural agricultural areas transmits the parasite that causes river blindness. Typically, it takes many bites for a person to become infected. For this reason,

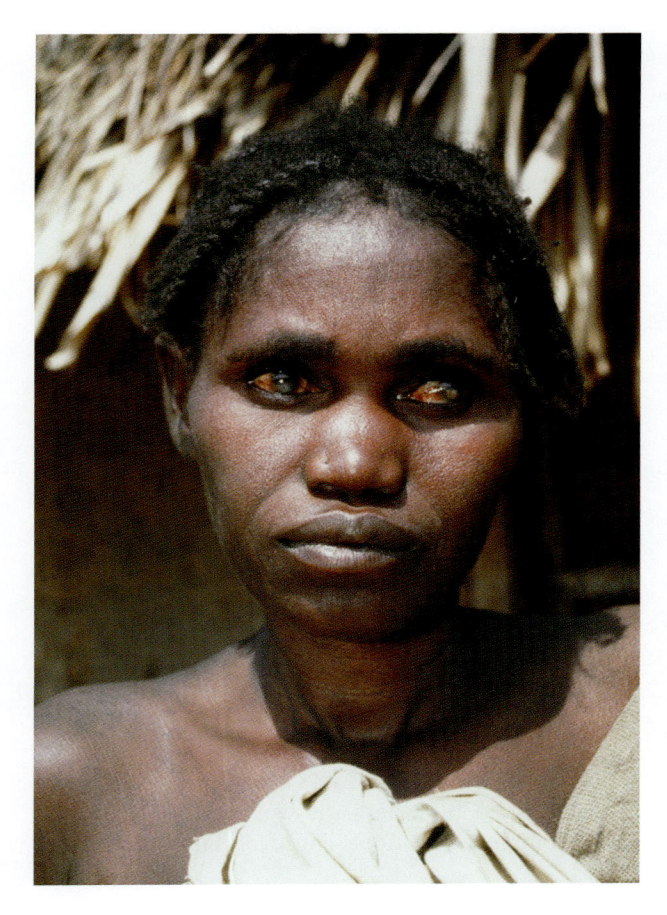

Young mother blinded by onchocerciasis ("river blindness").
(Andy Crump, TDR, World Health OrPhoto Researchers, Inc.)

beyond locals who live in these areas, researchers, missionaries, and members of the Peace Corps who stay in blackfly-infested areas for long periods are the most likely to be infected with *O. volvulus*.

Demographics

River blindness is found in 28 African countries, Yemen, and small, localized areas of six Central and South American countries. Ninety-nine percent of all infections occur in Africa. *O. volvulus* infects individuals independent of ethnicity, race, age, or sex. However, symptoms of those infected do vary depending on region. Although there is no clear understanding to why this is the case, one suspicion holds that it is due to genetic variations of the host.

Causes and symptoms

River blindness is a disease caused by infection with *O. volvulus*, a thread-shaped roundworm (a nematode), which is transmitted by the bite of a blackfly. The larvae of *O. volvulus* develop into the infective stage, called *L4*, inside the blackfly. It takes between 10 and 12 days for larvae to become infective for humans. *O. volvulus* is introduced into humans by the bite of an infected blackfly. Typically, it takes many bites for the person to become infected.

Larvae take between three months and one year to develop into adults. Female adult *O. volvulus* live coiled within subcutaneous nodules several inches in diameter and are 13–20 inches (33–50 cm) in length. Males live near females and are smaller, between 7 and 17 inches (19–42 cm). *O. volvulus* can live up to fourteen years inside the human body, and their larvae can live up to two years. Adult females produce up to 1,000 larvae each day. These larvae can begin to be detected in the skin between 10 and 20 months after the first infection.

Symptoms of river blindness vary depending on the region and person infected. Whereas some people experience no symptoms and no pain, others experience skin rashes, nodules under the skin, itchiness, and problems with vision. Itching and inflammation of the skin, caused by the immune system's reaction to dead larvae, can cause long-term damage. People with skin damage from *O. volvulus* are often said to have "leopard skin." Others may find that their skin becomes extremely thin, causing them to suffer from a condition called "hanging groin." Although not all nodules are painful, they are unattractive. Additionally, dead larvae that make their way to the eye can cause vision problems. At first, these problems are reversible; however, with time, the cornea becomes cloudy, and blindness can result. Inflammation of the optic nerve may occur also, resulting in blindness.

Diagnosis

The standard diagnosis for river blindness is a skin snip biopsy. This is done through removing 1–2 mg of skin by scraping with a scalpel. The skin sample is then kept at room temperature in a saline solution for about 24 hours. After 24 hours, a physician can use a microscope to see if any microfilariae have developed. For best results, six samples will be taken from various areas of the body such as the scapula, over the iliac crest, and from the lower extremities. This diagnosis is quite effective for later and high intensity infections. For infections that are under one year old or low in intensity, the results are limited, with only 20–50% accuracy.

Patients who have skin nodules caused by river blindness can be diagnosed through a nodulectomy. Additionally, slit lamp eye exams can be used to see microfilariae in people who have eye disease as a result of river blindness. There are other, less common, ways to test for river blindness; however, these methods are almost always used in research settings. Methods include a polymerase chain reactions test; a test using hybrid proteins; and various antibody tests, including an Ov16 card test and an ELISA-based test, which uses three types of antigens.

Treatment

Once a diagnosis is made, it is important that the infected individual be treated quickly in order to prevent any further health problems, including blindness. The most common and recommended treatment is ivermectin, a medicine that must be given every six months for the entire life span of the adult worms infecting the patient(about 14 years). Ivermectin kills larvae but does not kill adult worms. Another treatment, which does kill adult worms, is doxycycline. Doxycycline kills the bacteria, known as *Wolbachia*, on which adult *O. volvulus* worms live. Some physicians choose to treat infected patients with both drugs simultaneously. It is important that physicians check for *Loa loa*, another parasite found in the regions where river blindness is common, before beginning any type of drug treatment. *Loa loa* can cause severe side effects to the medications used in the treatment of river blindness.

Public health role and response

Although as of 2012, river blindness had not been blamed for any deaths, it can be debilitating for communities in infected areas. WHO estimated that blindness, as a result of river blindness, can reduce life expectancy by 4–10 years. Onchocerciasis is the second most common infectious cause of blindness, and it has been estimated that in West Africa, up to 10% of villagers may be blind as a result of river blindness.

Physical symptoms are not the only public health threat river blindness poses. Blackflies live near fast-flowing water and therefore often very fertile areas. These areas are sometimes abandoned due to fear of river blindness. People migrate away from these areas to higher ground, which they then clear for cultivation. Clearing vegetation in Africa frequently results in soil erosion and the formation of gullies that channel water during heavy rains. The moving water allows blackflies to breed, spreading the disease to the new area. The reappearance of river blindness results in still further human migration, until large areas of badly eroded land are left unpopulated and unproductive, and entire villages are abandoned. These changes cause severe socioeconomic problems for local villagers.

> **KEY TERMS**
>
> **Host**—The organism (such as a monkey or human) in which another organism (such as a virus or bacteria) is living.
>
> **Inflammation**—The body's response to tissue damage, including warmth, swelling, redness, and pain in the affected part.
>
> **Parasite**—An organism that lives in or with another organism, called the host, in parasitism, a type of association characterized by the parasite obtaining benefits from the host, such as food, and the host being injured as a result.
>
> **Skin snip biopsy**—A procedure in which a small amount of suspicious skin is removed and examined for evidence of the parasite *Onchocerca volvulus*.
>
> **Vector**—An animal carrier that transfers an infectious organism from one host to another. The vector that transmits Onchocerciasis to and from humans is the blackfly.

Organizations such as WHO, World Bank, United Nations Development Programme, and the Food and Agriculture Organization of the United Nations have worked together to control the reproduction of blackflies and the spread of river blindness. The first program, known as the Onchocerciasis Control Programme in West Africa, took place in seven West African countries beginning in 1974. The goal of the program was to control the spread of blackflies through the use of insecticide. The program continued until 2002 and reduced the risk of infection for millions of people. Beginning in 1988, Merck donated the drug ivermectin to help people infected with river blindness. This program continued, and in 2007, Merck made a pledge to make unlimited donations of ivermectin through 2020.

In 1995, African Program for Onchocerciasis Control was developed to help limit the spread of river blindness in the remaining areas of Africa where it is **endemic**. The program is run by affected communities who work together to deliver medication and monitor the spread of the disease. The program was set to run through 2015. A similar program, the Onchocerciasis Elimination Program for the Americas, was also taking place in affected areas of Central and South America.

> **QUESTIONS TO ASK YOUR DOCTOR**
>
> - What can I do to protect myself from being bitten by blackflies?
> - Once diagnosed with river blindness, how often must I take medication?
> - What are the symptoms of river blindness?

Prognosis

Although still a serious problem in areas where blackflies breed, the river blindness has been brought largely under control through the distribution of medicine and the control of the blackfly population. Those infected with river blindness who receive early and consistent treatment and medication can expect to experience few symptoms and keep their vision.

Prevention

There are many ways to lower the risk of being infected by river blindness. People can wear clothing that covers their entire bodies and use insect repellant to reduce the chance of being bitten by blackflies. Staying fewer than three months in areas with blackflies also greatly reduces the likelihood of becoming infected. On a larger scale, the major method of prevention of river blindness in humans is the control of the blackfly intermediate hosts and vectors. In Kenya, the larval stages of *S. neavei* have been killed by releasing dichlorodiphenyltrichloroethane (DDT) into streams where the blackflies breed and evolve. However, the waterways must be treated frequently to prevent the re-establishment of blackfly populations, and there have been serious questions raised over the safety of DDT. In West Africa, *S. damnosum* is more difficult to control, since the adults can fly considerable distances and can easily re-infect cleared sites from up to 60 miles (97 km) away.

Resources

WEBSITES

BIO Ventures for Global Health. "What Is Onchocerciasis (River Blindness)?" http://www.bvgh.org/Biopharmaceutical-Solutions/Global-Health-Primer/Diseases/cid/ViewDetails/ItemID/16.aspx (accessed September 24, 2012).

Centers for Disease Control and Prevention. "Parasites—Onchocerciasis (also known as River Blindness)." http://www.cdc.gov/parasites/onchocerciasis/disease.html (accessed September 24, 2012).

Medscape. "Onchocerciasis." http://emedicine.medscape.com/article/224309-overview#a0101 (accessed September 24, 2012).

World Health Organization. "Onchocerciasis Disease Information." http://www.who.int/tdr/diseases/oncho/info/en/index.html (accessed September 24, 2012).

ORGANIZATIONS

Centers for Disease Control and Prevention (CDC), 1600 Clifton Rd., Atlanta, GA 30333, (404) 639-3534, (800) 232-4636, inquiry@cdc.gov, http://www.cdc.gov.

Food and Agriculture Organization of the United Nations (FAO Headquarters), Viale delle Terme di Caracalla, Rome, Italy 00153, 39 06 570 53625, Fax: 39 06 5705 3699, AGN-Director@fao.org (Nutrition and Consumer Protection), http://www.fao.org.

Pan American Health Organization, 525 23rd St. NW, Washington, DC 20037, (202) 974-3000, Fax: (202) 974-3663, www.paho.org.

World Health Organization, Avenue Appia 20, Geneva 27, Switzerland 1211, +22 41 791 21 11, Fax: 22 41 791 31 11, info@who.int, http://www.who.int.

Tish Davidson, AM

Rivers and Harbors Act of 1899

Definition

The Rivers and Harbors Act of 1899, also known as the RHA and as the Refuse Act, is the oldest federal environmental law in the United States. The RHA authorized the U.S. secretary of the army to maintain freedom of navigation and to prevent obstruction in U.S. waters. The RHA prohibited the deposit or discharge from any ship or other floating craft or from shore installations, such as wharves, manufacturing establishments, or mills, of any refuse materials into a navigable U.S. water or its tributary. It also prohibited the deposit of any materials on the bank of any navigable water or its tributaries if navigation would be impeded. Exceptions could be granted for the construction of public works and activities taken for improvement of navigable waters.

The law provided for fines in the amounts of $500 to $2,500 for violations of the law's requirements, which were classified as misdemeanors, as well as imprisonment for 30 days to one year. The law also had a "bounty hunter" provision, which allowed that one-half of the fine would be paid to the person providing information that led to a conviction.

Description

Origins

Starting in 1870, there was a series of rivers and harbors acts passed by the U.S. Congress that provided funding for oversight of navigation, infrastructure, flooding, and other problems associated with the nation's waterways. In the 1880s and 1890s, the U.S. Army Corps of Engineers was directed by Congress through these acts to prevent dumping and filling of the nation's harbors. In 1892, in the Port of Pittsburgh, the corps took a grand jury on a tour of the harbor and obtained 50 indictments of firms dumping debris into the harbor. In 1893, at the direction of the corps, a community in Ohio was required to build an incinerator to burn refuse rather than dump it in the river, where the corps indicated that it obstructed navigation.

Approved on March 3, 1899, the RHA continued to address projects and activities in navigable waters and in harbor and river improvements and added on activities to control **water pollution**. This law was still used in the early 2000s to regulate the navigability of interstate waterways and harbors.

The U.S. Army Corps of Engineers was delegated the authority to implement Sections 9, 10, 13, and 14 of the RHA. The Army Corps of Engineers is an organization of the U.S. Army, headquartered in Washington, DC, that is responsible for providing engineering services, including the planning, design, construction, and operation of water resources and other civil works projects, designing and managing the construction of military facilities for the U.S. Army and the U.S. Air Force, and providing design and construction management support for other Defense and federal agencies. In 2012, the staff consisted of about 37,000 civilian and military personnel. The corps is commanded by the chief of engineers, who serves as a staff officer at the Pentagon.

Also involved in the implementation of the RHA is the secretary of the army. When the RHA passed in 1899, the position was referred to as the secretary of war, which was in the Department of War. On September 18, 1947, the secretary of the army replaced the secretary of war, and the Department of War became the Department of the Army within the newly created Department of Defense.

Purpose

The pollution-preventing sections of the RHA of 1899 include the following:

- Section 9 prohibits the construction of any dam or dike across any navigable water without the consent of Congress and approval of the plans by the Army Corps chief of engineers and the secretary of the army. If the navigable portions of the water body are entirely within a single state, the structure may be built under the authority of that state, as long as the plans are approved by the chief of engineers and the secretary of the army. Section 403 of Section 9 also provides an exclusion from criminalizing discharges of refuse "flowing from streets and sewers and passing therefrom in a liquid state."
- Section 10 prohibits alteration or obstruction of any navigable waters of the United States unless the work has been recommended by the chief of engineers and authorized by the secretary of the army. This section applies to the construction of any structure in or over any navigable water or the accomplishment of any work affecting the course, location, condition, or physical capacity of the navigable water.
- Section 13 provides that the secretary of the army may permit the discharge of refuse into navigable waters, if the chief of engineers determines that anchorage and navigation will not be harmed. Without a permit stipulating that there will be no harm, discharge of refuse is prohibited. This part of the RHA is referred to as the Refuse Act and remained in effect as of 2012, although the permit authority of the secretary of the army has been superseded by the permitting authority of the administrator of the U.S. Environmental Protection Agency and the states under Sections 402 and 405 of the Clean Water Act.
- Section 14 provides that the secretary of the army, on the recommendation of the chief of engineers, may grant permission for the temporary occupation or use of any sea wall, bulkhead, jetty, dike, levee, wharf, pier, or other work built by the United States. This permission is granted through real estate regulations.

Public health role and response

Since its passing, the RHA has been used, or attempted to have been used, to protect the environment and public health. In 1910, the corps used Section 13 to object to a proposed sewer in New York City. However, a judge ruled that pollution control should be left to the individual states. In 1911 the chief of engineers recommended that treatment facilities and dumping prohibitions should either be made compulsory or encouraged throughout the United States, but his suggestions were not implemented.

Andrew Franz, in an 2010 article published in the *Tulane Environmental Law Journal*, examined the history and impact of the RHA on the environmental and

KEY TERMS

Clean Water Act (CWA)—the U.S. environmental law that establishes the basic structure for regulating discharges of pollutants into the waters of the United States and for regulating quality standards for surface waters. The basis of the CWA was enacted in 1948 and was called the Federal Water Pollution Control Act, but the act was significantly reorganized and expanded in 1972. Clean Water Act became its common name with amendments in 1972.

Environmental impact statement (EIS)—A document required by the National Environmental Policy Act (NEPA) for certain actions "significantly affecting the quality of the human environment." An EIS, a tool for decision making, describes the positive and negative environmental effects of a proposed action and usually also lists one or more alternative actions that may be chosen instead of the action described in the EIS.

National Environmental Policy Act of 1969 (NEPA)—The environmental law that established a national policy promoting the enhancement of the environment and also established the President's Council on Environmental Quality. The purpose of NEPA is to ensure that environmental factors are weighted equally when compared to other factors in the decision making process undertaken by federal agencies.

Navigable waters—Waters that provide a channel for commerce and transportation of people and goods. Under U.S. law, bodies of water are defined according to their use. Navigable waters are used for business or transportation. The federal government has jurisdiction over navigable waters rather than states or municipalities. The federal government can determine how the waters are used, by whom, and under what conditions, and also has the power to alter the waters, such as by dredging or building dams. Generally a state or private property owner who is inconvenienced by such work has no remedy against the federal government unless state or private property itself is taken; if such property is taken, the laws of Eminent Domain would apply, which may lead to compensation for the landowner.

Pentagon—Headquarters of the U.S. Department of Defense, located in Arlington County, Virginia. The word *Pentagon* is often used to refer to the Department of Defense rather than the building itself.

U.S. Environmental Protection Agency (EPA)—An agency of the U.S. federal government that was created to protect human health and the environment by writing and enforcing regulations based on laws passed by Congress. The EPA was proposed by President Richard Nixon and began operation on December 2, 1970.

---

public health movement. In early RHA cases, the dumping of mud into tidal waters, the discharge of oil from vessels, and throwing of refuse into water, including boxes, baskets, garbage, and wrappers, were prosecuted. At the beginning of the 1960s, though, the U.S. Supreme Court endorsed a stronger enforcement of the RHA of 1899, and by 1972, when the Federal Pollution Control Act was passed, most criminal indictments for water pollution cases were initiated using the RHA.

In 1960 a Supreme Court decision in *U.S. vs. Republic Steel Corp.* interpreted that obstruction to navigation does include water pollution. The Court found that anything within the limits of the jurisdiction of the United States that tends to destroy the navigable capacity of a navigable waterway is prohibited by the RHA. Republic Steels' unpermitted discharge of industrial solid wastes (that is, iron production deposits) had reduced the depth of the Calumet River 4–9 feet and was considered an obstruction to the waterway. Republic Steel argued that the discharge was lawful due to the RHA's exemption of liquid sewage, but the Court said the liquid sewage exception was only for solids that would decompose in the water.

In 1966, the Supreme Court in the case of the *U.S. vs. Standard Oil Company*, defined the term *refuse* in the RHA as "all foreign substances and pollutants." Standard Oil had spilled jet fuel into a waterway, and the Court reasoned that unused oil had the same environmental effects as used oil, and so it was prohibited from discharge.

As a result of this 1966 ruling, it was clear that any person or corporation that did not have a permit to discharge anything into the water could be found criminally liable. In the decades since the RHA was passed, only 415 permits were requested. However, there were an estimated 40,000 industrial plants discharging effluent into navigable waters and thus subject to criminal indictment. During the early 1970s, cases continued to be tried under the RHA.

Also in the early 1970s, environmental groups and citizens used the "bounty hunter" provision, which allowed one-half of fines imposed upon a polluter to be given to the informer upon conviction to bring cases for trial under RHA. Most of the cases brought by bounty hunters were successful only if the federal government participated in the prosecution.

On December 23, 1970, a few weeks after the establishment of the U.S. **Environmental Protection Agency (EPA)**, President Richard Nixon announced that the RHA would be modified to improve the permitting process. However, the permitting process would depend greatly on industries to provide information on their effluent makeup. Also, the government was tasked to issue regulatory standards for several categories of industries, which was expected to take years. Violations of permits would be tried through civil suits and not through criminal suits. In 1971, the permitting plan was invalidated in *Kalur v. Resor*, which was brought by environmentalists who wanted to prevent the corps from issuing permits on the highly polluted Ohio River. The first ground of the case as declared by the Court was that the purpose of the Nixon permit plan was to undermine RHA's criminal provisions. The second ground was that the corps had not written an Environmental Impact Statement (EIS) for each application as required by the **National Environmental Policy Act** of 1969 (NEPA).

With the creation of the **EPA** and the passage of the Federal Water Pollution Control Act of 1972, known as the **Clean Water Act**, the use of the RHA as the dominant federal criminal law enforcement tool against water pollution decreased. From 1966 to 1970, over 400 RHA criminal indictments were filed; between July 1971 and December 1972, there were 169 RHA criminal indictments; in 1973, there were 57 cases, and in 1974 only 22 referrals. In 1976 the EPA stopped reporting on RHA cases, although it was still used in certain situations.

RHA's continued use includes use of its criminal penalty process because it is easier to undertake than a Clean Water Act (CWA) case, since conviction in an RHA case only requires proof of a discharge, rather than the expensive and time-consuming analysis of the effluent and the receiving waters that is required by the CWA. The RHA also criminally prohibits any kind of discharge (except for refuse "flowing from streets and sewers and passing from there in a liquid state") with the CWA cannot be used to criminalize nonpoint source dischargers, which include landfill and septic system polluters, agricultural pollutants, forestry activities, urban runoff, abandoned mines, and construction on sites smaller than five acres.

The EPA also uses the RHA for oil spills in waterways reported by the Coast Guard because the RHA has no liability limit for recovery of costs, whereas the CWA permits recovery only to the value of the boat or ship responsible for the spill.

Resources

PERIODICALS

Franz, Andrew. "Crimes Against Water: The Rivers and Harbors Act of 1899." *Tulane Environmental Law Journal* 23 (2010): 255–78.

ORGANIZATIONS

Environmental Protection Agency, 1200 Pennsylvania Ave. NW, Washington, DC 20460, (202) 272-0167, http://water.epa.gov.

Judith L. Sims

Rodents

Definition

Rodents are members of the order Rodentia, a sub-category of the class Mammalia. They consistute the largest category of mammals, making up about 40 percent of that class. Some familiar members of the order are beavers, guinea pigs, hamsters, mice, porcupines, rats, and squirrels.

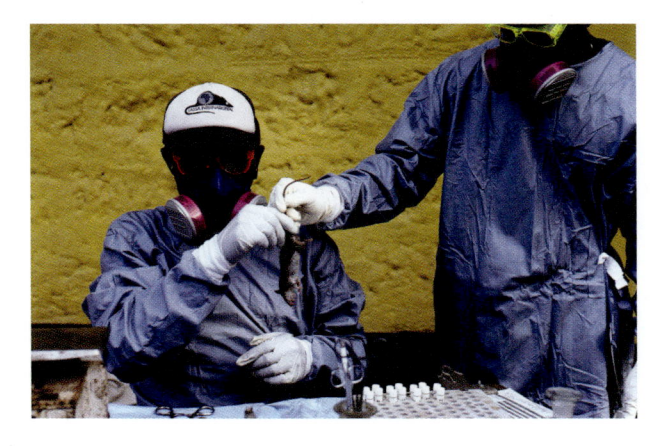

Public health workers prepare to dissect and examine a Mastomys Natalensis rat, which causes Lasso Fever, as soon as the rat is trapped in Kenema, Sierra Leone. (© Karen Kasmauski/CORBIS)

Description

The Rodentia consists of about 30 families and more than 2,000 species, making them the largest and most diverse of all mammalian species. They are found in every part of the world with the exception of Antarctica, New Zealand, and some oceanic islands. They range in size from the African pygmy mice (*Mus minutoides*), who weigh about 5 gm (0.2 oz) each, to the capybara (*Hydrochoerus hydrochaeris*), whose weight can exceed 70 kg (150 lb). The most common anatomical feature of rodents is the occurrence of a single pair of incisors in both the upper and low jaws. Each incisor is covered with a thick enamel layer on the front surface, and a softer, enamel-free surface on the back of the tooth. This arrangement makes it possible for the tooth to retain its chisel-like shape, appropriate for its primary activity of chewing and gnawing on tree bark and other plant material. The incisors continue to grow throughout the animal's lifetime, assuring that it has a cutting and grinding tool as long as it lives. This feature allows beavers to cut down large trees in a matter of hours and mice and rats to chew through house walls in a similarly short time.

An associated anatomical feature in rodents is the presence of a relatively large jaw and jaw muscles adapted to produce the chewing and gnawing action associated with the animal's dentition. The powerful muscles pull the lower jaw back and forth during chewing and gnawing. Most rodents are primarily herbivores, although some are carnivorous, with insects a popular secondary food. They have evolved a wide variety of lifestyles, ranging from the tree homes of flying squirrels to burrows of gophers and mole rats to aquatic capybaras.

Common diseases and disorders

Rodents are responsible for at least 35 human diseases worldwide. These diseases can be contracted in one of two ways, direct contact or indirect contact with a rodent. In the former case, a pathogen may be transmitted from a rodent to a human when a person comes into contact with saliva, feces, or urine from an infected animal. For example, one might accidentally rub against rodent feces or urine or inhale dust that contains small amounts of feces or urine. In some cases, a person might actually pick up a contaminated rodent, such as a pet rat or pet guinea pig that has become infected with a pathogen. The pathogen is then transmitted by accidental inhalation or ingestion of the pathogen or through contact with an open sore or wound in the skin. It some cases, a person may become infected as a result of being bitten by a rodent.

Some diseases that are transmitted directly from rodent to human are the following:

- Hantavirus pulmonary syndrome (HPS) is caused by a virus found in the saliva, feces, and urine of contaminated rodents, primarily the deer mouse (*Peromyscus maniculatus*). HPS is a relatively rare disease in the United States, with only 556 cases having been reported between 1993 and 2012. The disease begins with sneezing, coughing, and general respiratory distress, often resolving without treatment. It can become more serious, however, with about four out of ten cases of the diseases resulting in death. A related medical condition result from exposure to the hantavirus is hemorrhagic fever with renal syndrome (HFRS), which occurs in different forms in various parts of the world. Death rates from HFRS range from less than one percent to more than 15 percent, depending on the type of disease.

- Lassa fever occurs primarily in West Africa, where it is usually a mild infection that resolves without treatment. In about 20 percent of all cases, however, symptoms can rapidly grow more serious and, in some epidemics, the death rate has exceeded 50 percent.

- Leptospirosis is a worldwide disease caused by bacteria in the *Leptospira* genus. People infected with the disease are often asymptomatic, but in other instances, the bacteria can infect and damage the kidneys, meninges, respiratory system, and liver, sometimes resulting in death.

- Plague is perhaps the best known and most destructive of all infectious diseases known to humans. It is caused by the bacterium *Yersinia pestis*, which is transmitted by fleas that live on rodents. The precise symptoms associated with plague depend on the site of infection and the specific type of disease. Bubonic plague, for example, is characterized by fever, chills, headache, general weakness, and, most characteristically, by swollen and painful lymph nodes (buboes), that give the disease its name. Without treatment, a person rapidly becomes worse and may die within hours or days.

- Tularemia is a worldwide infectious disease caused by the bacterium *Francisella tularensis*. Humans can be exposed to the bacterium when they handle an animal that has been infected, by breathing dust that contains the bacterium, by absorbing the bacterium through open sores or wounds, or by being bitten by a parasite that lives on a rodent or other animal. The most common vectors for the bacterium in the United States are the dog tick (*Dermacentor variabilis*), wood tick (*Dermacentor andersoni*), and lone star tick (*Amblyomma americanum*).

Indirect disease transmission involves an intermediary stage between the rodent carrier of a disease and the ultimate human host for the pathogen that causes the disease. For example, **Lyme disease** is transmitted when a tick (in the United States, the blacklegged tick [or deer tick, *Ixodes scapularis*] or the western blacklegged tick [*Ixodes pacificus*]) bites a rodent whose blood is contaminated with the *Borrelia burgdorferi* bacterium. When the tick then later bites a human, it transmits that bacterium in its saliva to the human bloodstream. Some diseases that are transmitted indirectly from rodents to humans include the following:

- Babesiosis is caused by any one of a number of species in the genus Babesia. It is transmitted from a rodent, usually the white-footed mouse, *Peromyscus leucopus*, to a human, by way of a tick in the genus *Ixodes*. People with the disease are often asymptomatic and those with symptoms usually report nothing more serious than mild flu-like symptoms. For individuals with special health problems, such as HIV infection, symptoms may become more serious and the condition may actually be life-threatening.

- Cutaneous leishmaniasis is caused by a protozoa of the genus *Leishmania* that is usually transmitted from the wild woodrat *Neotoma spp.* to humans by way of a bite from a sand fly, such as *Phlebotomus papatasi*. The disease is realtively harmless that manifests as painless or mildly painful skin ulcer that generally resolve without treatment.

- Murine typhus is a form of typhus caused by the bacterium *Rickettsia typhi* transmitted most commonly from infected rats to humans by way of the *Xenopsylla cheopis* flea. The disease is relatively uncommon in the United States, but more common in parts of the world with poor sanitation, perhaps accounting for its common name of "jail fever."

- Rocky Mountain Spotted Fever (RMSF) is caused by the bacterium *Rickettsia rickettsii*, which is transmitted from wild rodents to humans through a bite from a tick such as the dog tick (*Dermacentor variabilis*), Rocky Mountain wood tick (*Dermacentor andersoni*), or brown dog tick (*Rhipicephalus sanguineus*. RMSF can be a very dangerous condition if not treated within the first eight days of infection, with death a potential outcome in such circumstances. After reaching a low of about two cases per million in the United States in the 1960s, the incidence of RMSF has increased to more than ten times that much (about 25 cases per million persons) in 2010. At the same time, the death rate from the disease has dropped to less than 0.5 percent.

> **KEY TERMS**
>
> **Asymptomatic**—Showing no signs or symptoms of a disease.
>
> **Incisor**—A tooth at the front of the mouth adapted for biting and gnawing.
>
> **Renal**—Having to do with the kidneys.
>
> **Rodenticide**—A chemical used to kill rodents.

- Western equine encephalitis (WEE) is caused by the Western equine encephalomyelitis virus, which is transmitted by a mosquito, usually *Aedes albopictus* or *A. japonicus*, that has previously bitten a ground squirrel or snowshoe hare infected by the virus. WEE is relatively rare in the United States, with a total of 639 confirmed cases since 1964. Symptoms of the disease range from mild flu-like traits to much more serious consequences that can end in death.

Every disease listed here has its own characteristic methods of diagnosis, treatment, and prognosis.

Diagnosis

A preliminary diagnosis of a rodent-related disease can often be made on the basis of characteristic signs and symptoms, along with a patient history that might reveal situations in which the patient may have been exposed to rodents or other disease-transmitting vectors. A confirmatory diagnosis often depends on bloodwork through which the causative agent can often be identified through microscopic analysis or other testing.

Treatment

Bacterial infections are most effectively treated by one or more antibiotics, the specific choice made being based on the infection involved. For example, the drugs of choice for treating babesiosis are atovaquone in conjunction with azithromycin or clinamycin and quinine. Treatment of cutaneous leishmaniasis generally makes use of pentavalent antimony (such as sodium stibogluconate) and treatment for RMSF usually makes use of doxycycline.

Prognosis

The prognosis for rodent-related diseases depends on a number of factors, most of important of which is the type of disease itself. Some infections may be asymptomatic and resolve by themselves without treatment in a matter of days or weeks. Other infections may or may not have as mild symptoms and may turn into life-threatening conditions without early and effective treatment. RMSF and WEE are two such conditions.

Prevention

Generally speaking, rodents tend to be a more serious source of disease in regions that lack adequate levels of **sanitation**. Garbage piles, for example, tend to attract rats and mice, who then become a primary host for pathogens responsible for a variety of human diseases. So the first recommendation in efforts to reduce rodent-associated disease is to maintain as high a level of sanitation as possible. In developed nations, where solid waste disposal, sewage treatment, and other sanitation procedures tend to be common, the problem of rodent control often becomes one for individual households or businesses. The **Centers for Disease Control and Prevention** (CDC) recommends a three-prong effort to control rodents in the home and the workplace. The three prongs are Seal Up! Trap Up! Clean Up!

The Seal Up! aspect of this progrm involves identifying apertures through which rodents can enter a building and sealing those apertures. Rodents are clever animals who will find and utilize openings almost anywhere, from cracks in basement walls to openings along roof lines. The Trap Up! aspect of the program refers, as the name suggests, to the use of traps to capture and kill rodents such as rats and mice. The CDC recommends traditional spring traps that kill a rodent rather than a live trap because the latter may allow the rodent to defecate or urinate within the building, leaving behind any pathogens that it may be carrying. Finally, the Clean Up! stage of the program emphasizes sanitary procedures that will discourage rodents from congregating near a building, procedures such as storing food in tight containers, keeping outdoor grills clean, hanging bird feeders at a distance from the main house, using a tightly fitting lid on garbage cans, and keeping composting devices at sufficient distance from the house to discourage rodents from entering the premises.

Rodenticides

Humans have been using a variety of chemicals for centuries in their efforts to bring the rodent population under control. At one time, the most popular rodenticides were compounds containing a heavy metal, such as arsenic or thallium. Somewhat later, chemists developed other compounds that acted by interrupting the normal blood clotting process in an animal, causing a rodent to begin hemorrhaging and eventually bleeding to death. The anticoagulant warfarin was once a popular ingredient in such products. Some objections were long raised to the use of such products believing that they were accompanied by severe pain and discomfort by the drugged animal, who often took days or weeks to die after ingesting the poison. Probably a more serious concern with such rodenticides was their potential for harm to humans who accidentally ingested the product.

As a result of these concerns, chemists have developed a second generation of rodenticides that, while still potentially unpleasant for the rodent, are safer for use in human environments. These products make use primarily of the poisons bromethalin, chlorophacinone, and diphacinone. The U.S. **Environmental Protection Agency (EPA)** has warned chemical manufacturers that rodenticides produced after June 4, 2011, that do not meet its new and higher standards for rodenticide safety will face the probability of action by the agency for removal of their older and more risky products.

> ## QUESTIONS TO ASK YOUR DOCTOR
>
> - Does our community have any type of public health program designed to reduce the risk of rodent-related diseases?
> - What rodent-related diseases should members of my family be concerned about?
> - What steps should I take if one of my children is bitten by our pet guinea pig?
> - Is there any way of knowing whether a pet rodent is infected with a pathogen that could be transmitted to a member of our family?
> - Do you recommend that children be allowed to have rodents as pets? Why or why not?

Resources

BOOKS

Padovan, Dennis. *Zoonotic Infections in North American Rodents*. Anacortes, WA: Corvus Publishing, 2010.

Suckow, Mark A., Karla A. Stevens, and Ronald P. Wilson, eds. *The Laboratory Rabbit, Guinea Pig, Hamster, and other Rodents*. Oxford, UK: Academic Press, 2012.

Triunveri, Alfeo, and Desi Scalise. *Rodents: Habitat, Pathology, and Environmental Impact*. Hauppage, NY: Nova Science, 2012.

PERIODICALS

Bolzoni, L., et al. "Effect of Deer Density on Tick Infestation of Rodents and the Hazard of Tick-borne Encephalitis. II: Population and Infection Models." *International Journal for Parasitology* 42, 4. (2012): 373–81.

Flanagan, M. L., et al. "Anticipating the Species Jump: Surveillance for Emerging Viral Threats." *Zoonoses and Public Health* 59, 3. (2012): 155–63.

Mascari, T. M., L. D. Foil, and R. W. Stout. "Laboratory Evaluation of Oral Treatment of Rodents with Systemic Insecticides for Control of Bloodfeeding Sand Flies (Diptera: Psychodidae)." *Vector-Borne and Zoonotic Diseases* 12, 8. (2012): 699–704.

Meerburg, B. G., G. R. Singleton, and A. Kijlstra. "Rodent-borne Diseases and Their Risks for Public Health." *Critical Reviews in Microbiology* 35, 3. (2009): 221–70.

Robie, Gordon S., Neil S. Lipman, and Virginia Gillespie. "Infectious Disease Survey of Mus Musculus from Pet Stores in New York City." *Journal of the American Association of Laboratory Animal Science* 51, 1. (2012): 37–41.

WEBSITES

"Diseases from Rodents." Centers for Disease Control and Prevention. http://www.cdc.gov/rodents/diseases/. (accessed on October 24, 2012).

"Diseases from Rodents, Pocket Pets, and Rabbits." Public Health. Seattle & King County. http://www.kingcounty.gov/healthservices/health/ehs/zoonotics/PocketPets.aspx. (accessed on October 24, 2012).

"Rodentia." Animal Diversity Web. http://animaldiversity.ummz.umich.edu/site/accounts/information/Rodentia.html. (accessed on October 24, 2012).

"Rodenticides." Environmental Protection Agency. http://www.epa.gov/pesticides/mice-and-rats/. (accessed on October 24, 2012).

ORGANIZATIONS

Centers for Disease Control and Prevention (CDC), 1600 Clifton Rd., Atlanta, GA 30333, (800) 232–4636, http://www.cdc.gov/cdc-info/requestform.html, http://www.cdc.gov.

David E. Newton, EdD

S

Safe Drinking Water Act (1974)

Definition

The Safe Drinking Water Act (SDWA) of 1974 is the main federal law that ensures the quality of drinking water in the Unites States.

Purpose

When implemented, the SDWA extended coverage of federal drinking water standards to all public water supplies. Previous standards, established by the U. S. **Public Health Service** beginning in 1914 and administered by the U.S. **Environmental Protection Agency (EPA)** since its creation in 1970, had legally applied only to water supplies serving interstate carriers (e.g., planes, ships, and rail cars engaged in interstate commerce). However, many states and municipalities complied with them on a voluntary basis.

Demographics

Under the SDWA, public water supplies were defined as publicly or privately owned community water systems having at least 15 connections or serving at least 25 year-round customers or noncommunity water supplies serving at least 25 nonresidents for at least 60 days per year.

Description

The SDWA required the **EPA** to promulgate primary drinking water regulations to protect public health and secondary drinking water regulations to protect the aesthetic and economic qualities of the water. The EPA was granted authority to regulate: 1) contaminants which may affect health (e.g., trace levels of carcinogenic chemicals that may or may not have an impact on human health); 2) compounds that react during water treatment to form contaminants; 3) classes of compounds (if more convenient than regulating individual compounds); and 4) treatment techniques, when it is not feasible to regulate individual contaminants (e.g., disinfection is required in lieu of standards on individual disease-causing microorganisms).

Recognizing the right and the responsibility of the states to oversee the safety of their own drinking water supplies, the SDWA authorized the EPA to grant primacy to states willing to accept primary responsibility for administering their own drinking water program. To obtain primacy, a state must develop a drinking water program meeting minimum federal requirements and must establish and enforce primary regulations at least as stringent as those promulgated by the EPA. States with primacy are encouraged to enforce the federal secondary drinking water regulations, but are not required to do so.

Other provisions of the SDWA authorized control of underground injection (e.g., waste disposal wells); required special protection of sole-source aquifers (those providing the only source of drinking water in a given area); authorized funds for research on drinking water treatment; required the EPA to conduct a rural water supply survey to investigate the quality of drinking water in rural areas; allocated funds to subsidize up to 75% of the cost of enlarging state drinking water programs; required utilities to publicly notify their customers when the primary regulations are violated; permitted citizens to file suit against the EPA or a state having primacy; and granted the EPA emergency powers to protect public health.

Results

Dissatisfied with the slow pace at which new regulations were being promulgated by the EPA, which had in 1983 initiated a process to revise the primary and secondary standards, Congress amended the SDWA in 1986. The 1986 amendments required the EPA:

- to set primary standards for nine contaminants within one year, 40 more within two years, 34 more within three years, and 25 more by 1991;
- to specify criteria for filtration of surface water supplies and disinfection of groundwater supplies;
- to require large public water systems to monitor for the presence of certain unregulated contaminants;
- to establish programs to demonstrate how to protect sole-source aquifers;
- to require the states to develop well-head protection programs;
- to issue, within 18 months, rules regarding injection of waste below a water source.

The 1986 SDWA amendments also prohibited the use of **lead** solder, flux, and pipe; authorized the EPA to treat Indian tribes as states, making them eligible for primacy and grant assistance; required the EPA to conduct a survey of drinking **water quality** on Indian lands; authorized the EPA to initiate enforcement action if a state fails to take appropriate action within 30 days; and increased both civil and criminal penalties for failure to comply with the SDWA.

Since 1986 was a congressional election year and every member of Congress wanted to go on record as having voted for safe drinking water, the amendments passed unanimously. However, Congress failed to provide federal funds to assist state programs in complying with the many new provisions of the SDWA. The average annual cost per state to comply with the SDWA by 1995 was estimated to be nearly $500 million.

Further amendments to SDWA were passed in 1996. The new amendments established a Drinking Water State Revolving Fund to finance state compliance costs for water treatment facilities, easier access to water quality information for consumers, and contamination prevention initiatives. The mandate for contaminant testing was changed to a risk-based prioritized system that granted the EPA the authority to decide whether or not to regulate a contaminant after completing a required review of five contaminants every five years. The amendments also called for specific risk assessments and final regulation of radon, arsenic, DBP/cryptosporidium, and sulfate.

The SDWA ranked the following drinking water standards as rule-making priorities:

- Arsenic: The SDWA required the EPA to revise the existing 50 parts per billion (ppb) standard for arsenic in drinking water; the EPA implemented a 10 ppb standard for arsenic in January 2001. After the Bush administration briefly withdrew the standard, the new rule 10 ppb standard was reaffirmed in February 2002. In 2010, the EPA asserted that some 13 million people in the United States had benefited from the reduction of arsenic concentrations in various U.S. public water systems, which were all required to be in compliance with the 10 ppb standard in 2006.
- Ground Water Rule: The EPA was directed to regulate the appropriate use of disinfection in ground water and of other components of ground water systems to ensure public health protection.
- Lead and copper: The EPA estimated that approximately 20% of human exposure to lead was attributable to lead in drinking water.
- Microbials and disinfection byproducts: The EPA considered that a major challenge for water suppliers was how to balance the risks from microbial pathogens and disinfection by-products.
- MTBE: MTBE (methyl-t-butyl ether) belongs to a group of chemicals commonly known as fuel oxygenates, and it replaced lead as an octane enhancer after 1979.
- Radionuclides: The EPA updated standards for radionuclides in drinking water.
- Radon: Radon is a naturally occurring radioactive gas associated with cancer and that may be found in drinking water and indoor air. The EPA developed a regulation to reduce radon in drinking water.

Research and general acceptance

In the summer of 2010, the EPA launched its new Drinking Water Strategy initiative. Touted by the EPA as a "national conversation" on how to best improve the nation's public drinking water supply, the Strategy encompassed four basic principles: determining which water contaminants might best be addressed within groups, instead of individually; developing new technologies to deal with broad categories of drinking water contaminants and doing so in the most economical ways feasible; applying multiple federal statues governing water supplies in the effort to improve drinking water safety; and finally, encouraging cooperation between the states and the appropriate federal agencies to share a larger variety of data compiled from monitoring public water systems.

Resources

BOOKS

Ertuo, Kudret, and Ilker Mirze, eds. *Water Quality: Physical, Chemical, and Biological Characteristics*. New York: Nova Science, 2010.

Langwith, Jacqueline, ed. *Water*. Detroit: Greenhaven Press, 2010.

Midkiff, Ken. *Not a Drop to Drink: America's Water Crisis (and What You Can Do)*. Novato, CA: New World Library, 2007.

Symons, James M., et al., eds. *Plain Talk About Drinking Water: Answers to Your Questions About the Water You Drink*. Denver, CO: American Water Works Association, 2010.

WEBSITES

Centers for Disease Control and Prevention. "Drinking Water." http://www.cdc.gov/healthywater/drinking/ (accessed August 16, 2012).

U.S. Environmental Protection Agency. "Water: Drinking Water." http://water.epa.gov/drink/ (accessed August 13, 2012).

World Health Organization. "Drinking Water." http://www.who.int/topics/drinking_water/en (accessed August 12, 2012).

World Health Organization. "Guidelines for Drinking-water Quality." http://www.who.int/water_sanitation_health/dwq/gdwq0506.pdf (accessed August 12, 2012).

ORGANIZATIONS

Water Environment Federation, 601 Wythe St., Alexandria, VA 22314-1994, Fax: (703) 684-2492, (800) 666-0206, http://www.wef.org.

Stephen J. Randtke
Stacey Chamberlin

Sanitation

Definition

Sanitation encompasses the measures, methods, and activities that prevent the transmission of diseases and ensure public health. Specifically, sanitation refers to the hygienic principles and practices relating to the safe collection, removal, and disposal of human excreta, refuse, and wastewater.

For a household, sanitation refers to the provision and ongoing operation and maintenance of a safe and easily accessible means of disposing of human excreta, garbage, and wastewater, and providing an effective barrier against waste-related and waterborne diseases.

Description

The problems that result from inadequate sanitation can be illustrated by the following events in history:

- 1700 B.C.: Ahead of his time by a few thousand years, the queen's megaron in the palace of Knossos of Crete had running water in the bathrooms. Although there is evidence of plumbing and sewerage systems at several ancient sites, including the cloaca maxima (or great sewer) of ancient Rome, their use did not become widespread until modern times.

- 1817: A major epidemic of cholera hit Calcutta, India, after a national festival. There is no record of exactly how many people were affected, but there were 10,000 fatalities among British troops alone. The epidemic then spread to other countries and arrived in the United States and Canada in 1832. The governor of New York quarantined the Canadian border in a vain attempt to stop the epidemic. When cholera reached New York City, people were so frightened they either fled or stayed inside, leaving the city streets deserted.

- 1854: The London physician John Snow (1813–1858) demonstrated that cholera deaths in an area of the city could all be traced to a common public drinking water pump that was contaminated with sewage from a nearby house. Although he could not identify the exact cause, he convinced authorities to close the pump.

- 1859: The British Parliament was suspended during the summer because of the stench coming from the Thames. As was the case in many cities at this time, storm sewers carried a combination of sewage, street debris and other wastes, and storm water to the nearest body of water. According to one account, the river began to "seethe and ferment under a burning sun."

- 1892: The comma-shaped bacterium that causes cholera was identified by German scientist and physician Robert Koch (1843–1919) during an epidemic in Hamburg. His discovery proved the relationship between contaminated water and the disease.

- 1939: Sixty people died in an outbreak of typhoid fever at Manteno State Hospital in Illinois. The cause was traced to a sewer line passing too close to the hospital's water supply.

- 1940: A valve that was accidentally opened caused polluted water from the Genesee River to be pumped into the Rochester, New York, public water supply system. About 35,000 cases of gastroenteritis and six cases of typhoid fever were reported.

- 1955: Water containing a large amount of sewage was blamed for overwhelming a water treatment plant and causing an epidemic of hepatitis in Delhi, India. An estimated one million people were infected.
- 1961: A worldwide epidemic of cholera began in Indonesia and spread to eastern Asia and India by 1964; Russia, Iran, and Iraq by 1966; Africa by 1970; and Latin America by 1991.
- 1968: A four-year epidemic of dysentery began in Central America resulting in more than 500,000 cases and at least 20,000 deaths. Epidemic dysentery is currently a problem in many African nations.
- 1993: An outbreak of cryptosporidiosis in Milwaukee, Wisconsin, claimed 104 lives and infected more than 400,000 people, making it, at the time, the largest recorded outbreak of waterborne disease in the United States.
- 2010: Ten months after an earthquake displaced more than one million people on the island of Haiti, a cholera outbreak began in one of the many rural tent cities, which lacked adequate sanitation and where survivors lived in cramped conditions. Despite efforts to extinguish the outbreak that had already taken the lives of over 500 people, Hurricane Tomas hit the island, flooding the contaminated water sources that initiated the outbreak and spread cholera to the heavily populated capital city of Port-Au-Prince.
- 2011: A cholera epidemic in the West African country of Ghana killed 60 people and infected nearly 4,000 after flooding the previous year contaminated the water sources.
- 2012: From the beginning of the year to August 24, the West African country of Sierra Leone recorded 12,456 cases of cholera, along with the death of 1.8% (224) of its population. The president of Sierra Leone declared the cholera epidemic a "humanitarian crisis."

Modern sanitation challenges: Pacific Islands

The problem of sanitation in developed countries, which have the luxury of adequate financial and technical resources, is more concerned with the consequences arising from inadequate commercial food preparation and the results of bacteria becoming resistant to disinfection techniques and antibiotics. Flush toilets and high-quality drinking water supplies have all but eliminated **cholera** and epidemic diarrheal diseases. However, in many developing countries, inadequate sanitation is still the cause of life-or-death struggles.

In 1992, the South Pacific Regional Environment Programme (SPREP) and a land-based pollutants inventory stated that the "disposal of solid and liquid wastes (particularly of human excrement and household garbage in urban areas), which have long plagued the Pacific, emerge now as perhaps the foremost regional environmental problem of the decade."

High levels of fecal coliform bacteria have been found in surface and coastal waters. The SPREP Land-Based Sources of Marine Pollution Inventory described the Federated States of Micronesia's sewage pollution problems in striking terms: The prevalence of water-related diseases and **water quality** monitoring data indicate that the sewage pollutant loading to the environment is very high. A waste quality monitoring study was unable to find a single clean, uncontaminated site in the Kolonia, Pohnpei, area.

Many central wastewater treatment plants constructed with funds from the U.S. **Environmental Protection Agency (EPA)** in Pohnpei and in Chuuk States have failed due to lack of trained personnel and funding for maintenance.

In addition, septic systems used in some rural areas are said to be of poor design and construction, and pour-flush toilets and latrines—which frequently overflow in heavy rains—are more common. Over-the-water latrines are found in many coastal areas, as well.

In the Marshall Islands, signs of eutrophication—excess water plant growth due to too many nutrients—resulting from sewage disposal are evident next to settlements, particularly urban centers. According to a draft by the Marshall Islands NEMS, "one-gallon blooms occur along the coastline in Majuro and Ebeye, and are especially apparent on the lagoon side adjacent to households lacking toilet facilities." Stagnation of lagoon waters, reef degradation, and fish kills resulting from the low levels of oxygen have been well documented over the years. Additionally, red tides **plague** the lagoon waters adjacent to Majuro.

There is significant groundwater pollution in the Marshall Islands as well. The Marshall Island **EPA** estimates that more than 75% of the rural wells tested are contaminated with fecal coliform and other bacteria. Cholera, typhoid, and various diarrheal disorders occur.

With very little industry present, most of these problems are blamed on domestic sewage, with the greatest contamination problems believed to be from pit latrines, septic tanks, and the complete lack of sanitation facilities for 60% of rural households. As is often the case, poor design and inappropriate placement of these systems are often identified as the cause of contamination problems. In fact, even the best of these systems in the most favorable soil conditions allow significant amounts of nutrients and pathogens into the surrounding environment, and the soil characteristics and high water table typically found on atolls significantly inhibit treatment. In addition, the lack of proper maintenance, due to a lack of equipment to pump out septic tanks, is likely to have degraded the performance of these systems even further.

Forty percent of the population in the Republic of Palau is served by a secondary sewage treatment plant in the state of Koror, which is generally thought to provide adequate treatment. However, the Koror State government has expressed concern over the possible contamination of Malakal Harbor, into which the plant discharges. Also, some low-lying areas served by the system experience periodic back-flows of sewage that run into mangrove areas, due to mechanical failures with pumps and electrical power outages. In other low-lying areas not covered by the sewer system, septic tanks and latrines are used, which also overflow, affecting marine water quality.

Rural areas primarily rely on latrines, causing localized marine contamination in some areas. Though there have been an increasing number of septic systems installed as part of a rural sanitation program funded by the United States, there is anecdotal evidence that they may not be very effective. Many of the septic tank leach fields may not be of adequate size. In addition, a number of the systems are not used at all, as some families prefer instead to use latrines as the actual toilets and enclosures are not provided with the septic tanks as part of the program.

Wastewater problems also result from agriculture. According to the EPA, pig waste is considered to be a more significant problem than human sewage in many areas.

Because sanitation has become a social responsibility, national, state and local governments have adopted regulations that, when followed, should provide adequate sanitation for the governed society. However, some of the very technologies and practices that were instituted to provide better health and sanitation were later found to be contaminating ground and surface waters. For example, placing chlorine in drinking water and wastewater to provide disinfection, was found to produce carcinogenic compounds called trihalomethanes and dioxin. Collecting sanitary waste and transporting them along with industrial waste to inadequate treatment plants costing billions of dollars has failed to provide adequate protection for public health and environmental security.

Demographics

About 90% of people without access to adequate sanitation facilities live in 29 countries of the world. Most of these countries are located in sub-Saharan Africa and South Asia. Countries without adequate sanitation facilities include Iraq, Jordan, Malaysia, Morocco, Niger, and Rwanda. Overall, the largest numbers of these people live in India and China. In the 2000s, these two countries had over 800 million and 600 million people, respectively, without access to sanitation facilities.

Purpose

The main purpose of adequate sanitation for all of the world's peoples is to reduce the amount of disease that is caused by inadequate sanitation facilities. By saving lives, improving health conditions, and raising living standards around the world, especially in developing countries, people will have a better chance at surviving and contributing to society. Specifically, improved sanitation facilities are shown to increase a country's gross domestic product (GDP). Consequently, good sanitation is an important health, humanitarian, and economic factor for the world's countries.

Common diseases and disorders

Common diseases that are caused by sanitation and water-related problems include:

- Arsenicosis: This disorder is caused by the long-term presence of arsenic in naturally contaminated drinking water sources. It causes painful skin lesions that can eventually turn into cancers of the bladder, kidney, lungs, and skin.
- Cholera: This disease is caused by an acute bacterial infection within the intestinal tract, which causes diarrhea that can lead to dehydration and death.
- Diarrhea: This condition is caused by numerous microorganisms such as bacteria and protozoans, and viruses. It causes water and electrolyte loss within the body, which leads to dehydration and in some cases death.
- Fluorosis: This disorder is caused by high concentrations of fluoride that commonly occurs naturally in groundwater. It can lead to bone disease.
- Guinea worm disease: This disease, also known as Dracunculiasis, is caused by contaminated drinking water containing the Dracunculus larvae. It can cause debilitating ulcers.
- HIV/AIDS: The human immunodeficiency virus infection/acquired immunodeficiency syndrome causes increased health risk in people who have inadequate water and sanitation facilities. People infected with HIV/AIDS have compromised immune systems are less able to combat infections from inadequate water and sanitation facilities than healthy individuals.

EDWIN CHADWICK (1800–1890)

Edwin Chadwick was a progressive thinking man. He studied law in London, and in 1832, he was asked by the prime minister to participate in the Royal Commission of Enquiry on the English Poor Laws. The Commission worked with Parliament, and the Poor Law Amendment Act was passed. Chadwick was credited with writing almost a third of the published report.

London experienced influenza and typhoid epidemics in 1837 and 1838, and Chadwick determined that the city's unsafe sanitation practices directly impacted health conditions. His findings were outlined in a 1842 report entitled *The Sanitary Conditions of the Labouring Population*.

This report explained that the government needed to take a greater role in public health reform and sanitary conditions. Chadwick proposed changes for the environment, including indoor bathrooms in each house, and a sewage disposal system that transferred sewage to farmlands for fertilizer. However, these changes were refuted. People that benefitted from the poor health conditions (landlords, water companies) effectively blocked these ideas.

Even though his efforts were thwarted, Chadwick believed in his cause. He continued to fight for environmental legislation changes.

- Intestinal worms: Parasitic worms, such as roundworms, hookworms, and whipworms live in soil contaminated with human feces and infect humans who eat contaminated foods. These infections can lead to such maladies as malnutrition, anemia, and retarded growth.
- Malaria: This disease is caused by parasites carried on mosquitoes, which bite humans. Its symptoms include high fevers, shaking chills, flu-like symptoms, and anemia. If left untreated, malaria is fatal.
- Schistosomiasis: This disease is caused by parasitic worms that penetrate the skin of people swimming, bathing, or washing in contaminated waters. The infection can eventually cause damage to the bladder, intestines, liver, and lungs.
- Trachoma: This infection is caused by unsafe water sources that introduce infection into the eye. It can cause blindness.
- Typhoid: This disease is caused by bacteria that are ingested with contaminated food or water. It can cause such symptoms as headache, loss of appetite, and nausea.

Stable ecosystems model

Increasingly, the solution seems to be found in methods and practices that borrow from the stable ecosystems model of waste management. That is, there are no wastes, only resources that need to be connected to the appropriate organism that requires the residuals from one organism as the nutritional requirement of another. New waterless composting toilets that destroy human fecal organisms while they produce fertilizer are now the technology of choice in the developing world and have also found a growing niche in the developed world. Wash water, rather than being disposed of into ground and surface waters, is now being used for irrigation. The combination of these two ecologically engineered technologies provides economical sanitation, eliminates pollution, and creates valuable fertilizers for plants, while reducing the use of potable water for irrigation and toilets.

Simple hand washing is the most important measure in preventing disease transmission. Hand washing breaks the primary connection between surfaces contaminated with fecal organisms and the introduction of these pathogens into the human body. The use of basic soap and water, not exotic disinfectants, when practiced before eating and after defecating may save more lives than all of the modern methodologies and technologies combined.

Public health role and response

One of the targets for the Millennium Development Goals (MDGs) of the United Nations is to reduce by half the proportion of people without access to basic sanitation by the year 2015. However, because progress has been slower than expected the United Nations General Assembly declared that 2008 would be the "International Year of Sanitation" in order to help increase awareness of the problem of inadequate sanitation in many parts of the world.

Other goals and targets for sanitation by the United Nations (as part of the Johannesburg Plan of Implementation) include:

- Development of innovative financing and partnership mechanisms
- Assurance that, by the year 2025, sanitation coverage is achieved in all rural areas
- Improvement in sanitation in public institutions, especially schools

- Integration of sanitation into water resources management strategies
- Promotion of affordable and socially and culturally acceptable technologies and practices
- Promotion of safe hygiene practices
- Strengthened existing information networks

Prognosis

According to the **World Health Organization** (WHO), every year unsafe drinking water and the lack of basic sanitation kills at least 1.6 million children under the age of five years. At the beginning of 2005, 1.1 billion people did not have adequate access to an improved source of drinking water. Of these people, 84% lived in rural areas. In addition, the WHO reported that approximately 40% (2.6 billion) of the world's population did not have access to a toilet and were forced to defecate in open or unsanitary places such as in fields, forests, and bodies of water.

As of 2005, sanitation was about twice as prevalent in urban areas as it was in rural ones. Sanitation levels in urban areas had increased by about one percentage point, from 79% to 80%, from 1990 to 2004. This improvement resulted in approximately 770 million people gaining improved sanitation conditions in urban areas, where improved sanitation refers to the ability to manage feces at the household level. The WHO stated in its report *Meeting the MDG Drinking Water and Sanitation Target*, "extending basic drinking water and sanitation services to periurban and slum areas to reach the poorest people is of the utmost importance to prevent outbreaks of cholera and other water-related diseases in these often overcrowded places." WHO estimated that, if current trends held through 2015, in that year 1.7 billion people in rural areas would still not have access to improved sanitation.

Prevention

The prevention of diseases that can be transmitted through human waste can be attained by isolating such waste through adequate sanitation and hygiene practices. Such diseases include waterborne diseases (which contaminate drinking water), fecal-borne diseases (which occur when humans come into physical contact with feces), and hookworm (whose eggs can be acquired from contacting infected soil).

According to the report *Progress on Sanitation and Drinking-water, 2010 Update*, by the Joint Monitoring Programme for Water Supply and Sanitation, which is conducted by the WHO and the United Nations Children's Fund (**UNICEF**), improved sanitation facilities are those that "hygienically separates human excreta from human contact." The following are ways to provide improved sanitation facilities to peoples of the world without adequate sanitation and thus help to prevent unsanitary conditions:

> **KEY TERMS**
>
> **Dioxins**—Any of numerous by-products of various industrial processes, which are regarded as extremely toxic. These dioxins or dioxin-like compounds include polychlorinated dibenzo-p-dioxins (PCDDs), polychlorinated dibenzofurans (PCDFs), and polychlorinated biphenyls (PCBs).
>
> **Electrolyte**—A compound that is separated into ions within a solution.
>
> **Red tide**—A brownish-red coloration in seawater that is caused by increased plant-based plankton.

- using a composting toilet
- connecting to a piped sewer system
- connecting to a septic system
- using a flush toilet
- using flush/pour-flush to a pit latrine
- using a pit latrine with slab
- ventilating an improved pit (VIP) latrine

Resources

BOOKS

Davis, Mackenzie Leo. *Introduction to Environmental Engineering*. Dubuque, IA: McGraw-Hill, 2008.

Eaton, Andrew D., and M. A. H. Franson. *Standard Methods for the Examination of Water & Wastewater*. Washington, DC: American Public Health Association, 2005.

Hempel, Sandra. *The Strange Case of the Broad Street Pump: John Snow and the Mystery of Cholera*. Berkeley: University of California Press, 2006.

Juuti, Petri S., Tapio S. Katko, and Heikki S. Vuorinen. *Environmental History of Water: Global Views on Community Water Supply and Sanitation*. London: IWA, 2007.

Prakash, Anjal, V. S. Saravanan, and Jayati Choubey, eds. *Interlacing Water and Human Health: Case Studies from South Asia*. New Delhi: Sage, 2012.

Russell, David L. *Practical Wastewater Treatment*. New York: Wiley-Interscience, 2006.

WEBSITES

Division for Social Development, Department of Economic and Social Affairs, United Nations. "Sanitation." http://www.un.org/esa/dsd/susdevtopics/sdt_sanitation.shtml (accessed September 19, 2012).

The Independent Staff. "World's Poor to Wait 200 Years for Sanitation." http://www.independent.co.uk/news/world/politics/worlds-poor-to-wait-200-years-for-sanitation-6261623.html (accessed September 19, 2012).

Joint Monitoring Programme (JMP) for Water Supply and Sanitation, WHO and UNICEF. "Progress on Drinking Water and Sanitation: 2012 Update." http://www.wssinfo.org/documents-links/documents/ (accessed September 19, 2012).

Sanitation Updates. "Cholera Epidemic Kills 60 in Ghana." http://sanitationupdates.wordpress.com/2011/03/18/cholera-epidemic-kills-60-in-ghana/ (accessed September 19, 2012).

United Nations Children's Fund. "Water, Sanitation and Hygiene." http://www.unicef.org/wash/index_wes_related.html (accessed September 19, 2012).

World Health Organization. "Cholera." http://www.who.int/entity/mediacentre/factsheets/fs107/en/index.html (accessed September 19, 2012).

World Health Organization. "Cholera in Sierra Leone (Update 24 August 2012)." http://www.afro.who.int/en/clusters-a-programmes/dpc/epidemic-a-pandemic-alert-and-response/outbreak-news/3668-cholera-in-sierra-leone-update-24-august-2012.html (accessed September 19, 2012).

World Health Organization. "Global Analysis and Assessment of Sanitation and Drinking Water." http://www.who.int/water_sanitation_health/en/ (accessed September 19, 2012).

World Health Organization. "Meeting the MDG Drinking-Water and Sanitation Target." http://www.who.int/water_sanitation_health/monitoring/jmpfinal.pdf (accessed September 19, 2012).

World Health Organization. "Sanitation." http://www.who.int/topics/sanitation/en/ (accessed September 19, 2012).

ORGANIZATIONS

Centers for Disease Control and Prevention, 1600 Clifton Rd., Atlanta, GA 30333, (800) 232-4636, cdcinfo@cdc.gov, http://www.cdc.gov.

Environmental Protection Agency, 1200 Pennsylvania Ave. NW, Ariel Rios Bldg., Washington, DC 20460, (202) 272-0167, http://www.epa.gov.

Environmental Research Foundation, PO Box 160, New Brunswick, NJ 08908, (732) 828-9995, erf@rachel.org, http://www.rachel.org.

World Health Organization, Avenue Appia 20, Geneva, Switzerland 1211 27, 41 22 791-2111, Fax: 41 22 791-3111, cdcinfo@cdc.gov, http://www.who.int/en.

Carol Steinfeld
William A. Atkins, B.B., B.S., M.B.A.

SARS *see* **Severe acute respiratory syndrome**

Save the Children

Definition

Save the Children is a nongovernmental organization (NGO) made up of 30 member organizations focused on the protection of children's rights around the world.

Purpose

Save the Children is committed to the protection of human rights for children around the world, both domestically and in developing countries. The organization focuses on promoting education, combating hunger, reducing childhood mortality, improving access to health care, and improving economic opportunities. Save the Children also provides emergency assistance in areas affected by natural disaster, war, and other humanitarian crises.

Demographics

Save the Children is made up of Save the Children Alliance member-country organizations in 30 countries on six continents. In 2010, efforts reached over 100 million children in over 120 countries. In 2011, the largest expenditures went toward South and Central Asia and East Africa with 22% of expenditures each. Other geographical areas of focus included domestic programs (18% of expenditures), South East and East Asia (9%), and West and Central Africa (9%).

Description

Through programs in over 120 countries, the member organizations of Save the Children work together to make lasting changes that improve the lives of children around the world. This work includes providing education, economic, and healthcare opportunities to children both domestically and in developing countries. Each member organization has its own staff stationed both in home offices and international ones. Save the Children is also focused on training locals in target aid areas to become members of ongoing projects to help their own communities. In 2011, Save the Children had over two million supporting members and raised over $1.6 billion.

Origins

Save the Children was founded by sisters Eglantyne Jebb and Dorothy Buxton in the United Kingdom in May 1919. The organization originated in response to the many children in Austria and Eastern Europe dying of hunger after the World War I. The first relief effort was focused on providing food to starving children in Austria.

At the start, Save the Children was not intended as a permanent organization, but as the number of emergencies and the need grew, Save the Children became a permanent support organization. As the organization's work increased, so did fundraising efforts.

Although Buxton became less involved in Save the Children after the initial foundation period, Jebb became known for her new and effective fundraising efforts. These included using page-length advertisements in newspapers and filming Save the Children activities in disaster areas. Jebb was also recognized for her focus on the human rights of children around the world. During the 1920s, the League of Nations adopted her "Declaration of the Rights of the Child," and these same ideas became the basis of the United Nations Convention Rights of the Child that went into force in September 1990.

Although Jebb died in 1928, her vision continued. The 1930s witnessed an expansion of Save the Children's work into Africa and Asia. Save the Children had projects to support children facing both hardship and war, including the World War II and the Korean War. Branches and member organizations of Save the Children were present from the beginning of the organization. Save the Children groups continued to open around the world, including in Canada (1921), the United States (1932), South Africa (1944), Mexico (1972), India (1988), and Brazil (1991). In 2011, Save the Children International was launched in order to centralize and coordinate implementation of oversea projects among member organizations.

Save the Children has been working around world to protect children's rights, improve educational opportunities, combat hunger, and decrease the number of child deaths. As of 2012, Save the Children had 30 member-country organizations and was present in over 120 countries, impacting millions of children each year.

Results

Together, Save the Children member organizations successfully improved the lives of millions of children around the world. The organization estimates that its efforts reach as many as 100 million children each year. Current major focus areas include child protection, education, children's rights, HIV/AIDS prevention, and emergency aid in humanitarian crises. Additionally, between 2005 and 2012, Save the Children conducted multiple worldwide campaigns, including Rewrite the Future, EVERY ONE, and Every Beat Matters. Each of these campaigns has a specific theme.

Rewrite the Future was launched 2005 with the goal of giving children in areas affected by armed conflict equal and quality education. The campaign was considered successful, giving 1.4 million children access to school and benefiting more than 10.6 million children in 20 countries through educational programs. The campaign was completed at the end of 2010.

The EVERY ONE campaign began in 2009, with the goal of decreasing child mortality by two-thirds by 2015. The program is active in 50 countries, with a special emphasis on countries with high child mortality rates. By 2011, Save the Children and its partners had trained almost 180,000 health workers and reached over 50.4 million women and children, putting the program on track to reach its goals.

Every Beat Matters, begun in August 2012, focused on keeping children healthy around the world by ending preventable childhood deaths. The project received attention through its partnership with the music group One Republic, that wrote the song "Feel Again," inspired by the heartbeats of children in Malawi and Guatemala. Proceeds from song sales go toward the Every Beat Matters campaign.

Research and general acceptance

Worldwide, Save the Children is a trusted and well-supported charity. The United States branch of Save the Children is approved through May 2013 by the Better Business Bureau as meeting standards in all 20 investigated areas, including board oversight, truthful materials, and detailed expense breakdowns. Facts and statistics developed by Save the Children Alliance members are considered reliable in their assessment of children's conditions in countries around the world.

The charity has been criticized for having certain partners, such as its partnership with the Coca-Cola Company. In September 2012, Save the Children received negative publicity when it was ordered to leave Pakistan and was accused of being a cover for the United States Central Intelligence Agency (CIA). Save the Children stated that it had no connection to the CIA and that the accused doctor in the matter had never worked for the organization. Many of these criticisms are short lived, and they are few in number compared to the numerous positive reports Save the Children receives.

Resources

BOOKS

Mahood, Linda. *Save the Children (International Organizations)*. Mankato, MN: Weigl, 2003.

Nault, Jennifer. *Feminism and Voluntary Action: Eglantyne Jebb and Save the Children, 1876–1928*. New York: Palgrave Macmillan, 2009.

WEBSITES

Forbes. "The 200 Largest U.S. Charities List: Save the Children." http://www.forbes.com/lists/2011/14/charities-11_Save-the-Children-Federation_CH0147.html (accessed October 12, 2012).

Save the Children Every One. "Facts Campaigning to Save Children's Lives." http://www.savethechildren.net/sites/default/files/Report2012LowresARTWORKsingles.pdf (accessed October 10, 2012).

Save the Children. "Our Finances." http://www.savethechildren.net/about-us/our-finances (accessed October 10, 2012).

Save the Children. "Program Areas." http://www.savethechildren.org/site/c.8rKLIXMGIpI4E/b.6153013/k.9328/Program_Areas.htm (accessed October 12, 2012).

ORGANIZATIONS

Save the Children (United Kingdom), 1 St. John's Lane, London, UK EC1M 4AR, 44 20 7012 6400, supporter.care@savethechildren.org.uk, http://www.savethechildren.org.uk.

Save the Children (United States), 54 Wilton Rd., Westport, CT 06880, (203) 221-4030, (800) 728-3843, twebster@savechildren.org, http://www.savethechildren.org.

Tish Davidson, AM

Schistosomiasis

Definition

Schistosomiasis, also known as bilharziasis or snail fever, is primarily a tropical parasitic disease caused by the larvae of one or more of five types of flatworms or blood flukes known as schistosomes. The name bilharziasis comes from Theodor Bilharz, a German pathologist, who identified the worms in 1851.

Description

Infections associated with worms present some of the most universal health problems in the world. In fact, only **malaria** accounts for more diseases than schistosomiasis. The **World Health Organization** (WHO) estimates that 200 million people are infected and 120 million display symptoms. Another 600 million people are at risk of infection. Schistosomes are prevalent in rural and outlying city areas of 74 countries in Africa, Asia, and Latin America. In Central China and Egypt, the disease poses a major health risk.

There are five species of schistosomes that are prevalent in different areas of the world and produce somewhat different symptoms:

- *Schistosoma mansoni* is widespread in Africa, the Eastern Mediterranean, the Caribbean, and South America and can only infect humans and rodents.
- *S. mekongi* is prevalent only in the Mekong river basin in Asia.
- *S. japonicum* is limited to China and the Philippines and can infect other mammals, in addition to humans, such as pigs, dogs, and water buffalos. As a result, it can be harder to control the disease caused by this species.
- *S. intercalatum* is found in central Africa.
- *S. haematobium* occurs predominantly in Africa and the Eastern Mediterranean.

Intestinal schistosomiasis, caused by *Schistosoma japonicum*, *S. mekongi*, *S. mansoni*, and *S. intercalatum*, can lead to serious complications of the liver and spleen. Urinary schistosomiasis is caused by *S. haematobium*.

It is difficult to determine how many individuals die of schistomiasis each year because death certificates and patient records seldom identify schistosomiasis as the primary cause of death. Mortality estimates vary related to the type of schistosome infection but are generally low. For example, the estimated annual death rate from infection with *S. mansoni* is 2.4 per 100,000.

Causes and symptoms

All five species are contracted in the same way, through direct contact with fresh water infested with the free-living form of the parasite known as cercariae. The building of **dams**, irrigation systems, and reservoirs, and the movements of refugee groups introduce and spread schistosomiasis.

Eggs are excreted in human urine and feces and, in areas with poor **sanitation**, contaminate freshwater sources. The eggs break open to release a form of the parasite called miracidium. Freshwater snails become infested with the miracidium, which multiply inside the snail and mature into multiple cercariae that the snail ejects into the water. The cercariae, which survive outside a host for 48 hours, quickly penetrate unbroken skin, the lining of the mouth, or the gastrointestinal tract. Once inside the human body, the worms penetrate the wall of the nearest vein and travel to the liver where they grow and sexually mature. Mature male and female worms pair and migrate either to the intestines or the bladder where egg production occurs. One female worm may lay an average of 200 to 2,000 eggs per day for up to twenty years. Most eggs leave the blood stream and body through the intestines. Some of the eggs are not excreted, however, and can lodge in the tissues. It is the presence of these eggs, rather than the worms themselves, that causes the disease.

Early symptoms of infection

Many individuals do not experience symptoms. If infection is present, it usually takes four to six weeks for symptoms to appear. The first symptom of the disease may be a general ill feeling. Within twelve hours of infection, an individual may complain of a tingling sensation or light rash, commonly referred to as "swimmer's itch," due to irritation at the point of entrance. The rash that may develop can mimic scabies and other types of rashes. Other symptoms can occur two to ten weeks later and can include fever, aching, cough, diarrhea, or gland enlargement. These symptoms can also be related to avian schistosomiasis, which does not cause any further symptoms in humans.

Katayama fever

Another primary condition, called Katayama fever, may also develop from infection with these worms, and it can be very difficult to recognize. Symptoms include fever, lethargy, the eruption of pale temporary bumps associated with severe itching (urticarial) rash, liver and spleen enlargement, and bronchospasm.

Intestinal schistosomiasis

In intestinal schistosomiasis, eggs become lodged in the intestinal wall and cause an immune system reaction called a granulomatous reaction. This immune response can lead to obstruction of the colon and blood loss. The infected individual may have what appears to be a potbelly. Eggs can also become lodged in the liver, leading to high blood pressure through the liver, enlarged spleen, the build-up of fluid in the abdomen (ascites), and potentially life-threatening dilations or swollen areas in the esophagus or gastrointestinal tract that can tear and bleed profusely (esophageal varices). Rarely, the central nervous system may be affected. Individuals with chronic active schistosomiasis may not complain of typical symptoms.

Urinary tract schistosomiasis

Urinary tract schistosomiasis is characterized by blood in the urine, pain or difficulty urinating, and frequent urination and are associated with *S. haematobium*. The loss of blood can lead to iron deficiency anemia. A large percentage of persons, especially children, who are moderately to heavily infected experience urinary tract damage that can lead to blocking of the urinary tract and bladder cancer.

Diagnosis

Proper diagnosis and treatment may require a **tropical disease** specialist because the disease can be confused with malaria or typhoid in the early stages. The healthcare provider should do a thorough history of travel in **endemic** areas. The rash, if present, can mimic scabies or other rashes, and the gastrointestinal symptoms may be confused with those caused by bacterial illnesses or other intestinal **parasites**. These other conditions will need to be excluded before an accurate diagnosis can be made. As a result, clinical evidence of exposure to infected water along with physical findings, a negative test for malaria, and an increased number of one type of immune cell, called an eosinophil, are necessary to diagnose acute schistosomiasis.

Eggs may be detected in the feces or urine. Repeated stool tests may be required to concentrate and identify the eggs. Blood tests may be used to detect a particular antigen or particle associated with the schistosome that induces an immune response. Persons infected with schistosomiasis may not test positive for six months, and as a result, tests may need to be repeated to obtain an accurate diagnosis. Blood can be detected visually in the urine or with chemical strips that react to small amounts of blood.

Sophisticated imaging techniques, such as ultrasound, computed tomography scan (CT scan), and magnetic resonance imaging (MRI), can detect damage to the blood vessels in the liver and visualize polyps and ulcers of the urinary tract, for example, that occur in the more advanced stages. *S. haematobium* is difficult to diagnose with ultrasound in pregnant women.

Treatment

The use of medications against schistosomiasis, such as praziquantel (Biltricide), oxamniquine, and metrifonate, has been shown to be safe and effective. Praziquantel is effective against all forms of schistososmiasis and has few side effects. This drug is given in either two or three doses over the course of a single day. Oxamniquine is typically used in Africa and

> **KEY TERMS**
>
> **Ascites**—The condition that occurs when the liver and kidneys are not functioning properly and a clear, straw-colored fluid is excreted by the membrane that lines the abdominal cavity (peritoneum).
>
> **Cercariae**—The free-living form of the schistosome worm that has a tail, swims, and has suckers on its head for penetration into a host.
>
> **Miracidium**—The form of the schistosome worm that infects freshwater snails.

South America to treat intestinal schistosomiasis. Metrifonate has been found to be safe and effective in the treatment of urinary schistosomiasis. Patients are typically checked for the presence of living eggs at three and six months after treatment. If the number of eggs excreted has not significantly decreased, the patient may require another course of medication.

Prognosis

If treated early, prognosis is very good and complete recovery is expected. The illness is treatable, but people can die from the effects of untreated schistosomiasis. The severity of the disease depends on the number of worms, or worm load, in addition to how long the person has been infected. With treatment, the number of worms can be substantially reduced, and the secondary conditions can be treated. The goal of the World Health Organization is to reduce the severity of the disease rather than to completely stop transmission of the disease. There is, however, little natural immunity to reinfection. Treated individuals do not usually require retreatment for two to five years in areas of low transmission. The World Health Organization has made research to develop a vaccine against the disease one of its priorities.

Prevention

Prevention of the disease involves several targets and requires long-term community commitment. Infected patients require diagnosis, treatment, and education about how to avoid reinfecting themselves and others. Adequate healthcare facilities need to be available, water systems must be treated to kill the worms and control snail populations, and sanitation must be improved to prevent the spread of the disease.

To avoid schistosomiasis iwhen visiting endemic areas, individuals ought to take the following precautions:

- Contact the CDC for current health information on travel destinations.
- Upon arrival, ask an informed local authority about the infestation of schistosomiasis before being exposed to freshwater in countries that are likely to have the disease.
- Do not swim, stand, wade, or take baths in untreated water.
- Treat all water used for drinking or bathing. Water can be treated by letting it stand for three days, heating it for five minutes to around 122°F (around 50°C), or filtering or treating water chemically, with chlorine or iodine, as with drinking water.

> **QUESTIONS TO ASK YOUR DOCTOR**
>
> - In what regions of the world that we might visit for a vacation is schistosomiasis likely to be a health problem?
> - Does the federal government issue health alerts for regions such as these?
> - Are there preparations we should make before leaving for a vacation in such areas?
> - What is the long-term risk if we should contract schistosomiasis on a foreign trip?

- Should accidental exposure occur, infection can be prevented by hastily drying off or applying rubbing alcohol to the exposed area.

Resources

BOOKS

Bogitsh, Burton J., Clint E. Carter, and Thomas N. Oeltmann. *Human Parasitology*, 4th ed. New York: Academic Press, 2012.

Secor, W. Evan, and Daniel G. Colley, eds. *Schistosomiasis*. New York: Springer, 2010.

PERIODICALS

Gryseels, B. "Schistosomiasis" *Infectious Disease Clinics of North America* 26, no. 2 (2012): 383–97.

Nour, Nawal M. "Schistosomiasis: Health Effects on Women." *Obstetrics and Gynecology* 3, no. 1 (2010): 28–32.

Siddiqui, A. A., B. A. Siddiqui, and L. Ganley-Leal. "Schistosomiasis Vaccines." *Human Vaccines* 7, no. 11 (2011): 1192–97.

WEBSITES

Gonya, Lenna. "Symptoms and Treatment of Schistosomiasis." Helium. http://www.helium.com/items/2101285-symptoms-and-treatment-of-schistosomiasis (accessed September 21, 2012).

Gray, Darren J., et al. "Diagnosis and Management of Schistosomiasis." http://www.ncbi.nlm.nih.gov/pmc/articles/PMC3230106/pdf/bmj.d2651.pdf (accessed on September 21, 2012).

"Schistosomiasis." PubMed Health. http://www.ncbi.nlm.nih.gov/pubmedhealth/PMH0002298/ (accessed September 21, 2012).

ORGANIZATIONS

Centers for Disease Control and Prevention, 1600 Clifton Rd., Atlanta, GA 30333, (800) CDC-INFO (232-4636), cdcinfor@cdc.gov, http://www.cdc.gov.

World Health Organization, Avenue Appia 20, 1211 Geneva 27, Switzerland, +22 41 791 21 11, Fax: +22 41 791 31 11, info@who.int, http://www.who.int.

Ruth E. Mawyer, RN

Severe acute respiratory syndrome (SARS)

Definition

Severe acute respiratory syndrome (SARS) is the first emergent and highly transmissible viral disease to appear during the twenty-first century. SARS is a potentially life-threatening disease. It is caused by a virus of the Coronaviridae family. The Coronaviridae family of **viruses** is also responsible for many common colds. SARS, however, is far more serious than a cold.

Description

The first reported case of SARS was traced to a November 2002 case in Guangdong province, China. By mid-February 2003, Chinese health officials tracked more than 300 cases, including five deaths in Guangdong province from what was at the time described as an acute respiratory syndrome. Many flu-causing viruses have previously originated from Guangdong Province because of cultural and exotic cuisine practices that bring animals, animal parts, and humans into close proximity along with limited **sanitation**. In such an environment, pathogens can more easily mutate and make the leap from animal hosts to humans. The first cases of SARS showed high rates among Guangdong food handlers and chefs.

Chinese health officials initially remained silent about the outbreak, and no special precautions were taken to limit travel or prevent the spread of the disease. The world health community, therefore, had no chance to institute testing, isolation, and quarantine measures that might have prevented the subsequent global spread of the disease.

On February 21, Jianlun Liu, a 64-year-old Chinese physician from Zhongshan hospital (later determined to have been a "super-spreader,"—a person capable of infecting unusually high numbers of contacts) traveled to Hong Kong to attend a family wedding despite the fact that he had a fever. Epidemiologists subsequently determined that, Liu passed on the SARS virus to other guests at the Metropole Hotel where he stayed, including an American businessman en route to Hanoi, three women from Singapore, two Canadians, and a Hong Kong resident. Liu's travel to Hong Kong and the subsequent travel of those he infected allowed SARS to spread from China to the infected travelers' destinations.

Johnny Chen, the American businessman, grew ill in Hanoi, Vietnam, and was admitted to a local hospital. Chen infected 20 health care workers at the hospital including noted Italian epidemiologist Carlo Urbani who worked at the Hanoi **World Health Organization** (WHO) office. Urbani provided medical care for Chen and first formally identified SARS as a unique disease on February 28, 2003. By early March, 22 hospital workers in Hanoi were ill with SARS.

Unaware of the problems in China, Urbani's report drew increased attention among epidemiologists when coupled with news reports in mid-March that Hong Kong health officials had also discovered an outbreak of an acute respiratory syndrome among health care workers. Unsuspecting hospital workers had admitted the Hong Kong man infected by Liu to a general ward at the Prince of Wales Hospital because it was assumed he had a typical severe pneumonia—a fairly routine admission. The first sign that clinicians were dealing with an unusual illness came from the observation that hospital staff, and those determined to have been in close proximity to the infected persons had become ill. There were still no health notices from China of increasing illnesses and deaths due to SARS.

After many of the Hong Kong hosptial staff became ill, Hong Kong authorities decided that those experiencing flu-like symptoms would be given the option of self-isolation, with family members allowed to remain confined at home or in special camps. Compliance checks were conducted by police.

One of the most intriguing aspects of the early Hong Kong cases was a cluster of more than 250 SARS cases that occurred in a group of high-rise apartment buildings—many **housing** health care workers—that provided evidence of a high rate of secondary transmission. Epidemiologists conducted extensive investigations to rule out the hypothesis that the illnesses were related to some form of local contamination (e.g., sewage, bacteria in the ventilation system). Rumors began that the illness was due to cockroaches or **rodents**, but no scientific evidence supported the hypothesis that the disease pathogen was carried by insects or animals.

One of the Canadians infected in Hong Kong, Sui-Chu Kwan, return to Toronto, Ontario, and died in a Toronto hospital on March 5. As in Hong Kong, because there was no alert from China about the SARS outbreak, Canadian officials did not initially suspect that Kwan had been infected with a highly contagious virus, until Kwan's son and five health care workers showed similar symptoms. By mid-April, Canada reported more than 130 SARS cases and 15 fatalities.

Public health role and response

Faced with reports that provided evidence of global dissemination, on March 15, 2003, the World

DR. CARLO URBANI (1956–2003)

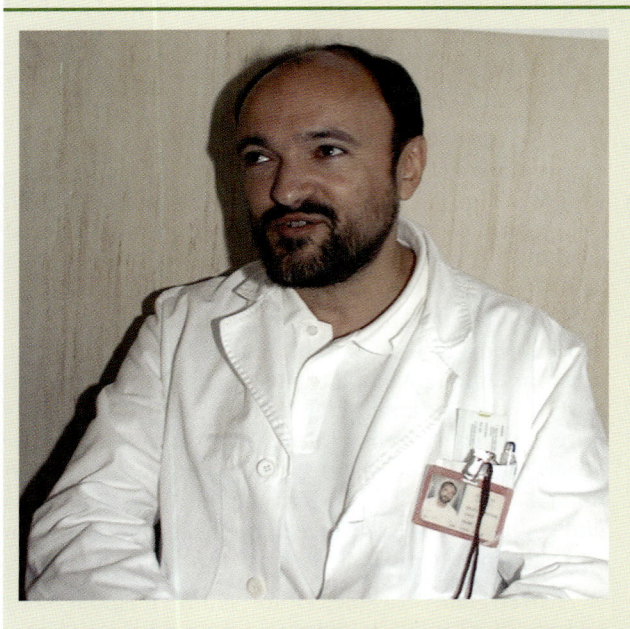

Dr. Carlo Urbani, an Italian epidemiologist, died due to complications from Severe Acute Respiratory Syndrome (SARS), the very disease he helped to identify and control. In February 2003, Urbani was serving as Vietnam's infectious disease specialist within the World Health Organization (WHO) when he was alerted to an atypical case of pneumonia. Urbani immediately identified and conveyed the seriousness of the disease, and worked with health professionals and government officials to establish protective measures. Efforts such as global communication/awareness, quarantining patients, and thorough screening of international travelers paid off. By June 2003, the number of new SARS cases had diminished enough that WHO stopped their daily reports on the disease.

Dr. Urbani's global involvement in infectious diseases began in the 1980s, with parasitic disease control. He was passionate about his work, taking an active role in identifying and treating diseases, as well as educating people. In March 2003, Dr. Urbani's wife expressed her concerns about his constant exposure to deadly diseases, such as SARS. Urbani insisted that he continue his active role in epidemiology, no matter the threat to his health. Days later, he died. He was 46 years old.

Italian Dr. Carlo Urbani, 46, the first doctor to recognize the then unfamiliar disease SARS (Severe Acute Respiratory Syndrome), Bangkok, Thailand, 2003. *(AP Images/Guido Picchio.)*

Health Organization (WHO) took the unusual step of issuing a travel warning that described SARS as a "worldwide health threat." WHO officials announced that SARS cases, and potential cases, had been tracked from China to Singapore, Thailand, Vietnam, Indonesia, Philippines, and Canada. Although the exact cause of the "acute respiratory syndrome" had not, at that time, been determined, WHO officials issuance of the precautionary warning to travelers bound for Southeast Asia about the potential SARS risk served as notice to public health officials about the potential dangers of SARS.

WHO was initially encouraged that isolation procedures and alerts were working to stem the spread of SARS, as some countries that had reported small numbers of cases experienced no further dissemination to hospital staff or others in contact with SARS victims. However, in some countries, including Canada, where SARS cases occurred before WHO alerts, SARS continued to spread beyond the isolated patients.

WHO officials responded by recommending increased screening and quarantine measures that included mandatory screening of persons returning from visits to the most severely affected areas in China, Southeast Asia, and Hong Kong.

In early April 2003, WHO took the controversial additional step of recommending against non-essential travel to Hong Kong and Guangdong Province in China. The recommendation, sought by infectious disease specialists, was not controversial within the medical community, but caused immediate concern regarding the potentially widespread economic impacts.

Mounting reports of SARS showed an increasing global dissemination of the virus. By April 9, the first confirmed reports of SARS cases in Africa reached WHO headquarters, and eight days later, a confirmed case was discovered in India.

The outbreak of SARS lasted from November 2002 through July 2003. The last reported cases occurred in China in 2004. As of mid-2012, no additional cases of SARS have been reported anywhere in the world.

State governments within the United States have a general authority to set and enforce quarantine conditions for threats to public health. At the federal level, the Centers for Disease Control and Prevention (CDC) Division of Global Migration and Quarantine is empowered to detain, examine, or conditionally release (release with restrictions on movement or with a required treatment protocol) individuals suspected of carrying certain listed **communicable diseases**, incouding SARS.

Demographics

During the 2002–2003 SARS outbreak, about 8,000 people were infected, including many health care workers, and 774 deaths were reported (9.6% of reported cases). The majority of cases occurred in mainland China, followed by Hong Kong, Taiwan, and Singapore. There were 251 cases and 43 deaths in Canada and none in the United States.

Causes and symptoms

SARS is caused by a virus that is transmitted from person to person predominantly through the air by the aerosolized droplets of virus-infected material. The incubation period ranges from about 2–7 days. Patients appear to be contagious only when they develop fever and other symptoms. However, the **Centers for Disease Control and Prevention** (CDC) recommends individuals remain in isolation for 10 days after the fever is gone as a precaution against spreading the disease.

The initial symptoms of SARS are non-specific flu-like symptoms of fever, headache, malaise, dry cough. Infected patients then typically spike a fever of 100.4°F (38°C) or higher as they develop a deep cough, shortness of breath, and difficult or painful breathing. SARS often fulminates (reaches it maximum progression) in a severe pneumonia that can cause respiratory failure and death.

In mid-April 2003, Canadian scientists at the British Columbia Cancer Agency in Vancouver announced that they that sequenced the genome of the coronavirus most likely to be the cause of SARS. Within days, scientists at the Centers for Disease Control (CDC) in Atlanta, Georgia, offered a genomic map that confirmed more than 99% of the Canadian findings.

The genetic map was generated from studies of viruses isolated from SARS cases. The particular coronavirus mapped had a genomic sequence of 29,727 nucleotides—average for the family of coronavirus that typically contain between 29,000–31,000 nucleotides.

Proof that the coronavirus map was the specific virus responsible for SARS eventually came from animal testing. Rhesus monkeys were exposed to the virus via injection and inhalation and then monitored to determine whether SARS-like symptoms developed. Sick animals were examined for histological pathology (i.e., an examination of the tissue and cellular level for signs of illness) similar to findings in human patients.

KEY TERMS

Mutate—To make a permanent change in the genetic material that may alter a trait or characteristic of an individual or manifest as disease and can be transmitted to offspring.

Other tests, including polymerase chain reaction (PCR) testing helped positively match the specific coronavirus present in the lung tissue, blood, and feces of infected animals to the exposure virus.

Diagnosis

To be diagnosed with SARS the individual must have

- a temperature of 100.4°F (38°C) or higher
- symptoms of lower respiratory tract illness such as cough, difficulty breathing, and shortness of breath
- x-ray evidence of pneumonia
- symptoms that cannot be explained by any other illness

Blood cultures, Gram stains, chest radiographs, and tests for other viral respiratory pathogens such as influenza A and B may be done to rule out other illnesses. If SARS is suspected, samples are forwarded to state/local public health departments and/or the CDC for coronavirus antibody testing.

Treatment

As of mid-2012, no specific treatments or therapies had been developed to treat SARS. Antibiotics are ineffective against the SARS and all other viruses. Antiviral medications may be used, but their effectiveness remains unproven. Supportive therapy, such as the administration of fluids, oxygen, ventilation, and fever control are the only available treatments.

Prognosis

Based on a single past outbreak, about 10% of infected individuals would be expected to die from complications of SARS.

Prevention

As of mid-2012, isolation and quarantine remain the best tools to prevent the spread of SARS. Both procedures seek to control exposure to infected individuals or materials. Isolation procedures are used with patients with a confirmed illness. Quarantine rules and

> **QUESTIONS TO ASK YOUR DOCTOR**
>
> - How would I find out about any new cases of SARS that may develop?
> - I travel frequently to Southeast Asia, especially to China. What is your assessment of the SARS infection situation in that area?

procedures apply to individuals who are not currently ill, but have been exposed to the illness (e.g., been in the company of an infected person or come in contact with infected materials).

Isolation and quarantine both act to restrict movement and to slow or stop the spread of disease within a community. Depending on the illness, patients placed in isolation may be cared for in hospitals, specialized health care facilities, or in less severe cases, at home. In some cases, isolation and quarantine are voluntary; however, isolation and quarantine can be compelled by federal, state, and some local law.

Should another SARS outbreak occur, people who must travel should review travel advisories issued by WHO and the CDC. Preventative measures such as frequent hand washing and avoidance of large crowds should be followed rigorously. Likewise, family members caring for suspected and/or confirmed SARS patients should wash hands frequently, avoid direct contact with the patient's bodily fluids, and monitor their own possible development of symptoms closely.

Resources

BOOKS

Abraham, Thomas. *Twenty-first Century Plague: The Story of SARS.* Baltimore, MD: Johns Hopkins University Press, 2005.

WEBSITES

Centers for Disease Control and Prevention (CDC). Severe Acute Respiratory Syndrome (SARS) February 12, 2012 [accessed June 26, 2012]. http://www.cdc.gov/sars/index.html

Severe Acute Respiratory Syndrome. MedlinePlus. February 29, 2012 [accessed June 26, 2012]. http://www.nlm.nih.gov/medlineplus/severeacuterespiratorysyndrome.html

Trivedi, Manish N. Severe Acute Respiratory Syndrome. Medscape.com [accessed June 26, 2012]. http://emedicine.medscape.com/article/237755-overview

ORGANIZATIONS

National Institute of Allergy and Infectious Diseases Office of Communications and Government Relations, 6610 Rockledge Drive, MSC 6612, Bethesda, MD 20892-6612, (301) 496-5717, (866) 284-4107 or TDD: (800)877-8339 (for hearing impaired), Fax: (301) 402-3573, http://www3.niaid.nih.gov.

United States Centers for Disease Control and Prevention (CDC), 1600 Clifton Road, Atlanta, GA 30333, (404) 639-3534, 800-CDC-INFO (800-232-4636). TTY: (888) 232-6348, inquiry@cdc.gov, http://www.cdc.gov.

World Health Organization, Avenue Appia 20, 1211 Geneva 27, Switzerland, +22 41 791 21 11, Fax: +22 41 791 31 11, info@who.int, http://www.who.int.

Brenda Wilmoth Lerner
Tish Davidson, AM

Seveso, Italy

Definition

Accidents in which large quantities of dangerous chemicals are released into the environment are seemingly inevitable in the modern world. In fact, toxic chemicals are produced in such large volumes today that it would be a surprise if such accidents never occurred. One of the most infamous accidents of this kind occurred at Seveso, Italy, a town near Milan in the Lombardy region in Italy, on July 10, 1976. This industrial accident resulted in the exposure of its residents to 2,3,7,8-tetrachlorodibenzo-p-dioxin (TCDD), an ingredient within the chemical commonly known as dioxin, a poisonous and carcinogenic substance.

Description

Hoffman-LaRoche, a small Swiss chemical manufacturing firm, operated a plant at Seveso for the production of hexachlorophene, a widely used disinfectant, for use in pesticides and herbicides. Specifically, the company ICMESA (Industrie Chimiche Meda Societá Azionaria), a subsidiary of Givaudan, owned the plant, which was itself a subsidiary of Hoffmann-La Roche (Roche Group). One of the raw materials used in this process is 2,4,5-trichlorophenol (2,4,5-TCP). At one point in the operation—at approximately 12:37 p.m. local time on July 10, 1976—a vessel containing 2,4,5-TCP exploded, releasing the carcinogenic chemical into the atmosphere as a toxic vapor. A cloud 100–160 feet (30–50 meters) high escaped from the plant and then drifted downwind. It eventually covered an area about 2,300 feet (700 meters) wide and 1.2 miles (2 kilometers) long.

The area most affected by the chemical exposure—the one that contained the highest concentration of contaminated soil—contained over 700 residents. Further out, an area with a lower soil contamination concentration contained about 4,700 residents, and still further out with an even lower concentration of contaminated soil was a population of about 31,800. Following the accident, several thousand farm and wild animals died. The rest of the farm animals were slaughtered to prevent their meat from entering the food chain. Fifteen children were hospitalized with skin inflammation. Just over 400 adults were also found to have skin lesions.

Chloracne, a skin rash resembling acne, was the leading medical problem caused by the disaster. Over 190 cases involved skin inflammation or rashes. Other disorders that occurred included peripheral neuropathy (damage to nerves of the peripheral nervous system) and hepataic enzyme induction (drug-induced liver injury). Most studies of medical impairments were inconclusive, such as for neurological problems, reproductive effects, cancer, cardiovascular conditions, and respiratory diseases.

Risk factors

Although 2,4,5-TCP is a skin irritant, it was not this chemical that caused concern. Instead, it was an impurity in 2,4,5-TCP, the compound 2,3,7,8-tetrachlorodibenzo-p-dioxin, that caused alarm. This compound, one of a family known as dioxins, is one of the most toxic chemicals known to science. It occurs as a byproduct in many manufacturing reactions in which 2,4,5-TCP is involved, especially when the reaction temperature is high. Experts estimated that 7–35 pounds (3–16 kilograms) of dioxin were released into the atmosphere as a result of the Seveso explosion.

Demographics

In addition to the city of Severso, which had a population of about 17,000 residents at the time of the disaster, other nearby communities were affected. These included Barlassina (with a population of about 6,000), Bovisio-Masciago (11,000), Cesano Maderno (34,000), Desio (33,000), and Meda (19,000).

Although exposures to dioxins had occurred in the past, they were minor occurrences. This one was a major event, one that warranted evacuating residents. People living closest to the Hoffman-LaRoche plant were evacuated from their homes and the area was closed off. About 5,000 nearby residents were allowed to stay but were subsequently prohibited from raising crops or farm animals.

Causes and symptoms

Damage to plants and animals in the exposed area was severe. Thousands of farm animals died or had to be destroyed. More than 2.5 tons (225 kilograms) of contaminated soil were removed before planting could begin again. Short- and long-term effects on human health, however, were relatively modest.

Common diseases and disorders

In the months following the accident, 176 individuals were found to have chloracne, an inflammation of the skin caused by chlorine-based chemicals. An additional 137 cases of the condition were found in a follow-up survey six months after the accident.

Some people claimed that exposed women had higher rates of miscarriage and of deformed babies, but local authorities were unable to substantiate these claims. No human lives were lost in the accident.

Treatment

Over 600 people were evacuated from their residences as the result of being exposed to dioxin at Seveso, and upwards of 2,000 people were treated for dioxin poisoning.

Public health role and response

Within six months of the accident, a plan to decontaminate and restore the affected area had been completed. That plan was implemented in the spring of 1977. By June 1977, over 200,000 people were being monitored for adverse health effects from the incident. An international team, including biostatisticians, epidemiologists, toxicologists and pathologists, from the International Steering Committee began a scientific assessment of the situation. With its 1983 report *The Work of the International Steering Committee for the Study of the Health Effects of the Seveso Accident: Its Methodology, Its Issues and Its Conclusions*, the committee concluded that no human effects other than 193 cases of chloracne occurred within the Seveso disaster.

Prognosis

The Seveso chemical exposure incident is increasingly seen as a lucky escape, where a potentially catastrophic release caused relatively little damage.

Prevention

The outcome at Seveso has often been linked with numerous scientific studies and standardized industrial safety regulations. In addition, a set of innovative public policies for managing industrial disasters, known as the Seveso Directive, within the European Union was also implemented. After a series of accidents, in 2003 the EU industrial safety regulations were substantially

> **KEY TERMS**
>
> **Carcinogenic**—Cancer causing.
>
> **Chloracne**—A skin rash that resembles acne, which is caused by repeated contact with chlorinated hydrocarbons.
>
> **Dioxins**—Any of numerous by-products of various industrial processes, which are regarded as extremely toxic. These dioxins or dioxin-like compounds include polychlorinated dibenzo-p-dioxins (PCDDs), polychlorinated dibenzofurans (PCDFs), and polychlorinated biphenyls (PCBs).

updated (Severso II Directive) to strength monitoring and enforcement provisions. In 2012, the Seveso III Directive was implemented to take into account changes in chemical classifications, provide better access to citizens about local chemical risks, and implement stricter safety standards for inspections of plants containing dangerous chemicals. The resulting directive applied to about 10,000 industrial organizations in Europe where potentially dangerous chemical substances were used or stored in large quantities. According to the European Commission, "The Seveso Directive obliges Member States to ensure that operators have a policy in place to prevent major accidents. Operators handling dangerous substances above certain thresholds must regularly inform the public likely to be affected by an accident, providing safety reports, a safety management system and an internal emergency plan. Member States must ensure that emergency plans are in place for the surrounding areas and that mitigation actions are planned. Account must also be taken of these objectives in land-use planning."

Resources

BOOKS

Gunn, Angus M. *Encyclopedia of Disasters: Environmental Catastrophes and Human Tragedies*. Westport, CT: Greenwood Press, 2008.

Hites, Ronald A., and Jonathan D. Raff. *Elements of Environmental Chemistry*. Hoboken, NJ: Wiley and Sons, 2012.

Schecter, Arnold, ed. *Dioxins and Health: Including Other Persistent Organic Pollutants and Endocrine Disruptors*. Hoboken, NJ: John Wiley and Sons, 2012.

Spiro, Thomas G, Kathleen L. Purvis-Roberts, and William M. Stigliani. *Chemistry of the Environment*. Mill Valley, CA: University Science Books, 2012.

WEBSITES

Center for Environmental Research and Children's Health. "Seveso Women's Health Study." http://cerch.org/research-programs/seveso/ (accessed September 20, 2012).

European Commission. "Chemical Accidents (Seveso III)—Prevention, Preparedness and Response." http://ec.europa.eu/environment/seveso/index.htm (accessed September 20, 2012).

ORGANIZATIONS

American Association of Poison Control Centers, (800) 222-1222, http://www.aapcc.org.

Center for Environmental Research and Children's Health (University of California at Berkeley), 1995 University Ave., Ste. 265, Berkeley, CA 94720-7392, (510) 643-9598, Fax: (510) 642-9083, cerch@berkeley.edu, http://cerch.org.

National Toxicology Program (National Institute of Environmental Health Sciences), PO Box 12233, Research Triangle Park, NC 27709, http://ntp.niehs.nih.gov.

World Health Organization, Avenue Appia 20, Geneva, Switzerland 1211 27, 41 22 791-2111, Fax: 41 22 791-3111, cdcinfo@cdc.gov, http://www.who.int/en.

David E. Newton, EdD
William A. Atkins, BB, BS, MBA

Shigellosis

Definition

Shigellosis is an infection of the intestinal tract caused by a group of bacteria called *Shigella*. The major symptoms are diarrhea, abdominal cramps, fever, and severe fluid loss (dehydration). Four different species of the genus *Shigella* can affect humans; of these, *S. dysenteriae* generally produces the most severe attacks, and *S. sonnei* the mildest. The other two species of *Shigella* include *S. boydii* and *S. flexneri*. Shigella is also sometimes called Marlow syndrome.

Description

The bacteria are named in honor of Kiyoshi Shiga (1871–1957), a Japanese physician and microbiological researcher, who discovered the organism in 1897. In the 2010s, Shigellosis is a well-known cause of traveler's diarrhea and illness throughout the world. The organisms making up *Shigella* are extremely infectious bacteria and ingestion of just 10 organisms is enough to cause severe diarrhea and dehydration. Shigeliosis accounts for 10% to 20% of all cases of diarrhea worldwide. In any given year, it is estimated to infect from 90 million to over 140 million persons and to kill at least 100,000 people but sometimes upwards to 600,000. Children and the elderly in developing

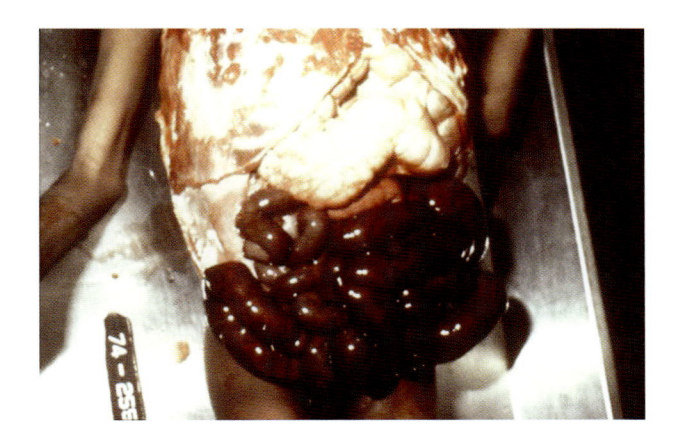

This man developed necrosis of the intestines due to a Shigellosis infection resulting in his death. (CDC/Dr. Eugene Gangaroa)

countries are most at risk. The most serious form of the disease is called dysentery, which is characterized by severe watery (and often blood- and mucous-streaked) diarrhea, abdominal cramping, rectal pain, and fever. *Shigella* is only one of several organisms that can cause dysentery, but the term bacillary dysentery is usually another name for shigellosis.

Most deaths are in less-developed or developing countries, but even in the United States, shigellosis can be a dangerous and potentially deadly disease. The common way to transmit shigellosis is person-to-person contact, primarily hand-to-mouth such as shaking hands with someone and then putting a finger into one's mouth. Being a contagious disease, shigellosis can be spread by air, blood, blood transfusions, coughing, fecal-oral, mother-to-fetus, needles, saliva, sexual contact, and surface contact. Poor hygiene, overcrowding, and improper storage of food are leading causes of infection. The following statistics show the marked difference in the frequency of cases between developed and less-developed countries; in the United States, the disease harms upwards to 30,000 individuals each year, or about 10 cases per 100,000 of the population. On the other hand, infection in some areas of South America is 1,000 times more frequent. Shigellosis is most common in children below the age of 5 years and occurs less often in adults over 20 years.

One major outbreak from shigellosis occurred in Zaire in 1994. According to the World Health Organization (WHO), between 500,000 and 800,000 Rwandan refugees had escaped into the northern Kivu region of Zaire. However, they contracted the infection and within one month about 20,000 of them had died from dysentery caused by *S. dysenteriae* type 1.

Risk factors

Shigellosis is almost never found in animals, except for humans and other primates like monkeys and chimpanzees. The organism is frequently found in water polluted with human feces, which usually is found in poor and undeveloped countries of the world. Children are at higher risk than other groups of humans because they are less likely to perform common hygiene practices, such as washing of the hands after a bowel movement.

The species *Shigella sonnei* accounts for over two-thirds of the shigellosis in the United States. *Shigella flexneri* makes up for almost all of the rest. The other species of *Shigella* are rare in the United States; however, they occur much more frequently in the developing world. In fact, the species *S. dysenteriae* type 1 causes deadly epidemics in many developing regions and nations.

Demographics

Between 10,000 and 30,000 cases of shigellosis are reported annually in the United States. Because mild cases of the disease are not diagnosed as shigellosis, the real number of infections has been estimated to be as high as twenty times greater. Shigellosis is more common in the months of summer than in winter ones. In the United States, young children from the age of two to four years are most likely to contract shigellosis. The spread of the disease is often reported in child-care facilities and in families with several children. In developing countries, especially the poorest ones, the presence of shigellosis is much more common and is usually present in various degrees in most villages and other community settings.

Causes and symptoms

Shigella shares several of the characteristics of a group of bacteria that inhabit the intestinal tract. *Escherichia coli* (*E coli*), another cause of food-borne illness, can be mistaken for *Shigella* both by physicians and laboratory personnel. Careful testing is needed to assure proper diagnosis and treatment.

Shigella organisms are very resistant to the acid produced by the stomach, and this allows them to easily pass through the gastrointestinal tract and infect the colon (large intestine). The result is a colitis that produces multiple ulcers, which can bleed. *Shigella* also produces a number of toxins (such as Shiga toxin) that increase the amount of fluid secretion by the intestinal tract. This fluid secretion is a major cause of diarrhea symptoms.

Shigella infection spreads through food or water contaminated by human waste. Sources of transmission are:

- contaminated milk, ice cream, vegetables and other foods, which often cause epidemics
- household contacts (40% of adults and 20% of children will develop an infection from such a source)
- poor hygiene and overcrowded living conditions
- day care centers
- sexual practices that lead to oral-anal contact, directly or indirectly

Symptoms can be limited to only mild diarrhea or can progress to full-blown dysentery. Dehydration results from the large fluid losses due to diarrhea, vomiting, and fever. Inability to eat or drink worsens the situation.

In developed countries, most infections are of the less severe type and are often due to *S. sonnei*. The period between infection and symptoms (incubation period) varies from one to seven days. Shigellosis can last from a few days to several weeks, with an average of seven days.

Complications

Areas outside the intestine can be involved, including:

- nervous system (irritation of the meninges or meningitis, encephalitis, and seizures)
- kidneys (producing **hemolytic-uremic syndrome** or HUS, which leads to kidney failure)
- joints (leading to an unusual form of arthritis called **Reiter's syndrome**)
- skin (rash)

One of the most serious complications of this disease is HUS, which involves the kidney. The main findings are kidney failure and damage to red blood cells. As many as 15% of patients die from this complication, and half of the survivors develop chronic kidney failure, which requires dialysis.

Another life-threatening condition is toxic megacolon. Severe inflammation causes the colon to dilate or stretch, and the thin colon wall may eventually tear. Certain medications (particularly those that diminish intestinal contractions) may increase this risk but this interaction is unclear. Clues to this diagnosis include sudden decrease in diarrhea, swelling of the abdomen, and worsening abdominal pain.

Diagnosis

Shigellosis is one of the many causes of acute diarrhea. Culture (growing the bacteria in the laboratory) of freshly obtained diarrhea fluid is the only way to be certain of the diagnosis. However, even this is not always positive, especially if the patient is already on antibiotics. *Shigella* are identified by a combination of their appearance under the microscope and various chemical tests. These studies take several days but quicker means to recognize the bacteria and its toxins are being developed.

Treatment

The first aims of treatment are to keep up nutrition and avoid dehydration. Ideally, a physician should be consulted before starting any treatment. Antibiotics may not be necessary, except for the more severe infections. Many cases resolve before the diagnosis is established by culture. Medications that control diarrhea by slowing intestinal contractions can cause problems and should be avoided by patients with bloody diarrhea or fever, especially if antibiotics have not been started.

Rehydration

The World Health Organization (WHO) has developed guidelines for a standard solution taken by mouth and prepared from ingredients readily available at home. This Oral Rehydration Solution (ORS) includes salt, baking powder, sugar, orange juice, and water. Commercial preparations, such as Pedialyte, are also available. For many patients with mild symptoms, this is the only treatment needed. Severe dehydration usually requires intravenous fluid replacement.

Antibiotics

In the early and mid-1990s, researchers began to realize that not all cases of bacterial dysentery needed antibiotic treatment. Therefore, these drugs are indicated only for treatment of moderate or severe disease, as found in the tropics. Choice of antibiotic is based on the type of bacteria found in the geographical area and on laboratory results. Recommendations include ampicillin, sulfa derivatives such as Trimethoprim-Sulfamethoxazole (TMP-SMX) sold as Bactrim, or fluoroquinolones (such as Ciprofloxacin, which is not approved by the U.S. Food and Drug Administration for use in children due to risk of permanent musculoskeletal system injury, except in cases when safe or effective alternatives are not available).

KEY TERMS

Antibiotic—A medication that is designed to kill or weaken bacteria.

Anti-motility medications—Medications such as loperamide (Imodium), dephenoxylate (Lomotil), or medications containing codeine or narcotics which decrease the ability of the intestine to contract. These may worsen the condition of a patient with dysentery or colitis.

Carrier state—The continued presence of an organism (bacteria, virus, or parasite) in the body that does not cause symptoms but is able to be transmitted and infect other persons.

Colitis—Inflammation of the colon or large bowel, which has several causes. The lining of the colon becomes swollen and ulcers often develop. The ability of the colon to absorb fluids is also affected and diarrhea often results.

Dialysis—A form of treatment for patients with kidneys that do not function properly. The treatment removes toxic wastes from the body that are normally removed by the kidneys.

Dysentery—A disease marked by frequent watery bowel movements, often with blood and mucus, and characterized by pain, urgency to have a bowel movement, fever, and dehydration.

Fluoroquinolones—A group of antibiotics that have had good success in treating infections with many gram-negative bacteria, such as *Shigella*. One drawback is that they should not be used in children under 17 years of age because of possible effects on bone and cartilage growth.

Food-borne illness—A disease that is transmitted by eating or handling contaminated food.

Meninges—Outer covering of the spinal cord and brain. Infection is called meningitis, which can lead to damage to the brain or spinal cord and lead to death.

Oral Rehydration Solution (ORS)—A liquid preparation developed by the World Health Organization that can decrease fluid loss in persons with diarrhea. Originally developed to be prepared with materials available in the home, commercial preparations have come into use.

Stool—Passage of fecal material; a bowel movement.

Traveler's diarrhea—An illness due to infection from a bacteria or parasite that occurs in persons traveling to areas where there is a high frequency of the illness. The disease is usually spread by contaminated food or water.

Public health role and response

Cases of shigellosis should be reported at the state level. The states then report to the national level, to the U.S. Centers for Disease Control and Prevention (CDC). Public health laboratories throughout the United States survey and analyze foodborne infections. Public health laboratories contribute to the surveillance and analysis of foodborne infections, such as shigelosis. A national network of public health and food regulatory agency laboratories exist throughout the United States. For additional information on this network, go to PulseNet (http://www.cdc.gov/pulsenet/). The network consists of local health departments, state health departments, and federal agencies, specifically the CDC, United States Department of Agriculture (USDA) Safety and Inspection Service (FSIS), and the Food and Drug Administration (FDA)

Prognosis

Many patients with mild infections do not need specific treatment and will recover completely. In those with severe infections, antibiotics will decrease the length of symptoms and the number of days bacteria appear in the feces. In rare cases, an individual may fail to clear the bacteria from the intestinal tract; the result is a persistent carrier state. This may be more frequent in AIDS (Acquired Immune Deficiency Syndrome) patients. Antibiotics are about 90% effective in eliminating these chronic infections.

In patients who have suffered particularly severe attacks, some degree of cramping and diarrhea can last for several weeks. This is usually due to damage to the intestinal tract, which requires some time to heal. Since antibiotics can also produce a form of colitis, this must be considered as a possible cause of persistent or recurrent symptoms.

Prevention

Shigellosis is an extremely contagious disease; good hand washing techniques and proper precautions in food handling will help in avoiding the spread of infection. Children in day care centers need to be reminded about hand washing during an outbreak to

> **QUESTIONS TO ASK YOUR DOCTOR**
>
> - What type of germ produces shigellosis?
> - How can infections involving shigellosis be diagnosed?
> - How will I be treated for shigellosis?
> - Will I completely recover from shigellosis?
> - How can I prevent getting shigellosis?
> - What are the long-term consequences of such an infection?
> - How do people catch shigellosis?
> - Where do I learn more about shigellosis?

minimize spread. *Shigellosis* in schools or day care settings almost always disappears when holiday breaks occur, which sever the chain of transmission.

Traveler's diarrhea (TD)

Shigella accounts for about 10% of diarrhea illness in travelers to Mexico, South America, and the tropics. Most cases of TD are more of a nuisance than a life-threatening disease. However, bloody diarrhea is an indication that *Shigella* may be responsible.

In some cases though, aside from ruining a well-deserved vacation, these infections can interrupt business conference schedules and, in the worst instances, lead to a life-threatening illness. Therefore, researchers have tried to find a safe and effective way of preventing TD. One of the best means of prevention is to follow closely the rules outlined by the WHO and other groups regarding eating fresh fruits, vegetables, and other foods.

One safe and effective method of preventing TD is the use of large doses of Pepto-Bismol or other such antidiarrheal medicines. Tablets are now available, which are easier for travel; usage must start a few days before departure. Patients should be aware that bismuth subsalicylate (the active ingredient in Pepto-Bismol) will turn bowel movements black.

Antibiotics have also proven to be highly effective in preventing TD. They can also produce significant side effects; therefore, a physician should be consulted before use. Like Pepto-Bismol, antibiotics need to be started before beginning travel.

Resources

BOOKS

Brachman, Philip S., and Elias Abrutyn, editors. *Bacterial Infections of Humans: Epidemiology and Control.* New York: Springer Science and Business Media, 2009.

Dworkin, Mark S., editor. *Outbreak Investigations Around the World: Case Studies in Infectious Disease Field Epidemiology.* Sudbury, MA: Jones and Bartlett, 2010.

Shannon, Joyce Brennfleck, editor. *Contagious Diseases Sourcebook: Basic Consumer Health Information about Diseases Spread from Person to Person.* Detroit: Omnigraphics, 2010.

PERIODICALS

Clemens, John, Karen Kotloff, and Kay Bradford "Generic Protocol to Estimate the Burden of Shigella Diarrhoea and Dysenteric Mortalit." *World Health Organization: Department of Vaccines and Biologicals* May 1999.

WEBSITES

Generic Protocol to Estimate the Burden of Shigella Diarrhea and Dysenteric Mortality. World Health Organization. (May 1999). http://www.who.int/vaccines-documents/DocsPDF99/www9947.pdf (accessed June 28, 2012).

PulseNet. Centers for Disease Control and Prevention. http://www.cdc.gov/pulsenet/ (accessed July 8, 2012).

Shigella. World Health Organization. http://www.who.int/topics/shigella/en/ (accessed June 28, 2012).

Shigellosis. Centers for Disease Control and Prevention. (November 16, 2009). http://www.cdc.gov/nczved/divisions/dfbmd/diseases/shigellosis/#how_common (accessed June 28, 2012).

Shigellosis. WebMD. (February 8, 2011). http://www.webmd.com/a-to-z-guides/shigellosis-topic-overview (accessed June 28, 2012).

Todar, Kenneth. *Shigella and Shigellosis.* Todar's Online Textbook of Bacteriology. (February 21, 2012). http://textbookofbacteriology.net/Shigella.html (accessed June 28, 2012).

ORGANIZATIONS

Centers for Disease Control and Prevention, 1600 Clifton Rd., Atlanta, GA 30333, (800) 232-4636, cdcinfo@cdc.gov, http://www.fda.gov/.

Food and Drug Administration, 10903 New Hampshire Ave., Silver Spring, MD 20993, (888) 463-6332, http://www.fda.gov/.

United States Department of Agriculture, 1400 Independence Ave. W, Washington, D.C. 20250 (202) 720-2791, (800) 232-4636, cdcinfo@cdc.gov, http://usda.gov/.

World Health Organization, Avenue Appia 20, Geneva, Switzerland 1211 27, 41 22 791-2111, Fax: 41 22 791-3111, cdcinfo@cdc.gov, http://www.who.int/en/.

David Kaminstein, MD
William A. Atkins, BB, BS, MBA

Sick building syndrome

Definition

Sick building syndrome (SBS) is a term applied to an indoor environment that causes its occupants to become ill. The syndrome is usually associated with indoor air pollutants, although it has often been difficult to associate the symptoms with specific pollutants. Other issues such as poor building management and work-place stress may also be factors. **Indoor air quality** (IAQ) health problems fall into three categories: SBS, building-related illnesses (BRI), and **multiple chemical sensitivity**. Of the three, SBS accounts for about 75% of all IAQ complaints.

Description

Indoor air is a health hazard in about 30% of all buildings, according to the **World Health Organization** (WHO). The **Environmental Protection Agency (EPA)** lists IAQ fourth among top environmental health threats. The problem of SBS is of increasing concern to employees and occupational health specialists, as well as landlords and corporations who fear the financial consequences of illnesses among tenants and employees, respectively. Respiratory diseases attributed to SBS account for about 150 million lost workdays each year, $59 billion in indirect costs, and $15 billion in medical costs.

Sick building syndrome was first recognized in the 1970s around the time of the energy crisis and the move toward conservation. Because heating and air conditioning systems accounted for a major portion of energy consumption in the United States, buildings were sealed for energy efficiency. In these buildings, occupants depend on mechanical systems rather than open windows for outside air and ventilation. There are three methods in which outside air can enter a building, including infiltration, natural ventilation, and mechanical ventilation. Infiltration occurs when outside air enters a building through cracks around windows, floors, doors, and walls. Natural ventilation occurs through open doors or windows. For mechanical ventilation, outdoor-vented fans for heating, venting, and air conditioning systems (HVAC) bring outside air in and move inside air out. A building that is well-insulated and sealed for energy efficiency, referred to as a tight building, can seal in and create contaminants.

According to the U.S. **Environmental Protection Agency (EPA)**, SBS is strongly identified when the following situations are present:

- Symptoms are associated with the time spent in a particular building or part of a building.
- Symptoms disappear when the individual is not in a building causing such symptoms.

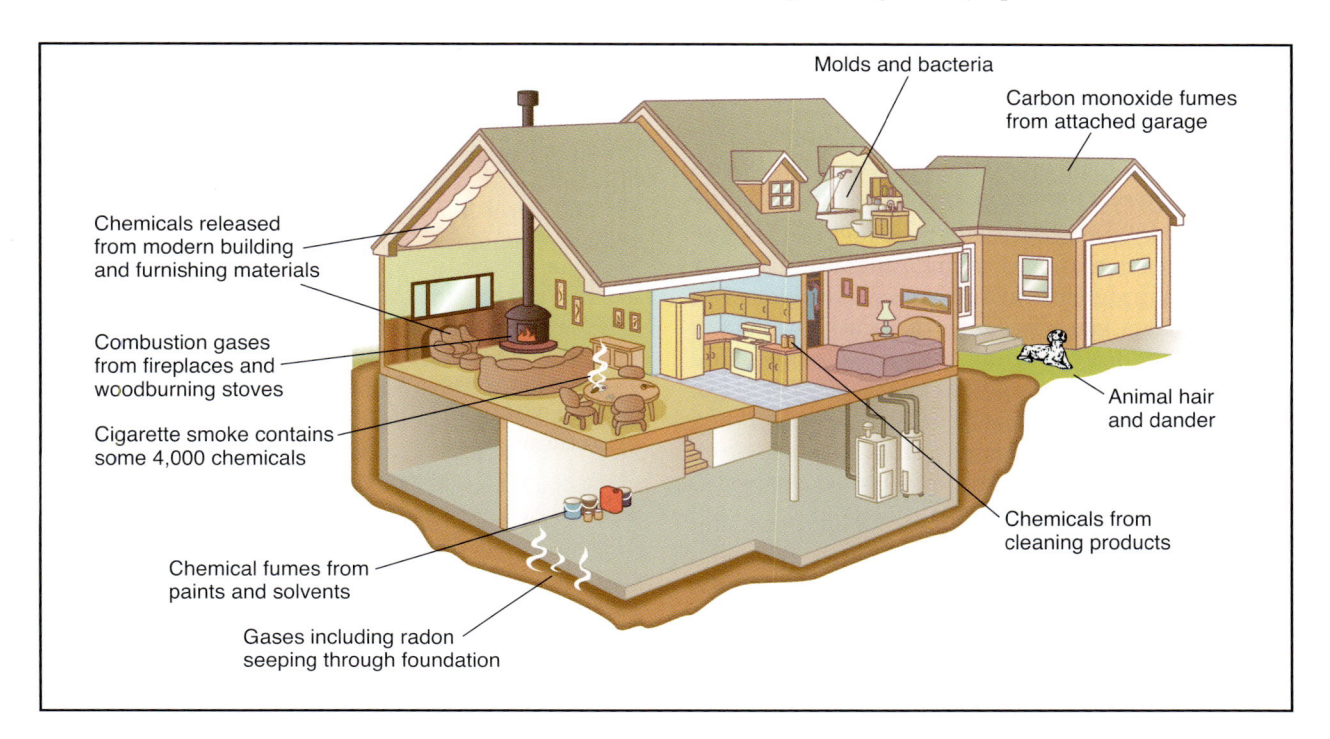

(Illustration by Electronic Illustrators Group. © 2013 Cengage Learning.)

- Symptoms recur seasonally (such as when a building is heated or cooled).
- Coworkers or other individuals within the particular building note similar symptoms.

Demographics

Sick building syndrome occurs when individuals occupying a certain building report similar acute health problems that seem to be related directly to the time spent in the building. No specific illness or cause is identified, and the problems may be concentrated in a particular room or area or may be widespread throughout the building.

Causes and symptoms

According to the Environmental Protection Agency, SBS is caused by four major factors:

- biological contaminants: bacteria, molds, pollen, and viruses accumulated in ducts, humidifiers, drain pans, and other sources where water has collected
- chemical contaminants from indoor sources: primarily from adhesives, carpeting, cleaning supplies, copy machines, manufactured wood products, and upholstery that emit volatile organic compounds, including formaldehyde; other contributing factors, including tobacco smoke and combustion products such as carbon monoxide, nitrogen dioxide, and other particles from unvented kerosene and gas space heaters, fireplaces, gas stoves, and woodstoves
- chemical contaminants from outdoor sources: primarily from motor vehicle exhaust and from plumbing vents and building exhausts (such as bathrooms and kitchens) that enter the building through poorly located air intake vents, windows, and other openings
- inadequate ventilation: heating, ventilating, and air conditioning systems that do not effectively distribute air throughout a building; the American Society of Heating, Refrigerating and Air-Conditioning Engineers recommends a minimum flow of 15 cubic feet per minute (cfm) of outdoor air per person in a home and 20 cfm per person in office spaces in order to maintain the health and comfort of occupants.

Common symptoms of SBS include dizziness, skin irritation, headaches, fatigue, dry cough, sneezing, nausea, hoarseness of voice, allergies, **asthma** attacks, cold, flu-like symptoms, difficulty concentrating, and irritations of the eyes, nose and throat. In addition, many people have more general symptoms, including personality changes, hypersensitivity reactions, and odor and taste sensations. Symptoms are caused by a range of contaminants including volatile organic compounds (VOC), which are chemicals that turn to gas at room temperature and are given off by paints, adhesives, caulking, vinyl, telephone cable, printed documents, furniture, and solvents. Most common VOCs are **benzene** (C_6H_6) and chloroform ($CHCl_3$), both of which have been shown to be carcinogenic. Formaldehyde (CH_2O) in building materials is also an indoor irritant. However, the concentrations of VOCs at which SBS is observed are usually well below the concentrations at which the common symptoms would be expected.

Biological agents such as **viruses**, bacteria, fungal spores, algae, pollen, **mold**, and dust mites add to the problems. These are produced by water-damaged carpet and furnishing or standing water in ventilation systems, humidifiers, and flush toilets.

Carbon dioxide (CO_2) levels increase as the number of people in a room increases, and too much can cause occupants to suffer hyperventilation, headaches, dizziness, shortness of breath, and drowsiness, as does carbon monoxide (CO) and the other toxins from cigarette smoke.

Schoolchildren are considered more vulnerable to SBS because schools typically have more people per room breathing the same stale air. Their size, childhood allergies, and asthmas increase their vulnerability.

Diagnosis

The diagnosis for SBS is difficult because a specific illness or cause cannot be easily identified by the medical community.

> ## KEY TERMS
>
> **Carbon monoxide**—With the chemical formula CO (where C stands for carbon, and O for oxygen), a colorless, odorless, and tasteless gas that is toxic to humans in higher than normal concentrations.
>
> **Nitrogen dioxide**—With the chemical formula NO_2 (where N stands for nitrogen, and O for oxygen), a reddish-brown toxic gas that is one of several nitrogen oxides.
>
> **Toxins**—Any type of poison made by humans or introduced into the environment by human activity, such as insecticides.
>
> **Volatile organic chemicals**—Any organic chemicals with a high vapor pressure at ordinary, room-temperatures.

Treatment

Sick buildings can be treated by updating and cleaning ventilation systems regularly and using air cleaners and filtration devices. Also, plants spaced every 100 square feet (9.3 square meters) in offices, homes, and schools have been shown to filter out pollutants in recycled air.

A simple survey of the indoor environment can detect many SBS problems. Each room should have an air source; if windows cannot be opened, every room should have a supply vent and exhaust vent. The vents should be cleaned regularly. A tissue can be place at each vent opening to check that air is circulating through the system. The tissue should blow out at a supply vent and be pulled in at an exhaust vent. Vents should not be blocked by partitions, file cabinets, or boxes. Supply and exhaust vents should be more than a few feet apart. Dead spaces where air stagnates and pollutants build up should be renovated. Printing and copying machines should be moved away from people and should be given adequate exhaust. The ventilation system should be checked every season for verification of full operation.

Public health role and response

The EPA enforces laws on outdoor **air pollution** but not for indoor air except for some **smoking** bans. Yet almost every pollutant, according to the EPA, is at higher levels indoors than outdoors. Help in detecting and correcting SBS is available from the National Institute of Occupational Safety and Health (NIOSH), the federal agency responsible for conducting research and making recommendations for safe and healthy work standards. The EPA and the NIOSH have developed a Building Air Quality Action plan with guidelines for improving and maintaining IAQ in public and commercial buildings.

Prognosis

The prognosis for sick building syndrome is generally good if the cause of the disorder can be identified. However, because its symptoms vary widely and no one specific illness is easily identified, the diagnosis of SBS may be lengthy.

Prevention

Important factors that can prevent and control SBS are:

- increased ventilation and air distribution
- routine maintenance of HVAC systems and replacement of water-damaged flooring and ceiling tiles

> **QUESTIONS TO ASK YOUR DOCTOR**
>
> - How common is sick building syndrome?
> - Is SBS real or imaginary?
> - Will I be taken seriously if I say I have SBS?
> - Where can I acquire more information about SBS?
> - Can you diagnosis my problem if I think I have SBS? If so, can you treat me?
> - What can I do to minimize my symptoms of SBS?
> - Will medicines help?

- use of open office designs and indoor plants along with skylights and scheduled filter cleaning
- education of residents and workers on the importance of ventilation
- support of legislation that bans smoking inside buildings

Resources

BOOKS

Abdul-Wahab, Sabah A, ed. *Sick Building Syndrome: In Public Buildings and Workplaces.* Berlin: Springer, 2011.

Bluyssen, Philomena M. *The Indoor Environment Handbook: How to Make Buildings Healthy and Comfortable.* London: Earthscan, 2009.

Larsen, Laura, ed. *Environmental Health Sourcebook.* Detroit: Omnigraphics, 2010.

May, Jeffrey C. *My Office Is Killing Me! The Sick Building Survival Guide.* Baltimore: Johns Hopkins University Press, 2006.

Natelson, Benjamin H. *Your Symptoms Are Real: What to Do When Your Doctor Says Nothing Is Wrong.* Hoboken, NJ: John Wiley, 2008.

Pall, Martin L. *Explaining "Unexplained Illnesses": Disease Paradigm for Chronic Fatigue Syndrome, Multiple Chemical Sensitivity, Fibromyalgia, Post-Traumatic Stress Disorder, Gulf War Syndrome, and Others.* New York: Harrington Park Press, 2007.

Preston, Flora. *Convenient, "Safe" and Deadly: The True Costs of Our Chemical Lifestyle.* Lanark, ONT: Health Risk Navigation, 2006.

Sutton, Amy L. *Allergies Sourcebook: Basic Consumer Health Information About Allergic Disorders, such as Anaphylaxis.* Detroit: Omnigraphics, 2007.

WEBSITES

Centers for Disease Control and Prevention. "Indoor Environmental Quality." (November 28, 2011). http://www.cdc.gov/niosh/topics/indoorenv/ (accessed September 21, 2012).

Environmental Illness Resource. "Sick Building Syndrome (SBS)." (March 19, 2011). http://www.ei-resource.org/illness-information/related-conditions/sick-building-syndrome-(sbs)/ (accessed September 21, 2012).
Environmental Protection Agency. "Building Air Quality: A Guide for Building Owners and Facility Managers." http://www.epa.gov/iaq/largebldgs/baqtoc.html (accessed September 21, 2012).
Environmental Protection Agency. "Consumer's Guide to Radon Reduction." http://www.epa.gov/radon/pubs/consguid.html (accessed September 21, 2012).
Environmental Protection Agency. "Indoor Air Facts No. 4 (revised) Sick Building Syndrome." (February 1999). http://www.epa.gov/iaq/pdfs/sick_building_factsheet.pdf (accessed September 21, 2012).
Environmental Protection Agency. "Indoor Air: Publications and Resources." http://www.epa.gov/iaq/pubs/ (accessed September 21, 2012).
Joshi, Sumedha M. "The Sick Building Syndrome." National Center for Biotechnology Information. (August 2008). http://www.ncbi.nlm.nih.gov/pmc/articles/PMC2796751/ (accessed September 21, 2012).

ORGANIZATIONS

Agency for Toxic Substances and Disease Registry, Centers for Disease Control and Prevention, 4770 Buford Hwy. NE, Atlanta, GA 30341, (800) 232-4636, http://www.atsdr.cdc.gov.
American Academy of Environmental Medicine, 6505 E Central Ave., No. 296, Wichita, KS 67206, (316) 684-5500, Fax: (316) 684-5709, administrator@aaemonline.org, http://aaemonline.org.
Environmental Protection Agency, 1200 Pennsylvania Ave., NW, Ariel Rios Bldg., Washington, DC 20460, (202) 272-0167, http://www.epa.gov.
National Institute of Occupational Safety and Health, Centers for Disease Control and Prevention, 1600 Clifton Rd., Atlanta, GA 30333, (800) 232-4636, cdcinfo@cdc.gov, http://www.cdc.gov/niosh.
Occupational Safety and Health Organization, U.S. Department of Labor, 200 Constitution Ave. NW, Washington, DC 20210, (800) 321-6742, http://www.osha.gov.

Linda Rehkopf

Sierra Club

Definition

The Sierra Club is a nonprofit organization dedicated to protecting the planet. It is one of the largest grassroots organizations in the United States.

Purpose

The Sierra Club was developed to help people explore, enjoy, and protect the planet. It promotes responsible use of Earth's ecosystems and natural resources in order to protect the environment and develop a sustainable future for the planet.

Description

The Sierra Club is one of the nation's foremost conservation organizations and has worked for over 100 years to preserve "the wild places of the earth." It has a total of 64 chapters in the United States, including one in each state and Puerto Rico, with the exception of California, which has 13 chapters. There are also two Sierra Club chapters in Canada, organized under the Sierra Club Canada. Although the Sierra Club is involved with many environmental issues, main goals for 2012 included, Beyond Oil, Beyond Coal, Beyond Gas, Protect America's Waters, and Resilient Habitats.

As of November 2012, Michael Brune was the executive director of the more than 600,000-member organization. In addition to members, the Sierra Club has around 500 paid staff members who work in the club's national headquarters in California or the club's lobbying office in Washington DC. The Sierra Club also publishes the bimonthly magazine for members *Sierra Magazine* and produces a weekly half-hour radio show *Sierra Club Radio*.

Origins

The Sierra Club was founded in 1892 by author and wilderness explorer John Muir, who helped lead the fight to establish Yosemite **National Park**. Muir was elected the group's first president and led the group's first goal, to preserve the Sierra Nevada mountain chain. Since then, the club has worked to protect dozens of other national treasures.

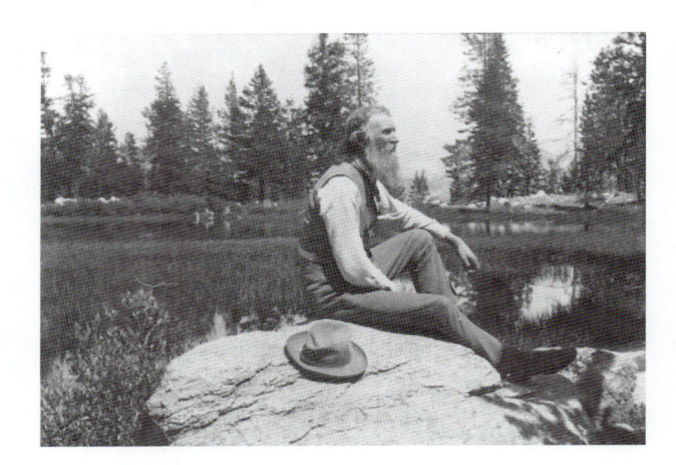

John Muir *(The Library of Congress.)*

Results

The club has helped secure many conservation victories. The preservation of Mount Rainier was one of the Sierra Club's earliest achievements, and in 1899 Congress made that area a national park. The group also helped to establish Glacier National Park in 1910. The Sierra Club supported the creation of the National Park Service in 1916 and in 1919 began a campaign to halt the indiscriminate cutting of redwood trees.

The Sierra Club also worked to create such national parks as Kings Canyon, Olympic, and Redwood, national seashores such as Point Reyes in California and Padre Island in Texas, as well as the Jackson Hole National Monument. Additionally, the club campaigned to expand Sequoia and Grand Teton national parks. In the 1960s, the Sierra Club helped to secure such legislative victories as the Wilderness Act in 1964, the establishment of the National Wilderness Preservation System, and the expansion of the Land and Water Conservation Fund in 1968.

By 1970, the Sierra Club had 100,000 members, with chapters in every state, and the group took advantage of growing public support for the environment to accelerate progress toward conserving the U.S. natural heritage. The **National Environmental Policy Act** was passed by Congress that year, and the **Environmental Protection Agency (EPA)** was created. Later, the club helped defeat a proposal to build a fleet of polluting supersonic transports, and it organized the Sierra Club Legal Defense Fund. In 1976, the club's lobbying efforts sped passage of the Bureau of Land Management (BLM) Organic Act, which increased governmental protection for an additional 459 million acres (185 ha).

One of the most important victories for the Sierra Club came in 1980, when a year-long campaign culminated in passage of the Alaska National Interest Conservation Act, establishing 103 million acres (41.6 million ha) as either national parks, monuments, refuges, or wilderness areas. Superfund legislation also was enacted to clean up the nation's abandoned toxic waste sites.

The decade of the 1980s, however, was a difficult one for conservationists. With James Watt as secretary of interior under President Ronald Reagan and Ann Gorsuch Burford as **EPA** administrator, the Sierra Club was placed in a defensive position. The group focused mainly on preventing environmentally destructive projects and legislation—for example, blocking the MX missile complex in the Great Basin (1981), preventing weakening of the **Clean Air Act**, and stopping BLM from cropping 1.5 million acres (607,030 ha) from its wilderness inventory in 1983. Despite government interference, pressure from the public and from Congress helped the club continue its record of positive accomplishments.

In 1990, after years of grassroots lobbying, a compromise Clean Air Act was reauthorized, strengthening safeguards against **acid rain** and **air pollution**. Projects in the first decade of the twenty-first century included protecting the remaining ancient forests of the Pacific Northwest; preventing oil and gas drilling in the 1.5- million-acre (607,030-ha) Arctic National Wildlife Refuge in Alaska; securing wilderness and park areas in California, Colorado, Idaho, Montana, Nebraska, North Carolina, South Dakota, New Mexico, and Utah; and campaigning for energy conservation and reducing carbon emissions to combat global warming.

General acceptance

The Sierra Club had an estimated 600,000 members in 2012, down from its peak of 780,000 members in 2004. It was considered one of the "big ten" U.S. conservation organizations. An extensive professional staff is required to operate this complex organization, and members tend to have little influence over club policy at the national level. Some radical activists have criticized mainline organizations of this kind for being too conservative, too comfortable in their relationship to established powers, and too willing to compromise basic principles in order to maintain power and prestige. Supporters of the club argue that a spectrum of environmental organizations is desirable and that different organizations can play useful roles.

Resources

BOOKS

Goldstein, Natalie. *John Muir*. New York: Chelsea House, 2011.

WEBSITES

Barringer, Felicity. "Q. & A.: Michael Brune, Executive Director of the Sierra Club." http://green.blogs.nytimes.com/2012/04/17/a-q-a-with-the-sierra-clubs-michael-brune (accessed October 30, 2012).

Sierra Club. "The Goals of the Sierra Club's Climate Recovery Partnership." http://www.sierraclub.org/goals (accessed October 30, 2012).

Sierra Club. "Sierra Club Chapters." http://www.sierraclub.org/chapters (accessed October 30, 2012).

Sierra Club. "Sierra Club History." http://www.sierraclub.org/history (accessed October 30, 2012).

ORGANIZATIONS

Sierra Club, 85 Second St., 2nd Fl., San Francisco, CA 94105, (415) 977-5500, Fax: (415) 977-5797, information@sierraclub.org, http://www.sierraclub.org.

Sierra Club Canada, 412-1 Nicholas St., Ottawa, Canada Ontario K1N 7B7, 1(613) 241-4611, 1(888) 810-4204, http://www.sierraclub.ca.

Lewis G. Regenstein
Tish Davidson, AM

Silicosis

Definition

Silicosis is a progressive disease that belongs to a group of lung disorders called pneumoconioses. Silicosis is marked by the formation of lumps (nodules) and fibrous scar tissue in the lungs and is caused by exposure to inhaled particles of silica, mostly from quartz in rocks, sand, and similar substances.

Description

Silicosis is the oldest known occupational lung disease. It was first described in 1705 in stonecutters. An estimated 2 million workers in the United States are employed in occupations at risk for the development of silicosis. These include miners, foundry workers, stonecutters, potters and ceramics workers, sandblasters, tunnel workers, and rock drillers. Risk of developing silicosis increases with increasing years of exposure.

Silicosis is mostly found in adults over 40 years of age. It has four forms:

- Chronic: Chronic silicosis may take 15 or more years of exposure to develop. There is only mild impairment of lung functioning. Chronic silicosis may progress to more advanced forms.
- Complicated: Patients with complicated silicosis have noticeable shortness of breath, weight loss, and extensive formation of fibrosis in the lungs. These patients are at risk for developing tuberculosis (TB).
- Accelerated: This form of silicosis appears after 5–10 years of intense exposure. The symptoms are similar to those of complicated silicosis. Patients in this group often develop rheumatoid arthritis and other autoimmune disorders.
- Acute: Acute silicosis develops within 6 months to 2 years of intense exposure to silica. The patient loses a great deal of weight and is constantly short of breath. These patients are at severe risk of TB.

KEY TERMS

Alveoli—The small air sacs located at the ends of the breathing tubes of the lung, where oxygen normally passes from inhaled air through the membranes into the capillaries and the bloodstream.

Bronchoscopy—A procedure in which a fiber optic instrument called a bronchoscope is inserted in the airways allowing the physician to inspect the linings of the airways.

Fibrosis—A condition characterized by the presence of scar tissue or collagen proliferation in tissues to the extent that it replaces normal tissues.

Pneumoconiosis (plural, pneumoconioses)—Any chronic lung disease caused by inhaling particles of silica or similar substances that lead to loss of lung function.

Silica—A substance (silicon dioxide) occurring in quartz sand, sandstone, flint, and agate and other rocks. It is used in certain processes, such as making glass or pottery and scouring and grinding powders.

Causes and symptoms

The precise mechanism that triggers the development of silicosis is still unclear. What is known is that particles of silica dust get trapped in alveoli in the lungs where air exchange takes place. White blood cells called macrophages enter the alveoli, ingest the silica, and die. The resulting inflammation attracts other macrophages to the region. The nodule forms when the immune system forms fibrous tissue to seal off the reactive area. The disease process may stop at this point or speed up and destroy large areas of the lung. The **fibrosis** may continue even after the worker is no longer exposed to silica.

Early symptoms of silicosis include shortness of breath after exercising and a harsh, dry cough. Patients may have more trouble breathing and cough up blood as the disease progresses. Congestive heart failure can give their nails a bluish tint. Patients with advanced silicosis may have trouble sleeping and experience chest pain, hoarseness, and loss of appetite. Silicosis patients are at high risk for TB and should be checked for the disease during the doctor's examination.

Diagnosis

Diagnosis of silicosis is based on the following:

- occupational history
- chest x rays. These usually show small round opaque areas in chronic silicosis; the round areas are larger in complicated and accelerated silicosis.
- bronchoscopy
- lung function tests. The severity of the patient's symptoms does not always correlate with x-ray findings or lung function test results.

Treatment

Symptom management

There is no cure for silicosis. Therapy is intended to relieve symptoms, treat complications, and prevent respiratory infections. It includes careful monitoring for signs of TB. Respiratory symptoms may be treated with bronchodilators, increased fluid intake, steam inhalation, and physical therapy. Patients with severe breathing difficulties may be given oxygen therapy or placed on a mechanical ventilator. Acute silicosis may progress to complete respiratory failure. Heart-lung transplants are the only hope for some patients.

Patients with silicosis should call their doctor for any of the following symptoms:

- tiredness or mental confusion
- continued weight loss
- coughing up blood
- fever, chest pain, breathlessness, or new unexplained symptoms

Lifestyle changes

Patients with silicosis should be advised to quit **smoking**, prevent infections by avoiding crowds and persons with colds or similar infections, and receive vaccinations against influenza and pneumonia. They should be encouraged to increase their exercise capacity by keeping up regular activity and to pace themselves with their daily routine.

Prognosis

Silicosis is currently incurable. The prognosis for patients with chronic silicosis is generally good. Acute silicosis, however, may progress rapidly to respiratory failure and death.

Prevention

Silicosis is a preventable disease. In the United States, the **National Institute for Occupational Safety and Health** (NIOSH) standard for exposure to inhalable silica is 0.05 mg/m3, whereas the **Occupational Safety and Health Administration** (OSHA) has set a permissible exposure limit slightly higher at 10 mg/m3. These workplace rules have substantially decreased the number of cases of silicosis in American workers.

Other preventive occupational safety measures are:

- controls to minimize workplace exposure to silica dust
- substitution of substances—especially in sandblasting—that are less hazardous than silica
- clear identification of dangerous areas in the workplace
- informing workers about the dangers of overexposure to silica dust, training them in safety techniques, and giving them appropriate protective clothing and equipment

Coworkers of anyone diagnosed with silicosis should be examined for symptoms of the disease. The state health department and OSHA or the Mine Safety and Health Administration (MSHA) must be notified whenever a diagnosis of silicosis is confirmed.

QUESTIONS TO ASK YOUR DOCTOR

- What can I do to slow the progress of silicosis?
- How are you going to monitor the progress of my disease?
- Does silicosis put me at high risk for developing other respiratory diseases?
- Do you know of any support groups for people with silicosis?
- What should I tell my family about my disease?

Resources

BOOKS

Rosner, David, and Gerald Markowitz. *Deadly Dust: Silicosis and the On-going Struggle to Protect Workers' Health.* Ann Arbor: University of Michigan Press, 2006.

Tarlo, Susan, Paul Cullinan, and Benoit Nemery, eds. *Occupational and Environmental Lung Diseases: Diseases from Work, Home, Outdoor and Other Exposures.* Hoboken, NJ: Wiley, 2010.

WEBSITES

MedlinePlus Encyclopedia. "Silicosis." http://www.nlm.nih.gov/medlineplus/ency/article/000134.htm (accessed September 18, 2012).

National Center for Biotechnology Information. "Resources for Silicosis." http://www.ncbi.nlm.nih.gov/sites/ga?disorder=Silicosis (accessed September 18, 2012).

National Institute for Occupational Safety and Health (NIOSH). "Silica." Centers for Disease Control and Prevention. http://www.cdc.gov/niosh/topics/silica (accessed September 18, 2012).

Varkey, Basil. "Silicosis." Medscape Reference. http://emedicine.medscape.com/article/302027-overview (accessed September 18, 2012).

ORGANIZATIONS

Centers for Disease Control and Prevention (CDC), 1600 Clifton Rd., Atlanta, GA 30333, (404) 639-3534, (800) 232-4636; TTY: (888) 232-6348, inquiry@cdc.gov, http://www.cdc.gov.

Mine Safety and Health Administration, 4015 Wilson Blvd., Arlington, VA 22203, (877) 778-6055, MSHAhelpdesk@dol.gov, http://www.msha.gov.

National Center for Biotechnology Information, 8600 Rockville Pike, Bethesda, MD 20894, (301) 496-2475, http://www.ncbi.nlm.nih.gov.

Occupational Safety & Health Administration, 200 Constitution Ave. NW, Washington, DC 20210, http://www.osha.gov.

Maureen Haggerty
Tish Davidson, AM

Skin cancer

Definition

Non-melanoma skin cancer is a malignant growth of the external surface or epithelial layer of the skin.

Demographics

Skin cancers are the most common type of cancer by far in the United States. Approximately 800,000 to 900,000 new cases of basal cell skin cancer are diagnosed each year. Squamous cell skin cancers are diagnosed less frequently with 200,000 to 300,000 new cases diagnosed annually. The number of new cases of non-melanoma skin cancers is increasing each year. This increase is attributed to improved detection capabilities, increased exposure to the sun, and increase in the lifespan of the general population. Most of the time, basal cell and squamous cell skin cancers are not fatal. The American Cancer Society reports a decline of about 30% in deaths from skin cancer between 1980 and 2010.

Description

Risk factors

Exposure to sunlight is documented as the main cause of more than 1 million cases of non-melanoma skin cancers diagnosed each year in the United States. Incidence increases for those living where direct sunshine is plentiful, such as near the equator.

Ultraviolet B (UVB) rays are thought to cause most basal cell and squamous cell skin cancers. Ultraviolet A (UVA) rays may also directly cause some skin cancers. In addition to sunlight, overexposure to UVB rays can occur from the use of tanning booths and beds and from sunlamps.

People who are at highest risk for the development of skin cancer include individuals who have fair skin and light-colored eyes and who freckle or burn easily when exposed to UVB rays.

Other individuals at high risk include older adults because exposure increases over time. Males are two to three times as likely to develop skin cancer as females. Exposure to chemicals such as arsenic, industrial tar, coal, paraffin, and certain types of oil can lead to skin cancer. Other risk factors include a history of **smoking**, a history of previous skin cancer, and history of illnesses, diseases, or conditions which impair immunity.

Skin cancer is the growth of abnormal cells capable of invading and destroying other associated skin cells. Skin cancer is often subdivided into either **melanoma** or non-melanoma. Melanoma is a dark-pigmented, usually malignant tumor arising from a skin cell capable of making the pigment melanin (a melanocyte). Melanomas can also develop from benign tissue such as moles. Non-melanoma skin cancer most often originates from the outermost skin surface as a squamous cell carcinoma or from cells in the basal layer, the deepest part of the epidermis. Cancers of the latter type are termed basal cell carcinomas. Basal cell and squamous cell skin cancers may also be referred to as keratinocyte cancers.

Other types of skin cancers that occur less frequently are: Merkel cell carcinoma, Kaposi sarcoma, cutaneous lymphoma, skin adenexal tumors, and various types of sarcomas. Combined, the incidence of all of these rarer types of non-melanoma skin cancer account for less than 1% of skin cancer.

Basal cell carcinoma affects the skin's basal layer and has the potential to grow progressively larger, although it rarely spreads to distant areas (metastasizes). Basal cell carcinomas account for 80% of skin cancers (excluding melanoma), whereas squamous cell cancer makes up about 20%. Basal cell cancer tends to

KEY TERMS

Autoimmune—Pertaining to an immune response by the body against one of its own tissues or types of cells.

Curettage—The removal of tissue or growths by scraping with a curette.

Dermatologist—A physician specializing in the branch of medicine concerned with skin.

Electrodesiccation—To make dry, dull, or lifeless with the use of electrical current.

Lesion—A patch of skin that has been infected or diseased.

Topical—Referring to a medication or other preparation applied to the skin or the outside of the body.

---

recur, with approximately 50% of people diagnosed with basal cell cancer developing a new skin cancer within five years. Squamous cell carcinoma is a malignant growth of the external surface of the skin. Squamous cell cancers metastasize at a rate of 2% to 6%, with up to 10% of lesions affecting the ear and lip. Squamous cell carcinomas appear to be more aggressive than basal cell cancers.

Causes and symptoms

Cumulative sun exposure is considered a significant risk factor for non-melanoma skin cancer. There is evidence suggesting that early, intense exposure causing blistering sunburn in childhood may also play an important role in the cause of non-melanoma skin cancer. Basal cell carcinoma most frequently affects the skin of the face, with the next most common sites being the ears, the backs of the hands, the shoulders, and the arms. It is prevalent in both sexes and most common in people over 40.

About 1% to 2% of all skin cancers develop within burn scars; squamous cell carcinomas account for about 95% of these cancers, with 3% being basal cell carcinomas and the remainder malignant melanomas.

Basal cell carcinomas usually appear as small skin lesions that persist for at least three weeks. This form of non-melanomatous skin cancer looks flat and waxy with the edges of the lesion translucent and rounded. The edges also contain small fresh blood vessels. An ulcer in the center of the lesion gives it a dimpled appearance. Basal cell carcinoma lesions vary from 4 to 6 millimeters in size, but can slowly grow larger if untreated.

Squamous cell carcinoma also involves skin exposed to the sun, such as the face, ears, hands, or arms. This form of non-melanoma is also most common among people over 40. Squamous cell carcinoma is characterized by a small, scaling, raised bump on the skin with a crusting ulcer in the center, but without pain and itching. The lesion may also appear as flat, reddish, slow-growing patches.

Basal cell and squamous cell carcinomas can grow more easily when people have a suppressed immune system because they are taking immunosuppressive drugs or are exposed to **radiation**. Some people must take immunosuppressive drugs to prevent the rejection of a transplanted organ or because they have a disease in which the immune system attacks the body's own tissues (autoimmune illnesses); others may need radiation therapy to treat another form of cancer. Because of this, individuals taking immunosuppressive drugs or receiving radiation treatments should undergo complete skin examination at regular intervals. If proper treatment is delayed and the tumor continues to grow, tumor cells can spread (metastasize) to muscle, bone, nerves, and possibly the brain.

Diagnosis

Examination

To diagnose skin cancer, clinicians must carefully examine the lesion and ask the patient about how long it has been there, whether it itches or bleeds, and other questions about the patient's medical history. Lymph nodes in the vicinity of the suspicious lesion will be palpated.

The patient may be referred to a dermatologist for a more comprehensive examination. The dermatologist may use a device known as a dermatoscope to visualize spots on the skin more clearly.

Procedures

If skin cancer cannot be ruled out, a sample of tissue is removed and examined under a microscope (a biopsy). A definitive diagnosis of squamous or basal cell cancer can only be made with microscopic examination of the tumor cells. Once skin cancer has been diagnosed, the stage of the disease's development is determined. The information from the biopsy and staging allows the physician and patient to plan for treatment and possible surgical intervention.

Treatment

Traditional

A variety of treatment options are available for those diagnosed with non-melanoma skin cancer. Some carcinomas can be removed by cryosurgery, the process of freezing with liquid nitrogen. Uncomplicated and previously untreated basal cell carcinoma of the trunk and arms is often treated with curettage and electrodesiccation, which is the scraping of the lesion and the destruction of any remaining malignant cells with an electrical current. Removal of a lesion layer-by-layer down to normal margins (Mohs' surgery) is an effective treatment for both basal and squamous cell carcinoma. Removal of larger tumors may require skin grafting and reconstructive surgery.

Treatments for non-melanoma skin cancer also include photodynamic therapy (PDT), topical chemotherapy in which the anticancer drug is applied to the lesion as an ointment or as a cream, laser surgery, and the use of drugs such as imiquimod and interferon. These drugs are classified as immune response modifiers. The drugs work to boost the body's immune system to help decrease the size of the lesion and sometimes are effective in eliminating the skin cancer altogether.

Radiation therapy is best reserved for older, debilitated patients or when the tumor is considered inoperable.

Prognosis

Both squamous and basal cell carcinoma are curable with appropriate treatment, although basal cell carcinomas have a higher rate of recurrence. Early detection remains critical for a positive prognosis. Although it is rare for basal cell carcinomas to metastasize, metastases can rapidly lead to death if the tumor cells invade the eyes, ears, mouth, or the membranes covering the brain.

Prevention

Not all skin cancers can be prevented. However, there are ways to reduce risk for skin cancer. Avoiding exposure to the sun reduces the incidence of non-melanoma skin cancer. Sunscreen and sunblock preparations provide protection against both UVA and UVB rays. These preparations should also be rated with a sun protection factor (SPF) of 30 or higher. They should be applied 30 minutes before going outdoors and then reapplied every two hours and after swimming. Other recommended practices are to wear a hat, sunglasses, and clothing to shield the skin from sun damage. The lips should be protected by wearing lip balm with sunscreen.

Other strategies include avoiding the outdoors during times of maximum UV effects which is typically between the hours of 10 A.M. until 4 P.M. especially on days when the UV index is high. People can check online at www.epa.gov/sunwise/uvindex.html to determine the UV index in their area on any particular day. Avoiding tanning beds, tanning booths, and sunlamps is also strongly recommended. Adults should consider applying protective wear for children. Such wear is designed to cover the child from the neck to the knees with sun-protective fabric.

People should examine their skin monthly for unusual lesions, especially if previous skin cancers have been experienced.

Resources

BOOKS

Hendi, Ali, and Juan Carlos Martinez. *Atlas of Skin Cancers: Practical Guide to Diagnosis and Treatment.* New York: Springer, 2011.

Rigel, Darrel S., et al. *Cancer of the Skin: Expert Consult.* 2nd ed. Philadelphia: Saunders, 2011.

PERIODICALS

Cafardi, J. A., et al. "Prospects for Skin Cancer Treatment and Prevention: The Potential Contribution of an Engineered Virus." *Journal of Investigative Dermatology* 131, no. 3 (2011): 559–61.

Lomas, A., et al. "A Systematic Review of Worldwide Incidence of Nonmelanoma Skin Cancer." *British Journal of Dermatology* 166, no. 5 (2012): 1069–80.

Patel, R. V., A. Frankel, and A. Goldenberg. "An Update on Nonmelanoma Skin Cancer." *Journal of Clinical and Aesthetic Dermatology* 4, no. 2 (2011): 20–7.

Tan, S., C. Sinclair, and P. Foley. "Running Behind a Tourist: Leisure-related Skin Cancer Prophylaxis." *British Journal of Dermatology* 167, Suppl. 2 (2012): 70–5.

ORGANIZATIONS

American Academy of Dermatology (AAD), PO Box 4014, Schaumburg, IL 60168, (866) 503-7546, MRC@aad.org, http://www.aad.org.

American Cancer Society, 250 Williams St., Atlanta, GA 30303, (800) 227-2345, http://www.cancer.org.

National Cancer Institute (NCI), 6116 Executive Blvd., Ste. 300, Bethesda, MD 20892-8322, (800) 422-6237, http://www.cancer.gov/global/contact/email-us, http://www.cancer.gov.

Skin Cancer Foundation, 149 Madison Ave., Ste. 901, New York, NY 10016, (212) 725-5176, http://www.skincancer.org/contact-us, http://www.skincancer.org.

Jeffrey P. Larson, RPT
Ken R. Wells
Melinda Granger Oberleitner, RN, DNS, APRN, CNS

Sleeping sickness

Definition

Sleeping sickness (also called trypanosomiasis) is an infection caused by *Trypanosoma* protozoa; it is passed to humans through the bite of the tsetse fly. If left untreated, the infection progresses to death within months or years.

Description

Protozoa are single-celled organisms considered to be the simplest life form in the animal kingdom. The protozoa responsible for sleeping sickness are a variety that bears numerous flagella (hair-like projections from the cell that help the cell to move). These protozoa exist only on the continent of Africa. The type of protozoa causing sleeping sickness in humans is referred to as the *Trypanasoma brucei* complex, which can be divided further into Rhodesian (Central and East African) and Gambian (Central and West African) subspecies.

The Rhodesian variety lives within antelopes in savanna and woodland areas, and it causes no problems with the antelope's health. The protozoa are then acquired by tsetse flies when they bite and suck the blood of an infected antelope or cow.

Within the tsetse fly, the protozoa cycle through several different life forms; ultimately they migrate to the salivary glands of the tsetse fly. Once the protozoa are harbored in the salivary glands, they are ready to be deposited into the bloodstream of the fly's next source of a blood meal.

Humans most likely to become infected by Rhodesian trypanosomes are people such as game wardens and visitors to game parks in East Africa, who may be bitten by a tsetse fly that has fed on game (antelope) carrying the protozoa. The Rhodesian variety of sleeping sickness causes a much more severe illness, with even greater likelihood of eventual death than the Gambian form.

The Gambian variety of *Trypanosoma* thrives in tropical rain forests throughout Central and West Africa; it does not infect game or cattle and is primarily a threat to people dwelling in such areas, rarely infecting visitors.

Causes and symptoms

The first sign of infection with the trypanosome may be a sore appearing at the site of the tsetse fly bite about two to three days after the person was bitten. Redness, pain, and swelling occur but are often ignored by the patient.

DAVID BRUCE (1855–1931)

David Bruce was born in Melbourne, Australia, on May 29, 1855, to Scottish immigrants. Bruce's family moved back to Scotland when he was five years old. Bruce attended the University of Edinburgh where he studied natural history and medicine. Following graduation, he accepted a position working with a doctor. In 1883, Bruce married Mary Elizabeth Steele who would help him with his work throughout his life.

In 1884, Bruce began to study the disease called Malta or Mediterranean fever when he and Mary were stationed in Malta with the Army Medical Service. Using a microscope, Bruce discovered that the disease was caused by a microccus that grew in the individual's spleen. The organism responsible for this disease was ultimately isolated by Bernhard L. F. Bang. In 1905, Bruce led a scientific team that discovered that the soldiers who contracted the disease had ingested the milk of infected goats. The disease disappeared when the soldiers quit drinking goat's milk. Many physicians began calling the disease brucellosis in honor of Bruce's discoveries. Bruce also conducted research in Africa where he found that the tsetse fly could infect humans, as well as animals, with the nagana disease. Ultimately, his work would prove that sleeping sickness was caused by the tsetse fly.

In 1903, Bruce became the director of the Royal Society's Sleeping Sickness Commission and, in 1908, he was knighted. He served as commandant of the Royal Army Medical College after he and his wife returned to England. Bruce died on November 20, 1931.

Stage I illness

Two to three weeks later, Stage I disease develops as a result of the protozoa's being carried through the blood and lymph circulation of the host. This systemic (meaning that symptoms affect the whole body) phase of the illness is characterized by a fever that rises quite high then falls to normal, then spikes (rises rapidly). A rash with intense itching may be present, and headache and mental confusion may occur. The Gambian form, in particular, includes extreme swelling of lymph tissue, with enlargement of both the spleen and liver, and greatly swollen lymph nodes. Winterbottom's sign is classic of Gambian sleeping sickness and consists of a visibly swollen area of lymph nodes located behind the ear and just above the base of the neck. During this stage, the heart may be affected by a severe inflammatory reaction, particularly when the infection is caused by the Rhodesian variety of trypanosomiasis.

Many of the symptoms of sleeping sickness are actually the result of attempts by the patient's immune system to get rid of the invading organism. The heightened activity of the cells of the immune system results in damage to the patient's own organs, anemia, and leaky blood vessels. These leaks in the blood vessels ultimately help to spread the protozoa throughout the afflicted person's body.

One reason for the intense reaction of the immune system to the presence of the trypanosomes also provides the reason why the trypanosomes survive so well despite the efforts of the immune system to eradicate them. The protozoa causing sleeping sickness are able to rapidly change specific markers (unique proteins) on their outer coats. These kinds of markers usually serve to stimulate the host's immune system to produce immune cells that will specifically target the marker, allowing quick destruction of those cells bearing the markers. Trypanosomes, however, are able to express new markers at such a high rate of change that the host's immune system is constantly trying to catch up.

Stage II illness

Stage II sleeping sickness involves the nervous system. Gambian sleeping sickness, in particular, has a clearly delineated phase in which the predominant symptoms involve the brain. The patient's speech becomes slurred, mental processes are slow, and the patient sits and stares for long periods of time or sleeps. Other symptoms resemble Parkinson's disease, including imbalance when walking, slow and shuffling gait, trembling of the limbs, involuntary movements, muscle tightness, and increasing mental confusion. Untreated, these symptoms eventually lead to coma and then to death.

Diagnosis

Diagnosis of sleeping sickness can be made by microscopic examination of fluid from the original sore at the site of the tsetse fly bite. Trypanosomes will be present in the fluid for a short period following the bite. If the sore has already resolved, fluid can be obtained from swollen lymph nodes for examination. Other methods of trypanosome diagnosis involve culturing blood, lymph node fluid, bone marrow, or spinal fluid. These cultures are then injected into rats, which develop blood-borne protozoa infection that can be detected in blood smears within one to two weeks. However, this last method is effective only for the Rhodesian variety of sleeping sickness.

KEY TERMS

Immune system—The network of tissues and cells throughout the body that is responsible for ridding the body of any invaders, such as viruses, bacteria, and protozoa.

Protozoa—Single-celled organisms considered to be the simplest life form in the animal kingdom.

Treatment

Without treatment, sleeping sickness will lead to death. Unfortunately, however, those medications effective against the *Trypanosoma brucei* complex protozoa all have significant potential side effects for the patient. Suramin, eflornithine, pentamidine, and several drugs that contain arsenic (a chemical which in higher doses is highly poisonous to humans) are all effective antitrypanosomal agents. Each of these drugs, however, requires careful monitoring to ensure that the drugs themselves do not cause serious complications such as fatal hypersensitivity (allergic) reaction, kidney or liver damage, or inflammation of the brain.

Prevention

Prevention of sleeping sickness requires avoiding contact with the tsetse fly. Insect repellents and clothing that covers the limbs to the wrists and ankles are advisable. Public health measures have included drug treatment of humans who are infected with one of the *Trypanosoma brucei* complex. As of 2012 there were no immunizations to prevent the acquisition of sleeping sickness.

Resources

BOOKS

Zeibig, Elizabeth. *Clinical Parasitology: A Practical Approach*, 2nd ed. Philadelphia: W. B. Saunders, 2012.

PERIODICALS

Brun, R., et al. "Human African Trypanosomiasis." *Lancet* 375, no. 9709 (2010): 148–59.

Malvy, D., and F. Chappuis. "Sleeping Sickness." *Clinical Microbiology and Infection* 17, no. 7 (2011): 986–95.

WEBSITES

Odero, Randy O. "African Trypanosomiasis (Sleeping Sickness)." http://emedicine.medscape.com/article/228613-overview (accessed September 24, 2012).

"Parasites: African Trypanosomiasis (also known as Sleeping Sickness)." Centers for Disease Control and Prevention. http://www.cdc.gov/parasites/sleepingsickness/index.html (accessed September 24, 2012).

"Trypanosomiasis, African." World Health Organization. http://www.who.int/topics/trypanosomiasis_african/en/ (accessed September 24, 2012).

ORGANIZATIONS

Centers for Disease Control and Prevention, 1600 Clifton Rd., Atlanta, GA 30333, (800) 232-4636, cdcinfor@cdc.gov, http://www.cdc.gov.

Rosalyn Carson-DeWitt, MD

Smallpox

Definition

Smallpox is an infection caused by the variola virus (either of two variants, Variola major or variola minor), a member of the poxvirus family. Throughout history, smallpox has been a greatly feared disease because it was responsible for worldwide epidemics that resulted in large numbers of deaths. In 1980, the **World Health Organization** (WHO) announced that an extensive program of **vaccination** against the disease had resulted in the complete eradication of the virus with the exception of samples of stored virus in two laboratories.

Description

The first appearance of smallpox is unknown in the medical community. Smallpox probably evolved from a rodent virus anywhere from 16,000 to 79,000 years ago. Two clades (organisms with a common ancestor) evolved. The variola major stain spread outward from Asia 400–1,500 years ago. A second clade, found on the North and South American continents and West Africa, was known to exist roughly 1,400–6,500 years ago.

Smallpox is strictly an infection of human beings. Animals and insects do not contract or carry the virus in any form. Most infections are caused by contact with a person who has developed the characteristic skin lesions (pox) of the disease, although a person with a less severe infection (not symptomatic or diagnosable in the usual way) can unknowingly spread the virus.

Risk factors

Because smallpox was eradicated in 1980, there are no risk factors for contracting smallpox in the natural environment. However, scientists and technicians working in laboratories and facilities with the smallpox virus do have a minimal risk of contracting smallpox. Other risks, though slight, include having the smallpox virus stolen from laboratories that are holding it and its being used as a biological weapon.

Demographics

Vaccinations for smallpox began in the early 1800s. According to WHO, an estimated 50 million cases of smallpox occurred worldwide in the early 1950s. By the mid-1960s that number dropped to between 10 and 15 million. In 1967, WHO launched an intense plan to eradicate smallpox, which continued to present serious health consequences for about 60% of the world's population. The global campaign to eradicate smallpox successfully decreased the area in which the infection was present. The last two outbreaks of smallpox occurred in Yugoslavia, in 1972; and in India, in 1974, where 15,000 people died of the infection. By 1977, the last natural case of smallpox occurred in Somalia, Africa. In 1980, the World Health Assembly made the official pronouncement that smallpox was eradicated from the planet.

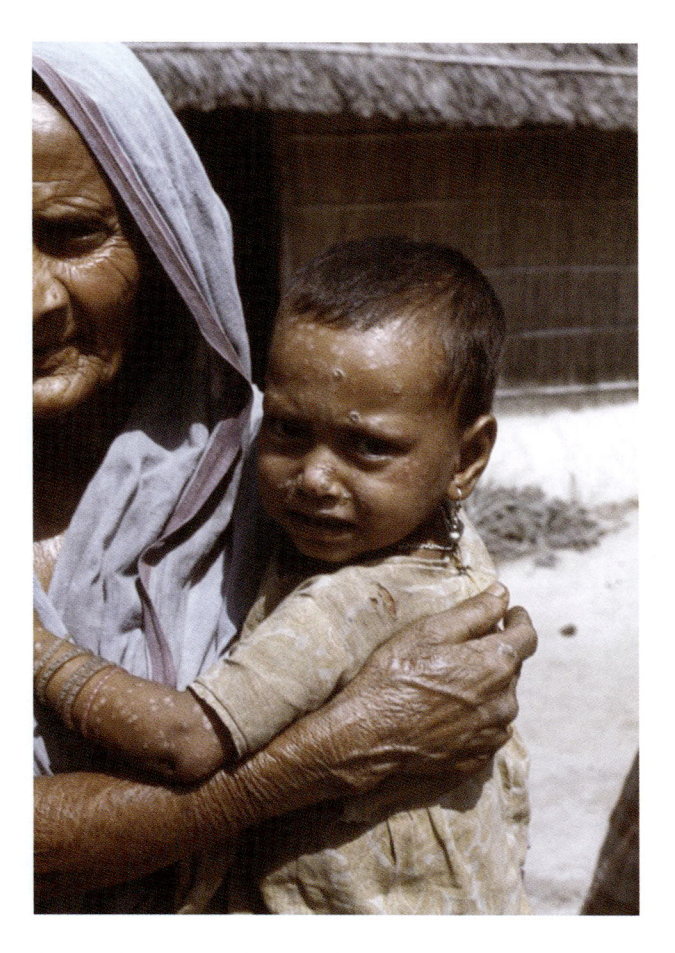

A Bengali woman holidng a child with smallpox in a Bangladesh village during the early 1970s worldwide smallpox eradication campaign. *(CDC/Jean Roy)*

GALE ENCYCLOPEDIA OF ENVIRONMENTAL HEALTH

Causes and symptoms

Smallpox is a relatively contagious disease, which accounts for its ability to cause massive epidemics. The variola virus is acquired from direct contact with individuals infected with the disease, from contaminated air droplets, and even from objects used by a person with smallpox (books, blankets, utensils). The respiratory tract is the usual entry point for the variola virus into a human being.

After the virus enters the body, there is a 12- to 14-day incubation period during which the virus multiplies, although no symptoms are recognizable. After the incubation period, symptoms appear abruptly and include fever, chills, and muscle aches. Two to three days later, a bumpy rash begins appearing first on the face and forearms. The rash progresses—ultimately reaching the chest, abdomen, and back. Seven to ten days after the rash appears, the patient is most infectious. The individual bumps (papules) fill with clear fluid and eventually become pus-filled over the course of 10 to 12 days. These pox eventually scab over, each leaving a permanently scarred pock or pit when the scab drops off.

Initially, the smallpox symptoms and rash appear similar to chickenpox. However, unlike chickenpox, smallpox lesions develop at the same rate so that they are all visible in the same stage. Another major difference is that smallpox occurs primarily on the face and extremities, whereas chickenpox tends to be concentrate on the face and trunk area.

Complications such as bacterial infection of the open skin lesions, pneumonia, or bone infections are the major causes of death from smallpox. A severe and quickly fatal form, called sledgehammer smallpox, occurs in 5–10% of patients and results in massive, uncontrollable bleeding (hemorrhage) from skin lesions, as well as from the mouth, nose, and other areas of the body. This form is very infectious and usually fatal five to seven days after onset.

Fear of smallpox comes from both the epidemic nature of the disease as well as from the fact that no therapies have ever been discovered to either treat the symptoms of smallpox or shorten the course of the disease.

Diagnosis

In modern times, a diagnosis of smallpox is made using an electron microscope to identify virus in fluid from the papules, urine, or in the patient's blood prior to the appearance of the papular rash.

EDWARD JENNER (1749–1823)

The first successful vaccine was Edward Jenner's smallpox vaccine, which not only saved lives and eliminated the threat of smallpox as an epimedic, but paved the way for inoculations to become common practice. During his smallpox research, Jenner created the term "virus". For these reasons, Jenner is known as the inventor of vaccination and the pioneer of virology.

Edward Jenner improved the existing inoculation process—an arduous routine where healthy people were infected with smallpox pustules. Jenner realized that some patients were resistant to the smallpox disease. He realized patients resistant to smallpox had previously contracted a specific strain of cowpox.

On May 14, 1796, Jenner created a cowpox vaccination using a pustule from a milkmaid suffering from the disease. He used this to inoculate an eight-year-old boy, who subsequently contracted cowpox and recovered in days. Jenner inoculated the boy with smallpox on July 1, 1796. As he had hoped, the inoculation had no effect.

Jenner's passion allowed inoculations to become a common preventative practice. He would work with vaccination research and development throughout the remainder of his life.

Treatment

No treatments have been developed to halt progression of the disease. Treatment for smallpox is only supportive, meaning that it is aimed at keeping a patient as comfortable as possible. Antibiotics are sometimes administered to prevent secondary bacterial infections.

Public health role and response

As of 2012, two laboratories (the U.S. **Centers for Disease Control and Prevention** [CDC] in Atlanta, Georgia, and the Russian State Centre of Virology and Biotechnology [VECTOR] in Koltsovo, Novosibirsk Region) officially retain samples of the smallpox virus. These samples, as well as stockpiles of the smallpox vaccine, are stored because some level of concern exists that another smallpox virus could undergo genetic changes (mutate) and cause human infection. There is also the minute chance that smallpox virus could escape from the laboratories where it is stored. For these reasons, surveillance continues of various animal groups that continue to be infected with **viruses** related to the variola virus, and large quantities of vaccine are stored in different countries around the world so that response to any future threat by the smallpox virus can be swift and effective.

Of greatest concern is the potential use of smallpox as a biological weapon. Since 1980, when the WHO announced smallpox had been eradicated, essentially no one has been vaccinated against the disease. Individuals vaccinated prior to 1980 are believed to be susceptible as well because immunity only lasts 15–20 years. These circumstances, along with the nature of smallpox to spread quickly from person to person, could lead to devastating consequences.

The United States and Russia are the only two countries to officially house remaining samples of the virus. However, it is believed that other countries, such as Iraq, may have obtained samples of the smallpox virus during the Cold War (1947–1991) through their association with the Soviet Union. It is also possible that scientists with access to the virus may have sold their services and knowledge to other governments.

On June 22 and 23, 2001, four U.S. organizations (CSIS—Center for Strategic and International Studies, Johns Hopkins Center for Civilian Biodefense Studies, ANSER—Analytic Services Inc., and MIPT—Memorial Institute for the Prevention of Terrorism) presented a fictitious scenario of the U.S. response to a deliberate introduction of smallpox titled *Dark Winter*. This exercise demonstrated that if such an event were to occur, the United States would be ill prepared on several fronts. The primary concern is an inadequate supply of vaccine, which is essential to preventing disease development in exposed persons. Between 1997 and 2001, two companies were contracted to produce additional smallpox vaccines for both military and civilian use. Through these contracts, an additional 40 million doses were made available for civilian use as of 2005. Studies were also conducted to determine if existing vaccines can be diluted in order to increase the number of doses available for immediate use. Results from a very small group of volunteers tested in 2000 found that at one-tenth strength, the existing smallpox vaccines are approximately 70% effective. In late 2001, a new study began evaluating the effectiveness of the vaccine at one-fifth strength. In 2004, the European Commission (EC) reviewed two U.S. dilution studies at one-fifth strength. It concluded that "diluting vaccine would be inadvisable." The EC states that the dilution would "increase the risk of ineffective inoculations." In addition, WHO stated that it would not consider diluting any of its stockpile of vaccine because of the risks associated with dilution.

In the event that smallpox is reintroduced into the current population, it will be imperative that doctors immediately recognize the symptoms and isolate the individual to prevent further spread of the disease. Prompt vaccination of any persons who had contact with the patient is also necessary to prevent additional cases of smallpox from developing. Controlling and containing spread of this disease is critical for prevention of a world-wide epidemic that would have a devastating impact on current populations.

> ### KEY TERMS
>
> **Endemic**—Occurring naturally and consistently in a particular area.
>
> **Epidemic**—Occurs when the number of cases of a disease exceeds the usual or average (endemic) number for an area or region. These may occur as a large cluster of cases all occurring at about the same time within a specific community or region.
>
> **Eradicate**—To completely do away with something, eliminate it, end its existence.
>
> **Hemorrhage**—Bleeding that is massive, uncontrollable, and often life-threatening.
>
> **Lesion**—The tissue disruption or the loss of function caused by a particular disease process.
>
> **Papules**—Firm bumps on the skin.
>
> **Pox**—A pus-filled bump on the skin.
>
> **Vaccine**—A preparation using a noninfectious element or relative of a particular virus or bacteria that is administered with the intention of halting the progress of an infection, or completely preventing it.

Prognosis

Approximately one in three patients die from smallpox, with the more severe, hemorrhagic form nearly 100% fatal. Patients who survive smallpox infection nearly always have multiple areas of scarring at the site of each pock.

Prevention

From about the tenth century in China, India, and the Americas, it has been noted that individuals who had even a mild case of smallpox could not be infected again. Writings from all over the world account different ways in which people tried to prevent smallpox. Material from people mildly ill with smallpox (fluid or pus from the papules, scabs over the pox) was scratched into the skin of people who had never had the illness, in an attempt to produce a mild reaction and

> **QUESTIONS TO ASK YOUR DOCTOR**
>
> - Should I be worried about smallpox if I travel to a developing country?
> - How dangerous is the threat of smallpox as a terrorist attack?
> - Is smallpox contagious before a rash appears?
> - Is there any treatment for smallpox?
> - If the vaccine for smallpox is ever given to the public, how is the vaccine given?
> - Are diluted doses of smallpox vaccine as effective as the undiluted form?
> - What is the smallpox vaccine made of?
> - Is it possible to get smallpox from the vaccination?

its accompanying protective effect. These efforts often resulted in full-fledged smallpox, and probably served only to help effectively spread the infection throughout a community. In fact, such crude smallpox vaccinations were against the law in Colonial America.

In 1798, English physician and scientist Edward Jenner (1749–1823) published a paper in which he discussed his important observation that milkmaids who contracted a mild infection of the hands (called cowpox, and caused by a relative of the variola virus) appeared to be immune to smallpox. Jenner created an immunization against smallpox using the pus found in the lesions of cowpox infection. Jenner's paper led to much work in the area of vaccinations and ultimately resulted in the creation of a very effective vaccination against smallpox that utilized the vaccinia virus, another close relative of variola. The term vaccination is derived from *vacca*, Latin for cow and related to the cowpox link. Later, the term was applied to other vaccinations.

In 1967, WHO began its attempt to eradicate the smallpox virus worldwide. The methods used in the program were simple:

- Careful surveillance for all smallpox infections worldwide, to allow for quick diagnosis and immediate quarantine of patients.
- Immediate vaccination of all contacts diagnosed with infection, in order to interrupt the virus' usual pattern of infection.

WHO's program was extremely successful, and the virus was declared eradicated worldwide in May 1980.

Resources

BOOKS

Brachman, Philip S., and Elias Abrutyn, eds. *Bacterial Infections of Humans: Epidemiology and Control*. New York: Springer Science and Business Media, 2009.

Dworkin, Mark S., ed. *Outbreak Investigations Around the World: Case Studies in Infectious Disease Field Epidemiology*. Sudbury, MA: Jones and Bartlett, 2010.

Shannon, Joyce Brennfleck, ed. *Contagious Diseases Sourcebook: Basic Consumer Health Information about Diseases Spread from Person to Person*. Detroit: Omnigraphics, 2010.

PERIODICALS

Broad, William J. "U.S. Acts to Make Vaccines and Drugs Against Smallpox." *The New York Times*, October 9, 2001: D1–2.

Gouvras G. "Policies in Place Throughout the World: Action by the European Union." *International Journal of Infectious Diseases* 8, Suppl 2 (Oct 2004): S21–30.

Miller, Judith, and Sheryl Gay Stolberg. "Sept. 11 Attacks Led to Push for More Smallpox Vaccine." *The New York Times*, October 22, 2001: A1.

WEBSITES

Constantine, Alex. *The Path to 9/11 (Part Five): DARK WINTER/ANSER, CSIS & Other Main Players Stage a Terror Drill in Preparation for Black Tuesday & Anthrax Attacks*. Constantine Report. May 25, 2008. http://www.constantinereport.com/allposts/the-path-to-911-part-five-dark-winteranser-csis-other-main-players-stage-a-terror-drill-in-preparation-for-black-tuesday-anthrax-attacks/ (accessed October 13, 2012).

Smallpox: Surveillance and Investigation. Centers for Disease Control and Prevention. March 19, 2012. http://www.bt.cdc.gov/agent/smallpox/surveillance/ (accessed October 13, 2012).

Smallpox. World Health Organization. (2012). http://www.who.int/topics/smallpox/en/ (accessed October 13, 2012).

ORGANIZATIONS

U.S. Centers for Disease Control and Prevention, 1600 Clifton Rd., Atlanta, GA 30333, (800) 232-4636, cdcinfo@cdc.gov, http://www.cdc.gov/.

U.S. Food and Drug Administration, 10903 New Hampshire Ave., Silver Spring, MD 20993, (888) 463-6332, http://www.fda.gov.

World Health Organization, Avenue Appia 20, Geneva, Switzerland 1211 27, 41 22 791-2111, Fax: 41 22 791-3111, http://www.who.int/en/.

Rosalyn Carson-DeWitt, MD
William A. Atkins, BB, BS, MBA

Smog

Definition

Smog is the term chosen by the Glasgow (Scotland) public health official Henry Antoine Des Voeux at the beginning of the twentieth century to describe the smoky fogs that characterized coal-burning cities of the time. The word, formed by combining the words smoke and fog, has persisted as a description of this type of urban atmosphere. It has frequently been used to describe photochemical smog, the haze that became a characteristic of the Los Angeles Basin (in southern California) from the 1940s. Smog is sometimes even used to describe **air pollution** in general, even where there is not a reduction in visibility at all. However, the term is most properly used to describe the two distinctive types of pollution that dominated the atmospheres of late-nineteenth-century London and other industrial cities in England, known as winter smog, and twentieth-century Los Angeles, called summer smog.

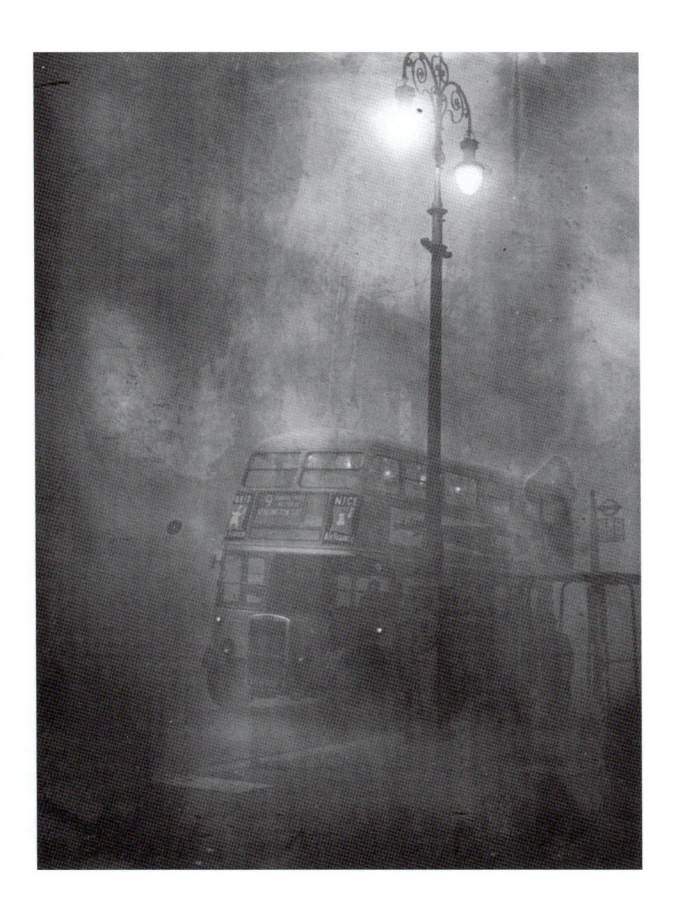

A London bus makes its way along Fleet Street in heavy smog, 6th December 1952. *(Edward Miller/Keystone/Hulton Archive/Getty Images)*

Description

Smog can be described by using two prominent real-life examples:

- Nineteenth-century London, England, smog, which resulted from a combination of windless cold, wet weather, causing fog, and emissions from coal-burning factories. This kind of smog recurred in 1952.
- The Los Angeles (California) Basin summer smog is considered modern smog, or a type of air pollution derived from hot weather coupled with the exhaust of internal combustion engines from motorized vehicles and the fumes from industrial plants. These exhausts and fumes react in the atmosphere with sunlight to form secondary pollutants, which then combine with primary pollutant emissions to make photochemical smog.

Nineteenth-century London smog

The city of London (United Kingdom [U.K.]) burned almost 20 million tons (18 million metric tons) of coal annually by the end of the nineteenth century. In addition to what was used in factories, much coal was burned in domestic hearths, and the smoke and sulfur dioxide produced barely rose from the chimneys above the housetops. Only a few rather inaccurate measurements of the pollutant concentrations in the air were made in the nineteenth century, although they hint at concentrations much higher than what scientists might expect in London today.

The smog of nineteenth-century London took the form of dense, vividly colored fogs. The smog was frequently so dense that torches were provided at door entries for people to use to find their way to waiting carriages or to their homes on foot. It is said that visibility became so restricted that fingers on an outstretched arm were invisible. The fog that rolled over window sills and into rooms became such an integral part of what people know as Victorian London that almost any Sherlock Holmes story mentions it. (Scottish author and physician Sir Arthur Conan Doyle (1859–1930) created the fictional detective Sherlock Holmes.)

With London's high humidity and frequent fog, smoke particles from coal-burning formed a nucleus for the condensation of vapor into large fog droplets. This water also served as a site for chemical reactions, in particular the formation of sulfuric acid. Sulfur dioxide dissolved in fog droplets, perhaps aided by the presence of alkaline material such as ammonia or coal ash. Once in solution the sulfur was oxidized, a process often catalyzed by the presence of dissolved metallic ions such as iron and manganese. Dissolution and oxidation of sulfur dioxide gave rise to sulfuric

GALE ENCYCLOPEDIA OF ENVIRONMENTAL HEALTH

acid droplets, and it was sulfuric acid that made the smog so damaging to the health of Londoners.

London's severe smog occurred throughout the last decades of the nineteenth century. British-Canadian detective writer Robert Barr (1849–1912) even published *The Doom of London* at the turn of the century, which saw the entire population of London eliminated by an apocalyptic fog.

Twentieth-century London smog

Many residents of Victorian London recognized that the fogs increased death rates, but the most infamous twentieth-century incident occurred in 1952, when a slow-moving anti-cyclone stalled the air over the city. On the first morning, the fog was thicker than many people could ever remember. By the afternoon people noticed the choking smell in the air and started experiencing discomfort. Those who walked about in the fog found their skin and clothing filthy after just a short time. At night, the treatment of respiratory cases was running at twice its normal level. The situation continued for four days.

It was difficult to describe exactly what had happened, because primitive air pollution monitoring equipment could not cope with high and rapidly changing concentrations of pollutants, but it has been argued that for short periods the smoke and sulfur dioxide concentrations may have approached ten thousand micrograms per 1.3 cubic yards (1 cubic meters).

While London smog conditions generally improved with the decades of the twentieth century, such was not the case between December 5 and December 9, 1952, when the Great Smog of '52 or Big Smoke, as it was called, occurred. During these four days, windless cold weather combined with factory emissions to render visibility practically nil. Pea-soup conditions were not unusual for London, but these conditions were proven to be unusually severe. Later medical reports found that about four thousand people had died prematurely, probably because of the air pollution. The government, barraged with questions, set up an investigative committee, and its findings eventually served as the basis for the U.K. **Clean Air Act** of 1956. This law was gradually adopted through many towns and cities of the United Kingdom and was seen by many as a model piece of legislation. In addition, wide use of electricity in homes reduced, if it did not completely eliminate, the use of coal-burning heaters, a chief source of urban smoke.

Los Angeles summer smog

Photochemical smog is sometimes called summer smog, because unlike the classical London type, this smog is more typical in summer, often because it requires long hours of sunshine to build up. When photochemical smog was first noticed in Los Angeles, California, in the United States, people believed it to be much the same as the smog of London and Pittsburgh, Pennsylvania. Early attempts at control looked largely at local industry emissions. The automobile was eliminated as a likely cause because of low concentrations of sulfur in the fuel and the fact that only minute amounts of smoke were generated.

It was some time before Dutch biochemist Arie Jan Haagen-Smit (1900–1977) recognized that damage to crops in the Los Angeles area arose not from familiar pollutants, but from a reaction that takes place in the presence of petroleum vapors and sunlight. His observations focused unwelcome attention on the automobile as an important factor in the generation of summer smog.

The Los Angeles basin proved an almost perfect place for generating smog of this type. It had a huge number of cars and heavy commuter traffic, long hours of sunshine, gentle sea breezes to help pollutants accumulate up against the mountains, and high level inversions preventing the pollutants from dispersing vertically.

Studies through the 1950s revealed that the smog was generated through a photolytic cycle. Sunlight split nitrogen dioxide into nitric oxide and atomic oxygen that could subsequently react and form **ozone** (O_3). This was the key pollutant that clearly distinguished the Los Angeles smog from that occuring in London. Although the highly reactive ozone reacts rapidly with nitric oxide, converting it back into nitrogen dioxide, organic radicals produced from petroleum vapor react with nitric oxide very quickly. The nitrogen dioxide is again split by the sunlight, leading to the formation of more ozone. The cycle continues to build ozone concentrations to higher levels throughout the day.

The nitrogen oxide-ozone cycle is just one of many processes initiated in a smog of this kind. The photochemically active atmosphere contains a great number of reactive molecular fragments that lead to a range of complex organic compounds. Some of the hydrocarbon molecules of petroleum vapor are oxidized to aldehydes or ketones, such as acrolein or formaldehyde, which are irritants and suspected carcinogens. Some oxygenated fragments of organic molecules react with the nitrogen oxides present in the atmosphere. The best-known product of these reactions is peroxyacetyl nitrate, often called **PAN**, one of a class of nitrated compounds causing eye irritation experienced in summer smog.

The reactions that were recognized in the Los Angeles smog are now known to occur over wide areas of the industrialized world. The production of smog of this kind is not limited to urban or suburban areas but may occur for many hundreds of miles to the lee of cities using large quantities of liquid fuel. The importance of hydrocarbons in sustaining the processes that generate photochemical smog has given rise to control policies that recognize the need to lower the emission of hydrocarbons into the atmosphere. Hence, these policies have emphasized the use of catalytic converters and low volatility fuels as part of air pollution control strategies.

Demographics

Summer smog occurs in areas where heavy traffic involving motorized vehicles are present, along with climate conditions that include high temperatures (during the summer months) and calm winds. Serious smog problems exist in many metropolitan areas around the world. In the United States, smog exists in California from San Francisco in the north to San Diego in the south. On the East Coast, smog exists from above Boston, Massachusetts, to Washington, DC. Many other large cities in the United States also experience smog. In fact, most U.S. cities with populations over 250,000 people have problems with smog. The U.S. **Environmental Protection Agency** reports that over half of all Americans live in areas where pollution levels, including smog, exceed U.S. air quality standards. In addition, Mexico City, Mexico, and Beijing, China, are two well-known cities that regularly experience smog conditions.

Causes and symptoms

Smog is caused by a series of photochemical reactions involving volatile organic compounds (VOCs), nitrogen oxides and sunlight. These complex reactions form ground-level ozone, which produce smog. Pollutants from power plants, factories, motorized vehicle exhaust, and consumer products help to form smog. Smog can cause symptoms respiratory problems such as dyspnea (difficulty breathing), hypopnea (shallow breathing), hyperpnea (deep breathing), tachypnea (rapid breathing), and, in extreme cases, apnea (absence of breathing). Eye irritation is one symptom that is common to all smog-related illnesses.

Common diseases and disorders

Smog can cause such respiratory disorders as **asthma**, chronic **bronchitis**, and **emphysema**. People most susceptible to such respiratory problems—and thus who are at risk for smog conditions where they live—are:
- Children: especially active children who spend plenty of time playing outside in the summer when smog is present, and children who have asthma and other respiratory problems
- Adults: especially those who are active outside such as during work or while exercising when smog is present
- People with respiratory diseases: those with chronic respiratory ailments are more vulnerable to the effects of ozone; that is, they experience more serious symptoms and for longer periods
- People with unusual susceptibility to smog: those that are genetically more sensitive to ozone and other pollutants than are other people
- Elderly people: generally, older people are more susceptible to respiratory diseases, have more chronic diseases and ailments, and have a weaker immune system than do younger people, which all contribute to being more vulnerable to smog

> **KEY TERMS**
>
> **Cap and trade**—Part of environmental policy that uses a mandatory cap on emissions while providing flexibility on how to comply with the rules.
>
> **Carbon monoxide**—With the chemical formula CO (where C stands for carbon, and O for oxygen), a colorless, odorless, and tasteless gas that is toxic to humans in higher than normal concentrations.
>
> **Fossil fuels**—Any type of fuel, such as coal, natural gas, peat, and petroleum, derived from the decomposed remains of prehistoric plants and animals.
>
> **Nitrogen dioxide**—With the chemical formula NO_2 (where N stands for nitrogen, and O for oxygen), a reddish-brown toxic gas that is one of several nitrogen oxides.
>
> **Sulfur dioxide**—With the chemical formula SO_2 (where S stands for sulfur, and O for oxygen), a toxic gas with a strong, irritating smell; in nature it is released from spewing volcanoes and it is also released by human-producing industrial processes.

Public health role and response

Federal and state governments in the United States promote many solutions to smog. Laws encourage automobile manufacturers to develop motorized vehicles that produce fewer emissions. Chemical companies are being regulated and inspected more carefully given that they produce potentially harmful substances that can produce health risks to humans and other living creatures.

The U.S. **Environmental Protection Agency (EPA)** uses the Air Quality Index (AQI) to communicate to the public the pollution levels in different parts of the country. For example, ozone concentrations above 125 parts per billion are stated as "very unhealthy." The AQI is based on five pollutants: ground-level ozone, carbon monoxide, nitrogen dioxide, particulate matter, and sulfur dioxide.

The **EPA** also maintains the National Ambient Air Quality Standards (**NAAQS**) as part of its directive under the U.S. Clean Air Act of 1963. This Act and the NAAQS were created to protect human health from the adverse effects of pollutants.

Prognosis

In July 2010, the Environmental Protection Agency proposed the Cross-State Air Pollution Rule (CSAPR) to protect the health of Americans by reducing the air emissions of sulfur dioxide (SO_2) and nitrogen oxides (NO_x). The EPA estimated that from 2012 (the year the rule would go into effect) to 2014, the transport rule would reduce power-plant emissions of SO_2 and NO_x by 64% and 35%, respectively. However, in August 2012, the U.S. Court of Appeals struck down the EPA transport rule, saying the EPA overstepped its authority in requiring states to excessively reduce their emissions of pollutants. Consequently, the EPA reverted to its 2005 Clean Air Interstate Rule (CAIR). The CAIR covers 27 eastern states and the District of Columbia by using a cap-and-trade system to reduce the pollutants of sulfur dioxide and nitrogen oxides. One of the goals of this rule is to provide solutions to the problem of pollution drifting from one state to another from the emissions of power plants.

Prevention

Air pollution may be prevented only if individuals and businesses stop using toxic substances that cause air pollution in the first place. This change would require the cessation of all fossil fuel-burning processes, from industrial manufacturing to home use of air conditioners. This is a very unlikely scenario at the present. However, smog can be diminished by reducing the amount of air pollution. This can be done by reducing the use of all toxic substances that cause air pollution. With current technology, this would involve reducing the use of fossil fuel-burning processes. The use of more efficient and less polluting fossil fuel-burning devices is possible. Motor vehicles are a major source of pollution, so converting to cleaner running internal combustion engines or replacing such engines with cleaner running motors (such as electric) is one way to reduce smog. Driving fewer miles with existing motor vehicles or carpooling are other ways to cut down on smog. Using public transportation rather than individual vehicles also reduces smog conditions in major metropolitan areas. Instead of using coal to generate electricity, wind turbines, solar energy, geothermal, and other cleaner forms of electricity-generating means can help to reduce smog.

Many organizations have formed to reduce smog. For instance, the Galveston-Houston Association for Smog Prevention (GHASP) was formed to "persuade government and corporate officials to prevent smog." According to the GHASP website, the organization "seeks to accomplish its mission by being the most credible advocate for clean air in the Houston region; by supporting efforts to educate the public; and by directly engaging government officials, community leaders, the media and industry on regional air pollution issues."

Resources

BOOKS

Feinstein, Stephen. *Solving the Air Pollution Problem: What You Can Do*. Berkeley Heights, NJ: Enslow, 2011.

Franchetti, Matthew John, and Defne Apul. *Carbon Footprint Analysis: Concepts, Methods, Implementation, and Case Studies*. Boca Raton, FL: CRC Press, 2013.

Gold, Susan Dudley. *Clean Air and Clean Water Acts*. New York: Marshall Cavendish Benchmark, 2012.

Holloway, Ann M., and Richard P. Wayne. *Atmospheric Chemistry*. Cambridge, UK: Royal Society of Chemistry, 2010.

Manahan, Stanley E. *Environmental Chemistry*. Boca Raton, FL: CRC Press, 2010.

Phalen, Robert F., and Robert N. Phalen. *Introduction to Air Pollution Science: A Public Health Perspective*. Burlington, MA: Jones & Bartlett Learning, 2013.

Schumann, Ulrich, ed. *Atmospheric Physics*. Berlin: Springer, 2012.

Tiwary, Abhishek, and Jeremy Colls. *Air Pollution: Measurement, Modelling and Mitigation*. London: Routledge, 2010.

QUESTIONS TO ASK YOUR DOCTOR

- Am I susceptible to the health effects of smog?
- How can smog be harmful to me?
- What are the health risks associated smog?

WEBSITES

Citizens' Environmental Coalition. "Galveston/Houston Association for Smog Prevention." http://www.cechouston.org/2006/03/07/galvestonhouston-association-for-smog-prevention/ (accessed September 20, 2012).

Environmental Protection Agency. "Air Pollutants." http://www.epa.gov/oar/airpollutants.html (accessed September 10, 2012).

Environmental Protection Agency. "Air Quality and Public Health." http://www.epa.gov/oia/air/pollution.htm (accessed September 10, 2012).

Environmental Protection Agency. "Clean Air Interstate Rule (CAIR)." http://www.epa.gov/airmarkets/progsregs/cair/index.html (accessed September 21, 2012).

Environmental Protection Agency. "Cross-State Air Pollution Rule (CSAPR)." http://www.epa.gov/airtransport/ (accessed September 20, 2012).

Environmental Protection Agency. "National Ambient Air Quality Standards (NAAQS)." http://www.epa.gov/air/criteria.html (accessed September 10, 2012).

Hopey, Don. "U.S. Court Strikes Down Federal Pollution Regulation." Pittsburgh Post-Gazette.com. http://www.post-gazette.com/stories/news/environment/us-court-strikes-down-federal-pollution-regulation-649927/ (accessed September 10, 2012).

McIntyre, Douglas. "The 10 Cities with the World's Worst Air." DailyFinance.com. http://www.dailyfinance.com/2010/11/29/10-cities-with-worlds-worst-air/ (accessed September 10, 2012).

Nolen, Janice. "5 Steps to Clean Up Air Pollution." Scientific American. http://www.scientificamerican.com/article.cfm?id=5-steps-to-clean-up (accessed September 10, 2012).

ThinkQuest. "Smog." http://library.thinkquest.org/26026/Environmental_Problems/smog.html (accessed September 20, 2012).

ORGANIZATIONS

American Lung Association, 1301 Pennsylvania Ave. NW, Ste. 800, Washington, DC 20004, (202) 785-3355, Fax: (202) 452-1805, (800) 621-8335, http://www.lung.org.

Environmental Protection Agency, 1200 Pennsylvania Ave. NW, Ariel Rios Bldg., Washington, DC 20460, (202) 272-0167, http://www.epa.gov.

Peter Brimblecombe, PhD
William A. Atkins, BB, BS, MBA

Smoking

Definition

Smoking is the inhalation of the smoke of burning tobacco encased in cigarettes, pipes, and cigars. Casual smoking is the act of smoking only occasionally, usually in a social situation or to relieve stress. A smoking habit is a physical addiction to tobacco products. Many health experts now regard habitual smoking as a psychological addiction with serious health consequences.

Description

Nicotine is the active ingredient in tobacco. In smoking, it is inhaled into the lungs, where most of it stays. The rest passes into the bloodstream, reaching the brain in about 10 seconds and dispersing throughout the body in about 20 seconds. The United States **Food and Drug Administration** (FDA) has asserted that cigarettes and smokeless tobacco should be considered nicotine delivery devices.

Depending on the circumstances and the amount consumed, nicotine can act as either a stimulant or a tranquilizer. This can explain why some people report that smoking gives them energy and stimulates their mental activity, while others note that smoking relieves anxiety and relaxes them. The initial "kick" that comes from smoking results in part from the drug's stimulation of the adrenal glands and resulting release of epinephrine into the bloodstream. Epinephrine causes several physiological changes: it temporarily narrows the arteries, raises the blood pressure, raises the levels of fat in the blood, and increases the heart rate and flow of blood from the heart. Some researchers think epinephrine release contributes to smokers' increased risk of high blood pressure.

When a person smokes, he or she is ingesting a lot more than nicotine. Smoke from a cigarette, pipe, or cigar is made up of many additional toxic chemicals, including tar and carbon monoxide. Tar is a sticky substance that forms into deposits in the lungs, causing lung cancer and respiratory distress. Carbon monoxide limits the amount of oxygen that the red blood cells can convey throughout your body. Also, it may damage the inner walls of the arteries, which allows fat to build up in them.

Besides tar, nicotine, and carbon monoxide, tobacco smoke contains 4,000 different chemicals. More than 200 of these chemicals are known to be toxic. Nonsmokers who are exposed to tobacco smoke also take in these toxic chemicals. They inhale the smoke exhaled by the smoker as well as sidestream smoke—the smoke from the end of the burning cigarette, cigar, or pipe. Sidestream smoke is more toxic than exhaled smoke. When a person smokes, many toxic chemicals remain in the lungs, so the exhaled smoke contains fewer poisonous chemicals. This smoke is dangerous even for a nonsmoker.

Some brands of cigarettes are advertised as "low tar," but no cigarette is safe. If smokers switch to a low-tar cigarette, they are likely to inhale longer and more deeply to get the chemicals their body craves. A smoker has to quit the habit entirely in order to improve his health and decrease the chance of disease.

Although some people believe chewing tobacco is safer, it also carries health risks. People who chew tobacco have an increased risk of heart disease and mouth and throat cancer. Pipe and cigar smokers have increased health risks as well, even though these smokers generally do not inhale as deeply as cigarette smokers do. These groups have not been studied as extensively as cigarette smokers. There is some evidence that they may be at a slightly lower risk of cardiovascular problems but a higher risk of cancer and various types of circulatory conditions.

Risk factors

Socioeconomic factors play a role in who is likely to begin smoking. Two major indicators are low income and low level of education. In addition, people who live with smokers or who come from families where smoking is considered acceptable are more likely to begin smoking.

Researchers think that genetic factors may contribute substantially to developing a smoking habit. Several twin studies have led to estimates of 46–84% heritability for smoking. It is thought that some genetic variations affect the speed of nicotine metabolism in the body and the activity level of nicotinic receptors in the brain.

Demographics

According to the **Centers for Disease Control and Prevention** (CDC), in 2010 (data reported in 2012), 19.3% of Americans over age 18 (more than 45.3 million people) were smokers. Men comprised 21.5% of smokers while 17.3% of women smoked. From ages 18–64, the rate of smoking is about 21%, but the rate drops drastically after age 65 to 9.5%.

In the United States, more Native Americans smoke than any other racial or ethnic group (31.4%), while Asian Americans smoke the least (9.2&%). The more education a person has, the less likely he or she is to smoke. About 45.2% of adults who have obtained a GED diploma smoke compared to 6.2% of people with a postgraduate college degree.

The highest rates of smoking are found in the Southeast and Midwest. Utah has the lowest rate of smoking (9.1%) and West Virginia the highest (26.8%). Substantially more people whose incomes fall below the poverty level smoke than those whose incomes are at or above the poverty level.

Causes and symptoms

No one starts smoking intending to become addicted to nicotine. It is not known how much nicotine may be consumed before the body becomes addicted. However, once smoking becomes habitual, the smoker faces a lifetime of health risks.

Smoking risks

Smoking is recognized as the leading preventable cause of death in the United States. According to the CDC, each year smoking causes approximately 443,000 deaths and secondhand smoke contributes to almost 50,000 more. Smoking causes more deaths than human immunodeficiency virus (HIV), illegal drug use, alcohol use, motor vehicle injuries, suicides, and murders combined. Smokers live on average 12 years less than non-smokers. In addition people who smoke have an increased chance of developing cancer of the lung, esophagus, lips and mouth, larynx, pancreas, kidney, urinary bladder and cervix (women); increased likelihood of developing chronic respiratory diseases such as **emphysema**, **asthma**, and chronic **bronchitis**; and cardiovascular disease, such as heart attack, high blood pressure, stroke, and atherosclerosis (narrowing and hardening of the arteries). The risk of stroke is especially high in women who take oral contraceptives (birth control pills).

Smoking can damage fertility, making it harder to conceive, and it can interfere with the growth of the fetus during pregnancy. It accounts for an estimated 14% of premature births and 10% of infant deaths. There is some evidence that smoking may cause impotence in some men.

Because smoking affects so many of the body's systems, smokers often have vitamin deficiencies and suffer oxidative damage caused by free radicals. Free radicals are molecules that steal electrons from other molecules, turning the other molecules into free radicals and destabilizing the molecules in the body's cells.

Recent research reveals that passive smokers, or those who unavoidably breathe in second-hand tobacco smoke, have an increased chance of many health problems such as lung cancer and asthma, and in children, sudden infant death syndrome.

Smokers' symptoms

Smokers are likely to exhibit a variety of symptoms that reveal the damage caused by smoking. A nagging morning cough may be one sign of a tobacco habit. Other symptoms include shortness of breath, wheezing, and frequent occurrences of respiratory illness, such as bronchitis. Smoking also increases fatigue and decreases the smoker's sense of smell and taste. Smokers are more likely to develop poor circulation, with cold hands and feet and premature wrinkles.

Sometimes the illnesses that result from smoking come on silently with little warning. For instance, coronary artery disease may exhibit few or no symptoms. At other times, there will be warning signs, such as a hacking cough that brings up phlegm or blood—a sign of lung cancer.

Withdrawal symptoms

A smoker who tries to quit may expect one or more of these withdrawal symptoms: nausea, constipation or diarrhea, drowsiness, loss of concentration, insomnia, headache, nausea, and irritability.

Diagnosis

Smokers know they smoke. They do not need a doctor to tell them they are addicted. However, because it is hard to quit smoking, it may be wise for a smoker to turn to a healthcare practitioner for help. For the greatest success in quitting and to help with the withdrawal symptoms, the smoker should talk over a treatment plan with his doctor or alternative practitioner. Often, the smoker will have a general physical examination to gauge general health status and uncover any smoking-related health problems along with developing a smoking cessation treatment plan.

Treatment

Research shows that most smokers who want to quit benefit from the support of other people. It helps to quit with a friend or to join a group such as those organized by the American Cancer Society. These groups provide support and teach behavior modification methods that can help the smoker quit. The smoker's physician can often refer him to such groups or to a psychotherapist who has experience treating people who are trying to quit smoking.

For those who do quit, the benefits to health are worth the effort. Once a smoker quits, the health effects are immediate and dramatic. After the first day, oxygen and carbon monoxide levels in the blood return to normal. At two days, nerve endings begin to grow back and the senses of taste and smell revive. Within two weeks to three months, circulation and breathing improve. After one year of not smoking, the risk of heart disease is reduced by 50%. After 15 years of abstinence, the risks of health problems from smoking virtually vanish. A smoker who quits for good often feels better, with less fatigue and fewer respiratory illnesses.

Nicotine replacement

It is very difficult to simply stop smoking. The greatest success rate in quitting smoking is achieved by people who seek help with the withdrawal symptoms. Common smoking cessation aides provide nicotine replacement therapy in the form of gum, patches, nasal sprays, and oral inhalers. These are available by prescription or over the counter. A health care provider can give advice on how to use them.

Nicotine replacement therapies release a small amount of nicotine into the bloodstream, satisfying the smoker's physical craving for nicotine. Over time, the amount of nicotine is decreased (e.g., the amount of nicotine gum the smoker chews or the strength of the nicotine patch is decreased). This helps wean the smoker from nicotine slowly, eventually beating his addiction to the drug. However, if the person begins smoking again while using a nicotine replacement therapy, nicotine overdose may cause serious health problems.

Drugs therapy

The prescription drug Zyban (bupropion hydrochloride) is an antidepressant that has shown success in helping smokers quit. This drug contains no nicotine and was originally developed as an antidepressant. It is unclear exactly how bupropion works to suppress the desire for nicotine. A five-year study of bupropion reported that the drug has a very good record for safety and effectiveness in treating tobacco dependence. Its most common side effect is insomnia, which can also result from nicotine withdrawal.

Varenicline (Chantix) was approved by the FDA in 2006 for treatment of smoking addiction. The drug reduces the desire for nicotine by stimulating the same receptors in the brain as nicotine, but more weakly, thus reducing the craving for nicotine. The drug is approved for use in people over age 18 for 12 weeks. In 2011, a study found that the drug increased the risk of serious cardiovascular events. As of mid-2012, the drug is still available and research on side effects continues.

Alternative treatment

A wide range of alternative and complementary treatments help some smokers stop smoking. These include hypnotherapy, herbs, acupuncture, and meditation. Many people use these treatments in addition to, rather than as a substitute for nicotine replacement or drug therapy.

Hypnotherapy

Hypnotherapy helps the smoker achieve a trance-like state, during which the deepest levels of the mind are accessed. A session with a hypnotherapist may begin with a discussion of whether the smoker really wants to and truly is motivated to stop smoking. The therapist will explain how hypnosis can reduce the stress-related symptoms that sometimes come with quitting smoking.

Often the therapist will discuss the dangers of smoking with the patient and begin to "reframe' the patient's thinking about smoking. Many smokers are convinced they cannot quit and the therapist can help persuade them that they can change this behavior. These suggestions are then repeated while the smoker is under hypnosis. The therapist may also suggest while the smoker is under hypnosis that his feelings of worry, anxiety, and irritability will decrease.

In a review of 17 studies of the effectiveness of hypnotherapy, the percentage of people treated by hypnosis who still were not smoking after six months ranged from 4–8%. In programs that included several hours of treatment, intense interpersonal interaction, individualized suggestions, and follow-up treatment, success rates were above 50%.

Aromatherapy

One study demonstrated that inhaling the vapor from black pepper extract may reduce symptoms associated with smoking withdrawal. Other essential oils can be used for relieving the anxiety a smoker often experiences while quitting.

Herbs

A variety of herbs may help smokers reduce their cravings for nicotine, calm their irritability, and even reverse the oxidative cellular damage done by smoking. Lobelia, sometimes called Indian tobacco, has historically been used as a substitute for tobacco. It contains a substance called lobeline, which decreases the craving for nicotine by bolstering the nervous system and calming the smoker. In high doses, lobelia can cause vomiting but the average dose—about 10 drops per day—should pose no problems.

To reduce the oral fixation supplied by a nicotine habit, a smoker can chew on licorice root (the plant, not the candy). Licorice is good for the liver, which has a major role in the body's detoxification process. Licorice also acts as a tonic for the adrenal system, which helps reduce stress. As an added incentive, if a smoker smokes a cigarette after chewing on licorice root, the cigarette tastes like burned cardboard.

Other botanicals that may help repair free-radical damage to the lungs and cardiovascular system are those high in flavonoids, such as hawthorn, gingko biloba, and bilberry, as well as antioxidants such as vitamin A, vitamin C, zinc, and selenium.

Acupuncture

This ancient Chinese method of healing often is used to help diminish addictions, including smoking.

KEY TERMS

Antioxidant—Any substance that reduces the damage caused by oxidation, such as the harm caused by free radicals.

Chronic bronchitis—A smoking-related respiratory illness in which the membranes that line the bronchi, or the lung's air passages, narrow over time. Symptoms include breathlessness, wheezing, and a morning cough that brings up phlegm.

Emphysema—An incurable, smoking-related disease, in which the air sacs at the end of the lung's bronchi become weak and inefficient. People with emphysema often first notice shortness of breath, repeated wheezing, and coughing that brings up phlegm.

Epinephrine—A nervous system hormone stimulated by the nicotine in tobacco. It increases heart rate and may raise smokers' blood pressure.

Flavonoid—A food chemical that helps to limit oxidative damage to the body's cells and protects against heart disease and cancer.

Free radical—An unstable molecule that causes oxidative damage by stealing electrons from surrounding molecules, thereby disrupting activity in the body's cells.

Nicotine—The addictive ingredient of tobacco, which acts on the nervous system and is both stimulating and calming.

Nicotine replacement therapy—A method of weaning a smoker away from both nicotine and the oral fixation that accompanies a smoking habit by giving the smoker smaller and smaller doses of nicotine in the form of a patch or gum.

Sidestream smoke—The smoke that is emitted from the burning end of a cigarette or cigar or that comes from the end of a pipe. Along with exhaled smoke, it is a constituent of second-hand smoke.

The acupuncturist will use hair-thin needles to stimulate the body's *qi*, or healthy energy. Acupuncture is a sophisticated treatment system based on revitalizing qi, which supposedly flows through the body in defined pathways called meridians. According to acupuncture theory, in an individual with an addiction, qi is not flowing smoothly and needs to be unblocked.

Vitamins

Smoking depletes vitamin C in the body, which may leave it more susceptible to infections. Vitamin C helps to prevent or reduce free-radical damage by acting as an antioxidant in the lungs. Smokers may need Vitamin C in higher dosage than nonsmokers.

Fish in the diet supplies Omega-3 fatty acids, which are associated with a reduced risk of chronic obstructive pulmonary disease (emphysema or chronic bronchitis) in smokers. Omega-3 fats also provide cardiovascular benefits as well as an anti-depressive effect. Vitamin therapy does not reduce nicotine craving but it can help modify some of the damage created by smoking.

Public health role and response

The United States has committed massive amounts of money to public health campaigns to get people to stop smoking. One of the goals of Healthy People 2020, a set of health targets for Americans issued every ten years, is to reduce the number of smokers to 12% of the population. As of 2012, it appears unlikely that this goal will be met.

In addition to federal public health campaigns to eliminate smoking, individual states have developed anti-smoking programs. California has been one of the leaders in aggressively working to reduce the rate of smoking among its residents. Besides public health campaigns and public service announcements, many states and cities have passed strict anti-smoking ordinances that forbid smoking in public buildings such as restaurants, airports, and schools. Some of these laws have been extended to include outdoor areas such as public parks.

Aside from government activity, the marketplace reinforces the message that smoking is harmful by charging smokers more for health and life insurance. Many private companies have introduced smoking cessation programs at work as a way of reducing the cost of health care for their employees.

Prevention

The best way to prevent health problems associated with smoking is to not start. However, quitting,

> ## QUESTIONS TO ASK YOUR DOCTOR
>
> - Can you refer me to a self-help group for stopping smoking?
> - In your experience, what works best - nicotine patch, gum, lozenge, or inhaler?
> - I have tried nicotine replacement therapy without complete success. Should I consider prescription drug therapy?
> - How long will I continue to crave cigarettes?
> - I work in a bar where smoking is permitted. How concerned should I be about the effects of secondhand smoke on my health?

even if one has been a heavy smoker, provides substantial health benefits. For people who already smoke, some successful aids in quitting include:

- Have a plan and set a definite quit date.
- Get rid of all the cigarettes and ashtrays at home or in your desk at work.
- Do not allow others to smoke in your house.
- Tell your friends and neighbors that you are quitting. Doing so helps make quitting a matter of pride.
- Chew sugarless gum or eat sugar-free hard candy to redirect the oral fixation that comes with smoking. This will prevent weight gain, too.
- Eat as much as you want but only low-calorie foods and drinks. Drink plenty of water. This may help with the feelings of tension and restlessness that quitting can bring. After 8–12 weeks, you will lose much of your craving for tobacco and can return to your usual eating habits.
- Stay away from social situations that prompt you to smoke. Dine in the nonsmoking section of restaurants.
- Spend the money you save not smoking on an occasional treat for yourself.

Resources

BOOKS

Bevins, Rick A., and Anthony R. Caggiula. *The Motivational Impact of Nicotine and Its Role in Tobacco Use*. Nebraska Symposium on Motivation. New York: Springer, 2008.

Kuhar, Michael. *The Addicted Brain: Why We Abuse Drugs, Alcohol, and Nicotine*. Upper Saddle River, NJ: FT Press, 2012.

WEBSITES

Centers for Disease Control and Prevention (CDC). "Smoking and Tobacco Use." May 8, 2012 [accessed June 27, 2012]. http://www.cdc.gov/tobacco.

"Smoking." MedlinePlus undated [accessed June 27, 2012]. http://www.nlm.nih.gov/medlineplus/smoking.html

Murphy, Timothy D. "Passive Smoking and Lung Disease." Medscape.com March 5, 2012 [accessed June 27, 2012]. http://emedicine.medscape.com/article/1005579-overview

National Institutes of Health (NIH). "Smoking." February 20, 2012 [accessed June 27, 2012]. http://health.nih.gov/topic/Smoking.

Office of the Surgeon General. "Tobacco." 2012 [accessed June 27, 2012]. http://www.surgeongeneral.gov/tobacco.

"Quitting Smoking." MedlinePlus undated [accessed June 27, 2012]. http://www.nlm.nih.gov/medlineplus/quittings moking.html

ORGANIZATIONS

American Cancer Society, 1599 Clifton Rd., NE, Atlanta, GA 30329, (404) 320-3333, (800) ACS-2345, http://www.cancer.org.

American Lung Association, 1301 Pennsylvania Ave., NW Suite 800, Washington, DC 20004, (212) 315-8700, (800)LUNG-USA [(800) 548-8252]

National Institute on Drug Abuse, 6001 Executive Boulevard, Room 5213, Bethesda, MD 20892-9561, (301) 443-1124; en espanole (240) 221-4007, information@nida.nih.gov, http://drugabuse.gov/nidahome.html.

United States Centers for Disease Control and Prevention (CDC), 1600 Clifton Road, Atlanta, GA 30333, (404) 639-3534, 800-CDC-INFO (800-232-4636). TTY: (888) 232-6348, inquiry@cdc.gov, http://www.cdc.gov.

World Health Organization, Avenue Appia 20, 1211 Geneva 27, Switzerland, +22 41 791 21 11, Fax: +22 41 791 31 11, info@who.int, http://www.who.int.

Barbara Boughton
Tish Davidson, AM

Snail fever *see* **Schistosomiasis**

Soil Conservation Act (1935)

Definition

The Soil Conservation Act of 1935 was enacted on April 27, 1935, and established the Soil Conservation Service, which sought to "control floods, prevent impairment of reservoirs and maintain the navigability of rivers and harbors, protect public health, public lands and relieve unemployment."

Purpose

The act gave farmers monetary subsidies to plant vegetation other than commercial crops in an attempt to correct the depletion of nutrients in the soil that had occurred as a result of overfarming. The law was written in response to the dust storms of the early 1930s, which caused significant ecological and agricultural damage to prairie land in what is commonly thought to be the worst man-made ecological disaster in U.S. history.

Description

History

In the 1930s, significant damage was done to agricultural productivity in the Midwest in an event known as the Dust Bowl, during which time soil was swept off the fields into dust clouds that destroyed crops and reduced land productivity. Before this act was adopted, farmers had no reason to conserve land, and the economic incentive to produce as much food as possible to sell at market drove the agricultural industry to use all available land for growing, rather than letting fields rest or rotating crops. The farming methods of the time showed little consideration for the quality of the soil, which eventually became thin and nutrient-poor.

Amendments

In March 1936, the Soil Conservation and Domestic Allotment Act was enacted, which provided for farmers to reduce production in an effort to conserve nutrients in the soil. It strengthened protections for sharecroppers and tenant farmers (landlords had previously not been required to share the subsidy with those who worked the land) and reduced the crop surplus. Additional measures were taken to educate farmers on how to use their land without causing further soil degradation.

The Soil and Water Resources Conservation Act of 1977 provided the U.S. Department of Agriculture (USDA) with broad strategic assessment and planning authority to strengthen the conservation, protection, and enhancement of soil, water, and related natural resources nationwide. Furthermore, these changes allowed the federal government to assess the status of resources on nonfederal land and evaluate programs and policies.

Results

Four years after the initial act was adopted recorded wind-inflicted soil erosion was reduced by 65%. The act was widely praised and touted by the White House as urging farmers to be socially minded and to do something for all instead of themselves.

Resources

WEBSITES

Glass, A. "FDR Signs Soil Conservation Act, April 27, 1935." http://www.politico.com/news/stories/0410/36362.html(accessed October 17, 2012).

National Resources Conservation Service. "Soil and Water Resources Conservation Act (RCA)." U.S. Department of Agriculture. http://www.nrcs.usda.gov/wps/portal/nrcs/main/national/technical/nra/rca(accessed October 17, 2012).

Roosevelt, F. D. "Statement on the Signing the Soil Conservation and Domestic Allotment Act. Washington, DC: March 1, 1936." http://www.presidency.ucsb.edu/ws/index.php?pid = 15254 (accessed October 17, 2012).

Alyson C. Heimer, MA

Spanish influenza *see* **Flu pandemics**

Sulfur exposure

Definition

Sulfur exposure refers to events in which a human, other animal, or plant is exposed to the element sulfur or one of its compounds. The compound of primary health interest is sulfur dioxide (SO_2). The element's name is spelled *sulphur* in Europe and many other parts of the world.

Description

Sulfur is a nonmetallic chemical element in the oxygen family of elements. It occurs naturally in Earth's surface as the native element (S), as a sulfide mineral such as pyrite (iron sulfide) or cinnabar (**mercury** sulfide), or as a sulfate mineral such as gypsum (calcium sulfate) or barite (barium sulfate). Sulfur is the 17th most abundant element in Earth's crust and the 10th most abundant element in the universe. In pure form, it is a soft, bright yellow solid with a melting point of 115.21°C and a boiling point of 444.6°C. It is not a particularly reactive element, but it does burn easily to produce sulfur dioxide gas (SO_2). Sulfur dioxide has the sharp, suffocating odor characteristic of a burning match. Under certain conditions, sulfur dioxide can be further oxidized to produce the gas sulfur trioxide (SO_3), from which sulfuric acid is made. Sulfur also combines with hydrogen to form hydrogen sulfide (H_2S), with its own characteristic "rotten-egg" odor. Sulfur is also a minor, but essential, component of some important biochemical compounds, including two amino acids, cysteine and methionine. It is about the seventh most abundant element in the human body, with a concentration about the same as that of potassium and chlorine: 0.2 percent.

> **KEY TERMS**
>
> **Ambient**—Relating to surrounding conditions.
> **Acaracide**—A pesticide used to kill or disable arachnids.
> **Carcinogenic**—Tending to cause cancer.
> **Mutagenic**—Tending to cause mutations.
> **Teratogenic**—Tending to cause birth defects.

Risk factors

Sulfur occurs naturally in locations where molten rock and its by-products are carried to Earth's surface, as around the rim of a volcano or adjacent to geysers and hot springs. Very large reserves of natural sulfur may also occur in domes similar to veins of coal beneath the Earth's surface. At one time, these domes were mined by a procedure known as the Frasch process in which steam and hot water were pumped into a vein of sulfur and the molten element forced to the surface. The sulfur thus produced was very pure, but the cost of the technology eventually became greater than that of other methods for the production of sulfur, and is no longer used to any great extent today.

Compounds of sulfur, particularly sulfur dioxide and hydrogen sulfide, typically occur in combination with elemental sulfur in the natural world. Very large amounts of sulfur dioxide and sulfur trioxide are now produced by industrial activities. (Environmental scientists often refer to the two gases together as "oxides of sulfur.") The largest single source of sulfur dioxide produced by human activity (about three-fourths of all the gas thus released into the atmosphere) comes from fossil-fuel-burning power plants. Coal, oil, and natural gas all contain small amounts of elemental sulfur and sulfur compounds. When these fuels are burned in an industrial process, the sulfur is converted primarily to sulfur dioxide, which then tends to escape into the atmosphere through emission systems. An additional 20 percent of all sulfur dioxide produced by human actions comes from a variety of industrial processes. The extraction of metals from their ores and the combustion of high sulfur fuels by locomotives, large ships, and non-road equipment account for the remaining fraction of sulfur dioxide produced by human activity.

Elemental sulfur is also released into the environment as a result of human activity, primarily as a pesticide. Sulfur has been used for this purpose for at least two millennia, and it continues to be popular for use with certain types of crops and certain types of pests. For example, sulfur sprays are used on a number of commercial fruit and vegetable crops to control the growth of ticks, mites, and other arachnids.

Effects on public health

Elemental sulfur is thought to have few significant acute or chronic health effects on humans. Inhalation of sulfur dust may cause a burning sensation and cough, followed by a sore throat, while a deposit of sulfur dust on the skin may produce redness and burning. Sulfur dust in the eyes may result in a burning sensation, pain or discomfort, and short-term blurred vision, while ingestion of the dust can cause intestinal upset and distress. All of these symptoms disappear fairly readily, however, when exposure to sulfur dust ends.

Almost everyone is exposed to sulfur dioxide at some concentration in their daily lives. In the United States, largely due to governmental regulations, the atmospheric level of sulfur dioxide has been decreasing, from about 70 ppb (parts per billion) in 1965 to about 2.5 ppb in 2010. At current levels, sulfur dioxide exposure is likely to produce relatively modest health effects in humans, largely respiratory discomfort manifested as coughing, sneezing, and sore throat. These effects have little effect on the average person and can be a source of concern only for individuals with other respiratory problems, such as chronic **asthma**, or the elderly. Sulfur dioxide exposure is more of a concern to individuals who are exposed to higher concentrations of the gas, such as workers employed in industry where sulfur dioxide is used or produced, such as certain mining operations, paper manufacture, production or use of fertilizers and pesticides, and the production or use of food preservatives. Others who may be at risk for exposure to sulfur emissions include individuals who live in the vicinity of such plants and industrial operations. In the case of very high exposures to sulfur dioxide, respiratory effects may lead to very serious health problems which can include death from respiratory failure. Such circumstances are rare, however, and can be traced almost entirely to industrial accidents in which very large volumes of sulfur dioxide gas are produced over a very short period of time. No evidence is available to suggest that sulfur dioxide is carcinogenic, mutagenic, or teratogenic.

Public health role and response

The U.S. **Environmental Protection Agency (EPA)** has established standards for safe exposure to sulfur dioxide. The primary standard is for an exposure of no more than 75 ppb over a period of one hour, while the secondary standard is for an exposure to no more than 500 ppb over a three hour period, no more than once a year. The primary standard is designed to protect all Americans against deleterious health effects of sulfur dioxide, including those with special health problems and the elderly. The secondary standard is designed to protect individuals against all possible effects of the gas on all aspects of the environment, including damage to plants, other animals, physical structures, and atmospheric visibility.

Diagnosis

Blood tests are available for providing a differential diagnosis for sulfur dioxide poisoning, but signs and symptoms, along with recent patient history of possible exposure to the gas, are usually adequate to obtain a diagnosis for the condition.

Treatment

Primary treatment for all cases of sulfur exposure is removal of the patient from exposure to the gas, providing access to clean air as quickly as possible. Skin irritation can best be dealt with by thorough washing of the exposed area with soap and water. Ingestion of the gas typically requires no special treatment, although rehydration and electrolyte supplementation may be needed in the most severe cases.

Precautions

The primary method for avoiding health problems associated with sulfur dioxide exposure is to restrict to the extent possible one's exposure to the gas. This precaution is not a problem for most people since ambient

---

QUESTIONS TO ASK YOUR DOCTOR

- Given that we live in a large, busy, urban area, are there ever circumstances in which our family might be at risk for sulfur dioxide health-related problems?
- Are there first aid procedures or materials of which we should be aware in case of unexpected exposure to sulfur, sulfur dioxide, or other compounds of sulfur?
- What are the chances that my child may be exposed to harmful concentrations of sulfur in her high school science classes?
- I have heard that sulfur has certain health benefits. Would it be advisable for me to take a sulfur supplement to gain those benefits in my own life?

sulfur dioxide concentrations are so low. Individuals who work at locations where sulfur dioxide concentrations may be higher than average may require specialized protective equipment, such as a full-face mask, gloves, clothing that covers as much of their bodies as possible, and respirators or plant equipment that removes sulfur dioxide from the work atmosphere.

Prognosis

As noted above, health problems arising out of exposure to sulfur dioxide generally clear up when a person is removed to a source of clean air. Large-scale release of sulfur dioxide may required specialized medical treatment, but should also result in relatively rapid recovery.

Resources

BOOKS

Compton, Brian W. *Sulfur Dioxide: Properties, Applications and Hazards.* New York: Nova Science, 2011.

Richards, Gary F., and Tabatha E. Jones. *Revised Sulfur Dioxide Air Quality Standard: Costs & Benefits.* Hauppauge, NY: Nova Science, 2012.

Rom, William N. *Environmental Policy and Public Health: Air Pollution, Global Climate Change, and Wilderness.* San Francisco: Jossey-Bass, 2012.

Schmalensee, Richard, and R. N. Stavins. *The SO2 Allowance Trading System: The Ironic History of a Grand Policy Experiment.* Cambridge, MA: National Bureau of Economic Research, 2012.

PERIODICALS

Kelly, Frank J., et al. "Monitoring Air Pollution: Use of Early Warning Systems for Public Health." *Respirology* 17, 1 (2012): 7–19.

Namdeo, A., A. Tiwary, and E. Farrow. "Estimation of Age-related Vulnerability to Air Pollution: Assessment of Respiratory Health at Local Scale." *Environment International* 37, 5 (2011): 829–37.

Takeshita, Takayuki. "Global Scenarios of Air Pollutant Emissions from Road Transport through to 2050." *International Journal of Environmental Research and Public Health* 8, 7 (2011): 3032–62.

Wickham, L. "The Revised US National Standard for Sulfur Dioxide." *Air Quality and Climate Change* 45, 4 (2011): 12–14.

WEBSITES

"Chapter 7.4: Sulfur Dioxide." World Health Organization. http://www.euro.who.int/__data/assets/pdf_file/0020/123086/AQG2ndEd_7_4Sulfurdioxide.pdf. Accessed on October 25, 2012.

"Public Health Statement." Agency for Agency for Toxic Substances and Disease Registry. http://www.atsdr.cdc.gov/toxprofiles/tp116-c1.pdf. Accessed on October 25, 2012.

"Sulfur." PAN Pesticides Database. http://www.pesticideinfo.org/Detail_Chemical.jsp?Rec_Id=PC34501. Accessed on October 25, 2012.

"Sulfur Dioxide." Environmental Protection Agency. http://www.epa.gov/airquality/sulfurdioxide/index.html. Accessed on October 25, 2012.

ORGANIZATIONS

Environmental Protection Agency (EPA), Ariel Rios Bldg., 1200 Pensylvania Ave. NW, Washington, DC, 20460, (202) 272–0167, http://publicaccess.supportportal.com/ics/support/ticketnewwizard.asp?style=classic, http://www.epa.gov/.

David E. Newton, EdD

Sunstroke *see* **Heat disorders**

Superfund Amendments and Reauthorization Act (1986)

Definition

The Superfund Amendment and Reauthorization Act (SARA), commonly referred to as the Superfund, targets areas in the United States that require environmental clean up. The Superfund emphasizes the importance of remedial actions, specifically those that reduce the volume, toxicity, or mobility of hazardous substances, pollutants and contaminants. Targets for long-term remedial actions are listed on the National Priorities List, which is revised each year.

Purpose

Congress initially authorized **Comprehensive Environmental Response, Compensation, and Liability Act (CERCLA)** legislation in 1980 to clean up abandoned dump sites in the United States that contained **hazardous waste**. The activities mandated under **CERCLA** were to be administered by the **Environmental Protection Agency (EPA)**. The program was reauthorized in 1986 by SARA. Several provisions of CERCLA were changed or clarified.

Demographics

Superfund sites identified in the original legislation were virtually ignored during the early 1980s. Several key **EPA** officials resigned after they were charged with mismanaging the monies allocated by the original legislation. The EPA attempted to speed cleanup of contaminated sites, but progress was still too slow for critics, some members of Congress, and many citizens. When the program expired in September 1985, the cleanup activities at more than 200 sites were delayed for lack of funds. Concern about hazardous waste sites continued. This pressure on Congress was sufficient to facilitate reauthorization of CERCLA.

The Superfund was originally financed by a tax on receipt of hazardous waste and by a tax on domestic refined or imported crude oil and chemicals. The SARA reauthorization increased funding from $1.6 billion to $8.5 billion over five years. It also authorized the use of contributions from potentially responsible parties (persons who had created the environmental hazards or who currently owned the land where former dump sites were located). However, SARA declined to place the full financial burden of cleanup on oil and chemical companies. Funding is obtained from a broad-based combination of business and public contributions.

Results

As of August 2012, some 1,304 sites were on the National Priorities List, and 59 new sites were proposed. Between the advent of the NPL and that date, 360 sites were delisted.

Over 40,000 uncontrolled waste sites have been reported to U.S. federal agencies. Factors used to rank the severity of reported sites include the type, quantity, and toxicity of the substance(s) found at the site, as well as the number of people likely to be exposed, the pathways of exposure, and the vulnerability of the groundwater supply at the site. If a site poses immediate threats such as the risk of fire or explosion, the EPA may initiate short-term actions to remove those threats before actual cleanup begins.

Research and general acceptance

Critics charge that the number of hazardous waste sites nationwide is still underreported. Many states have developed their own programs to supplement the federal Superfund.

Under SARA guidelines, the **Agency for Toxic Substances and Disease Registry** performs health assessments at Superfund sites. This program, administered by the **Centers for Disease Control and Prevention**, also lists hazardous substances found on sites, prepares toxicological profiles, identifies gaps in research on health effects, and publishes findings.

Resources

BOOKS

Macey, G., and J. Z. Cannon, eds. *Reclaiming the Land: Rethinking Superfund Institutions, Methods, and Practices.* Berlin: Springer, 2006.

WEBSITES

U.S. Environmental Protection Agency. "National Priorities List." March 2, 2012. http://www.epa.gov/superfund/sites/npl/ (accessed August 16, 2012).

U.S. Environmental Protection Agency. "Superfund: Cleaning Up the Nation's Hazardous Wastes Sites." July 19, 2012. http://www.epa.gov/superfund/index.htm (accessed August 16, 2012).

ORGANIZATIONS

Environmental Protection Agency, 1200 Pennsylvania Ave. NW, Washington, DC 20460, (202) 272-0167, http://water.epa.gov.

L. Fleming Fallon, Jr, MD, DrPH
Stacey Chamberlin

Suppurative fasciitis *see* **Necrotizing fasciitis**

Swimming advisories

Definition

Swimming advisories are warnings that are issued to the public from government authorities responsible for testing of recreational fresh and salt waters that contact with beach water could cause illness. An advisory follows the results of testing that reveals potentially harmful levels of bacteria.

Description

Typically, water monitoring assesses levels of coliform bacteria (bacteria found in several environments, including feces) and sometimes more specifically *Escherichiacoli*, a type of bacteria found exclusively in feces, as a means of detecting the presence of feces in recreational waters. Since coliforms and *E.coli* do not survive for very long outside of the intestinal tract, their detection in water is an indication of recent fecal contamination. As a result, local authorities restrict use of water for recreational activities when the bacteria level exceeds standards for safe use.

The bacteria that are tested for are indicators of fecal pollution. They are used for testing because they can be detected quickly and inexpensively. Their presence in the water does not necessarily pose a health danger, since the coliforms may not be disease-causing. However, other bacteria in feces (such as species of

Salmonella, Vibrio, and Shigella) can be dangerous. As well, disease-causing **viruses** can be present in feces.

Common diseases and disorders

A beach may be closed when the level of water contamination poses a definite health risk. Mildly polluted water can cause conditions such as a headache, sore throat, or vomiting. Highly polluted water can cause hepatitis, **cholera**, and **typhoid fever**.

People are at risk when they swim or come into contact with polluted water. The risk of illness increases when a person swallows water. Furthermore, direct exposure to water sometimes causes skin and eye infections.

Resources

WEBSITES

United States Environmental Protection Agency (EPA). "Human Health: Advisories: Swimming Advisories." http://www.epa.gov/ebtpages/humaadvisoriesswimmingadvisories.html (accessed October 16, 2010).

Liz Swain

Swine flu *see* **H1N1 influenza A (2009)**

Synergistic gangrene *see* **Necrotizing fasciitis**

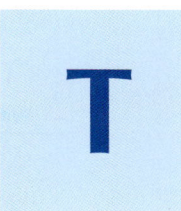

Talcosis

Definition

Talcosis belongs to a group of pulmonary dust disorders collectively called pneumoconioses. In these diseases, nodules form in the lungs as the result of inhaling dust. More commonly, talcosis arises from the injection of talc during illicit drugs abuse.

Description

Talc is the mineral magnesium sulfate hydroxide. In its solid form, it is called soapstone. In loose form, it is known as talcum powder and is used to absorb moisture. Talc is used in, among other things, the manufacture of plastics, paints, ceramics, cosmetics, and as filler for some pharmaceutical drugs manufactured in oral tablet (pill) form. As of 2011, China was the world's leading producer of talc, but the mineral is abundant and mined in many other countries, including South Korea, India, Finland, France, and the United States.

Talcosis was recognized as a lung disease over 100 years ago. When inhaled, talc causes a disease quite similar to the more common lung disease **silicosis**. However, beginning in the 1960s, a new cause of talcosis began to appear. Talc is used as filler in some drug tablets. Intravenous drug abusers sometimes crush tablets, mix them with water, and inject the mixture into a vein. Talc particles do not dissolve in water. Instead, they travel through the circulatory system lodging in blood vessels and the lungs, causing talcosis.

Risk factors

Babies who inhale baby powder containing talc are at risk for developing acute talcosis, a condition in which the cilia lining the airways stop working and the air passages fill up with mucus. Other people at risk for talcosis are miners, stonecutters, ceramics workers, sandblasters, tunnel workers, rock drillers, and individuals who work in industries where talc is used during the manufacturing process. Intravenous drug abusers who inject multiple drugs derived from crushed and powdered pills are at highest risk. People who snort cocaine that has been cut with talc are also at risk for developing talcosis. Risk increases with the frequency of exposure.

Demographics

It is difficult to determine how many people may have talcosis. Inhaled talcosis is uncommon, especially in countries where workplace health and safety rules regulate the amount of particulate matter to which workers can be exposed. Individuals working in industries using or making talc tend not to develop symptoms until they are in their 40s and 50s. Talcosis in intravenous drug users usually is diagnosed only on autopsy, as these individuals tend to die young and from other causes.

Causes and symptoms

The exact mechanism by which talcosis develops is not completely understood. When talc dust get trapped in alveoli in the lungs where air exchange takes place, white blood cells called macrophages enter the alveoli, ingest the talc, and die. The resulting inflammation attracts other macrophages to the region. Granulomas form when the immune system makes fibrous tissue to seal off the reactive area. The disease process may stop at this point or speed up and destroy large areas of the lung. The **fibrosis** may continue even after the individual no longer is exposed to talc.

When tablets containing talc are crushed and injected by intravenous drug abusers, the particles can become trapped in the lungs or the arteries, especially the pulmonary artery that leads to the lungs. Macrophages are drawn to the sites to wall off the talc particles. Granulomas then form in the blood vessels, as well as in the lung. Blood pressure in the pulmonary artery may increase to dangerously high levels (pulmonary hypertension).

KEY TERMS

Alveoli—The small air sacs located at the ends of the breathing tubes of the lung, where oxygen normally passes from inhaled air through the membranes into the capillaries and the bloodstream.

Bronchoscopy—A procedure in which a fiber optic instrument called a bronchoscope is inserted in the airways allowing the physician to inspect the linings of the airways.

Cilia—Tiny, hair-like projections from a cell. In the respiratory tract, cilia beat constantly in order to move mucus and debris up and out of the respiratory tree, in order to protect the lung from infection or irritation by foreign bodies.

Fibrosis—A condition characterized by the presence of scar tissue or collagen proliferation in tissues to the extent that it replaces normal tissues.

Granuloma—A small nodule that forms when immune system cells called macrophages gather to wall off foreign material in the body. Granulomas are a specialized type of inflammation that can occur many places in the body.

Pneumoconiosis (plural, pneumoconioses)—Any chronic lung disease caused by inhaling particles of silica or similar substances that lead to loss of lung function.

QUESTIONS TO ASK YOUR DOCTOR

- What can I do to slow my talcosis?
- How are you going to monitor the progress of my disease?
- Does talcosis put me at higher risk for developing other respiratory diseases?
- How much exercise is appropriate for someone with my condition?
- What should I tell my family about my disease?

Symptoms of talcosis can include shortness of breath after exercising and a harsh, dry cough. Individuals may have more trouble breathing and cough up blood as the disease progresses. They are also at higher risk for developing other respiratory diseases. Intravenous drug abusers also may have elevated blood pressure in the pulmonary artery.

Diagnosis

A diagnosis of talcosis may be made based on the following:

- occupational history
- chest x rays
- bronchoscopy
- lung function tests

Treatment

There is no cure for talcosis. Treatment involves therapy to relieve symptoms, treat complications, and prevent respiratory infections. Respiratory symptoms may be treated with bronchodilators to expand the airwatys, increased fluid intake, steam inhalation, and physical therapy. Patients with severe breathing difficulties may be given oxygen therapy or placed on a mechanical ventilator. Drugs may help to control high blood pressure.

A second aspect of treatment involves lifestyle changes. Individuals with talcosis should stop **smoking**, work to prevent infections by avoiding crowds and persons with colds or similar infections, and receive vaccinations against influenza and pneumonia. They should be encouraged to keep up regular activity and learn to pace themselves with their daily routine. Intravenous drug abusers should receive treatment for their addiction.

Prognosis

The degree which talcosis impairs daily life and the rate at which it progresses to respiratory failure vary considerably. Talcosis is only one of many health problems intravenous drug abusers face, so its effect is often difficult to discern.

Prevention

Talcosis is a preventable disease. In the United States, the **National Institute for Occupational Safety and Health** (NIOSH) and the **Occupational Safety and Health Administration** (OSHA) set standards limiting the amount of particulate matter to which workers may be exposed. These workplace rules have substantially decreased the number of cases of inhaled talcosis in American workers.

Other preventive measures include:

- using baby powder and cosmetics that do not contain talc
- clearly identifying dangerous areas in the workplace

- informing workers about the dangers of overexposure to talc dust, training them in safety techniques, and giving them appropriate protective clothing and equipment
- avoiding injecting drugs intended to be taken by mouth

Resources

PERIODICALS

Bhadra, Krish, and Benjamin T, Suratt. "Drug-induced Lung Diseases: A State-of-the-art Review." *Journal of Respiratory Diseases* 30, no 1 (2009). http://jrd.consultantlive.com/display/article/1145425/1372109 (accessed September 10, 2012).

Restrepo, Carlos, et al. "Pulmonary Complications from Cocaine and Cocaine-based Substances: Imaging Manifestations." *RadioGraphics*, 27 (July 2007): 941–56. http://radiographics.rsna.org/content/27/4/941.long (accessed September 10, 2012).

WEBSITES

Centers for Disease Control and Prevention. "Research on Long-term Exposure: Talk Miners and Millers (Talc)." http://www.cdc.gov/niosh/pgms/worknotify/Talc.html (accessed September 10, 2012).

MedlinePlus. "Talcum Powder Poisoning." http://www.nlm.nih.gov/medlineplus/ency/article/002719.htm (accessed September 10, 2012).

ORGANIZATIONS

Centers for Disease Control and Prevention, 1600 Clifton Rd., Atlanta, GA 30333, (800) 232-4636, cdcinfor@cdc.gov, http://www.cdc.gov.

Mine Safety and Health Administration, 4015 Wilson Blvd., Arlington, VA 22203, (877) 778-6055, MSHAhelpdesk@dol.gov, http://www.msha.gov.

National Toxicology Program, PO BOX 12233, MD K2-03, Research Triangle Park, NC 27709, (919) 541-3345, http://ntp.niehs.nih.gov.

U.S. Food and Drug Administration, 10903 New Hampshire Ave., Silver Spring, MD, USA 20993-0002, (888) INFO-FDA (463-6332), http://www.fda.gov.

Tish Davidson, AM

Teratogen

Definition

An environmental agent that can cause abnormalities in a developing organism resulting in either fetal death or congenital abnormality.

Description

The human fetus is separated from the mother by the placental barrier, but the barrier is imperfect and permits a number of chemical and infectious agents to pass to the fetus. Well known teratogens include (but are not limited to) alcohol, excess vitamin A, excess retinoic acid, the rubella virus, and high levels of ionizing **radiation**. Perhaps the best-known teratogenic agent is the drug thalidomide, which in the 1950s and 1960s induced severe limb abnormalities, known as phocomelia, in children whose mothers were prescribed the drug to relieve morning sickness.

Thesaurosis

Definition

Thesaurosis is a putative medical condition that may result from overexposure to very small particles of plastic found in hair sprays. The condition is also known as *storage disease* due to the apparent tendency of the plastic particles to become stored in the pulmonary system.

Description

Pulmonary thesaurosis was first described in a 1958 paper by three researchers, M. Bergmann, I. J. Flance, and H. T. Blumenthal. (The term *thesaurosis* in general is used to describe conditions in which particles are stored within various body parts.) The researchers reported on two individuals who presented to a medical provider with unexplained respiratory problems. Chest x rays showed the presence of small (about one millimeter in diameter) particles lodged throughout the reticuloendothelial system of the lungs. They hypothesized that small particles of the plastic poly(vinylpolypyrrolidone) (PVP) suspended in hair spray had entered the respiratory system and become lodged in its smaller passageways. Over the next decade other researchers reported on about 30 more cases of a condition that appeared to match the original description of Bergman and colleagues of pulmonary thesaurosis. By the early 1960s, the possibility of a respiratory condition caused by excessive exposure to hair spray became more widely known among the general public, and some individuals and groups were calling for regulation of hair spray use both among professional cosmetologists and hairdressers, and also among the general public. By the early 1960s, a number of professional organizations and regulatory agencies had begun studies of pulmonary thesaurosis, including the Medical Research Council in the United Kingdom and the National Heart, Lung and Blood Institute and the American Thoracic Society in the United States.

KEY TERMS

Pneumonitis—Inflammation of lung tissue.

Reticuloendothelial system—A group of cells located throughout the body that comprise part of the immune system with the ability to take up and sequester a variety of inert particles.

Sarcoidosis—The growth and development of small groups of inflammatory cells in various parts of the body. The cause of sarcoidosis is unknown.

QUESTIONS TO ASK YOUR DOCTOR

- To the best of your knowledge, does the use of hair sprays at home pose any type of health problem for my family?
- What can cosmetologists do to reduce their risk of respiratory diseases from the chemicals they use in their occupations?

Further research in the 1960s found relatively little clinical basis for a distinct disease that could be labeled pulmonary thesaurosis. Histological studies showed features of the condition similar to those associated with other conditions, such as pneumonitis and sarcoidosis. In addition, cases diagnosed as pulmonary thesaurosis were often characterized by significantly different signs and symptoms. By the early 1970s, then, a number of medical professionals had begun to question the existence of pulmonary thesaurosis as a unique disease. Some suggested that the symptoms attributed to the disease were, in fact, caused by other diseases and disorders. This uncertainty led to articles in the professional literature with titles such as "Thesaurosis: Illness or Illusion?" and "Thesaurosis—from Hairspray Exposure—a Nondisease." In December 1963, the Society of Cosmetic Chemists of Great Britain (SCC) issued its own assessment of the thesaurosis controversies. It said that "Surveys of personnel in hairdressing establishments both here and abroad, have failed to reveal evidence of lung disease resulting from the use of hair sprays. To date there is no valid evidence of pulmonary storage of hair spray materials in man. Accordingly the term 'hair spray thesaurosis' can no longer be regarded as a valid description of the published clinical cases." Other summaries of the research have come to similar conclusions.

SCC and other groups have based their conclusions primarily on two lines of evidence. First, the clinical conditions associated with thesaurosis by many researchers appear to be similar to those of sarcoidosis, suggesting that some factor other than hair spray use may be responsible for the conditions originally associated with plastic components of hair spray. Second, experiments with nonhuman animals in which hair spray components are intentionally introduced into the animals lungs fail to produce the symptoms or clinical features of thesaurosis supposedly associated with the condition. As a consequence, one of the most recent reviews of pulmonary thesaurosis came to the conclusion that the potential health hazard of aerosol cosmetics could not be determined.

Resources

BOOKS

Churg, Andrew, and Francis H. Y. Green. "Occupational Lung Disease." In William M. Thurlbeck and Andrew Churg, eds. *Pathology of the Lung*, 2nd ed. New York: Thieme Medical Publishers, 1994.

Doyon, Suzanne. "Hairdressers and Cosmetologists." In Michael Greenberg, Richard Hamilton, Scott Phillips, and Gayla J. McCluskey, eds. *Occupational, Industrial, and Environmental Toxicology*, 2nd ed. St. Louis: Mosby, 2003.

PERIODICALS

Bergmann, Martin. "Thesaurosis: Illness or Illusion?." *Chest* 64, 2. (1973): 153–54.

Kesavachandran, C., et al. "A Study of the Prevalence of Respiratory Morbidity and Ventilatory Obstruction in Beauty Parlour Workers." *Indian Journal of Occupational and Environmental Medicine* 10, 1. (2006): 28–31.

Renzetti, A. D., Jr., et al. "Thesaurosis—from Hairspray Exposure—a Nondisease. Validation Studies of an Epidemiologic Survey of Cosmetologists." *Environmental Research* 22, 1. (1980): 130–8.

Society of Cosmetic Chemists of Great Britain. "Report on the Present Position Regarding the Toxicology of Hair Sprays." *Journal of the Society of Cosmetic Chemists* 15. (1964): 45–50.

David E. Newton, EdD

Three Mile Island nuclear disaster

Definition

On March 28, 1979, a partial nuclear meltdown occurred at the Three Mile Island nuclear power plant near Middletown, Pennsylvania. During the accident

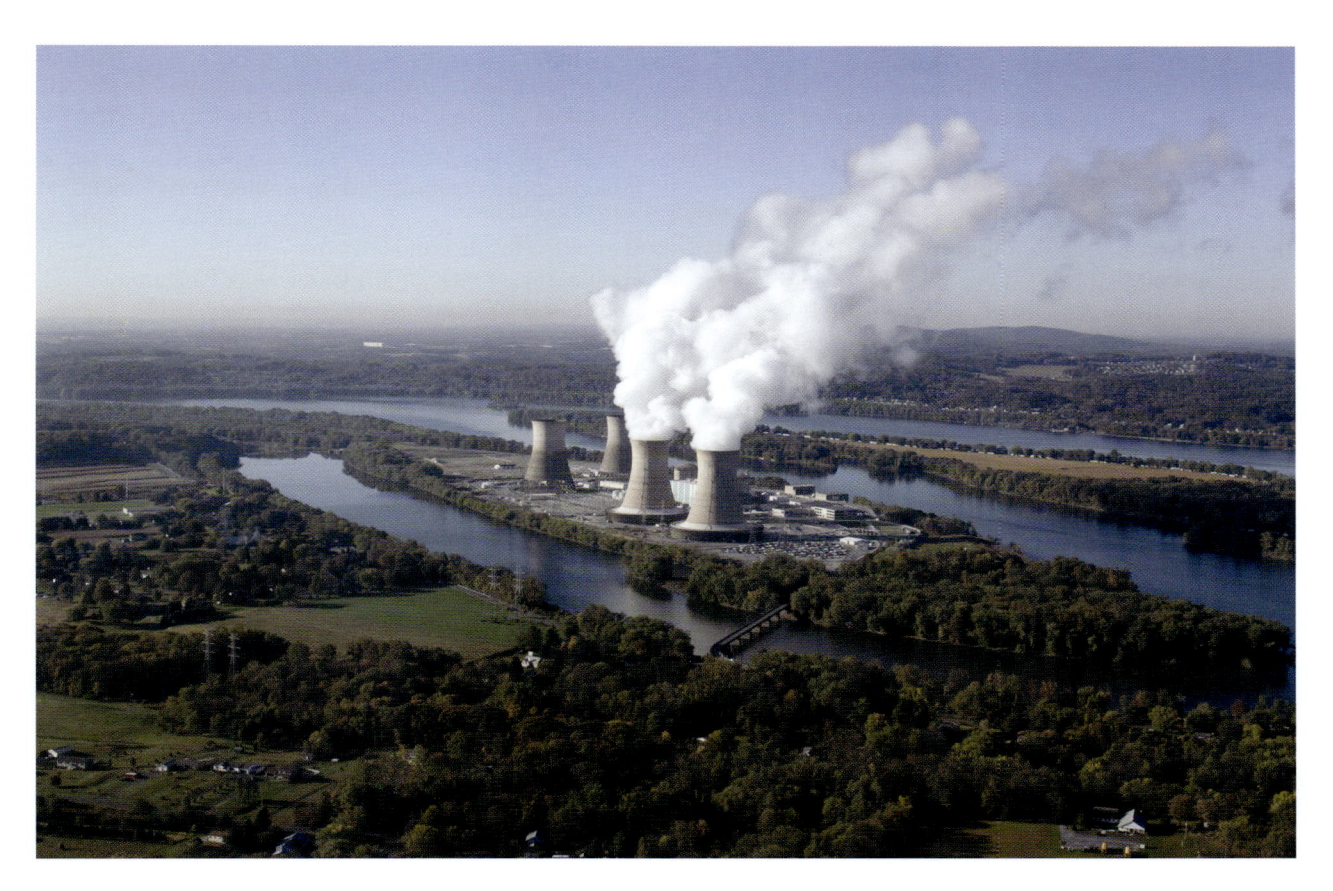

Three Mile Island nuclear power station. *(Dobresum/Shutterstock.com)*

small amounts of radioactive gases and radioactive iodine were released into the atmosphere. Although there were no deaths or injuries to plant workers or community members, it remains the most serious commercial nuclear power plant accident in U.S. nuclear power plant operating history.

Description

The accident at the Three Mile Island Unit 2 (TMI-2, one of two power plants at the site) began around 4:00 a.m. on March 28, 1979, as the plant experienced a failure in the secondary (non-nuclear) system of the plant. The main feedwater pumps stopped running, caused by either a mechanical or electrical failure that prevented the steam generators from removing heat. When the pumps stopped, the turbine and the reactor automatically shut down, which resulted in the pressure in the primary (nuclear) system of the plant increasing. A relief valve opened to release the excess pressure; however, this valve should have closed again when the pressure decreased, but it stayed open. Signals should have been sent to the operator to indicate that the valve was still open, but no such signal was received.

Cooling water escaped through the open valve, resulting in overheating of the reactor core. The reactor instrumentation, which did not include an instrument to measure coolant level in the core, did not make it clear to the operators that there was a loss of coolant, so they reduced the flow of coolant through the core, which resulted in the nuclear fuel overheating, whereby the tubes that hold the nuclear fuel pellets (zirconium cladding) ruptured and the fuel pellets began to melt. About one-half of the core in TMI-2 melted during the initial stages of the accident (although this was not known until 1985). However, a worse case accident did not occur, which would have been breaching of the containment building walls and release of large quantities of radiation into the environment.

The U.S. Nuclear Regulatory Commission (NRC) reacted within a few hours and sent inspectors and response teams to the site, although they did not know that the core had melted. Other agencies also responded, such as the U.S. Department of Energy, the U.S. Environmental Protection Agency, and Brookhaven National Laboratory. By 11 a.m. on March 28, all nonessential personnel left the plant, and monitoring of radiation levels in the atmosphere above the plant was being conducted using helicopters. By the evening of March 28, the reactor appeared to be stable, with the core flooded again and the temperature under control.

However, on March 30 (later known as Black Friday), confusion and rumors arose on the amount of radiation that had or could be released from the plant, which resulted in discussions between the NRC and the Pennsylvania governor, Richard Thornburgh, on whether the population near the plant should be evacuated. The decision was made to recommend that members of the population vulnerable to radiation, including pregnant women and pre-school-age children who lived within a 5-mile radius of the plant, leave the area. In response to the potential threats, about 140,000 people evacuated the area. Ninety-eight percent of the evacuees returned to their homes within three weeks.

Additional concerns arose on March 31 because of the presence of a large hydrogen bubble in the dome of the pressure vessel, the container that holds the reactor core. There were fears that the hydrogen bubble might burn or explode and rupture the pressure vessel. The core would then fall into the containment building and perhaps cause a breach of containment. On Sunday, April 1, it was determined that the bubble could not burn or explode because of the absence of oxygen in the pressure vessel. In addition, the operators had significantly reduced the size of the bubble.

On April 2, 1979, five days after the meltdown, the crisis at Three Mile Island was officially declared to be over. TMI - 2 was too badly damaged and contaminated to resume operations; the reactor was gradually deactivated and permanently closed. The reactor coolant system was drained, the radioactive water decontaminated and evaporated, radioactive waste shipped off-site to an appropriate disposal site, reactor fuel and core debris shipped off-site to a Department of Energy facility, and the remainder of the site was being monitored. When the operating license for the TMI-1 plant expires, both plants will be decommissioned. As of 2012, TMI-1 is licensed to operate until April 19, 2034.

Demographics

Based on many studies conducted by the NRC, the U.S. Environmental Protection Agency, the U.S. Department of Health, Education and Welfare (now Health and Human Services), the Department of Energy, and the State of Pennsylvania, the estimated average dose to about 2 million people in the area was only about 1 millirem. Exposure from a chest x-ray is about 6 millirem, and the natural background radiation dose in the area is about 100 to 125 millirem per year. The maximum dose to a person at the site boundary would have been less than 100 millirem.

In the aftermath of the accident, no possible adverse effects from radiation on human, animal, and plant life in the surrounding area could be directly correlated to the accident, although thousands of environmental samples of air, water, milk, vegetation, soil, and foodstuffs were collected and analyzed by various groups monitoring the area. The U.S. Environmental Protection Agency remained in the area for eight years, maintaining a field office to monitor the air. Only very low levels of radionuclides were found as a result of the accident.

Comprehensive investigative and assessment reports by several well-respected organizations concluded that in spite of serious damage to the reactor, most of the radiation was contained and that the radioactive release had little effect on the physical health of individuals or the environment. However, other studies reported that lung cancer and leukemia rates were two to ten times greater downwind of TMI than upwind and that infant mortality increased in downwind communities two years after the accident.

Causes

The accident was apparently caused by a combination of personnel error, design deficiencies, and component failures, although the definite proximate (or legal) cause of the meltdown remains unknown and no proof of negligence was ever uncovered. Examples of problems that occurred included reactor operators not trained to deal with accident conditions, and the NRC not having established effective communication channels with utilities. Once the accident occurred, the lines of authority were shown to be ill defined. The public received conflicting reports that caused panic and evacuations.

The Kemeny Commission, the presidential commission tasked with conducting a comprehensive investigation of the TMI accident, noted the type of valve that had stuck open had previously failed on eleven occasions in different nuclear power plants, nine of them in the open position, allowing coolant to escape.

Public health role and response

In the days after the accident, engineers, scientists and mechanics worked to minimize further release of radiation and to prevent a total meltdown of the core, while state and federal government officials tried to come up with emergency response measures. Initially

DR. HELEN CALDICOTT (1938–)

Dr. Helen Caldicott was born in Australia but moved to the United States to practice pediatric medicine in Boston. After the Three Mile Island nuclear accident in 1980, Caldicott left medicine. She felt strongly about the world's dependence on nuclear energy and devoted her career to researching and raising awareness on the dangers of nuclear power.

Caldicott was the founding president of the Physicians for Social Responsibility, a group devoted to educating people on the dangers of nuclear energy. She also created the Women's Action for Nuclear Disarmament (WAND), which works to divert government funding from nuclear-related items to social causes.

Dr. Caldicott's lecture to SUNY college students about the threat of nuclear weapons became a 1982 Academy-Award-winning short documentary film, entitled *If You Love This Planet*.

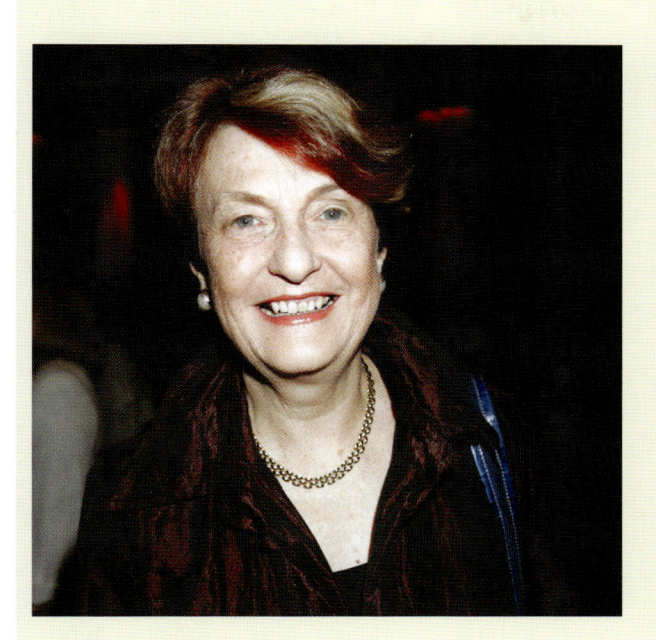

(Patrick Riviere/Getty Images.)

reports indicated no threats to the public, but later it was reported that the situation was more complex than initially thought. Two days after the accident, Governor Richard Thornburgh recommended that preschool children and pregnant women within five miles of the plant evacuate the area. Residents within a ten-mile radius were asked to stay at home, turn off their air-conditioners, and close their windows. Farmers were told to keep their animals under cover and eating stored feed.

The Kemeny Commission concluded that the major health effect of the accident appeared to have been on the mental health of the people living in the region of Three Mile Island and of the workers at TMI. There was immediate, short-lived mental distress produced by the accident among certain groups of the general population living within 20 miles of TMI. The highest levels of distress were found among adults living within 5 miles of TMI or with preschool children; and among teenagers living within 5 miles of TMI, with preschool siblings, or whose families left the area. Workers at TMI experienced more distress than workers at another plant studied for comparison purposes. This distress was higher among the nonsupervisory employees and continued in the months following the accident.

This accident highlighted the lack of preparedness for a nuclear power plant incident, and the resulting heightened awareness led to better preparedness plans by agencies responsible for public health and safety. These plans include:

- designation of agency in charge and who to call for help
- protection equipment and procedures for the responders
- guidance on how to triage patients
- decontamination procedures
- methods for transporting patients
- hospital responses and medical therapies

Prognosis

The TMI-2 cleanup took 11 years and cost about $1 billion. There were serious public relations consequences for nuclear power. Following the accident, the number of reactors under construction in the U.S. declined every year. At the time of the TMI accident, 129 nuclear power plants had been approved. Of those, only 53 (which were not already operating) were completed. Internationally, declines in nuclear power plant construction came as a result of the

KEY TERMS

Background radiation—The radiation in the natural environment, including cosmic rays and radiation from the naturally radioactive elements, both outside and inside the bodies of humans and animals. The usually quoted average individual exposure from background radiation is 300 millirem per year.

Cladding—The thin-walled metal tube that forms the outer jacket of a nuclear fuel rod. It prevents the corrosion of the fuel by the coolant and the release of fission products in the coolants. Aluminum, stainless steel and zirconium alloys are common cladding materials.

Containment—The gas-tight shell or other enclosure around a reactor to confine fission products that otherwise might be released to the atmosphere in the event of an accident.

Coolant—A substance circulated through a nuclear reactor to remove or transfer heat. The most commonly used coolant in the U.S. is water. Other coolants include air, carbon dioxide, and helium.

Core—The central portion of a nuclear reactor containing the fuel elements, and control rods.

Decontamination—The reduction or removal of contaminating radioactive material from a structure, area, object, or person. Decontamination may be accomplished by (1) treating the surface to remove or decrease the contamination; (2) letting the material stand so that the radioactivity is decreased by natural decay; and (3) covering the contamination to shield the radiation emitted.

Feedwater—Water supplied to the steam generator that removes heat from the fuel rods by boiling and becoming steam. The steam then becomes the driving force for the turbine generator.

Nuclear reactor—A device in which nuclear fission may be sustained and controlled in a self-supporting nuclear reaction. There are several varieties, but all incorporate certain features, such as fissionable material or fuel, a moderating material (to control the reaction), a reflector to conserve escaping neutrons, provisions for removal of heat, measuring and controlling instruments, and protective devices.

Pressure vessel—A strong-walled container housing the core of most types of power reactors.

Primary system—The cooling system used to remove energy from the reactor core and transfer that energy either directly or indirectly to the steam turbine.

Radiation—Particles (alpha, beta, neutrons) or photons (gamma) emitted from the nucleus of an unstable atom as a result of radioactive decay.

Secondary system—The steam generator tubes, steam turbine, condenser and associated pipes, pumps, and heaters used to convert the heat energy of the reactor coolant system into mechanical energy for electrical generation.

Steam generator—The heat exchanger used in some reactor designs to transfer heat from the primary (reactor coolant) system to the secondary (steam) system. This design permits heat exchange with little or no contamination of the secondary system equipment.

Turbine—A rotary engine made with a series of curved vanes on a rotating shaft. Usually turned by water or steam. Turbines are considered to be the most economical means to turn large electrical generators.

---

catastrophic Chernobyl nuclear power plant accident in 1986. In February 2012, the NRC approved construction and licensing of two new nuclear reactors at Plant Vogtle in Georgia, the first such approval in the U.S. since 1978.

The accident at Three Mile Island changed both the nuclear industry and the NRC. Public fear and distrust increased, NRC's regulations and oversight became broader and stronger, and management of the plants was scrutinized more carefully. The problems identified from careful analysis of the events during those days and the changes made in response to the analysis has reduced the risk to public health and safety.

Prevention

Changes to the U.S. nuclear power plant program to provide protection against future accidents that were made in response to the Three Mile Island accident, according the the NRC, include:

- upgrading and strengthening of plant design and equipment requirements. This includes fire protection, piping systems, auxiliary feedwater systems, containment building isolation, reliability of individual components (pressure relief valves and electrical circuit breakers), and the ability of plants to shut down automatically;
- identifying human performance as a critical part of plant safety, revamping operator training and

staffing requirements, followed by improved instrumentation and controls for operating the plant, and establishment of fitness-for-duty programs for plant workers to guard against alcohol or drug abuse;
- improved instruction to avoid the confusing signals that affected operations during the accident;
- enhancement of emergency preparedness to include immediate NRC notification requirements for plant events and an NRC operations center that is staffed 24 hours a day. Drills and response plans are now tested by licensees several times a year, and state and local agencies participate in drills with the Federal Emergency Management Agency and NRC;
- establishment of a program to integrate NRC observations, findings, and conclusions about licensee performance and management effectiveness into a periodic, public report;
- regular analysis of plant performance by senior NRC managers, who identify plants needing additional regulatory attention;
- expansion of NRC's resident inspector program, which was first authorized in 1977, whereby at least two inspectors live nearby and work exclusively at each plant in the U.S. to provide daily surveillance of licensee adherence to NRC regulations;
- expansion of performance-oriented as well as safety-oriented inspections, and the use of risk assessment to identify vulnerabilities of a plant to severe accidents;
- strengthening and reorganization of enforcement as a separate office within the NRC;
- the establishment of the Institute of Nuclear Power Operations (INPO), the industry's own policing group, and formation of what is now the Nuclear Energy Institute to provide a unified industry approach to generic nuclear regulatory issues, and interaction with NRC and other government agencies;
- installation of additional equipment by licensees to mitigate accident conditions, and monitor radiation levels and plant status;
- employment of major initiatives by licensees in early identification of important safety-related problems, and in the collection and assessment of relevant data so lessons of experience can be shared and quickly acted upon; and
- expansion of NRC's international activities to share enhanced knowledge of nuclear safety with other countries in a number of important technical areas.

Resources

BOOKS

Derkins, Susie. *The Meltdown at Three Mile Island*. New York: Rosen Publishing Group, 2003.

Dresser, P. D. *Nuclear Power Plants Worldwide*. Detroit, MI: Gale Research, 1993.

Ford, D. *Three Mile Island: Thirty Minutes to Meltdown*. New York: Penguin, 1983.

Geigenbaum, Aaron. *Emergency at Three Mile Island*. New York: Bearport, 2007.

Gray, M., and I. Rosen. *The Warming: Accident at Three Mile Island*. New York: W.W. Norton, 1982.

Moss, T. H., and D. L. Sills, eds. *The Three Mile Island Nuclear Accident: Lessons and Implications*. New York: Academy of Sciences, 1981.

Osif, Bonnie, A.; Anthony J. Baratta; and Thomas W. Conkling. *TMI 25 Years Later: The Three Mile Island Nuclear Power Plant Accident and its Impact*. University Park: Pennsylvania State University Press, 2006.

Walker, J. Samuel. *Three Mile Island: A Nuclear Crisis in Historical Perspective*. Berkeley: University of California Press, 2004.

WEBSITES

ThreeMileIsland.org, Dickinson College. http://www.threemileisland.org

Judith L. Sims

Times Beach

Definition

Times Beach is a town once located in St. Louis County, Missouri, southwest of St. Louis. The town was evacuated in 1983 because of dioxin contamination that made the region unsafe for human occupation. The even constituted the largest recorded exposure to date of humans to dioxin in U.S. history.

Description

In 1971, the town of Times Beach hired waste-hauler Russell M. Bliss to spray the streets of the town to keep down dust. Bliss used chemical wastes containing dioxin mixed with oil for this purpose from 1972 to 1976. Bliss obtained the mixture from waste oils and chemicals his company collected from service stations and industrial plants. Much of this toxic waste oil was sprayed on roads throughout Missouri.

Shortly after the spraying around Times Beach began, horses on local farms began dying. At one breeding stable, from 1971 to 1973, 62 horses died, as well as several dogs and cats. Soil samples were sent to the Centers for Disease Control (now the **Centers for Disease Control and Prevention** [CDC]) in Atlanta for analysis, and after three years of testing, the agency determined that dangerous levels of dioxin were present in the soil.

A decade after the spraying, the town experienced the worst flooding in its history. On December 5, 1982, the Meramec River flooded its banks and inundated the town, submerging homes and contaminating them and almost everything else in Times Beach with dioxin. This compound binds tightly to soil and degrades very slowly, so it was still present in significantly high levels ten years after being used on the roads as a dust suppressant. Following a CDC warning that the town had become uninhabitable, most of the families were temporarily evacuated. The U.S. **Environmental Protection Agency (EPA)** eventually agreed to buy out the town for about $33 million and relocate its inhabitants.

By 1983, federal and state officials had located about 100 other sites in Missouri where dioxin wastes had been improperly dumped or sprayed, with levels of the compound reaching as high as 1,750 ppb in some areas.

The former site of Times Beach is now Route 66 State Park, which has hiking and bicycling paths and a historic retelling of the evacuation of the town.

Effects on public health

At the time, the CDC considered soil dioxin levels of one part per billion (ppb) and above to be potentially hazardous to human health. Levels found in some areas of Times Beach reached 100 to 300 ppb and above. Dioxin is considered a very toxic chemical. Exposure to this chemical has been linked to cancer, miscarriages, genetic mutations, liver and nerve damage, and other health effects, including death, in humans and animals.

Common diseases and disorders

The contamination seemed to take a serious toll on the health of Times Beach residents. Town officials claimed that virtually every household in Times Beach experienced health disorders, ranging from nosebleeds, depression, and chloracne (a severe skin disorder) to cancer and heart disease. Almost all of the residents tested for dioxin contamination showed abnormalities in their blood, liver, and kidney functions.

Resources

BOOKS

Hernan, Robert Emmet. *This Borrowed Earth: Lessons from the Fifteen Worst Environmental Disasters Around the World.* New York: Palgrave Macmillan, 2010.

WEBSITES

"Ill-Fated Times Beach." http://www.legendsofamerica.com/mo-timesbeach.html (accessed September 21, 2012).

Leistner, Marilyn. "The Times Beach Story." http://www.greens.org/s-r/078/07-09.html (accessed September 21, 2012).

"Times Beach Site." http://www.epa.gov/region7/cleanup/npl_files/mod980685226.pdf (accessed September 21, 2012).

Lewis G. Regenstein

Tornado and cyclone

Definition

A tornado is a vortex or powerful whirling wind, often visible as a funnel-shaped cloud hanging from the base of a thunderstorm. In some places such storms are referred to as cyclones.

Description

It can be very violent and destructive as it moves across land in a fairly narrow path, usually a few hundred yards in width. Wind speeds are most often too strong to measure with instruments and are often estimated from the damages they cause. Winds have been estimated to exceed 350 miles per hour (563 kph). Very steep pressure gradients are also associated with tornados and contribute to their destructiveness. Sudden changes in atmospheric pressure taking place as the storm passes sometimes cause walls and roofs of buildings to explode or collapse.

Tornadoes most frequently occur in the United States in the central plains where maritime polar and maritime tropical air masses often meet, producing highly unstable atmospheric conditions conducive to the development of severe thunderstorms. Most tornados occur between noon and sunset, when late afternoon heating contributes to atmospheric instability.

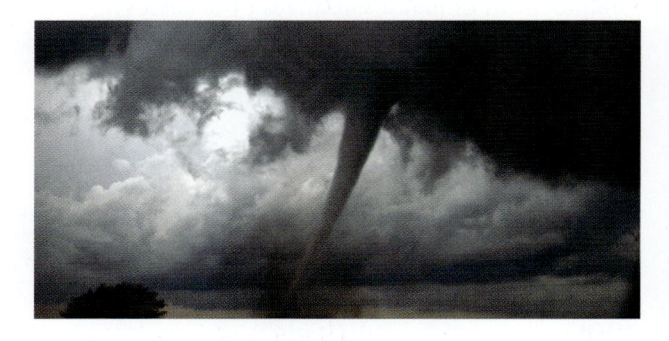

One of several tornadoes observed on May 3, 1999, in central Oklahoma. *(NOAA)*

JOPLIN, MISSOURI (MAY 22, 2011)

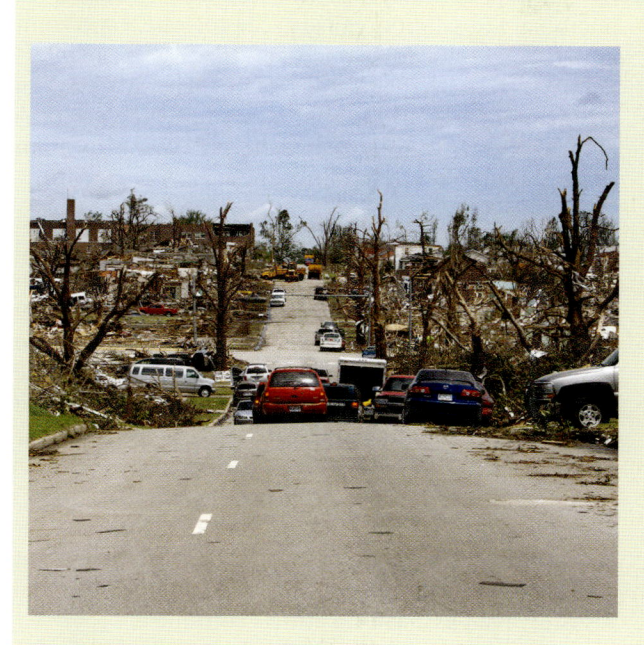

The tornado that struck Joplin, Missouri, holds the dubious distinction as the costliest single tornado in American history, generating over $2 billion in insurance claims. The massive tornado was classified an EF-5 on the Enhanced Fujita Scale, and the devastating winds exceeded 200 mph. With approximately 160 human casualties, it is also the deadliest American tornado on record since 1947.

Unfortunately, many casualties might have been avoided. A post-tornado survey conducted by the National Weather Service revealed that most people did not heed the tornado warnings and take cover, assuming they were false alarms. The National Weather Service is working to improve the tornado warning communication process.

Thirteen of the Joplin tornado survivors were diagnosed with a deadly fungal infection known as mucormycosis. This type of infection can be contracted during natural disasters, when victims have open wounds that are contaminated with dirt and decaying vegetation.

On May 22, 2011, Joplin, Missouri, was devastated by an EF-5 tornado. (© Ryan McGinnis / Alamy)

In addition to clashes between warm and cold fronts, tornadoes are often spawned by hurricanes and tropical storms. Global warming is expected to increase sea surface temperatures in the tropical regions of the world, which will increase the amount of energy in the oceans available for such storms. The result of this process could be an increase in the annual frequency of hurricanes, and an increase in their intensity (wind speed), with a consequential increase in both the number and strength of tornadoes they create. The process of tornado formation is, however, extremely complicated, so the influence of warmer ocean temperatures could be countered by the typical factors that disrupt formation and result in no net gain in frequency.

Toxic sludge spill in Hungary

Definition

In early October 2010, Hungary declared a state of emergency in three western counties after a massive and deadly industrial spill of highly alkaline, red-colored, toxic sludge from a ruptured industrial reservoir flooded nearby towns and flowed into tributaries leading to the Danube River.

Description

The industrial reservoir ruptured on October 4, 2010, releasing at least 35 million cubic feet (1 million cubic meters) of toxic mud-like waste created during the refining of bauxite into alumina. Bauxite is a naturally occurring mixture of aluminum hydroxide minerals. Often extracted by strip mining, bauxite is then mixed with industrial strength and highly caustic sodium hydroxide under high temperature (400°F, 200°C) and pressure to release alumina. Alumina is an industrially produced crystalline aluminum oxide used in smelting aluminum. Alumina is also used in many ceramic products. During filtering, a red mud or red sludge is removed to evaporation tanks or reservoirs. A precipitate containing aluminum hydroxide then forms as the filtered solution cools. The precipitate is then purified and heated again to form aluminum oxide. The red mud or red sludge typically has high concentrations of caustic, alkaline sodium hydroxide mixed with variable amount of silicon and titanium. The sludge may also be slightly radioactive and can contain varying concentrations of heavy metals such as arsenic, **lead**, **cadmium**, and chromium.

Effects on the environment

Efforts to contain the massive spill initially failed to prevent contaminated sludge from reaching the Danube, Europe's second longest river. Polluted runoff into feeder streams also thwarted containment efforts. Waterways near the broken reservoir, including streams near Kolontar, the village nearest the spill and about 45 miles (70 km) from the Danube, reported massive fish kills. Observers also reported massive kills in all forms of aquatic life in the Marcal River, a smaller river that flows into the Raba River, which in turn, flows into the Danube.

At the source of the spill, engineers and rescue workers recorded strongly alkaline pH scale readings of pH 12 to pH 13. The pH scale measurements relate the concentration of hydrogen ions (H+) in a solution to a logarithmic scale. The hydrogen ion concentration can be determined empirically and expressed as the pH. The pH scale ranges from 0 to 14, with 1 being the most acidic and 14 being the most basic. The pH scale is a logarithmic scale, and so each integer division differs by a factor of ten. For example, a solution that has a pH of 9 is ten times more basic than a solution with a pH of 8.

An acidic environment is rich in hydrogen ions, whereas a basic environment is relatively depleted of hydrogen ions and, in an aqueous environment, is rich in OH$^-$ ions. Mathematically, pH is calculated as the negative logarithm of the hydrogen ion concentration. For example, the hydrogen ion concentration of distilled water is 10^{-7} and hence, pure or distilled water has a pH of 7. In comparison, a pH of 0 corresponds to 10 million more hydrogen ions per unit volume, and a pH of 14 corresponds to one ten-millionth as many hydrogen ions per unit volume.

As the sludge mixed with water (with a neutral pH of 7), dilution reduced the highly alkaline sludge, By the time the sludge reached the Danube, investigators and environmental officials recorded pH levels of 9.4 in contaminants entering the river. The diluted sludge was more than 1000 times less alkaline than the sludge at the source. Investigators remained uncertain, however, as to the heavy metal content of the sludge.

Emergency response teams also poured plaster and vinegar (a dilute form of acetic acid) into the sludge as part of efforts to neutralize the deadly alkalinity.

The day after diluted sludge was detected in the Danube, sporadic losses of fish were reported. Water pH near areas where the Raba flows into the Danube measured 9.1. Fish and many forms of vegetation cannot survive in such alkaline conditions. Industrial pollution in the Danube routinely creates pH levels of 8.0 to 8.4.

Experts continued to test waters for impacts on microbial life. Microorganisms can tolerate a spectrum of pHs, while individual microbes usually have an internal pH close to that of distilled water. The surrounding cell membranes and external layers (e.g., the glycocalyx) help buffer the cell membrane and offer protection from pH extremes in the surrounding environment.

Engineers and government officials launched investigations to determine the reason the industrial waste reservoir collapsed. The industrial evaporation reservoir suffered a collapse in a section of one of the containment walls. Engineers worked for two days to repair the ruptured section. Just a week prior to the accident, Hungarian environmental authorities had declared the reservoir safe. The cause of the reservoir failure appears to have been a period of heavy rains that weakened the walls of the reservoir embankment. The threat of a second spill was averted with the construction of a second dam embankment, and the plant resumed production less than a week after the original disaster, even as clean up efforts continued.

Public health role and response

Ten deaths were attributed to the Hungarian spill, with between 120 and 150 people also treated for chemical burns and other injuries. Exposure to highly alkaline or acidic substances can result in chemical burns that manifest hours or days after exposure. Deep tissue burns are also possible.

By mid-October, **World Health Organization (WHO)** personnel, who continuously tested waters downstream of the spill, declared **water quality** to be adequate and within expected ranges of pollution established prior to the spill. Local drinking water supplies were also cleared for use. WHO officials announced plans for long-term monitoring for pH fluctuations and heavy metal contamination. Public health officials continued to warn against contact, inhalation or ingestion of the highly alkaline industrial sludge.

Resources

BOOKS

Yu, Ming-Ho, Humio Tsunoda, and Masashi Tsunoda. *Environmental Toxicology: Biological and Health Effects of Pollutants*, 3rd ed. Boca Raton, FL: CRC Press, 2011.

WEBSITES

"Hungarian Sludge Spills (2010)." http://topics.nytimes.com/top/reference/timestopics/subjects/h/hungarian_sludge_spill/index.html (accessed September 21, 2012).

"Hungary Toxic Sludge Spill an 'Ecological Catastrophe' Says Government." http://www.guardian.co.uk/world/2010/oct/05/hungary-toxic-sludge-spill (accessed September 21, 2012).

"Toxic Hungarian Sludge Spill Reaches River Danube." Reuters.http://www.reuters.com/article/2010/10/07/us-hungary-spill-idUSTRE69415O20101007 (accessed September 21, 2012).

ORGANIZATIONS

Environmental Protection Agency, 1200 Pennsylvania Ave. NW, Washington, DC 20460, (202) 272-0167, http://water.epa.gov.

World Health Organization, Avenue Appia 20, 1211 Geneva 27, Switzerland, 2241 791 21 11, Fax: 2241 791 31 11, info@who.int, http://www.who.int.

K. Lee Lerner

Toxic Substances Control Act (1976)

Definition

The Toxic Substances Control Act (TSCA), enacted in 1976, is a key law for regulating toxic substances in the United States.

Purpose

The TSCA authorizes the **Environmental Protection Agency (EPA)** to study the health and environmental effects of chemicals already on the market and new chemicals proposed for commercial manufacture. If the **EPA** finds these health and environmental effects to pose unreasonable risks, it can regulate, or even ban, the chemical(s) under consideration.

Description

Origins

The initiative to regulate toxic substances began in the early 1970s. In 1971, the Council on Environmental Quality produced a report on toxic substances. It concluded that existing health and environmental laws were not adequately regulating such substances. The report recommended that a new comprehensive law to deal with toxic substances be enacted. Among the problem substances that had helped to focus national concern on toxic substances were **asbestos**, chlorofluorocarbons (CFCs), Kepone (a pesticide), **mercury**, polychlorinated biphenyls (PCBs), and vinyl chloride. Research proved that these substances caused significant health and environmental problems, yet they were unregulated.

Demographics

Congressional debate on regulating toxic substances began in 1971. The Senate passed bills in 1972 and 1973 that were strongly supported by environmentalists and labor, but the House approach was more limited, in part because of chemical industry influence. The key difference between the two approaches was how much premarket review would be required before new chemicals could be introduced and marketed. Although none of the key stakeholders—the chemical industry, environmentalists, or labor—was entirely happy with the compromise bill of 1976, all three groups supported it.

Results

The approach adopted in TSCA is premarket notification, rather than the more rigorous premarket testing that is required before new drugs are introduced on the market. When a new chemical is to be manufactured or an existing chemical is to be used in a substantially different way, the manufacturer of the chemical must provide the EPA with premanufacture notification data at least 90 days before the chemical is to be commercially produced. The EPA then examines this data and determines if regulation is necessary for the new chemical or new use of an existing chemical. The agency can require additional testing by manufacturers if it deems the existing data insufficient. Until such data are available, the EPA has the option to ban or limit the manufacture, distribution, use, or disposal of the chemical. For new chemicals or new applications of existing chemicals, producers must demonstrate that the chemicals do not pose unreasonable risks to humans or the environment. The EPA can act quickly and with limited burden to prevent such new chemicals from being produced or distributed.

Between July 1979, when TSCA went into effect for new chemicals, and April 2002, the EPA received 23,486 new chemical notices. The agency determined that no action was necessary for nearly 90% of these chemicals. Of the 2,702 chemicals that required further action, 917 were never produced commercially due to EPA concerns. The remaining 1,785 chemicals were controlled through formal actions or negotiated agreements.

As of mid-2012, there were over 83,000 chemicals within the purview of TSCA. Although the law requires that the EPA examine each of these chemicals for its potential health and environmental risk, the volume of chemicals and lack of EPA resources has made such a task virtually impossible. Through 2000, the agency had examined almost 700 existing chemicals. Of the compounds on this list, the EPA determined that 370 chemicals required no further action. This was due to the fact that the chemical was no longer being manufactured, it was under study by another federal agency or industry, adequate data on the chemical existed, or exposure to the chemical was limited. The EPA issued rules to regulate 112 of these chemicals. The remaining chemicals were in various stages of testing and review.

TSCA created an Interagency Testing Committee (ITC) to help the EPA set priorities. The ITC designates which existing chemicals should be examined first. Once designated by the ITC, the EPA has one year to study the chemical and issue a ruling. The agency initially had difficulty meeting this one-year limit. In fact, the EPA was sued over its failure to meet the deadline and worked under a court schedule to test these identified chemicals. The record of the EPA has improved, but the agency continued to struggle to meet deadlines imposed by ITC due to budgetary and personnel shortages.

The EPA also identifies specific chemicals already in use for review. Unlike the policy with new chemicals, the EPA must demonstrate that existing chemicals warrant toxicity testing. Furthermore, if the EPA desires to regulate the chemical once it has been tested, it must pursue another complex course of action. By design, the regulation of existing chemicals is a lengthy and complicated process.

There are several options available to the EPA if it concludes that a new or existing chemical presents "an unreasonable risk of injury to health or the environment." The EPA can 1) prohibit the manufacture of the chemical by applying a rule or obtaining a court injunction; 2) limit the amount of the chemical produced or the concentration at which the chemical is used; 3) impose a ban or limit uses of the chemical; 4) regulate the disposal of the chemical; 5) require public notification of its use; and 6) require labeling and record keeping for the chemical. The EPA is required to use the least burdensome of these regulatory approaches for chemicals already in use.

There are several other important components to TSCA. First, the law requires strict reporting and record keeping by the manufacturers and processors of the chemicals regulated under the law. In addition to keeping track of the chemicals, these records include data on environmental and health effects. Second, TSCA is one of the few federal environmental laws that require environmental and health benefits to be balanced by economic and societal costs in the regulatory process. The act states that toxic substances should only be regulated when an unreasonable risk to people or the environment is present. Although "unreasonable risk" is not clearly defined in the language of the act, it does incorporate a concern for balancing costs and benefits.

Third, PCBs were singled out in the TSCA legislation. Although the manufacture of PCBs was prohibited by 1979, fewer than 1% of all PCBs in use up to that time were phased out. Despite the ban, a significant PCB problem still remains. One major problem is how to process the millions of pounds of PCBs abandoned by firms that went bankrupt in the 1980s. There is also concern about the safety of disposing PCBs. Environmentalists argued that PCB treatment required new legislation. In response, the EPA decided to issue stricter regulation under the TSCA to ensure the safe the transportation and final disposal of PCBs.

Fourth, TSCA contained provisions for private citizens, as opposed to the U.S. government, to file lawsuits. Under the TSCA rules, private citizens could sue companies for violation of the law. They could also sue the EPA for failure to implement TSCA in a timely manner. Fifth, certain materials are not covered by TSCA. These include ammunition and firearms; nuclear materials; tobacco; and chemicals used exclusively in cosmetics, drugs, food and **food additives**, and pesticides. These substances are regulated by other laws.

The scope of the law was expanded in 1986 by an amendment requiring asbestos hazards to be reduced in schools and in 1988 by an amendment providing grants and technical assistance to state programs that reduce indoor radon and assigning the regulation of genetically engineered organisms to TSCA. A 1990 amendment required accreditation of persons who inspect for asbestos-containing material in school, public, and commercial buildings, and the Residential Lead-Based Paint Hazard Reduction Act of 1992 introduced new requirements for the reduction of hazards associated with the inspection and abatement of lead-based paints.

In terms of existing chemicals, only one—PCBs—has been banned in the United States. Many chemicals in pesticides have been heavily regulated. A notable EPA action was prohibiting the use of chlorofluorocarbons (CFCs) as aerosol propellants. This occurred in March 1978.

Lack of action may be due in part to the costs involved in implementing such a complex regulatory program. It is also difficult to determine unreasonable risk in light of inadequate data and more general uncertainties. Most premarket notifications for new chemicals are not accompanied by test data. Rather, the EPA identifies potentially harmful chemicals by comparing the new chemical to existing chemicals for which data exists. If the EPA were to require more data for most new chemicals, in many cases the new chemicals might not be produced since the test costs would exceed the expected profit.

Research and general acceptance

The chemical industry and environmentalists have reached conflicting conclusions about the TSCA legislation. The chemical industry has argued that the EPA has required more testing than is scientifically needed and that the regulatory approach for new chemicals is overly burdensome. Environmentalists have criticized the EPA for its slow progress in examining existing chemicals, for requiring no health data for new chemicals, and for withholding much of the data for new chemicals to comply with the desire for confidentiality requested by chemical manufacturers.

Resources

BOOKS

Applegate, John, et al. *The Regulation of Toxic Substances and Hazardous Wastes*. 2nd ed. New York: Foundation Press, 2011.

Kumar, Dharti. *Nanomaterials: Toxicity, Health and Environmental Issues*. Weinheim, Germany: Wiley-VCH, 2006.

WEBSITES

U.S. Environmental Protection Agency. "Human Health: Toxicity." http://www.epa.gov/ebtpages/humatoxicity.html (accessed October 25, 2010).

U.S. Environmental Protection Agency. "Learn the Issues: Pesticides, Chemicals and Toxics." July 10, 2012. http://www.epa.gov/gateway/learn/pestchemtox.html (accessed August 13, 2012).

World Health Organization. "Intergovernmental Forum on Chemical Safety." WHO Programs and Projects. http://www.who.int/entity/ifcs/en (accessed August 13, 2012).

L. Fleming Fallon, Jr, MD, DrPH
Stacey Chamberlin

Toxicology

Definition

Toxicology is the scientific study of poisons or toxins. The National Library of Medicine describes toxicology as "the study of the adverse effects of chemicals or physical agents on living organisms." How these toxins affect humans and other animals is based on understanding these basic relationships.

Description

The study and classification of toxic substances goes back two thousand years to Dioscorides (AD 40–90), a Greek physician and pharmacologist who compiled a five-volume encyclopedia on medicinal plants and drugs called *De Materia Medica*. The Swiss physician and alchemist Theophrastus Philippus Aureolus Bombastus von Hohenheim, also known as Paracelsus (1493–1541), however, is said to be the father of the modern science of toxicology. Paracelsus wrote, "All things are poison, and nothing is without poison, the dose alone makes a thing not a poison." In other words, if poisoning is to be caused, an exposure to a potentially toxic chemical must result in a dose that exceeds a physiologically determined threshold of tolerance. Smaller exposures do not cause poisoning.

The dose of toxin is a crucial factor to consider when evaluating effects of a toxin. Small quantities of a substance like strychnine taken daily over an extended period of time might have little to no effect, while one large dose in one day could be fatal. In addition, some toxins may only affect a particular species of organism, such as pesticides and antibiotics killing insects and microorganisms with significantly less harmful effects on humans.

Organisms vary greatly in their tolerance of exposure to chemicals. Even within populations of the same species great variations in sensitivity can exist. In rare cases, some individuals may be extremely sensitive to particular chemicals or groups of similar chemicals, a phenomenon known as hypersensitivity. Organisms are often exposed to a wide variety of potentially toxic chemicals through medicine, food, water, and the atmosphere.

The study of the disruption of biochemical pathways by poisons is a key aspect of toxicology. Poisons affect normal physiology in many ways; but some of the more common mechanisms involve the disabling of enzyme systems, induction of cancers, interference with the regulation of blood chemistry, and disruption of genetic processes.

Toxic agents may be physical (for example, **radiation**), biological (for example, poisonous snake bite), or chemical (for example, arsenic) in nature. In addition, biological organisms may cause disease by invading the body and releasing toxins. An example of this process is tetanus, in which the bacterium *Clostridium* *tetani* releases a powerful toxin that travels to the nervous system.

Toxic agents may also cause systemic or organ-specific reactions in the body. Cyanide affects the entire body by interfering with the body's capacity for utilizing oxygen. **Lead** has three specific targets: the central nervous system, the kidneys, and the hematopoietic (blood-cell generating) system. The target is affected by the dose and route of the toxin. For example, the initial effects of a chemical may affect the nervous system; repeated exposure over time might cause chronic damage to the liver.

Function

Toxicology is a discipline with a growing number of subdisciplines as of 2012.

Environmental and occupational toxicology

The toxicologist employs the tools and methods of science to understand more completely the consequences of exposure to toxic chemicals. Toxicologists typically assess the relationship between toxic chemicals and environmental health by evaluating such factors as the following:

- Risk: To assess the risk associated with exposure to a toxic substance, toxicologists first measure the exposure characteristics and then compute the doses that enter the human body. Then they compare these numbers to derive an estimate of risk, sometimes based on animal studies. In cases where human data exist for a toxic substance, such as benzene, more straightforward correlations with human risk of illness or death are possible.
- Precautionary strategies: Given recommendations from toxicologists, government agencies sometimes decide to regulate a chemical based on limited evidence from animal and human epidemiological studies that the chemical is toxic.
- Clinical data: Some toxicologists devise new techniques and develop new applications of existing methods to monitor changes in the health of individuals exposed to toxic substances. For example, one academic research group in the United States has spent many years developing new methods for monitoring the effects of exposure to oxidants (for example, free radicals) in healthy and diseased humans.
- Epidemiological evidence: Another way to understand the environmental factors contributing to human illness is to study large populations that have been exposed to substances suspected of being toxic. Scientists then attempt to tie these observations to clinical data. Ecological studies seek to correlate exposure patterns with a specific outcome. Case-control studies compare groups of persons with a particular illness with similar healthy groups, and seek to identify the degree of exposure required to bring about the illness. Other studies may refine the scope of environmental factor studies; or, examine a small group of individuals in which there is a high incidence of a rare disease and a history of exposure to a particular chemical.
- Evidence of bioaccumulation: When a chemical is nonbiodegradable, it may accumulate in biosystems, resulting in very high concentrations accumulating in animals at the top of food chains. Such chlorinated pesticides as dieldrin and DDT, for example, have been found in fish in much greater concentrations than in the seawater where they swim.

Medical toxicology

Medical toxicology is recognized as a subspecialty by the American Board of Medical Specialties. Medical toxicologists may work in emergency departments, intensive care units, poison control centers, public health organizations, or pharmaceutical and government research facilities. Their work includes:

- Diagnosis and treatment of accidental or intentional drug overdoses, including over-the-counter as well as prescription medications.
- Evaluation of envenomations, ingestion of poisonous plants or mushrooms, and other forms of exposure to natural toxins.
- Diagnosis and treatment of adverse drug reactions.
- Health problems related to drugs of abuse, which may include assessment of contaminated drugs as well as medical and psychiatric disorders related to the consumption of such drugs.
- Education of other health professionals in the basic elements of medical toxicology.

Forensic toxicology

Forensic toxicology is the subdiscipline that assists with medicolegal investigations of poisoning, drug use, and suspicious deaths. Forensic toxicologists typically work with samples of hair, urine, blood, or other body fluids, various body tissues, and stomach contents. They may also evaluate or analyze pill bottles, other substance containers, syringes, drinking glasses, or similar objects found at the scene of the investigation. In addition, forensic toxicologists may be called on to serve as expert witnesses in courtroom proceedings.

Role in human health

Humans are exposed to complex mixtures of chemicals, many of which are synthetic and have been either deliberately or accidentally released into the environment. In some cases, people actively expose themselves to chemicals that are known to be toxic, such as those found in cigarettes, alcohol, or recreational drugs. Voluntary exposure to chemicals also occurs when people take medicines to deal with illness, use certain types of cosmetics and hair products, or when they choose to work in an occupation that involves routinely dealing with dangerous chemicals. Most exposures to potentially toxic chemicals are inadvertent, and involve living in an environment that is contaminated with small concentrations of pollutants, such as those associated with pesticide residues in food, lead from gasoline combustion, or sulfur dioxide and **ozone** in the urban atmosphere.

Drugs given to improve health can lead to toxicity even when given in appropriate doses. Conditions such as dehydration and other forms of physiological compromise can make the patient more vulnerable to toxicity. Drugs like acetaminophen, digoxin, lidocaine, and lithium are common examples of drugs with potentially toxic effects. Interactions of substances in the body may also produce toxic effects. For example, if two central nervous system depressants are taken at once, as in the case of combining alcohol and a benzodiazepine tranquilizer, the effects are additive and could lead to extreme depression of the central nervous system functions.

The health care system's role related to toxicology includes education and prevention as well as treatment of both acute and chronic effects of toxins. Such agencies as the **Food and Drug Administration** (FDA), the National Toxicology Program (NTP), the **Agency for Toxic Substances and Disease Registry** (ATSDR; part of the CDC), and the **Occupational Safety and Health Administration** (OSHA) work with health care and industry to offer guidelines and restrictions on the manufacture and use of pharmaceuticals, foods, cosmetics, and other substances.

Health care workers are involved by being aware of these regulations, and staying informed. They also provide education, such as, teaching new parents about the dangers of lead paint consumption by children, and help prevent exposure to toxins, such as tetanus **vaccination**, or monitoring for signs of lithium toxicity. The Poison Control Center uses nurses and other allied health workers to inform the public of immediate actions to take in the event of a poisoning emergency. Emergency interventions at the hospital include blood and urine tests, gastric lavage with administration of absorbent activated charcoal, and administration of antidotes when available.

> ### KEY TERMS
>
> **Antidote**—A substance that combats the effects of a poison or toxin.
>
> **Bioaccumulation**—The absorption of toxic chemicals by the tissues of a living organism.
>
> **Forensic**—Dealing with matters of interest to a court of law, whether criminal or civil proceedings.
>
> **Gastric lavage**—The act of emptying out the stomach via orogastric or nasogastric tube.

Common diseases and disorders

Toxicologists have ranked the most commonly encountered toxic chemicals in the United States. In descending order of frequency of encounter, they are as follows:

- Arsenic: Toxic exposure occurs mainly in the workplace, near hazardous waste sites, or in areas with high natural levels. A powerful poison, arsenic can, at high levels of exposure, cause death or illness.

- Lead: Toxic exposure usually results from breathing workplace air or dust or from eating contaminated foods. Children may be exposed to lead from eating lead-based paint chips or playing in contaminated soil. Lead damages the nervous system, kidneys, and the immune systems.

- Mercury: Toxic exposure results from breathing contaminated air, ingesting contaminated water and food, and possibly having dental and medical treatments. At high levels, mercury damages the brain, kidneys, and developing fetuses.

- Vinyl chloride: Toxic exposure occurs mainly in the workplace. Breathing high levels of vinyl chloride for short periods can produce dizziness, sleepiness, unconsciousness, and, at very high levels, death. Breathing vinyl chloride for long periods of time can give rise to permanent liver damage, immune reactions, nerve damage, and liver cancer.

- Benzene: Benzene is formed in both natural processes and human activities. Breathing benzene can produce drowsiness, dizziness, and unconsciousness. Long-term exposure affects the bone marrow and can produce anemia and leukemia.

> **QUESTIONS TO ASK YOUR DOCTOR**
>
> - Have you ever taken courses in toxicology as part of your training?
> - What should health professionals who are not specialists in toxicology know about it?
> - Have you ever consulted an occupational or medical toxicologist to diagnose and treat a patient?

- Polychlorinated biphenyls (PCBs: PCBs are mixtures of chemicals. They are no longer produced in the United States but remain in the environment. They can irritate the nose and throat and cause acne and rashes. They have been shown to cause cancer in animal studies.
- Cadmium: Toxic exposure to cadmium occurs mainly in workplaces where cadmium products are made. Other sources of exposure include cigarette smoke and cadmium-contaminated foods. Cadmium can damage the lungs, cause kidney disease, and irritate the digestive tract.

Resources

BOOKS

Barceloux, Donald G., ed. *Medical Toxicology of Drug Abuse: Synthesized Chemicals and Psychoactive Plants.* Hoboken, NJ: John Wiley and Sons, 2012.

Bingham, Eula, and Barbara Cohrssen, eds. *Patty's Toxicology*, 6th ed. Hoboken, NJ: John Wiley and Sons, 2012.

Lynch, Joshua J., and Kevin R. McGee. *Lippincott's Manual of Toxicology*. Philadelphia: Wolters Kluwer/Lippincott Williams and Wilkins Health, 2012.

Rao, Kalipatnapu N. *Forensic Toxicology: Medico-Legal Case Studies*. Boca Raton, FL: CRC Press, 2012.

PERIODICALS

Alavanja, M.C., and M.R. Bonner. "Occupational Pesticide Exposures and Cancer Risk: A Review." *Journal of Toxicology and Environmental Health, Part B: Critical Reviews* 15 (May 2012): 238–263.

Andersen, D., et al. "Validation of a Fully Automated Robotic Setup for Preparation of Whole Blood Samples for LC-MS Toxicology Analysis." *Journal of Analytical Toxicology* 36 (May 2012): 280–287.

Andresen, H., et al. "Fentanyl: Toxic or Therapeutic? Postmortem and Antemortem Blood Concentrations after Transdermal Fentanyl Application." *Journal of Analytical Toxicology* 36 (April 2012): 182–194.

Domingo, J.L. "Polybrominated Diphenyl Ethers in Food and Human Dietary Exposure: A Review of the Recent Scientific Literature." *Food and Chemical Toxicology* 50 (February 2012): 238–249.

Fragou, D., et al. "Atypical Antipsychotics: Trends in Analysis and Sample Preparation of Various Biological Samples." *Bioanalysis* 4 (May 2012): 961–980.

Livshits, Z., et al. "Wolf Spider Envenomation." *Wilderness and Environmental Medicine* 23 (March 2012): 49–50.

Maskell, P.D., et al. "Phenazepam: The Drug That Came in from the Cold." *Journal of Forensic and Legal Medicine* 19 (April 2012): 122–125.

McGill, M.R., et al. "The Mechanism Underlying Acetaminophen-induced Hepatotoxicity in Humans and Mice Involves Mitochondrial Damage and Nuclear DNA Fragmentation." *Journal of Clinical Investigation* 122 (April 2, 2012): 1574–1583.

Porter, W.H. "Ethylene Glycol Poisoning: Quintessential Clinical Toxicology; Analytical Conundrum." *Clinica Chimica Acta* 413 (February 18, 2012): 365–377.

Taylor, D.L., et al. "Indicators of Sediment and Biotic Mercury Contamination in a Southern New England Estuary." *Marine Pollution Bulletin* 64 (April 2012): 807–819.

WEBSITES

Agency for Toxic Substances and Disease Registry (ATSDR). Toxic Substances Portal. http://www.atsdr.cdc.gov/substances/index.asp (accessed May 17, 2012).

American College of Medical Toxicology (ACMT). "What Is Medical Toxicology?" http://www.acmt.net/overview.html (accessed May 16, 2012).

National Library of Medicine (NLM). NLM Toxicology Tutorials. http://sis.nlm.nih.gov/enviro/toxtutor.html (accessed May 17, 2012).

ORGANIZATIONS

Division of Toxicology and Environmental Medicine, 4770 Buford Hwy NE, Atlanta, GA, United States 30341, (800) CDC-INFO, cdcinfo@cdc.gov, http://www.atsdr.cdc.gov/.

American Association of Poison Control Centers (AAPCC), (800) 222-1222, info@aapcc.org, http://www.aapcc.org/dnn/Home.aspx.

American College of Medical Toxicology (ACMT), 10645 N. Tatum Blvd., Suite 200-111, Phoenix, AZ, United States 85028, (623) 533-6340, Fax: (623) 533-6520, info@acmt.net, http://www.acmt.net/.

American College of Toxicology (ACTOX), 9650 Rockville Pike, No. 3408, Bethesda, MD, United States 20814, (301) 634-7840, Fax: (301) 634-7852, http://www.actox.org/Home/tabid/726/Default.aspx.

Food and Drug Administration (FDA), 10903 New Hampshire Avenue, Silver Spring, MD, United States 20993, (888) INFO-FDA (463-6332), http://www.fda.gov/default.htm.

National Toxicology Program (NTP), P.O. Box 12233, MD K2-05, Research Triangle Park, NC, United States 27709, (919) 541-3419, http://ntp.niehs.nih.gov/.

Society of Forensic Toxicologists (SOFT), One MacDonald Center, 1 N. MacDonald Street, Suite 15, Mesa, AZ, United States 85201, (888) 866-SOFT (7638), office@soft-tox.org, http://soft-tox.org/.

Katherine Hauswirth, APRN
Rebecca J. Frey, PhD

Transmissible spongiform encephalopathies (TSEs) *see* **Creutzfeldt-Jakob disease**

Traveler's health

Definition

When people travel, their bodies take some time to adapt to a new destination, especially to food and water. In some foreign countries lax sanitary conditions exist, which may even compromise a traveler's health. Thus, the risk of getting sick is often increased when traveling. Drinking water in some developing countries may contain bacteria, **parasites**, and **viruses**, which can cause traveler's diarrhea (TD). Traveler's diarrhea, one of the more common ailments experienced during traveling, is the occurrence of multiple loose bowel movements in someone traveling to an area outside their usual surroundings, usually from temperate industrialized regions to tropical areas. The cause is almost always bacterial or viral infection acquired through ingesting contaminated food or water.

When people travel outside of the United States, especially to developing countries, they need vaccinations or preventative medicine for certain diseases found there that are not so common in developed countries. These diseases include **yellow fever**, typhoid, **cholera**, and **malaria**. Which vaccinations or preventative medicines are needed depends on the particular destination, the time of travel, the age of the traveler, the general health of the traveler, and other pertinent factors.

Description

Every year Americans travel to international locations. Some of these foreign regions make American travelers more susceptible to diseases and medical conditions that adversely affects their health. For instance, diarrhea is a disorder caused by numerous microorganisms such as bacteria, protozoans, and viruses. It brings about water and electrolyte loss within the body, which leads to dehydration and in some cases death. It is estimated that 20% to 50% of the 12 to 20 million travelers going from temperate industrialized countries to the tropics have their health compromised and, as a consequence, could develop TD. Fortunately, most of these episodes are brief. Nevertheless, about 40% of those affected need to rearrange their schedule, and 20% may be ill enough to remain in bed for some days.

The chance of winding up with TD is directly related to the destination; only about 8% of individuals visiting an industrialized country are affected, whereas at least half of those traveling to nonindustrialized regions become ill. It is also clearly related to the number of potentially contaminated foods or beverages consumed. Attention to recommended guidelines regarding **food safety** and **sanitation** can greatly decrease the risk of infection.

The health of travelers can also be compromised by other medical condition. The U.S. **Centers for Disease Control and Prevention** (CDC) lists numerous diseases that can affect humans while traveling. Its list is contained under its website heading "Diseases Related to Travel." The CDC list is lengthy. Below are a few of the more commonly known travel diseases:

- altitude illness
- cholera
- encephalitis
- malaria
- meningitis
- plague
- tuberculosis
- typhoid fever
- West Nile virus
- yellow fever

Cholera is an acute and often fatal intestinal disease that produces severe gastrointestinal symptoms. Caused by the bacterium *Vibrio cholera*, cholera is rarely present in industrialized countries. In fact, it was mostly absent from the United States during the twentieth century and into the twenty-first century. However, as of the early 2000s, cholera was still common in many parts of the world, including the Indian subcontinent and sub-Saharan Africa.

In another instance, malaria is caused by parasite-carrying mosquitoes. People with malaria often have flu-like symptoms, such as chills and fever. If left untreated, malaria can cause serious complications, including death. According to the CDC, in 2010, about 216 million cases of malaria occurred in the world. Of those, 655,000 people died, with over 90% of them dying in Africa.

Typhoid fever is a life-threatening illness caused by the bacterium *Salmonella enterica* serotype Typhi. It is usually transmitted through water or food that is contaminated by feces. The CDC estimates that about 22 million cases occur worldwide each year, with an associated 200,000 deaths. In the United States, about 300 cases occur each year, with most of those occurring among recent travelers abroad. The highest risks of getting typhoid fever occur among those people traveling to southern Asia, eastern Asia, Southeast Asia, Africa, the Caribbean, Central American, and South America.

Demographics

CDC estimates that 15% to 70% of international travelers coming back to the United States have a travel-related illness. Although most of these illnesses have only mild symptoms, others necessitate medical care. Most travelers become ill within 12 weeks after returning to the United States. However, some illnesses may not cause symptoms for as long as six to 12 months or even longer after exposure. For instance, symptoms of malaria may show up less than two weeks after traveling, but other malaria symptoms may take longer than six weeks to appear. Younger age groups, particularly students, are at greatest risk for having a health problems while traveling than are older people, probably because of where and what they eat. Individuals over 55 years of age and business travelers are at lower risk than are other people of getting diseases while traveling abroad because they are more apt to take precautions before and during travel. Those travelers on adventure vacations are at increased risk for TD, just because of the more risky nature of their vacation activities. People visiting friends and relatives in foreign countries are also at increased risk because they are less likely to seek pretravel advice, obtain vaccinations, or take other precautions before and during travel. Foods with the highest chance of transmitting disease, especially diarrhea and upset stomach, are uncooked vegetables, unpeeled fruits, meat, and seafood. Tap water and even ice can be dangerous unless its source is clean.

The CDC provides valuable information for travelers with regards to health alerts for common diseases found around the world. Its website "Travel Notices" provides important current information.

Causes and symptoms

The causes and symptoms of diseases caught by travelers are much varied due to the high number of such ailments that occur around the world. Some of the more common causes and symptoms are discussed below.

Causes

Causes of the diseases commonly associated with traveling vary depending on the specific medical problem. For accurate information on causes and their symptoms for diseases associated with traveling, people ought to refer to the CDC website "Diseases Related to Travel."

Bacterial infections are the most common cause of traveler's diarrhea. Viruses and occasional parasites also can be the cause. As for the bacteria involved, toxin producing types of *E. coli* (called enterotoxigenic) account for approximately 40% to 60% of cases, with *Campylobacter* and *Shigella* each reported in at least 10% of cases. In some studies, *Campylobacter* has accounted for almost half of the attacks, especially during cooler seasons of the year. The cause can vary depending on several factors, including the season and country visited. More than one organism can be found in 15% to 30% of cases, while none is identified in up to 40% of cases worldwide.

Rotaviruses and a parvovirus called Norwalk agent also are responsible for TD. *Giardia* is probably the most common parasite identified, although amoebas (*Entamoeba histolytica*), *Cryptosporidium*, and *Cyclospora* are found frequently.

Symptoms

Symptoms associated with TD usually start within a few days after arrival but can be delayed for as long as two weeks. Illness lasts an average of three to five days but sometimes longer. Cramping abdominal pain, lack of appetite, and diarrhea are the main complaints. In approximately 10% of patients, diarrhea turns bloody. Fever develops in about half of the cases. The presence of bloody bowel movements and fever usually indicates a more severe form of illness and makes *Shigella* a more likely cause. Medications that decrease the motility or contractions of the intestine, such as loperamide (Imodium) or diphenoxylate (Lomotil), should not be used when fever or bleeding occur.

Complications

Diarrhea varies from a few loose stools per day to ten or more. Dehydration and changes in the normal blood pH (acid-base balance) are the main dangers associated with TD. Signs of dehydration can be hard to notice, but increasing thirst, dry mouth, weakness or lightheadedness (particularly if worsening while standing), or a darkening/decrease in urination are suggestive. Severe dehydration and changes in the body's chemistry can lead to kidney failure and become life-threatening.

Another potential complication is toxic megacolon, in which the colon gradually stretches and its wall thins to the point where it can tear. The presence of a hole in the intestine leads to peritonitis and is fatal unless quickly recognized and treated.

Other complications related to TD can involve the nervous system, skin, blood, or kidneys.

Diagnosis

Some travel-related illnesses may not show themselves for days, weeks, months, or even years after travelers return to the United States. In all cases, medical professionals will diagnosis a traveler with a medical problem according to the presence of specific symptoms, the destination and region of the world traveled to (some diseases are more common in certain parts of the world than they are in others), and other related factors. They will want to know about the weeks and months leading up to travel, during travel, and those following travel. A complete physical examination and gathering of a comprehensive history of the patient will be conducted, along with any laboratory tests that are deemed necessary. In some cases, appropriate health officials may be notified, such as for **measles**, **tuberculosis**, and viral hemorrhagic fever. Further, a physician familiar in travel-related illnesses may be called in under special circumstances. For example, travelers to a tropical location may need a tropical medicine specialist to evaluate their illness.

According to the CDC, the following should be evaluated by the medical professional when diagnosing returning travelers with illnesses:

- activities associated with many people, such as mass gathering
- activities in fresh water, such as rafting, swimming, and wading
- adherence to the prevention of diseases, such as malaria, through vaccines and antibiotics (what is called chemoprophylaxis)
- adventure travel, especially spelunking (cave exploration)
- animal bites and scratches
- consumption of raw meat, seafood, or unpasteurized dairy products
- exposures to water
- immunization history
- hospitalizations and other medical care while traveling
- insect and arthropod bites, such as from mosquitoes and ticks
- previous medical history and medications
- sexual contacts
- tattoos, body piercing, and the use of shared razors
- travel duration
- travel itinerary
- types of accommodations
- use of bed nets, insect repellents, and other preventative measures

With regards to TD, the occurrence of diarrhea in an individual while traveling is very suggestive of traveler's diarrhea. Although there are other possible causes, these are less likely. In most instances, the specific organism responsible for the symptoms does not need to be identified, and the majority of patients need only rest and treatment to avoid potential complications.

When patients develop fever or bloody diarrhea, the illness is more serious and a specific diagnosis is needed. In those cases, or when symptoms last longer than expected, stool samples are obtained to identify the organism.

For this purpose, laboratories can either try to grow (culture) the organism or identify it with high-powered microscopes (electron microscopy) or with the use of special tests or stains. These can show parasites such as *Giardia, Amoeba, Cryptosporidium* and others in freshly obtained stool specimens. New techniques that involve identification of DNA (formally known as deoxyribonucleic acid; the characteristic material that controls reproduction and is unique for all individuals) of the various organisms also can be used in special circumstances.

Treatment

The best treatment for any diseases incurred while traveling, including TD, is prevention. Before traveling to foreign destination, individuals should schedule a visit with their family doctor or other health professional. The CDC recommends that a medical visit be set up at least four to six weeks before the trip. While there, individuals need to confirm that all vaccinations are administered that are recommended or required for travel to specific regions of the world. In many cases, it takes at least four weeks for vaccines to become effective within the body. In other cases, vaccines must be delivered gradually to the body, which may take over six weeks to complete. Which vaccinations are needed depends on a number of factors, including the destination, season of travel, age, health status, previous immunizations, and other important considerations. The CDC has three categories for vaccines: routine, recommended, and required. Routine vaccines protect people from diseases that are still common in many parts of the world but only rarely occur in the United States. The CDC provides recommended immunization schedules for adults, adolescents, children, and infants at its website.

Recommended vaccines also help to protect travelers from illnesses present in other parts of the world; however, they also prevent infectious diseases from being brought into the United States when travelers return from their trips. The CDC provides detailed information on specific destinations in the world at its website. Required vaccines are only those required by International Health Regulation. Yellow fever, for instance, is required for individuals who are traveling to some countries in sub-Saharan Africa and tropical countries of South America. The Saudi Arabian government requires a **vaccination** for meningococcal when individuals are traveling during the Hajj (an Islamic pilgrimage to Mecca).

In addition, individuals should discuss with their medical provider any illnesses or medical conditions that may make them more susceptible to diseases while traveling, such as diabetes or human immunodeficiency virus (HIV). People who are traveling with infants or children should be especially aware of the dangers associated with traveling to foreign countries. Women who are pregnant or breastfeeding should also be aware of such concerns.

For traveler's diarrhea, once it occurs, therapy is aimed at preventing or reducing dehydration and using antibiotics when needed. Fortunately, severe dehydration is unusual in patients with TD, but any fluid losses should be treated early with either fruit juices and clear fluids such as tea or broth, or with the recommended Oral Rehydration Solutions (ORSs) suggested by the **World Health Organization** (WHO). Persons traveling to known areas of infection should consult with their physician prior to departure and obtain appropriate instructions. For example, it may be advised to take along pre-prepared packets of ORS designed for easy mixing or commercial preparations such as Pedialyte, Ceralyte, and Ricelyte.

> **KEY TERMS**
>
> **Oral rehydration solution (ORS)**—A liquid preparation developed by the World Health Organization that can decrease fluid loss in persons with diarrhea. Originally developed to be prepared with materials available in the home, commercial preparations are available.

When nothing else is available, the following WHO recipe can be made up from household items and taken in small frequent sips:

- table salt: 1-3/4 teaspoon
- baking powder: 1 teaspoon
- orange juice: 1 cup
- water: 1 quart or liter

A debate occurred in the medical community over the amount of salt (sodium) in the WHO preparations; some physicians explained that the content is too much for use by well-nourished persons in developed countries. Therefore, these preparations should not be used for extended periods of time without consulting a physician.

Pepto-Bismol (bismuth subsalicylate preparation) is effective in both preventing and treating TD. For treatment once symptoms begin, the drug must be taken more frequently than when used for prevention. Bismuth subsalicylate preparation (1 ounce of liquid or two 262.5-milligram tablets every 30 minutes for eight doses) has been shown to decrease the number of bowel movements and shorten the length of illness. However, there is some concern about the large doses of bismuth in patients with kidney disease; therefore, patients should check with physicians before starting this or any other therapy. Patients should be aware that bismuth can turn bowel movements black.

Rifamixin (Normix), a drug for treating traveler's diarrhea, was approved by the U.S. **Food and Drug Administration** (FDA) in 2010. Medications designed to decrease intestinal motility and contractions such as loperamide (Imodium), diphenoxylate (Lomotil), or others are safest when used by those without fever or bloody bowel movements. The presence of either of these symptoms indicates a more severe form of colitis.

Antibiotics are usually not prescribed, because most cases of TD rapidly improve with minimal treatment. For patients in whom symptoms are especially severe (four or more stools per day or the onset of bloody diarrhea or fever), or those with compromised immune systems, antibiotics are indicated. Individuals with less severe attacks can be treated with either antimotility medications or bismuth subsalicylate.

Choice of an antibiotic should ideally be tailored to the most likely organism and then adjusted according to results of stool cultures. Trimethoprim-sulfamethoxazole (Bactrim) or ciprofloxacin (Cipro) are the antibiotics most often prescribed, but others are also used. The type and duration of treatment continues to be revised, and it is therefore extremely important that patients check with a physician prior to beginning treatment. In many instances, an antibiotic can be combined with an anti-motility agent to provide the quickest relief.

Public health role and response

The U.S. Centers for Disease Control and Prevention (CDC) provides a website just for travelers' health. Topics discussed at this website include health information for over 200 destinations worldwide, general information about vaccinations, the types of illnesses frequently occurring overseas, and locations of health clinics and health specialists found throughout the world. The CDC also provides "Your Survival Guide to Safe and Healthy Travel." It gives details on how to be proactive, prepared, and protected while traveling.

In the 2012, numerous CDC outbreak notices were issued around the world. As of October 2012, the latest outbreak notice occurred in Greece and involved malaria.

Prognosis

Most people who are treated promptly recover from illnesses associated with traveling. However, there are always exceptions. For instance, diagnosed cases of yellow fever result in death 5% to 10% of the time. Jaundice is an important indicator when individuals are infected with yellow fever.

Prevention

Hygienic sewage disposal systems in a community, good water treatment facilities, and proper personal hygiene are the most important factors in preventing many problems occurring with travelers. Immunizations are available for travelers who expect to visit countries where known public health problems are common. Some of these immunizations provide only short-term protection (for a few months), while others may be effective for several years. Efforts are being made to develop vaccines that provide a longer period of protection with fewer side effects from the vaccine itself. For instance, an effective yellow fever vaccine exists. Called the Arilvax vaccine, it is made from a weakened form of the yellow fever virus, strain 17D. In the United States, the vaccine is given only at Yellow Fever Vaccination Centers authorized by the U.S. **Public Health Service**. About 95% of vaccine recipients acquire long-term immunity to the yellow fever virus.

With regards to traveler's diarrhea, the best means of prevention is avoiding foods, beverages, and food handling practices that lead to infection with the organisms that cause TD. Drinking bottled water and using bottled water for brushing teeth, eating fruits that travelers peel themselves, and eating well-cooked, hot foods can help prevent illness.

One effective means to prevent TD is liquid Pepto-Bismol; this bismuth-containing compound has been shown to be very effective in reducing the incidence of TD. Tablets are available, which are easier to carry. Two tablets four times a day is recommended, but use should continue beyond three weeks.

Antibiotics can also prevent TD, but their use is controversial, unless it is absolutely necessary to avoid infection (such as in someone on an important business trip or who has a weakened immune system). There is the tendency for bacteria to become resistant to these medications if people use them excessively, and these drugs have side effects that can be worse than the effects of TD. The benefits and risks of antibiotic treatment should be carefully weighed.

QUESTIONS TO ASK YOUR DOCTOR

- What should I do to minimize my chances of getting sick while traveling to foreign countries?
- Are there any special precautions I should take before traveling anywhere internationally?
- What shots do I need if I decide to travel to a developing country in the world?
- Are there any unusual diseases I need to be concerned about when visiting my destination country?
- Should I be concerned about my traveler's health if I am visiting a developed country comparable to the United States?
- What should I do to if I have a medical condition while traveling?

Resources

BOOKS

Juuti, Petri S., Tapio S. Katko, and Heikki S. Vuorinen. *Environmental History of Water: Global Views on Community Water Supply and Sanitation.* London: IWA, 2007.

Prakash, Anjal, V. S. Saravanan, and Jayati Choubey, eds. *Interlacing Water and Human Health: Case Studies from South Asia.* New Delhi: Sage, 2012.

Shannon, Joyce Brennfleck, ed. *Contagious Diseases Sourcebook: Basic Consumer Health Information about Diseases Spread from Person to Person.* Detroit, MI: Omnigraphics, 2010.

Vincent, J. L. *Textbook of Critical Care.* Philadelphia: Elsevier/Saunders, 2011.

Wilder-Smith, Annelies, Eli Schwartz, and Marc Shaw, eds. *Travel Medicine: Tales Behind the Science.* Amsterdam: Elsevier, 2007.

WEBSITES

Batara, Vandana. "Typhoid Fever." Centers for Disease Control and Prevention. October 5, 2010. http://www.cdc.gov/nczved/divisions/dfbmd/diseases/typhoid_fever/ (accessed July 6, 2012).

"Country List: Yellow Fever Vaccination Requirements and Recommendations; and Malaria Situation." World Health Organization. http://www.who.int/ith/ITH2010countrylist.pdf (accessed July 7, 2012).

"Diarrheal Diseases." World Health Organization. http://www.who.int/vaccine_research/diseases/diarrhoeal/en/index7.html (accessed July 6, 2012).

Dugdale, David, and Jatin M. Vyas. "Yellow Fever." MedlinePlus. http://www.nlm.nih.gov/medlineplus/ency/article/001365.htm (accessed July 7, 2012).

"General Approach to the Returned Traveler." Centers for Disease Control and Prevention. November 8, 2011. http://wwwnc.cdc.gov/travel/yellowbook/2012/chapter-5-post-travel-evaluation/general-approach-to-the-returned-traveler.htm (accessed October 19, 2012).

"Global Analysis and Assessment of Sanitation and Drinking-water." World Health Organization. April 12, 2012. http://www.who.int/water_sanitation_health/en/ (accessed September 19, 2012).

"Progress on Drinking Water and Sanitation: 2012 Update." Joint Monitoring Programme (JMP) for Water Supply and Sanitation, WHO and UNICEF. http://www.wssinfo.org/documents-links/documents/ (accessed September 19, 2012).

"Sanitation." Division for Social Development, Department of Economic and Social Affairs, United Nations. http://www.un.org/esa/dsd/susdevtopics/sdt_sanitation.shtml (accessed September 19, 2012).

"Sanitation." World Health Organizationhttp://www.who.int/topics/sanitation/en/ (accessed September 19, 2012).

"Travelers' Health." Centers for Disease Control and Prevention. (April 12, 2012). http://wwwnc.cdc.gov/travel/ (accessed October 19, 2012).

"Water, Sanitation and Hygiene." UN Children's Fund. http://www.unicef.org/wash/index_wes_related.html (accessed September 19, 2012).

ORGANIZATIONS

Centers for Disease Control and Prevention, 1600 Clifton Rd., Atlanta, GA 30333, (800) 232-4636, cdcinfo@cdc.gov, http://www.cdc.gov.

National Institute of Allergy and Infectious Diseases, 1301 Pennsylvania Ave. NW, Ste. 800, Washington, DC 20004, (202) 785-3355, Fax: (202) 452-1805, info@lung.org, http://www.lung.org.

World Health Organization, Avenue Appia 20, 1211 Geneva 27, Switzerland, 2241 791 21 11, Fax: 2241 791 31 11, info@who.int, http://www.who.int.

David Kaminstein, MD
Teresa G. Odle
William A. Atkins, BB, BS, MBA

Tropical disease

Definition

Tropical disease is any disease that primarily occurs in tropical and subtropical regions. The term is commonly applied to any infectious disease that is **endemic** in hot, humid climates.

Description

Early explorers from northern climes catalogued the so-called exotic diseases that they encountered in the tropics, and there are hundreds of tropical diseases that are public health concerns. The **World Health Organization** (WHO) considers tropical diseases to include those diseases that are endemic in Africa, the eastern Mediterranean, Southeast Asia, the Western Pacific, and Latin America. However, tropical diseases are present in—and increasingly spreading to—temperate regions.

Many tropical disease are caused by **parasites**, bacteria, or **viruses** that are transmitted by insect bites. These insect vectors thrive in hot climates with heavy rainfall, whereas they tend to hibernate or die out in cold weather. Diverse tropical wildlife provide natural reservoirs for disease, many of which are zoonoses (animal diseases that can be transmitted to humans). Hotter temperatures may promote more efficient reproduction of pathogens, both inside and outside their hosts. Finally, tropical countries are among the poorest in the world, with few resources for preventing the establishment and spread of disease. Thus, tropical disease causes immense suffering throughout the developing world, sickening and killing, interfering with children's physical and cognitive development, keeping people from work and school, and perpetuating a cycle of poverty and disease.

Tropical diseases are usually referred to as neglected tropical diseases (NTDs) because they have been largely eradicated in the developed world. NTDs persist in poor countries, marginalized communities, and conflict zones. Throughout most of the twentieth century, resources were directed to infectious diseases in developed countries, to the neglect of tropical disease. As a result, there are few vaccines against tropical disease, and many NTDs are difficult to treat or incurable.

Risk factors

The primary risk factors for tropical disease are residing in or visiting an endemic area. Poverty, lack of access to clean water and **sanitation**, natural disasters, political instability, violent conflicts, and human displacement are all risk factors for tropical disease.

Demographics

At least one NTD is present in 149 countries and territories. At any given time, every low-income country in the world is affected by at least five NTDs, and some NTDs affect the southern United States, especially among the poor. Tropical disease is increasing worldwide and spreading beyond the tropics with international travel, human migration, deforestation, and warming global temperatures that allow disease agents and their vectors to invade higher altitudes and latitudes.

Malaria is the most serious tropical disease, infecting 300–500 million people every year in about 100 countries. More than one million people, especially African and Asian children under age five, die of malaria every year. About 50% of the world's population live in areas at risk for malaria. **Cholera** and other diarrheal diseases are the second leading cause of death among the planet's poor. Intestinal worms or helminthiasis and **schistosomiasis** (blood flukes from contaminated water) are also major causes of disease and death. About 120 million people have symptoms of schistosomiasis, and more than 200,000 people in sub-Saharan Africa die of the disease every year. Another 700 million are considered to be at risk. Growing population and demand for water are increasing transmission of schistosomiasis, and refugees and urban migration are spreading it to new areas. Dengue is considered the second most significant tropical disease after malaria, because of its global resurgence between 1980 and 2010. Dengue infects at least 50 million people every year, with more than 500,000 becoming seriously ill. In contrast to these widespread NTDs, some tropical diseases, such as **Ebola hemorrhagic fever**, Lassa fever, and Marburg virus are very rare, appearing only occasionally in sudden deadly outbreaks.

Causes and symptoms

Parasitic protozoans

Malaria is the most prevalent NTD caused by protozoans. Five different parasites of the genus *Plasmodium* cause malaria in different parts of the world. *Plasmodium* is transmitted by the bite of female *Anopheles* mosquitoes that feed on human blood. The parasites invade red blood cells, causing repeated cycles of fever, chills, and other symptoms.

Chagas or American trypanosomiasis is caused by the *Trypanosoma cruzi*. It is transmitted by a blood-sucking "assassin" or "kissing" bug that resembles a cockroach. Chagas infects up to eight million people in the Western Hemisphere, including about 300,000 in the United States, and is a major cause of heart failure and sudden death. Pregnant women can transmit it to their babies. Some experts have called Chagas "the new **AIDS** of the Americas," because its spread resembles the early spread of HIV, it has a long incubation period, and it is difficult or impossible to cure. African trypanosomiasis or **sleeping sickness** is caused by *Trypanosoma gambiense* and *Trypanosoma brucei* that are transmitted by tsetse flies.

Leishmaniasis is caused by *Leishmania* protozoa that are transmitted by tiny sand flies. Depending on the species, symptoms range from skin ulcers to more serious disease and even death. Leishmaniasis affects up to 12 million people worldwide and is increasing due to international travel, global conflicts, alterations in vector habitats, and susceptibility from HIV/AIDS and malnutrition.

Parasitic worms

Schistosomiasis is caused by *Schistosoma* trematodes (flatworms) in contaminated water. Freshwater snails are its natural reservoir. Many other kinds of trematodes—liver, lung, and intestinal flukes—cause foodborne trematodiases from consumed fish and other animals and even plants from contaminated waters. Tapeworms are intestinal parasitic flatworms transmitted through undercooked beef or pork. Cysticercosis is caused by pork tapeworm larvae, and neurocysticercosis is the most common parasitic disease of the central nervous system.

Roundworms—such as *Ascaris lumbricoides* that causes ascariasis, hookworms, and *Trichuris trichiura* that causes trichuriasis or whipworm disease—are transmitted through feces-contaminated soil. Toxicariasis is caused by roundworms that normally infect dogs and cats. Lymphatic filariasis is caused by thread-like filarial nematodes or roundworms that are spread between humans by mosquitoes. Loa loa is a filarial worm transmitted by deer flies. These worms cause elephantiasis—thickening of the skin and tissues. Lymphatic filariasis infects more than 120 million people. Onchocerciasis or **river blindness** is caused by a nematode transmitted by black flies. Approximately 18 million people have onchocerciasis infections, and about 300,000 have been permanently blinded by the disease. Dracunculiasis or guinea-worm disease is caused by drinking water contaminated with larvae of the nematode *Dracunculus medinensis*. The worms emerge through the skin causing painful blisters.

Bacterial diseases

Tuberculosis (TB), Buruli ulcer, and leprosy are caused by related species of *Mycobacterium*. Although TB is now rare in developed countries, more than one-third of the human population has been infected with the bacterium, and the disease is prevalent in the tropics. TB is communicable through aerosols and, if untreated, has a mortality of above 50%. Buruli ulcer causes severe skin ulcerations and can spread to the bone. Leprosy is a chronic infectious disease of the peripheral nerves and upper respiratory tract.

Treponematoses is a collective term for diseases such as yaws, endemic syphilis, and pinta that are caused by subspecies of the spirochete *Treponema pallidum* and primarily affect children. Yaws is transmitted through skin contact. Its incidence was reduced by 95% in the 1950s, but it is undergoing a resurgence in various parts of the world.

Other bacterial NTDs include:
- trachoma caused by *Chlamydia trachomatis*, which, if untreated, can lead to irreversible blindness
- cholera, caused by *Vibrio cholerae* that thrives in unsanitary conditions, such as refugee camps
- typhus, which is transmitted from rodents by fleas
- leptospirosis, caused by bacteria that infect humans and animals and that is often mistaken for another disease

Viral diseases

Dengue, caused by four related flaviviruses, is spread by infected female *Aedes* mosquitoes, the same mosquito that transmits **yellow fever**, which killed millions before the development of a vaccine in the 1930s. Dengue causes a range of symptoms from severe muscle and joint pain to hemorrhage, shock, and death.

Viral **hemorrhagic fevers** are potentially fatal NTDs caused by various RNA viruses. They are highly infectious, with symptoms that include fever, vomiting, gastrointestinal bleeding, and low blood pressure. They are caused by viruses in four different families:

- Flaviviruses, in addition to dengue and yellow fever viruses, include West Nile virus and an encephalitis virus spread by ticks.
- Arenaviruses are responsible for Lassa fever in Africa and South American hemorrhagic fevers. They are typically transmitted through rodent excrement.
- Phlebovirus, nairovirus, and hantavirus in the family Bunyaviridae cause, respectively, Rift Valley fever spread by mosquitoes, Crimean-Congo hemorrhagic fever spread by ticks, and hantavirus diseases spread by rodents.
- Filoviruses are responsible for deadly outbreaks of Marburg and Ebola in Africa, although their animal reservoirs have not been definitively identified.

Diagnosis

Tropical disease diagnosis may be straightforward where a disease is endemic and known outbreaks are occurring. However, many NTDs have similar symptoms and occur in regions with few health care workers. Migrants, emigrants, and travelers arrive with NTDs that local health care providers are unfamiliar with. Newer diagnostic tools are being developed for some NTDs to facilitate diagnoses in remote areas.

Treatment

Many NTDs can be treated with drugs; however, medications are not necessarily available or affordable to affected populations. Furthermore, some pathogens, such as malarial parasites and the TB bacterium, have developed resistance to commonly used drugs. Drug-resistant malaria often emerges within just a few years of new drug introductions. Chagas requires treatment with harsh drugs that must be taken for up to three months and are effective only in early stages of infection. Provided that they are accurately diagnosed, worm infestations, such as cysticercosis and toxocariasis, may be effectively treated with antiparasitic and anti-inflammatory drugs.

> **KEY TERMS**
>
> **Dengue**—Infectious disease caused by RNA flaviviruses and transmitted by *Aedes* mosquitoes.
>
> **Endemic**—Restricted or peculiar to a specific locale or region; especially a disease that is prevalent only in a particular population.
>
> **Epidemic**—Affecting many individuals in a community or population and spreading rapidly.
>
> **Helminthiasis**—Diseases caused by parasitic worms, including tapeworms, flukes, hookworm, *Ascaris*, and whipworm.
>
> **Hemorrhagic fever**—Viral diseases that are transmitted to humans by insects or rodents and are characterized by the sudden onset of fever, bleeding from internal organs, and shock.
>
> **Malaria**—A disease caused by parasites of the genus *Plasmodium* that infect red blood cells and are transmitted from infected to uninfected people by bites of anopheline mosquitoes; the single largest cause of illness and death worldwide.
>
> **Parasite**—An organism that survives by living with, on, or in another organism, usually to the detriment of the host.
>
> **Pathogen**—A causative agent of disease, such as a bacteria, virus, or parasite.
>
> **Protozoan**—A one-celled organism of the phylum or sub-kingdom Protozoa, including parasites that cause tropical disease.
>
> **Reservoir**—An animal species that harbors a virus, usually without symptoms of infection, and can transmit it to humans directly or via a vector.
>
> **Schistosomiasis**—A widespread disease caused by blood flukes (trematodes or flatworms) in the genus *Schistosoma* that are harbored by snails in contaminated water.
>
> **Vector**—An organism that can transmit infection from one organism or source to another, often a mosquito, tick, or rodent.
>
> **Zoonoses**—Diseases that can be transmitted from animals to humans under natural conditions.

Public health role and response

Some tropical countries, such as Brazil, that have been able to invest in public health and sanitation have had dramatic success in reducing or eliminating NTDs. Other countries have effectively interrupted the transmission of some NTDs. However, progress has been slow, and natural disasters and armed conflict increase the tropical disease burden. For example, cholera swept through the population in the aftermath of the 2010 earthquake in Haiti, due to overcrowding, poor sanitation, and limited access to clean food and water.

The World Health Organization (WHO), the U.S. **Centers for Disease Control and Prevention** (CDC), and other organizations work to reduce illness, disability, and death from NTDs. The CDC began a global campaign to eradicate guinea worm in 1980. At the time, there were about 3.5 million cases annually in 20—mostly African—countries, and an additional 120 million people were at risk through unsafe drinking water. By educating villagers and providing cloth and pipe water filters and larvicides to kill the fleas that transmit the disease, there had been a 99% reduction in guinea-worm infections by 2012. Guinea worm was on the verge of becoming the second human disease, after **smallpox**, to be completely eradicated. As of 2012, the CDC was focusing on soil-transmitted ascariasis, hookworm, and whipworm, lymphatic filariasis, onchocerciasis, schistosomiasis, and trachoma, since these diseases can be controlled or even eradicated by mass administration of safe and effective drugs. There is also an ongoing effort, led by the WHO and the Bill and Melinda Gates Foundation, to eradicate malaria, with short-term focus on new antimalarial drugs and a long-term aim of vaccine development.

Unfortunately, pharmaceutical companies have had little financial incentive for developing new diagnostic tests, drugs, and vaccines for NTDs that afflict poverty-stricken regions. However, new tropical disease institutes are focusing on research and development and training health care providers to recognize, diagnose, and treat NTDs. In part, this is a response to the increase in NTDs in the United States and other developed countries, both from immigration and from domestic transmission.

Prognosis

It is unlikely that tropical disease will ever be completely eradicated. With population growth, increased human migration, and **climate change**, NTDs are expected to spread, and new diseases will continue to emerge. However, with prevention and the development of new vaccines, diagnostic tools, and treatments, tropical disease could be controlled.

Prevention

Prevention is key to tropical disease control, and vector control is a major strategy. Draining wetlands reduces populations of insects and other vectors.

WHAT TO ASK YOUR DOCTOR

- Are you familiar with tropical disease?
- How can I protect myself from tropical disease?
- Are there vaccines or prophylactic medications that I should have before traveling to the tropics?
- How can I find out what tropical diseases are endemic to the areas I am traveling to?
- How do you test for tropical disease?

Insecticides can be used on bed nets, clothing, exposed skin, and insect habitats, and inside buildings. Wells and water filtration and treatment are necessary for eliminating waterborne parasites. Better sanitation helps control the spread of NTDs through human waste. The distribution of available vaccines, prophylactic drugs for preventing disease before and after exposure, and drugs for treating infections and infestations after they develop are important preventives measures. However, the most important goal is economic development—particularly investment in more productive subsistence farming—so that affected communities can afford to prevent and treat their own tropical disease.

Malaria and dengue are the targets of advanced biotechnological methods for vector control. Genetically modified Anopheles mosquitoes that are unable to bite or reproduce or that block development of the malaria parasite have been released into test environments. Likewise, although there is no vaccine or even an effective treatment for dengue, male *Aedes aegypti* mosquitoes have been genetically engineered so that newly hatched mosquitoes die.

Resources

BOOKS

Cochi, Stephen L., and Walter R. Dowdle. *Disease Eradication in the 21st Century: Implications for Global Health*. Cambridge, MA: MIT Press, 2011.

Hotez, Peter J. *Forgotten People, Forgotten Diseases: The Neglected Tropical Diseases and Their Impact on Global Health and Development*. Washington, DC: ASM, 2010.

Packard, Randall M. *The Making of a Tropical Disease: A Short History of Malaria*. Baltimore, MD: Johns Hopkins University Press, 2011.

Shah, Sonia. *The Fever: How Malaria Has Ruled Humankind for 500,000 Years*. New York: Sarah Crichton Books/Farrar, Straus, and Giroux, 2010.

Shore, William H. *The Imaginations of Unreasonable Men: Inspiration, Vision, and Purpose in the Quest to End Malaria*. New York: Public Affairs, 2010.

PERIODICALS

Brown, David. "Haiti Fights Disease One Mouth at a Time." *Washington Post*, October 1, 2012.

Brown, David. "New Study Doubles Estimate of Malaria Deaths." *Washington Post*, February 3, 2012.

Hotez, Peter J. "Tropical Diseases: The New Plague of Poverty." *New York Times*, August 19, 2012.

Nelson, Roxanne. "The Last Worm." *Scientific American* 307, no. 1 (July 2012): 24.

Specter, Michael. "The Mosquito Solution: Can Genetic Modification Eliminate a Deadly Tropical Disease?" *New Yorker* 88, no. 20 (July 9–16, 2012).

WEBSITES

Centers for Disease Control and Prevention. "Neglected Tropical Diseases." http://www.cdc.gov/globalhealth/ntd (accessed November 3, 2012).

Pigott, David C. "Viral Hemorrhagic Fevers." Medscape Reference. http://emedicine.medscape.com/article/830594-overview (accessed November 3, 2012).

"Tropical Diseases." World Health Organization. http://www.who.int/topics/tropical_diseases/en (accessed November 3, 2012).

ORGANIZATIONS

Bill and Melinda Gates Foundation, 500 Fifth Ave. N, Seattle, WA 98102, (206) 709-3100, info@gatesfoundation.org, http://www.gatesfoundation.org.

Global Fund to Fight AIDS, Tuberculosis, and Malaria, Geneva Secretariat, Chemin de Blandonnet 8, 1214 Vernier, Geneva, Switzerland, 41 58 791-1700, Fax: 41 58 791-1701, info@theglobalfund.org, http://www.theglobalfund.org/en.

U.S. Centers for Disease Control and Prevention, 1600 Clifton Rd., Atlanta, GA 30333, (800) CDC-INFO (232-4636), cdcinfor@cdc.gov, http://www.cdc.gov.

World Health Organization, Avenue Appia 20, 1211 Geneva 27, Switzerland, 2241 791 21 11, Fax: 2241 791 31 11, info@who.int, http://www.who.int.

Margaret Alic, PhD

Trypanosomiasis *see* **Sleeping sickness**

Tsunamis

Definition

Tsunamis are displacements of water that increase sea height and typically result in both a sea surge and large waves as the displaced water moves into the shore. Even without large waves, flooding from a tsunami can drive water inland, often causing major destruction in coastal regions. A tsunami can be caused by any event that rapidly displaces a large amount of water. Most

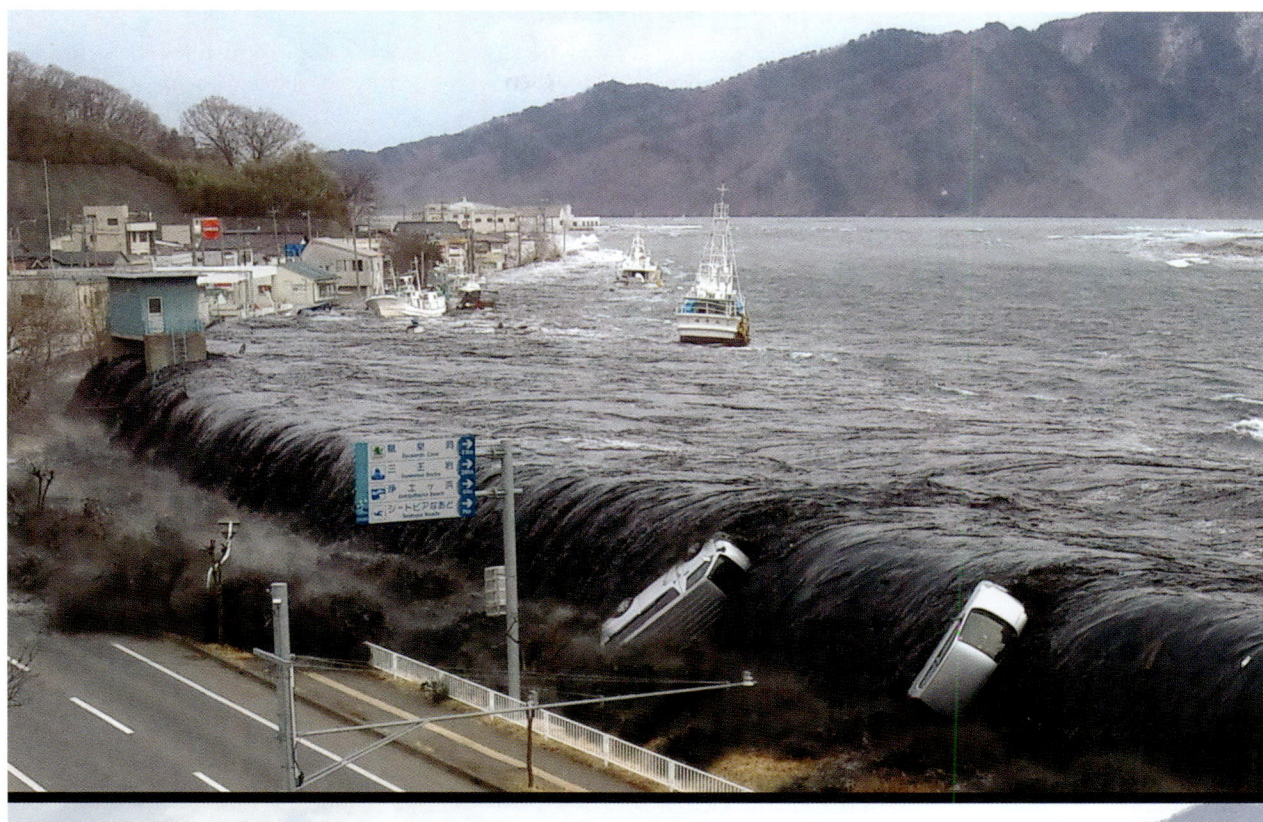

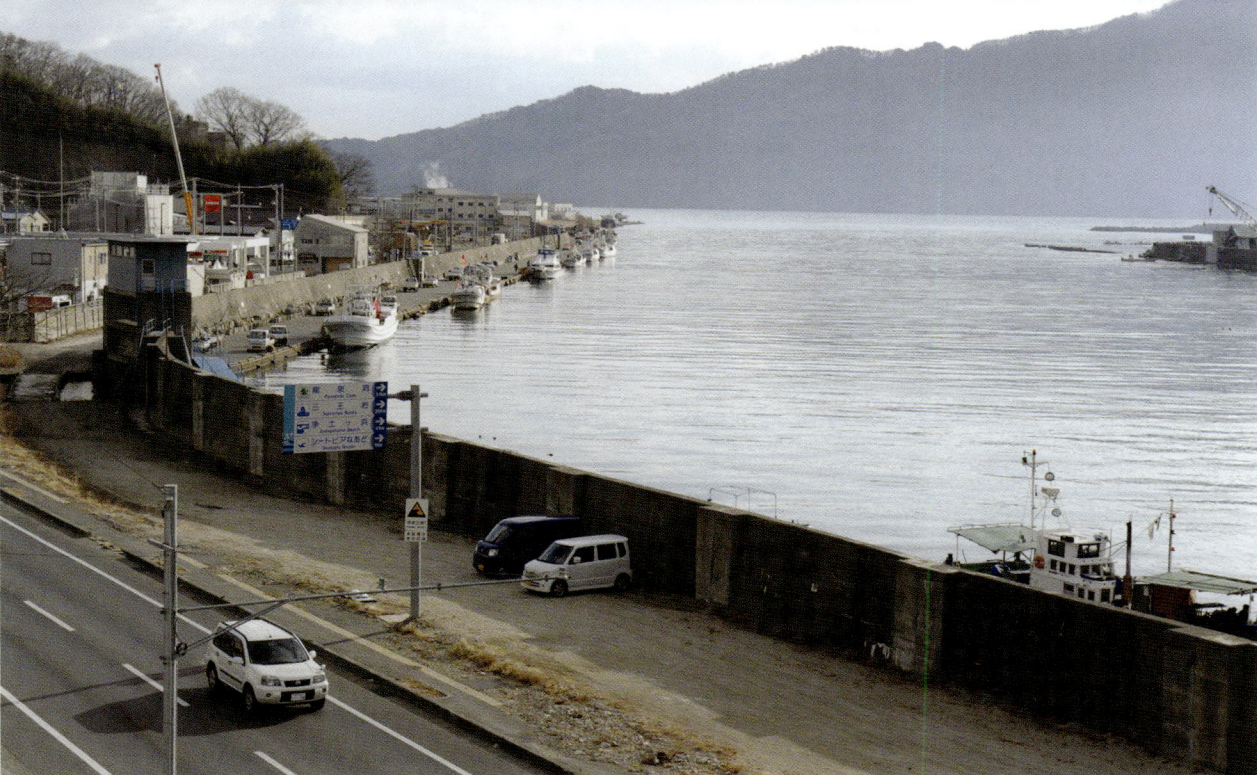

The image (top) was taken by a Miyako City official on March 11, 2011, of the tsunami breeching an embankment and flowing into the city of Miyako in Iwate prefecture. The same area (bottom) is photographed on January 16, 2012, nearly one year after the March 11 tsunami devastated the area. *(TORU YAMANAKA/AFP/Getty Images/Newscom)*

commonly, tsunamis occur as a result of underwater seismic activity, such as an earthquake.

Description

Though tsunamis are commonly termed tidal waves, this is an erroneous term; these potentially catastrophic waves have nothing to do with the tides. Tides are the up and down movements of the sea surface at the shore, and they are caused by the gravitational attraction of the moon and sun on our marine waters. Tides rarely cause major damage unless they are associated with a storm. Tsunamis, on the other hand, are caused by the movements of Earth's crustal plates, and they can cause major loss of life and property.

It has been known for several hundred years that tsunamis are caused by seismic movements of the ocean floor. Tsunamis occur most commonly during submarine earthquakes, underwater landslides, meteorite impacts, and volcanic eruptions. The sudden movement of Earth's crust caused by an underwater earthquake, for example, displaces or moves the water above it. This movement causes a high-energy wave to form, which then passes rapidly through the water.

Tsunamis are more common in the Pacific Ocean than in the other oceans of the world primarily because there is so much seismic activity at the perimeter of the Pacific Ocean, where crustal plates meet. Thus, this is the region where some of the world's most damaging tsunamis have occurred. Tsunamis also occur along the chain of Caribbean islands and in the Mediterranean. Both of these places, like the Pacific, are at the edges of Earth's crustal plates where earthquakes and other seismic activity are common. Areas that are 25 feet (7.6 m) or less above sea level and are within one mile of the coast are vulnerable to tsunamis.

A tsunami is composed of a very long series of waves (commonly referred to as a tsunami wave train), with a period (the time for one complete wave to pass a fixed point) ranging from ten minutes to two hours. These waves typically travel 500 to 600 miles per hour (800 to 1,000 km per hour). The speed of a tsunami is affected by water depth. In places where the ocean is 3.7 miles (6,000 m) deep, tsunamis can travel over 500 miles per hour (800 km per hour), but in shallow, coastal waters they slow down and their wave heights increase significantly.

It is almost impossible to feel a tsunami out at sea in deep water, but the form of the wave changes when it reaches shallow water. Because the water is shallower, the bottom of the wave begins to collide with the ocean bottom. The friction that results causes the wave to slow down from about 450 miles per hour (200 meters per second) in very deep ocean water to 49 miles per hour (22 meters per second) in water 164 feet (50 m) deep. While the front part of the wave has been reduced in speed, the part at sea is still moving in quickly. As a result, the energy of the wave is compressed. As the wave enters shallow water, like that in a bay, the crest rises. It quickly builds vertically as the wave moves onto the shore. This wall of water can be more than 100 feet (30.5 m) high in extreme cases. Because gravity is acting on this huge wall of water, it cannot support itself and crashes or breaks onto the land, similar to a normal breaker in the surf zone of a beach. However, the huge amounts of energy released by a breaking tsunami are many times greater and more destructive than an ordinary breaker, and the tsunami can destroy anything in its path. Hazards resulting from tsunamis include damage to buildings and structures, flooding, drinking water contamination, and gas-line or tank fires. The majority of deaths caused by tsunamis are a result of drowning.

In Japan, where some of the most destructive tsunamis have occurred, there have been cases in which whole fishing villages were devastated by tsunamis. Oddly, when these tsunamis occurred, fishermen at sea did not feel the wave as it passed right under them. They did not discover the disaster until they returned home and found their homes and villages destroyed. Because these villages were often located within shallow bays, and the fishermen, being at sea, did not experience the wave, they assumed that the tsunami arose within the bay or harbor. Therefore, these waves were referred to as tsunamis, which means "harbor wave" in Japanese.

Early warning systems

Tsunamis are capable of traveling hundreds of miles per hour in the ocean and rising over 100 feet (30.5 m) or more upon reaching the coast. About once in a decade, a major tsunami occurs. Of the tsunami events on record, 59 percent have occurred in the Pacific Ocean, 25 percent in the Mediterranean Sea, 12 percent in the Atlantic Ocean, and 4 percent in the Indian Ocean. Tsunamis can occur at any location along most of the U.S. coastline, but the most damaging tsunamis in the United States have affected the coasts of California, Oregon, Washington, Alaska, and Hawaii.

While scientists are not yet able to predict submarine seismic activity with much accuracy, they can easily measure such events when they occur, and they use this information to predict when destructive sea waves will occur. This early detection is extremely important in reducing loss of life and property. It became clear that a warning system was needed to monitor seismic activity throughout the Pacific Ocean after a very destructive tsunami hit Hawaii in 1946. As a result of the 1946 tsunami, the Pacific Tsunami Warning Center (PTWC) was established in 1948 which is the headquarters for the International Tsunami Warning System. The geographical and administrative center of this monitoring system is in Honolulu, Hawaii.

Under the early warning system, when an earthquake, underwater volcano, or landslide is sensed, scientists quickly pinpoint its location. If the seismic activity generates a wave, the change in the water height is measured at a nearby tide-measuring station, and the scientists can then accurately calculate the speed of the wave to determine when it will make landfall. The appropriate agencies can be alerted, and, if necessary, evacuations and other preparations can be made. This early warning system has been very successful in reducing the death toll associated with tsunamis. For example, when a large tsunami struck Hawaii in 1957, the early warning system prevented any tsunami-related deaths, despite the fact that the tsunami was over 26 feet (8 m) tall.

Before the warning systems existed, the first indication of an approaching tsunami was the rapid movement of water in a bay out to sea. This exposed areas of the bay bottom that were rarely or never exposed. The water that rushed offshore rose to build the huge crest of the wave that would crash down a few minutes later.

Despite the success of warning systems, early detection information sometimes results in warnings when no tsunamis occur. For example, not all seismic activity generates tsunamis. Many result from shallow focus earthquakes, where the actual point of crustal movement is close to the surface and major crustal movement is likely. Deep focus earthquakes, which can be very strong but often result in less crustal movement, are less likely to trigger tsunamis. It has been estimated that only one out of ten large underwater earthquakes causes damage. In addition, the chances of a tsunami hitting any one spot directly and causing major damage are relatively small because the energy in the form of the tsunami is not passed along equally in all directions. Finally, other factors may reduce or enhance the chances of a tsunami striking. For example, major tsunamis are rare in regions with wide continental shelves, such as the Atlantic Coast of the United States. A wide continental shelf is thought to both reflect the wave (with the energy being sent back out to sea) and absorb some of the energy of the wave through friction as it drags along the bottom. Thus, the early warning system, while essential, often gives false alarms.

Human impact of historic tsunamis

One of the most dramatic and destructive tsunamis occurred on August 27, 1883, when the volcanic island of Krakatoa, located in the Pacific Ocean between Sumatra and Java, Indonesia, exploded and disappeared in a massive volcanic eruption. The eruption was so immense that the sound of the volcanic explosion was heard 3,000 miles (4,827 km) away, and the dust that entered the atmosphere caused climate change and unusual sunsets for almost a year. The volcanic eruption generated a wall of water that reached over 98 feet (30 m) in height and caused catastrophic damage in coastal areas in the Sundra Strait. Of the more than 36,000 people who lost their lives due to the volcano, an estimated 90 percent were killed by the huge tsunami. The energy from the tsunami was still measurable after it had crossed the Indian Ocean, moved around the southern part of Africa, and headed north through the Atlantic Ocean into the English Channel.

In 1896, a major tsunami in Japan killed 27,000 people along the coast. In 1964, an earthquake in Alaska, and the resulting tsunami, caused major damage in some ports such as Kodiak and Seward. In addition, the tsunami traveled to the south, where four and a half hours later, despite warnings, it killed additional people and did major damage in Crescent City, California. A total of 119 people died, and damage to property amounted to over $100 million.

The tsunami of December 26, 2004 (known as the Indian Ocean Tsunami or Boxing Day Tsunami), which was generated by a very powerful earthquake off the west coast of Sumatra, is the worst tsunami in modern records, killing an estimated 230,000 people in 11 countries—with 170,000 deaths in Indonesia alone. There was no warning system in place for tsunamis in the Indian Ocean in 2004. Having an early warning system in place may have saved many lives. In 2006, the UN/International Strategy for Disaster Reduction (ISDR) project, Building Resilience to Tsunamis in the Indian Ocean, was established to strengthen methods of disaster risk reduction.

Since the Indian Ocean Tsunami in 2004, many smaller tsunamis have occurred. In March 2005, a tsunami resulting from an 8.7-magnitude earthquake struck the coast of Sumatra, killing 1,300 people. In 2006, a 3.3-yards (3-m) high tsunami generated by a 7.7-magnitude earthquake hit the West Java province of Indonesia, resulting in the deaths of an estimated 550 people. This tsunami caused damage in a 110-mile (177-km) coastal strip that had not been affected by the Indian Ocean Tsunami. Three minor tsunamis were reported in 2008, two in Indonesia and one in Japan.

On September 29, 2009, a tsunami raced ashore in the Samoan islands (composed of the Independent State of Samoa and American Samoa, a U.S. territory). That tsunami wiped out entire coastal villages and killed at least 150 people. The Pacific Tsunami Warning Center said a 8.3-magnitude earthquake, occurring at a depth of 20 miles (33 km) about 120 miles (190 km) from Apia in the Independent State of Samoa also sent small but measurable waves ashore as far away as New Zealand, Hawaii, and Japan.

Following the January 2010 earthquake in Haiti, the Pacific Tsunami Warning Center, which issues warnings worldwide, initially issued a tsunami warning for the area surrounding Haiti, but cancelled it shortly afterwards when no displacement of sea level was observed from the inland-centered earthquake.

In February 2010, a powerful 8.8-magnitude earthquake struck offshore Chile. Following the earthquake, alerts from the Pacific Tsunami Warning Center (PTWC) were quickly relayed to officials in Pacific rim nations. Close to the epicenter of the earthquake, on Chile's offshore islands and along the coastline, however, few tsunami warnings were issued. Minutes after the quake, tsunami waves swamped the island of Robinson Crusoe located off the Chilean coast. On the mainland, Chilean officials reported deadly tsunami waves swept into the port city of Talchahuano.

The surge of water generated by the earthquake off the Chilean coast ultimately resulted in much smaller tsunami waves than anticipated as they traveled across the Pacific Ocean. In Hawaii tsunami waves of less than 3 feet (1 meter) came ashore. Later the same day in Hokkaido, Japan, tsunami-generated waves of about 12 inches (30 centimeters) were observed.

The largest earthquake ever recorded, registering 9.5 on the Richter scale, occurred in 1960 in the same area as the 2010 Chilean quake and resulted in a Pacific-wide tsunami that arrived unannounced and generated waves up to 82 feet (25 meters) in height along the South American coast. Thousands of miles away from the epicenter of the 1960 earthquake, the tsunami carried walls of water 35 feet (10.6 meters) high.

Resources

BOOKS

Bachar, Kevin; Jaime Bernanke; Michael Carroll; et al. *Tsunami Killer Wave*. Washington, DC: National Geographic Society, 2005.

Krauss, Erich. *Wave of Destruction: The Stories of Four Families and History's Deadliest Tsunami*. New York: Rodale Books, 2005.

Stewart, Gail. *Overview Series—Catastrophe in Southern Asia: The Tsunami of 2004*. San Diego, CA: Lucent Books, 2005.

Tibballs, Geoff. *Tsunami: The Most Terrifying Disaster*. London: Carlton Publishing Group, 2005.

PERIODICALS

Kenneally, Christine. "Surviving the Tsunami." *Slate*, December 30, 2004.

WEBSITE

National Geographic Society. "Tsunami Safety Tips." http://environment.nationalgeographic.com/environment/natural-disasters/tsunami-safety-tips.html (accessed May 3, 2012).

Max Strieb

Tuberculosis

Definition

Tuberculosis (TB) is a chronic, potentially fatal contagious disease that most often affects the lungs but can affect other parts of the body. This infectious disease is caused by various strains of mycobacteria but usually by the tubercle bacillus (*Mycobacterium tuberculosis*). It causes small, round swellings (called tubercles) to form on mucous membranes. Tuberculosis is curable and preventable. However, as of 2012, TB is the second most fatal disease in the world; only HIV/AIDS kills more people annually.

Description

Tuberculosis caused widespread problems in the nineteenth and early twentieth centuries. In 1815, TB caused one in four deaths in England (considered the peak of fatalities in Europe), while it caused one in six deaths in France in 1918. Tuberculosis was commonly called consumption until well into the twentieth century. In 1882, the German microbiologist and physician Heinrich Hermann Robert Koch (1843–1910) isolated the tubercle bacillus (species name *Mycobacterium tuberculosis*) that causes the disease. The tubercle bacillus is transmitted when an infected person coughs or sneezes and another person breathes in the infected droplets. The disease is not spread through kissing or other physical contact.

Before antibiotics were discovered in the mid-1900s, the only means of controlling the spread of TB was to isolate patients in sanatoriums or hospitals limited to patients with TB. This practice continues in some countries. The reason for this pattern of treatment was

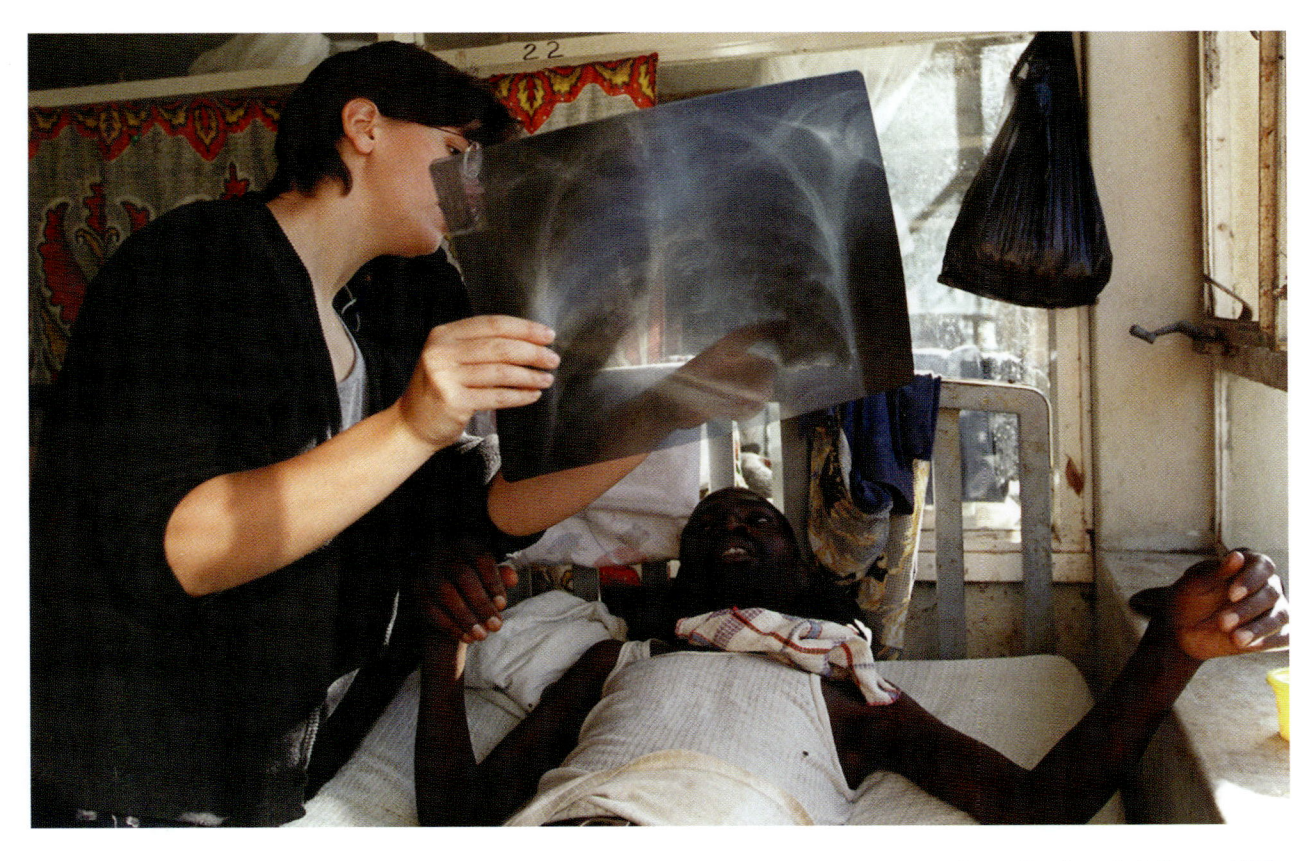

Dr. Diane Delongueville shows tuberculosis patient Elisha Unyango, an x ray of his chest, at Homa Bay hospital, Kenya, 2000, **photograph.** *(AP Images.)*

to separate the study of tuberculosis from mainstream medicine. Entire organizations were formed to study not only the disease as it affected individual patients, but also its impact on society. At the beginning of the twentieth century, more than 80% of the population in the United States was infected with TB before age 20, and tuberculosis was the single most common cause of death. By 1938, there were more than 700 specialized TB facilities in the United States.

History

Tuberculosis spread widely in Europe as the result of the industrial revolution in the late nineteenth century when many people moved to towns where they lived in crowded, unsanitary conditions. The disease became widespread somewhat later in the United States.

In the early 1940s, streptomycin was discovered and became the first antibiotic effective against *M. tuberculosis*. For the first time the infection began to be contained. Although other more effective anti-tuberculosis drugs that continue to reduce the number of TB cases have been developed in the past half-century, reports of active TB cases in the United States began to increase in the mid-1980s. This upsurge was in part a result of overcrowding and unsanitary conditions in the poor areas of large cities, prisons, and homeless shelters. Infected visitors and immigrants to the United States also contributed to the resurgence of TB. An additional factor was the **AIDS** epidemic. Individuals with HIV/AIDS are much more likely to develop tuberculosis because of their weakened immune systems than healthy individuals.

The number of reported TB cases in the United States peaked in 1993 and has since declined. New multidrug-resistant strains of TB (MDR TB) have become a major public health concern, with it being present in virtually all countries regularly surveyed by the **World Health Organization** (WHO). In the mid-2000s, health officials worldwide joined to work at preventing a drug-resistant form of the disease from becoming widespread. By 2007, WHO estimated that 13.7 million chronic, active cases of TB were present around the world.

In 2005, the U.S. **Centers for Disease Control and Prevention** (CDC) reported a record low number of

FLORENCE B. SEIBERT (1897–1991)

American biochemist Florence Barbara Seibert was born on October 6, 1897, in Easton, Pennsylvania, the second of three children. She was the daughter of George Peter Seibert, a rug manufacturer and merchant, and Barbara (Memmert) Seibert. At the age of three years she contracted polio. Despite her resultant handicaps, she completed high school, with the help of her highly supportive parents, and entered Goucher College in Baltimore, where she studied chemistry and zoology. She graduated in 1918, and then worked under the direction of one of her chemistry teachers, Jessie E. Minor, at the Chemistry Laboratory of the Hammersley Paper Mill in Garfield, New Jersey. She and her professor, having responded to the call for women to fill positions vacated by men fighting in World War I (1914–1918), coauthored scientific papers on the chemistry of cellulose and wood pulps.

A biochemist who received her doctoral degree (PhD) from Yale University in 1923, Seibert is best known for her research in the biochemistry of tuberculosis. She developed the protein substance used for the tuberculosis skin test. The substance was adopted as the standard in 1941 by the United States and a year later by the World Health Organization. In addition, in the early 1920s, Seibert discovered that bacteria in the distilled water used to make the protein solutions caused the sudden fevers that sometimes occurred during intravenous injections. She invented a distillation apparatus that prevented contamination. This research had great practical significance later when intravenous blood transfusions became widely used in surgery. Seibert authored or coauthored more than 100 scientific papers. Her later research involved the study of bacteria associated with certain cancers. Her many honors include five honorary degrees, induction into the National Women's Hall of Fame in Seneca Falls, New York (1990), the Garvan Gold Medal of the American Chemical Society (1942), and the John Elliot Memorial Award of the American Association of Blood Banks (1962). She died on August 23, 1991.

14,097 cases of active TB in the United States, of which 55% occurred in foreign-born individuals. However, the number of multi-drug resistant strains had increased 13.3% since 2000. The CDC estimated that in 2005 about 10 million people in the United States had latent (symptom-free) TB infections.

WHO estimates that about one-third of the world's population is infected with *M. tuberculosis*. Of those infected, between 5% and 10% will develop active TB. Among individuals who have HIV/AIDS infections, the rate is much higher. The greatest number of active TB infections per capita is found in sub-Saharan Africa where AIDS is epidemic. About one-third of infections occur in Southeast Asia. WHO estimates that TB caused about 1.6 million deaths worldwide in 2005. Although the rate per capita of active TB is declining worldwide, the absolute number of cases is increasing in many areas because of high population growth.

In 2010, approximately 8.8 million new cases were reported, along with about 1.4 million reported deaths associated with TB, mostly within developing countries of the world. In fact, over 95% of TB deaths occur in low-and middle-income countries. The countries of India and China accounted for about 40% of the world's reported cases of TB in 2010; while Africa reported 24% About 80% of the population in many Asian and African countries test positive for TB, while fewer than 10% do so in the United States. Between 2002 and 2008, the CDC reported that 27 outbreaks of TB involving 398 patients occurred in the United States. Twenty-four of the 27 outbreaks involved U.S.-born patients. One of the major features for nearly all cases was the presence of substance abuse.

The higher rates in developing countries is primarily due to higher rates of HIV infection and its corresponding development of AIDS as compared to developed countries. TB is the leading cause of death for people living with HIV, causing nearly one out of four deaths. However, WHO reports that the number of people contracting TB is decreasing slowly each year. Its Millennium Development Goal is to reverse the spread of TB by the year 2015.

Risk factors

People with heightened risks of contracting TB include the elderly, certain racial and ethnic groups, and people with various lifestyles.

THE ELDERLY. More than 60% of cases in the United States are diagnosed in people between the ages of 25 and 65 years. About one-quarter of TB cases newly diagnosed occur in people over the age of 65. Many elderly individuals developed TB after acquiring latent TB infection years earlier. As they age, their immune systems can no longer control the disease, and they develop active TB symptoms. In addition, elderly people living in nursing homes and other group facilities are often in close contact with others who may be infected.

RACIAL AND ETHNIC GROUPS. Higher rates of TB are found in the non-white population in the United States, but health researchers have reported that this is related to the socioeconomic status of these groups rather than to race-related biological factors. Individuals of lower socioeconomic status tend to live in more crowded conditions and have less access to health care than higher socioeconomic status individuals. These conditions encourage infection with *M. tuberculosis*.

As of 2012, TB continues to be a major health problem in the United States among certain immigrant groups that come from countries where TB infection is common. California, New York, Texas, and Florida—all states with large immigrant populations—accounted for almost half of all active TB cases. The most common countries of origin for foreign-born persons in the United States with active TB were Mexico, the Philippines, Vietnam, India, and China.

LIFESTYLE FACTORS. The high risk of TB in AIDS patients extends to those infected by HIV who have not yet developed clinical signs of AIDS but whose immune systems are weakened by the virus. People who take drugs that suppress the immune system (for example, transplant patients) are also at higher risk of becoming infected, as are people who have **silicosis**, a lung disease. Individuals who abuse alcohol, intravenous drug abusers, and the homeless are also at increased risk of contracting TB.

Demographics

People infected with TB have a 10% lifetime risk of falling ill with TB. Persons with compromised immune systems, such as people living with HIV, those with malnutrition or diabetes, or people who use tobacco, have a much higher risk of falling ill with TB. In fact, according to the WHO, people infected with HIV and TB are 21 to 34 times more likely to become sick with TB than people without those diseases. In addition, over 20% of TB cases worldwide are attributable to using tobacco products.

Causes and symptoms

The causes and symptoms of tuberculosis involve the way TB is transmitted into the body and its progression once inside. As TB develops inside the body, two common diseases can result: pulmonary tuberculosis and extrapulmonary tuberculosis. In addition, MDR TB has become a major concern in the world. Many similar diseases resemble tuberculosis.

Transmission

Tuberculosis spreads by droplet infection. When a person infected with *M. tuberculosis* exhales, coughs, or sneezes, tiny droplets of fluid containing tubercle bacilli are released into the air. People in close physical

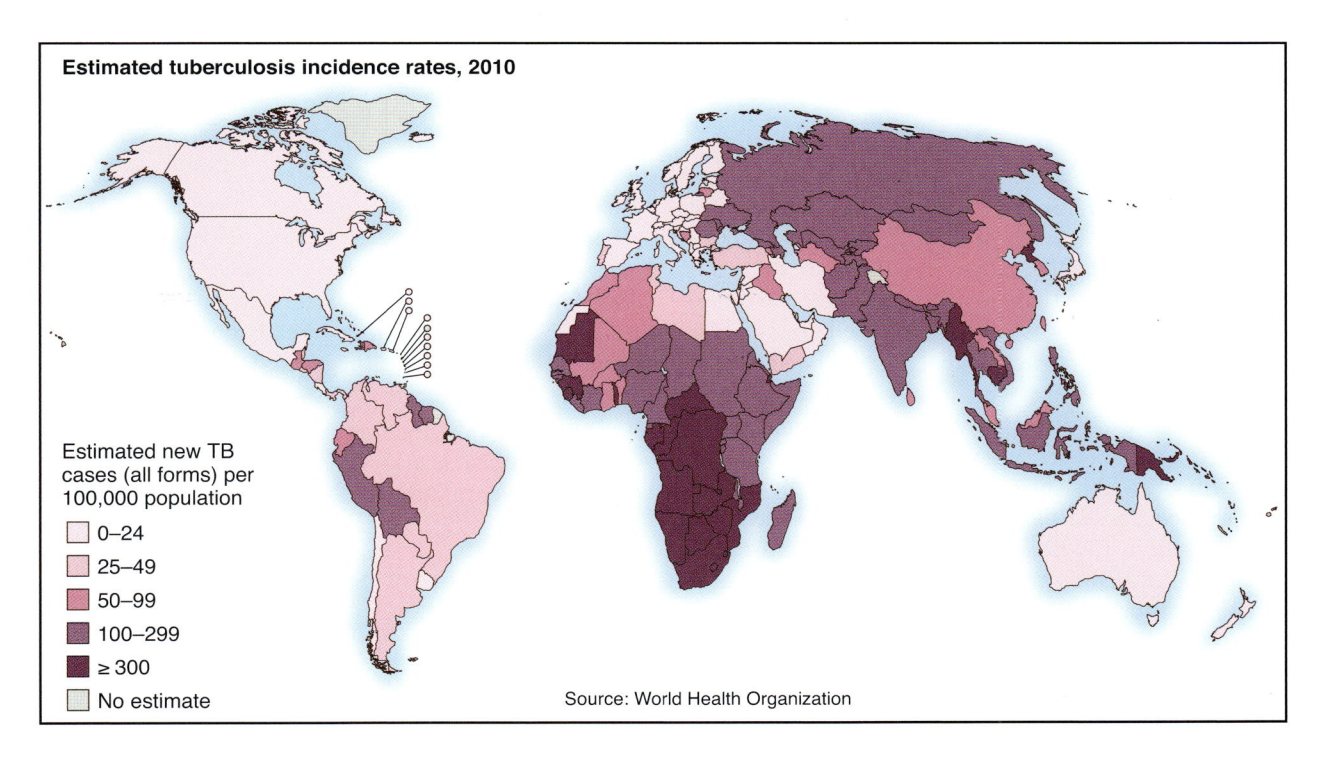

(Illustration by Electronic Illustrators Group. © 2012 Cengage Learning)

contact with the infected person inhale this fine mist. Tuberculosis is not highly contagious compared to some other infectious diseases. Close, frequent, or prolonged contact is needed to spread the disease. Most people do not develop TB even when exposed to a person with active TB. Unlike many other infections, TB is not passed on by contact with an infected individual's clothing, bed linens, dishes, or cooking utensils. The disease is not spread through kissing or other physical contact. The most important exception is pregnancy. The fetus of an infected mother may contract TB by inhaling or swallowing the bacilli in the amniotic fluid.

Progression

Once a person inhales *M. tuberculosis*, one of four things can happen:

- The person's immune system can kill the bacteria; TB infection does not result, and the person is not contagious.
- The bacteria can become dormant and never grow; thus, TB symptoms are not seen and the person is not contagious.
- The bacteria can become dormant for a period, then begin to grow; TB symptoms appear a long time after initial infection. The person is not contagious during the dormant period, then becomes contagious when symptoms appear.
- The bacteria multiplies immediately; active TB symptoms appear, and the person is contagious.

At least nine out of ten people infected with *M. tuberculosis* do not develop symptoms of TB, and their chest x-rays remain negative. These people have what is called a latent TB infection. They are not contagious; however, they do form a pool of infected individuals who may get sick later and then pass TB on to others. It is thought that more than 90% of cases of active tuberculosis come from this pool. In the United States, there are about 10 million people with latent TB infections. It is impossible to predict which individuals with latent TB infections will develop active TB. An estimated 5% of infected persons get sick within 12 to 24 months of being infected. Another 5% heal initially but, after years or decades, develop active TB either in the lungs or elsewhere in the body. On rare occasions, a previously infected person gets sick again after a later exposure to the tubercle bacillus.

Pulmonary tuberculosis

Pulmonary TB affects the lungs. Its initial symptoms are easily confused with those of other diseases. An infected person may initially feel vaguely unwell or develop a cough that could be blamed on **smoking** or a cold. A small amount of greenish or yellow sputum may be coughed up when the person gets up in the morning. In time, more sputum that is streaked with blood is produced. People who have pulmonary TB do not get a high fever, but they often have a low-grade one. The individual often loses interest in food and may lose weight. Chest pain is sometimes present. If the infection allows air to escape from the lungs into the chest cavity (pneumothorax) or if fluid collects in the pleural space (pleural effusion), the patient may have difficulty breathing. If a young adult develops a pleural effusion, the chance of tubercular infection being the cause is very high.

Before the development of effective TB drugs, many patients became chronically ill with increasingly severe lung symptoms. They lost a great deal of weight and developed a wasted appearance, hence the name consumption. This outcome is uncommon where modern treatment methods are available.

Extrapulmonary tuberculosis

Although the lungs are the major site of damage caused by tuberculosis, other organs and tissues in the body may be affected. The usual progression is for the disease to spread from the lungs to locations outside the lungs (extrapulmonary sites). In occasional cases, the first sign of disease appears outside the lungs. The tissues or organs that TB may affect include:

- Bones: TB is particularly likely to attack the spine and the ends of the long bones. Children are especially prone to spinal TB. If not treated, the spinal segments (vertebrae) may collapse and cause paralysis in one or both legs.
- Kidneys: Along with the bones, the kidneys are the most common site of extrapulmonary TB. There may be few symptoms even after part of a kidney is destroyed. TB may also spread to the bladder. In men, it may spread to the prostate gland and nearby structures.
- Female reproductive organs: The ovaries in women may be infected, and TB may spread from them to the peritoneum (the membrane lining the abdominal cavity).
- Abdominal cavity: TB peritonitis may cause pain ranging from the vague discomfort of stomach cramps to intense pain that may mimic the symptoms of appendicitis.
- Joints: Tubercular infection of joints causes a form of arthritis that most often affects the hips and knees. The wrist, hand, and elbow joints also may become painful and inflamed.

- Meninges: The meninges are tissues that cover the brain and the spinal cord. Infection of the meninges by the TB bacillus causes TB meningitis, a condition that is most common in young children but is especially dangerous in the elderly. Patients develop headaches, become drowsy, and eventually, comatose. Permanent brain damage results unless prompt treatment is given. Some patients with TB meningitis develop a tumor-like brain mass called a tuberculoma that causes stroke-like symptoms.
- Skin, intestines, adrenal glands, and blood vessels: All these parts of the body can be infected by *M. tuberculosis*. Infection of the wall of the body's main artery (the aorta) can cause it to rupture with catastrophic results. TB pericarditis occurs when the membrane surrounding the heart (the pericardium) is infected and fills up with fluid that interferes with the heart's ability to pump blood.
- Miliary tuberculosis: Miliary TB is a life-threatening condition that occurs when large numbers of tubercle bacilli spread throughout the body. Huge numbers of tiny tubercular lesions develop that cause marked weakness and weight loss, severe anemia, and gradual wasting of the body.

Multi drug-resistant tuberculosis (MDR TB)

In the twenty-first century, there is increasing concern about strains of *M. tuberculosis* that are resistant to the TB drugs that have brought the disease under control in the past half century. MDR TB is TB that fails to respond to at least two drugs, isoniazid (INH) and rifampin (RIF), which are routinely used to treat TB. In the United States, MDR TB, although rare, is on the rise. The CDC has developed a special group of experts to work with physicians who have patients with MDR TB. There is concern that drug-resistant TB could spread widely and cause a public health crisis. When alternate drug therapy fails to control MDR TB, lung surgery is the preferred treatment option.

Diseases similar to tuberculosis

There are many forms of mycobacteria other than *M. tuberculosis*, the tubercle bacillus. Some cause infections that may closely resemble tuberculosis, but they usually do so only when an infected person's immune system is defective. This occurs, for example, in some HIV-positive people. The most common mycobacteria that infect patients with HIV/AIDS are known as *Mycobacterium avium* complex (MAC). People infected by MAC are not contagious, but they may develop a serious lung infection that is highly resistant to antibiotics. MAC infections typically start with the patient coughing up mucus. The infection progresses slowly, but eventually blood is brought up in the sputum, and the patient has trouble breathing. In HIV/AIDS patients, MAC disease can spread throughout the body, with anemia, diarrhea, and stomach pain as common symptoms. Often these patients die unless their immune systems can be strengthened. Other mycobacteria grow in swimming pools and may cause skin infection. Some of them infect wounds and artificial body parts such as breast implants or mechanical heart valves.

Diagnosis

The standard screening test for TB is the tuberculin skin test. This test detects the presence of infection, not of active TB. Tuberculin is an extract prepared from cultures of *M. tuberculosis*. It contains proteins belonging to the bacillus (antigens) to which an infected person has been sensitized. When tuberculin is injected into the skin of an infected person, the area around the injection becomes hard, swollen, and red within one to three days.

Skin tests use a substance called purified protein derivative (PPD) that has a standard chemical composition and is therefore a good measure of the presence of tubercular infection. The PPD test is also called the Mantoux test. The Mantoux PPD skin test is not 100% accurate; it can produce false positive and false negative results. In other words, some people who have a skin reaction are not infected (false positive) and some who do not react are in fact infected (false negative). The PPD test is a highly useful screening test and is required in most states for children wanting to enter school. In addition, anyone who has suspicious findings on a chest x-ray or any condition that makes TB more likely should have a PPD test. People who are in close contact with a TB patient, those who come from a country where TB is common, all healthcare personnel, and persons living or working in institutions such as prisons should have a PPD test each year.

To verify the test results, a physician will order a chest x-ray and obtain a sample of sputum or a tissue sample (biopsy) for culture. Three to five sputum samples should be taken early in the morning. Culturing *M. tuberculosis* is useful for diagnosis because the bacillus has certain distinctive characteristics. Unlike many other types of bacteria, mycobacteria can retain certain dyes even when exposed to acid. This acid-fast property is characteristic of the tubercle bacillus.

Body fluids other than sputum can be used for a TB culture. If TB has invaded the brain or spinal cord, culturing a sample of spinal fluid will make the diagnosis. If TB of the kidneys is suspected because of pus or blood in the urine, culture of the urine may reveal a tubercular infection. Infection of the ovaries in women can be detected by inserting a tube with a light on its end (a laparoscope) into the area. Samples also may be taken from the liver or bone marrow to detect the tubercle bacillus.

For most people, a simple skin test is adequate to screen for TB. New advances in the diagnosis of TB use molecular techniques to speed the diagnostic process as well as improve its accuracy. As of 2012, molecular testing was being used more frequently in laboratories around the world. Molecular tests include a polymerase chain reaction to detect mycobacterial DNA in patient specimens; nucleic acid probes to identify mycobacteria in culture; restriction fragment length polymorphism analysis to compare different strains of TB for epidemiological studies; and genetic-based susceptibility testing to identify drug-resistant strains of mycobacteria.

Treatment

Treatment for tuberculosis includes supportive care, drug therapy, and surgery.

Supportive care

In the past, treatment of TB was primarily supportive. Patients were kept in isolation, encouraged to rest, and fed well. If these measures failed, the lung was collapsed surgically so that it could "rest" and heal. Surgical procedures are still used when necessary, but contemporary medicine relies on drug therapy as the mainstay of care. Given an effective combination of drugs, many patients with TB can be treated at home rather than in a sanatorium.

Drug therapy

Most patients with TB recover if given appropriate medication for a sufficient length of time. Three principles govern modern drug treatment of TB:

- Lowering the number of bacilli as quickly as possible. This minimizes the risk of transmitting the disease. When sputum cultures become negative, this has been achieved. Conversely, if the sputum remains positive after five to six months, treatment has failed.
- Preventing the development of drug resistance. For this reason, at least two different drugs and sometimes up to four are always given as initial treatment.
- Long-term treatment to prevent relapse.

Five drugs are most commonly used treat tuberculosis: isoniazid (INH, Laniazid, Nydrazid); rifampin (Rifadin, Rimactane); pyrazinamide (Tebrazid); streptomycin; and ethambutol (Myambutol). The CDC and the American Thoracic Society have developed standard regimens for treating TB in an effort to prevent the spread of drug resistant strains. For lung infections in non-immunocompromised people, the disease is usually treated with a regimen of rifampin and isoniazid (INH) for six months, supplemented in the first two months with pyrazinamide and sometimes ethambutol (or streptomycin in very young children). Because some strains of the disease are highly drug-resistant, cultures are grown from the patient's bacteria and tested with a variety of drugs to determine the most effective treatment, and alternate regimens may be determined to be more appropriate.

Except in cases of MDR TB, prolonged hospitalization is rarely necessary because most patients are no longer infectious after about two weeks of combination treatment. Follow-up involves monitoring side effects and monthly sputum tests. Of the five medications, INH is the most frequently used drug for both treatment and prevention. Hospitalization, isolation, and infectious control measures are required for individuals with MDR TB, which is a very serious disease both for the individual and from a public health standpoint. Most states have laws that allow individuals with TB to be hospitalized against their will for non-compliance with treatment.

Surgery

Surgical treatment of TB may be used if drugs fail to control the disease. There are three surgical treatments for pulmonary TB: pneumothorax, in which air is introduced into the chest to collapse the lung; thoracoplasty, in which one or more ribs are removed; and removal of a diseased lung, in whole or in part. Removal is usually required in the case of MDR TB. Individuals can survive with one healthy lung. Extrapulmonary TB may result in the need for other surgeries.

Public health role and response

Several national and international programs have been developed to address the public health concerns with TB. The Stop TB Partnership, which operates through a secretariat hosted by WHO, in Geneva, Switzerland, created the Global Plan to Stop Tuberculosis. The Plan aims to save 14 million lives between 2006 and 2015; thus, reducing the number of deaths and its incidence by 50% The Partnership is also working to reduce the global incidence of TB to less than one per million people by 2050, and to eliminate TB as a global public health problem in that same targeted year. In addition, the American Thoracic Society has

KEY TERMS

Bacillus Calmette-Guérin (BCG)—A vaccine made from a weakened bacillus similar to the tubercle bacillus that may help prevent serious pulmonary TB and its complications.

Mantoux test—Another name for the PPD test.

Miliary tuberculosis—The form of TB in which the bacillus spreads through all body tissues and organs, producing many thousands of tiny tubercular lesions. It is often fatal unless promptly treated.

Mycobacteria—A group of bacteria that includes *Mycobacterium tuberculosis*, the bacterium that causes tuberculosis, and other forms that cause related illnesses.

Pneumothorax—Air inside the chest cavity that may cause the lung to collapse. It is both a complication of pulmonary tuberculosis and a means of treatment designed to allow an infected lung to rest and heal.

Purified protein derivative (PPD)—An extract of tubercle bacilli that is injected into the skin to find out whether a person presently has or has ever had tuberculosis.

Sputum—Secretions produced in the lung and coughed up. A sign of illness, sputum is routinely used as a specimen for culturing the tubercle bacillus in the laboratory.

Tuberculoma—A tumor-like mass in the brain that sometimes develops as a complication of tuberculosis meningitis.

---

developed a tuberculosis classification system that is used primarily in the U.S. public health program.

Prognosis

Most patients recover from TB if the disease is diagnosed early and given prompt treatment with appropriate medications on a long-term regimen. The relapse rate is less than 4%. The exception is for those with MDR TB. When TB is multi drug-resistant, the prognosis depends largely on the ability to surgically remove all infected tissue. The outcome of surgery depends on where and how widespread the infected area is. Miliary TB is still fatal in many cases but is rarely seen in developed countries.

Prevention

The prevention of TB includes general measures, vaccinations, and prophylactic use of isoniazid.

General measures

General measures such as avoidance of overcrowded and unsanitary conditions are one aspect of prevention. Hospital emergency rooms and similar locations can be treated with ultraviolet light, which has an antibacterial effect. Regular skin testing is required in some jobs and of most children when they enter school and often again when entering college. Although screening does not prevent TB, it allows early treatment of those who are infected, reducing the likelihood that they will spread the disease.

Vaccination

Vaccination is a preventive measure against TB. A vaccine called BCG (Bacillus Calmette-Guérin, named after its French developers) is made from a weakened mycobacterium that infects cattle. Vaccination with BCG does not prevent infection by *M. tuberculosis*, but it does strengthen the immune system response and provide partial protection. BCG is used more widely in developing countries than in the United States. The effectiveness of vaccination is still being studied; it is not clear whether the vaccine's effectiveness depends on the population in which it is used or on variations in its formulation.

As of 2007, the first new TB vaccine in 80 years was in clinical trials in South Africa. The new vaccine known as MVA85A (modified vaccinia Ankara 85A), was developed by researchers at Oxford University, England, in response to increasing concern about the rise of MDR TB. This vaccine works with BCG vaccine to increase its effectiveness and produce a very strong immune system response. With phase I clinical trials completed, phase II clinical trials are ongoing in 2012, with a focus on whether the new vaccine actually prevents the disease. In one paper—*A Phase IIa Trial of the New TB Vaccine, MVA85A, in HIV and/or M. Tuberculosis Infected Adults*, published in January 2012 within the *American Journal of Respiratory and Critical Care Medicine*—the South Africa and United Kingdom researchers concluded, "MVA85A was safe and immunogenic in persons with HIV and/or M.tb infection. These results support further evaluation of safety and efficacy of this vaccine for prevention of TB in these target populations." Makers of the vaccine predict that even if clinical trials are successful, the vaccine will not predicted that even if clinical trials were successful, the vaccine would not be available on the market until about 2015.

Prophylactic use of isoniazid

INH can be given for the prevention and treatment of TB. INH is effective when given daily over a

> **QUESTIONS TO ASK YOUR DOCTOR**
>
> - Should I be worried about tuberculosis?
> - How dangerous is tuberculosis?
> - Is tuberculosis contagious before symptoms appear?
> - What symptoms should I be watching for with regards to TB?
> - Should I get tested for TB?
> - What should I do if I have a positive test for TB infection?
> - If I was exposed to someone with active TB disease, can I give TB to others?

period of six to 12 months to people in high-risk categories. INH appears to be most beneficial to persons under the age of 25 years. Because INH carries the risk of side effects (liver inflammation, nerve damage, changes in mood and behavior) in about one-fifth of people taking the drug, it is important to give it only to persons at special risk. The increase in MDR TB is causing some TB experts to re-evaluate preventative drug treatment.

High-risk groups for whom isoniazid prevention may be justified include:

- close contacts of TB patients, including health care workers
- newly infected patients whose skin test has turned positive in the past two years
- anyone who is HIV-positive with a positive PPD skin test; Isoniazid may be given even if the PPD results are negative if there is a risk of exposure to active tuberculosis
- intravenous drug users, even if they are negative for HIV
- persons with positive PPD results and evidence of old disease on their chest x-ray who have never been treated for TB
- patients who have an illness or are taking a drug that can suppress the immune system
- persons with positive PPD results who have had intestinal surgery; have diabetes or chronic kidney failure; have any type of cancer; or are more than 10% below their ideal body weight
- people from countries with high rates of TB who have positive PPD results
- people from low-income groups with positive skin test results
- persons with a positive PPD reaction who belong to high-risk ethnic groups (African Americans, Hispanics, Native Americans, Asians, and Pacific Islanders)
- householders who have lived with someone who has been diagnosed with an active TB infection

Resources

BOOKS

Cole, Stewart T., et al., eds. *Tuberculosis and the Tubercle Bacillus*. Washington, DC: ASM Press, 2005.

Magner, Lois N. *A History of Infectious Diseases and the Microbial World (Healing Society: Disease, Medicine, and History)*. Westport, CT: Praeger, 2009.

Mayho, Paul, and Richard Coker. *The Tuberculosis Survival Handbook*, 2nd ed. West Palm Beach, FL: Merit Publishing International, 2006.

World Health Organization. *Tuberculosis and Air Travel: Guidelines for Prevention and Control*. 3rd ed. Geneva 27, Switzerland: World Health Organization, 2008.

WEBSITES

Batara, Vandana. "Pediatric Tuberculosis." Medscape Reference. October 11, 2011. http://emedicine.medscape.com/article/969401-overview (accessed October 13, 2012).

"Florence B. Seibert." National Women's Hall of Fame. http://www.greatwomen.org/women-of-the-hall/search-the-hall-results/details/2/138-Seibert (accessed October 13, 2012).

"Global Tuberculosis Control 2011." World Health Organization. http://www.who.int/tb/publications/global_report/en/ (accessed October 13, 2012).

Herchline, Thomas E. "Tuberculosis." Medscape Reference. September 20, 2012. http://emedicine.medscape.com/article/230802-overview (accessed October 13, 2012).

Mitruka, Kiren, John Oeltmann, Kashef Ijaz, and Maryam Haddad. "Tuberculosis Outbreak Investigations in the United States, 2002–2008." *Emerging Infectious Diseases*. March 2011. http://wwwnc.cdc.gov/eid/article/17/3/10-1550_article.htm (accessed October 13, 2012).

Scriba, Thomas J., et al. "A Phase IIa Trial of the New TB Vaccine, MVA85A, in HIV and/or M. Tuberculosis Infected Adults." *American Journal of Respiratory and Critical Care Medicine* 185, no. 7 (April 1, 2012): 769–78. http://ajrccm.atsjournals.org/content/185/7/769.abstract?sid=8f1a92fc-06c0-4106-87cd-1709d3df8d4c (accessed October 13, 2012).

"Tuberculosis (TB)." Centers for Disease Control and Prevention. September 13, 2012. http://www.cdc.gov/tb/ (accessed October 13, 2012).

"Tuberculosis." World Health Organization. Fact sheet No. 104 (March 2012). http://www.who.int/mediacentre/factsheets/fs104/en/index.html (accessed October 13, 2012).

ORGANIZATIONS

American Lung Association, 1301 Pennsylvania Ave., NW, Ste. 800, Washington, D.C. 20004, (202) 785-3355, Fax: (202) 452-1805, info@lung.org, http://www.lung.org/.

American Thoracic Society, 25 Broadway, 18th Fl., New York, NY 10004, (212) 315-8600, Fax: (212) 315-6498, atsinfo@thoracic.org, http://www.thoracic.org/.

U.S. Centers for Disease Control and Prevention, 1600 Clifton Rd., Atlanta, GA 30333, (800) 232-4636, cdcinfo@cdc.gov, http://www.cdc.gov/.

World Health Organization, Avenue Appia 20, Geneva, Switzerland 1211 27, 41 22 791-2111, Fax: 41 22 791-3111, http://www.who.int/en/.

Tish Davidson, AM
Rebecca J. Frey, PhD
William A. Atkins, BB, BS, MBA

Typhoid fever

Definition

Typhoid fever is a severe infection caused by a bacterium, *Salmonella typhi*. *S. typhi* is in the same family of bacteria as the type spread by chicken and eggs, commonly known as salmonella poisoning or **food poisoning**. Unlike the bacteria that cause food poisoning, acquiring the *S. typhi* bacteria does not result in vomiting and diarrhea as the most prominent symptoms in humans. Instead, persistently high fever is the hallmark of *S. typhi* infection.

Description

As of 2012, according to the Mayo Clinic, over 21 million people around the world develop typhoid fever each year and 200,000 people died of the disease annually. Typhoid fever is passed from person to person through poor hygiene, such as incomplete or no hand washing after using the toilet. This allows *S. typhi* to enter the food and water supply. The bacteria are ingested and then they are passed into the stool and urine of infected patients. They may continue to be present in the stool of asymptomatic carriers—persons who have recovered from the symptoms of the disease but continue to carry the bacteria. This carrier state occurs in about 3% of all individuals who have recovered from typhoid fever. Persons who are carriers of the disease and who handle food can be the source of epidemic spread of typhoid. One such individual gave her name to the expression "Typhoid Mary," a name given to someone whom others avoid.

One of the largest outbreaks of typhoid fever occurred in 2004–2005 in the Democratic Republic of Congo. In 2004, according to the **World Health Organization**, 13,400 cases of typhoid fever were reported in the suburbs of Kimbanseke, Kikimi, Masina and Ndjili. Between October 1 and December 10, 2004, 615 cases of typhoid fever occurred with peritonitis, along with 134 deaths. The WHO stated that very poor sanitary conditions and a lack of drinking water were major causes of the outbreaks. Then, from September 2004 to January 11, 2005, the WHO reported that 42,564 cases and 214 deaths due to typhoid fever occurred in Kinshasa.

Natural disasters are also prime breeding grounds for typhoid fever. The January 2010 earthquake in Haiti displaced hundreds of thousands of people. Human and animal waste accumulated, which caused major diseases such as typhoid fever, **cholera**, and shigellosis to increase in frequency due to contaminated food and water. The dilapidated health system of Haiti worsened under the stress of these homeless people. Ian Greenwald, the chief medical officer for a Duke University team of doctors working in Haiti, is quoted in *The New York Times* article (February 19, 2010) *Poor Sanitation in Haiti's Camps Adds Disease Risk as saying*: "We're witnessing the setup for the spread of severe diarrheal illnesses in a place where the health system has collapsed and without a functioning sewage system to begin with."

Risk factors

Mayo Clinic states that the following are the major risk factors for typhoid fever:

- being a child (although their symptoms are generally milder than are the symptoms of adults)
- working or traveling to areas where typhoid fever is endemic (such as India, Southeast Asia, Africa, and South America)
- working as a clinical microbiologist handling *S. typhi* bacteria
- being in close contact with someone who is infected or has recently been infected with typhoid fever
- having an immune system that is weakened by medications such as corticosteroids or diseases such as human immunodeficiency virus/acquired immune deficiency syndrome (HIV/AIDS)
- drinking water contaminated by sewage that contains *S. typhi*

Demographics

According to the U.S. **Centers for Disease Control and Prevention** (CDC), about 400 Americans each year acquire typhoid, most of them while

MARY MALLON (1869–1938)

Mary Mallon was born in Cookstown, Ireland, on September 23, 1869, to Catherine Igo and John Mallon. As a teenager, Mallon left her parents and immigrated to New York to live with an aunt and uncle. Until 1906, when George A. Soper began to study an outbreak of typhoid fever in Long Island, little was known about Mallon.

Soper was called to identify possible causes of an eruption of typhoid fever at a summer house in Oyster Bay. After examining the food and water in a futile attempt to discover contaminants, Soper decided that a human carrier probably transmitted the disease. He soon learned that the cook, Mallon, had disappeared. He tracked Mallon to her new place of employment, expecting her cooperation in dealing with the matter. However, Mallon did not cooperate, and Soper eventually turned the case over to the New York City Department of Health. When Mallon was ultimately caught, she refused treatment and was held for three years as a threat to the public. In 1910, a judge granted her release with the stipulation that she not seek employment as a cook, since the disease was transmitted through food. Mallon agreed but, in 1915, an outbreak of typhoid at a hospital was, once again, linked to her. When Soper investigated this incident he learned that employees had nicknamed one of the cooks "Typhoid Mary."

After Mallon was found, she was taken into custody, and spent the rest of her life at Riverside Hospital. Mallon died on November 11, 1938.

---

traveling in developing countries. These areas include Asia, Africa, Latin America, the Caribbean, and Oceania. Although typhoid fever can be found in all those areas, 80% of cases worldwide are found in Bangladesh, China, India, Indonesia, Laos, Nepal, Pakistan, and Vietnam. Around 5% of those Americans who contract the illness abroad become chronic carriers. According to the National Institutes of Health (NIH), a study in the early 2010s found that "the cause of most cases of the disease that did not result from travel abroad could not be accounted for." The NIH stated that about 19% of typhoid cases in the United States (which did not occur while traveling abroad) occurred among groups of people. One of the largest recent outbreaks occurred from orange juice that was contaminated by a food handler. Forty-seven people were sickened from the outbreak in 1998. Typhoid fever is rare in industrialized countries with adequate sewage treatment facilities and clean water supplies.

Causes and symptoms

S. typhi must be ingested to cause disease. Transmission often occurs when a person in the carrier state does not wash hands thoroughly (or not at all) after defecation and serves food to others. This pathway is sometimes called the fecal-oral route of disease transmission. In countries where open sewage is accessible to flies, the insects land on the sewage, pick up the bacteria, and then contaminate food to be eaten by humans. In countries with poor sewage treatment facilities, sewage can contaminate the water supply and typhoid fever can spread by drinking contaminated water.

After being swallowed, the *S. typhi* bacteria enter the digestive tract where they are taken in by cells called mononuclear phagocytes. These phagocytes are cells of the immune system, whose job it is to engulf and kill invading bacteria and **viruses**. In the case of *S. typhi*, however, the bacteria are able to survive ingestion by the phagocytes, and multiply within these cells. This period of time, during which the bacteria are multiplying within the phagocytes, is the 10- to 14-day incubation period of typhoid fever. When huge numbers of bacteria fill an individual phagocyte, they spill out of the cell and into the bloodstream, where their presence begins to cause symptoms.

The presence of increasingly large numbers of bacteria in the bloodstream (bacteremia) is responsible for an increasingly high fever, which lasts throughout the four to eight weeks of the disease in untreated individuals. Other symptoms of typhoid fever include constipation (at first), nausea, extreme fatigue, headache, joint pain, and a rash across the abdomen known as rose spots.

The bacteria move from the bloodstream into certain tissues of the body, including the gallbladder and lymph tissue of the intestine (called Peyer's patches). The tissue's response to this invasion causes symptoms ranging from inflammation of the gallbladder (cholecystitis) to intestinal bleeding to actual perforation of the intestine. Perforation of the intestine refers to an actual hole occurring in the wall of the intestine, with leakage of intestinal contents into the abdominal cavity. This leakage causes severe irritation and inflammation of the lining of the abdominal cavity, which is called peritonitis. Peritonitis is a frequent cause of death from typhoid fever.

Other complications of typhoid fever include liver and spleen enlargement, sometimes so great that the

> **KEY TERMS**
>
> **Asymptomatic**—A state in which a person experiences no symptoms of a disease.
>
> **Bacteremia**—Bacteria in the blood.
>
> **Carrier**—A person who has a particular disease agent present within his or her body and can pass this agent on to others but who displays no symptoms of infection.
>
> **Epidemic**—A large number of cases of the same disease or infection all occurring within a short time period in a specific location.
>
> **Incubation period**—The time between when an individual becomes infected with a disease-causing agent and when symptoms begin to appear.
>
> **Mononuclear phagocyte**—A type of cell of the human immune system that ingests bacteria, viruses, and other foreign matter, thus removing potentially harmful substances from the bloodstream. These substances are usually then digested within the phagocyte.
>
> **Rose spots**—A pinkish rash across the trunk or abdomen that is a classic sign of typhoid fever.
>
> **Sickle cell disease**—An inherited disorder characterized by a genetic flaw in hemoglobin production. (Hemoglobin is the substance within red blood cells that enables them to transport oxygen.) The hemoglobin that is produced has a kink in its structure that forces the red blood cells to take on a sickle shape, inhibiting their circulation and causing pain. This disorder primarily affects people of African descent.

spleen ruptures or bursts; anemia, or low red blood cell count due to blood loss from the intestinal bleeding; joint infections, which are especially common in patients with sickle cell disease and immune system disorders; pneumonia caused by a bacterial infection (usually *Streptococcus pneumoniae*), which is able to take hold due to the patient's weakened state; heart infections; and **meningitis** and infections of the brain, which cause mental confusion and even coma. It may take a patient several months to recover fully from untreated typhoid fever.

Diagnosis

In some cases, the doctor may suspect the diagnosis if the patient has already developed the characteristic rose spots, or if he or she has a history of recent travel in areas with poor **sanitation**. The diagnosis is confirmed by a blood culture. Samples of a patient's stool, urine, and bone marrow can also be used to grow *S. typhi* in a laboratory for identification under a microscope. Cultures are the most accurate method of diagnosis. Blood cultures usually become positive in the first week of illness in 80% of patients who have not taken antibiotics.

Treatment

Antibiotics are the treatment of choice for typhoid fever. As of the early 2010s, commonly used drugs are ceftriaxone (Rocephin) and cefoperazone (Cefobid). Ciprofloxacin (Cipro, Proquin)) is sometimes given as follow-up therapy. It should be noted, that antibiotic resistance is common in *S. typhi*. Forty-three percent of samples of *S. typhi* collected from patients in the United States were resistant to at least one antibiotic. The antibiotic(s) used to treat typhoid fever is determined by the origin of the disease, sensitivity of cultures of the bacterium to specific antibiotics, and response to treatment.

Carriers of *S. typhi* must be treated even when they do not show any symptoms of the infection, because carriers are responsible for the majority of new cases of typhoid fever. Eliminating the carrier state is a difficult task. It requires treatment with one or even two different medications over a period of four to six weeks. The antibiotics most commonly given are ampicillin (Omnipen, Polycillin, Principen; sometimes given together with probenecid [Benemid]) and amoxicillin (Amoxicot, Amoxil, Dispermox, Moxatag). In the case of a carrier with gallstones, surgery may need to be performed to remove the gallbladder. This measure is necessary because typhoid bacteria are often housed in the gallbladder, where they may survive in spite of antibiotic treatment. In some patients, treatment with rifampin and trimethoprim-sulfamethoxazole is sufficient to eradicate the bacteria from the gallbladder without surgery.

Public health role and response

The U.S. Centers for Disease Control and Prevention (CDC) recommends that if one is traveling to a country where typhoid fever is common (generally outside of the United States, Canada, northern Europe, Australia, and New Zealand) or during epidemic outbreaks, then one should consider being vaccinated against typhoid. The CDC recommends that the **vaccination** should be completed at least one to two weeks before the date of departure so that the vaccine has sufficient time to take effect. In addition,

QUESTIONS TO ASK YOUR DOCTOR

- Should I be worried about typhoid fever?
- How dangerous is typhoid fever?
- Is typhoid fever contagious before symptoms appear?
- What symptoms should I be watching for with regards to typhoid?
- If I was exposed to someone with typhoid fever, can I give typhoid to others?
- What types of tests do I need?
- Are treatments available to help me recover from typhoid?
- How long will a full recovery take?
- When can I return to my daily routine?
- What are the possible causes for my symptoms?
- Am I at risk of any long-term complications?

the effectiveness of typhoid vaccinations typically last for several years. In addition, immunization is not always effective, so some health care provider may recommend taking electrolyte packets along on the trip in case one gets sick. In addition, always drink only boiled or bottled water and eat well-cooked foods while traveling.

The U.S. National Institutes of Health recommend that a health care provider should be summoned if a person has:

- any known exposure to typhoid fever
- been in an endemic area and symptoms of typhoid fever have developed
- had typhoid fever and the symptoms return
- developed severe abdominal pain, decreased urine output, or other new symptoms

Prognosis

The prognosis for recovery is good for most patients. In the era before effective antibiotics were discovered, about 12% of all typhoid fever patients died of the infection. Now, fewer than 1% of patients who receive prompt antibiotic treatment die. The mortality rate is highest in the very young and very old and in patients with malnutrition. The most ominous signs are changes in a patient's state of consciousness, including stupor or coma.

Prevention

Hygienic sewage disposal systems in a community, good water treatment facilities, and proper personal hygiene are the most important factors in preventing typhoid fever. Immunizations are available for travelers who expect to visit countries where *S. typhi* is a known public health problem. Some of these immunizations provide only short-term protection (for a few months), while others may be effective for several years. Efforts are being made to develop vaccines that provide a longer period of protection with fewer side effects from the vaccine itself. The most commonly reported side effects are flu-like muscle cramps and abdominal pain.

Resources

BOOKS

Emmeluth, Donald. *Typhoid Fever*. Philadelphia: Chelsea House, 2004.
Ray, Kurt. *Typhoid Fever*. New York: Rosen, 2001.
Shannon, Joyce Brennfleck, editor. *Contagious Diseases Sourcebook: Basic Consumer Health Information about Diseases Spread from Person to Person*. Detroit: Omnigraphics, 2010.
Wilder-Smith, Annelies, Eli Schwartz, and Marc Shaw, editors. *Travel Medicine: Tales Behind the Science*. Amsterdam: Elsevier, 2007.

WEBSITES

Batara, Vandana. *Typhoid Fever*. Centers for Disease Control and Prevention. (October 5, 2010). http://www.cdc.gov/nczved/divisions/dfbmd/diseases/typhoid_fever/ (accessed July 6, 2012).
"Diarrhoeal Diseases." World Health Organization. (February 2009). http://www.who.int/vaccine_research/diseases/diarrhoeal/en/index7.html (accessed July 6, 2012).
Romero, Simon. "Poor Sanitation in Haiti's Camps Adds Disease Risk." The New York Times. (February 19, 2010). http://www.nytimes.com/2010/02/20/world/americas/20haiti.html?_r=1 (accessed July 9, 2012).
"Typhoid Fever." Mayo Clinic. (April 9, 2010). http://www.mayoclinic.com/health/typhoid-fever/DS00538 (accessed July 6, 2012).
"Typhoid Fever." Medline Plus. (June 9, 2011). http://www.nlm.nih.gov/medlineplus/ency/article/001332.htm (accessed July 6, 2012).
"Typhoid fever." Medscape Reference. (September 21, 2011). http://emedicine.medscape.com/article/231135-overview (accessed July 6, 2012).
"Typhoid fever in Democratic Republic of the Congo." World Health Organization. (December 15, 2004). http://www.who.int/csr/don/2004_12_15/en/ (accessed July 6, 2012).
"Typhoid fever in the Democratic Republic of the Congo—Update." World Health Organization. (January 19, 2005). http://www.who.int/csr/don/2004_12_15/en/ (accessed July 6, 2012).

"Typhoid Vaccine—Oral Enteric-Coated Capsule." Medicine Net.com. http://www.medicinenet.com/typhoid_vaccine-oral_enteric-coated_capsule/article.htm (accessed July 6, 2012).

"Typhoid Vaccine: What You Need to Know." Centers for Disease Control and Prevention. (May 29, 2012). http://www.cdc.gov/vaccines/Pubs/vis/downloads/vis-typhoid.pdf (accessed July 6, 2012).

ORGANIZATIONS

Centers for Disease Control and Prevention, 1600 Clifton Rd., Atlanta, GA 30333, (800) 232-4636, cdcinfo@cdc.gov, http://www.fda.gov/.

National Institute of Allergy and Infectious Diseases, 1301 Pennsylvania Ave., N.W., Ste. 800, Washington, D.C. 20004, 1(202) 785-3355, Fax: 1(202) 452-1805, info@lung.org, http://www.lung.org/.

World Health Organization, Avenue Appia 20, Geneva, Switzerland 1211 27, 41 22 791-2111, Fax: 41 22 791-3111, cdcinfo@cdc.gov, http://www.who.int/en/.

Rosalyn Carson-DeWitt, MD
Tish Davidson, AM
Paul Checchia, MD
William A. Atkins, BB, BS, MBA

Typhus

Definition

Several different illnesses are called typhus; all of them are caused by one of the bacteria in the family Rickettsiae. Each illness occurs when the bacteria is passed to a human through contact with an infected insect.

Description

The first known description of typhus (probably epidemic typhus) occurred in the late 1480s and early 1490s while Spanish soldiers were fighting during the siege of Granada. Fever, rash, red spots (on their arms, back and chest), delirium, gangrenous sores, and decaying flesh were some of the common symptoms of typhus during this conflict. At the time, it was called disease gaol or jail fever. In 1760, the English government first called it typhus, from the Greek word "typhos". Meaning smoky or hazy, it described the state of mind of those people with the disease. Typhus continued to be a major problem in Europe over the next several centuries, most often due to the crowded and unsanitary living conditions commonly present. In the nineteenth century, many outbreaks occurred around the world. In the 1810s, large numbers of French troops under Napoleon died from typhus, and in the 1830s, hundreds of thousands of Americans and Irish died in several epidemics in the United States and Ireland.

By the early twentieth century, the cause of epidemic typhus was identified. In 1916 Brazilian physician Henrique da Rocha Lima (1879–1956) discovered its cause while performing typhus research in Germany. Millions of deaths were attributed to typhus in World War I (1914–1918) and World War II (1939–1945). After the second world war, the insecticide dichlorodiphenyltrichloroethane (DDT) was used to kill lice, which reduced the number of epidemics and limited their locations to Africa, the Middle East, Eastern Europe, and Asia.

The four main types of typhus are:

- epidemic typhus
- Brill-Zinsser disease
- endemic or murine typhus
- scrub typhus

These four diseases are somewhat similar, but they vary in terms of severity. The specific type of *Rickettsia* that causes the disease varies, as does the specific insect that carries the bacteria.

Epidemic typhus, sometimes called jail fever or louse-borne typhus, is caused by *Rickettsia prowazekii*, which is carried by body lice. When lice feed on a human, they may simultaneously defecate. When a person scratches the bite, the feces that carries the bacteria are scratched into the wound. Body lice are common in areas where there is overcrowding, poor **sanitation**, and poor hygiene. As a result, this form of typhus occurs simultaneously in large numbers of individuals living within the same community; that is, in epidemics. Epidemic typhus occurs when cold weather, poverty, war, and other disasters result in close living conditions that encourage the maintenance of a population of lice living among humans. Some medical historians have reported that the Great **Plague** of Athens in 430 B.C. may have been epidemic typhus. Epidemic typhus is now found in the mountainous regions of Africa, South America, and Asia.

Brill-Zinsser disease is a reactivation of an earlier infection with epidemic typhus. It affects people years after they have completely recovered from epidemic typhus. A weakening of a person's immune system (from aging, surgery, or illness) can cause the bacteria to gain hold again, causing illness. This disease tends to be extremely mild.

Endemic typhus is carried by fleas. When a flea lands on a human, it may defecate as it feeds. When a person scratches the itchy spot where the flea was

> **KEY TERMS**
>
> **Antibody**—Specialized cells of the immune system that recognize organisms that invade the body (such as bacteria, viruses, or fungi). Antibodies set off a complex chain of events designed to kill these foreign invaders.
>
> **Bioterrorism**—The use of disease microorganisms to intimidate or terrorize a civilian population.
>
> **Endemic**—Occurring naturally and consistently in a particular area.
>
> **Epidemic**—An outbreak of disease where the number of cases exceeds the usual (endemic) or typical number of cases.

feeding, the bacteria-laden feces are scratched into the skin causing infection. The causative bacteria is called *Rickettsia typhi*. Endemic typhus occurs most commonly in warm, coastal regions. In the United States, southern Texas and southern California have the largest number of cases.

Scrub typhus is caused by *Rickettsia tsutsugamushi*. Mites or chiggers carry the bacteria. As the mites feed on humans, they deposit the bacteria. Scrub typhus occurs commonly in the southwest Pacific, Southeast Asia, and Japan. It is a very common cause of illness in people living in or visiting these areas. It occurs more commonly during the wet season.

Risk factors

The risk factors for getting typhus include living in or visiting areas where it is endemic, such as coastal cities where rodent and insect (such as lice, mites, fleas, and ticks) populations are high and in close contact with people, and areas where hygiene is degraded such as within poverty-stricken regions, disaster zones, homeless camps, and other similar places. Typhus is most often contracted during the spring and summer months.

As of 2012, the International Association for Medical Assistance to Travellers identified the following countries as having increased risks for typhus: Bolivia, Burundi, Colombia, Eritrea, Ethiopia, Guatemala, Kenya, Mexico, Peru, Rwanda, and Somalia.

Demographics

Since World War II, large outbreaks of typhus have occurred primarily in three African countries: Burundi, Ethiopia and Rwanda. In Ethiopia, the number of cases reported annually has ranged between 7,000 and 17,000.

In 1996, for example, Burundi reported 3,500 cases and that number increased to 20,000 for the period from January to March 1997. In the first two decades of the twenty-first century, the **World Health Organization** (WHO) reported that typhus kills about 0.2 people per million per year.

Causes and symptoms

The four varieties of typhus cause similar types of illnesses, though they vary in severity.

Epidemic typhus causes fever, headache, weakness, and muscle aches. It also causes a rash composed of both spots and bumps. The rash starts on the back, chest, and abdomen, then spreads to the arms and legs. The worst complications involve swelling in the heart muscle (carditis) or brain (encephalitis). Without treatment, this type of typhus can be fatal.

Brill-Zinsser disease is quite mild, resulting in about a week-long fever and a light rash similar to that of the original illness.

Endemic typhus causes about 12 days of high fever, with chills and headache. A light rash may occur.

Scrub typhus causes a wide variety of effects. The main symptoms include fever, headache, muscle aches and pains, cough, abdominal pain, nausea and vomiting, and diarrhea. Some patients experience only these symptoms, while others also develop a rash that can be flat or bumpy. The individual spots develop crusty black scabs. Other patients develop a more serious disease, in which encephalitis, pneumonia, and swelling of the liver and spleen (hepatosplenomegaly) occur.

Diagnosis

Numerous tests exist to determine the reactions of a patient's antibodies (immune cells in the blood) to the presence of certain viral and bacterial markers. For instance, a complete blood count (CBC) may show anemia and low platelets. Blood tests for typhus may show: low level of albumin, high level of typhus antibodies, low sodium level, moderately high liver enzymes, and mild kidney failure. When the antibodies react in a particular way, it suggests the presence of a rickettsial infection. Many tests require time for processing, so practitioners frequently begin treatment without completing tests, simply on the basis of a patient's symptoms.

Treatment

The antibiotics tetracycline or chloramphenicol are used for treatment of each of the forms of typhus. Other antibiotics used for typhus include azithromycin and doxycycline. Tetracycline is taken orally. It is usually not prescribed for children because it can permanently stain their teeth. Besides antibiotics, patients with epidemic typhus may also require oxygen and intravenous fluids. Prompt treatment with one of these antibiotics usually will cure most cases of typhus. Without treatment, typhus can be fatal. The death rate for untreated epidemic typhus varies from 10% for younger people to 40% for older ones.

Public health role and response

Outbreaks of typhus are limited in developed countries like the United States but the disease has the potential to re-emerge. In undeveloped and developing countries, the disease is still responsible for major outbreaks. Typhus killed approximately 100,000 people during the civil war in Burundi, which lasted from 1993 to 2005.

WHO published the report *Outbreak Surveillance and Response in Humanitarian Emergencies* in 2012. The report notes that humanitarian crises that result in large populations of displaced people gathering in one location where there are infrastructure issues (refugee camps) are cause for increased spread of infectious diseases. Diseases that may remain contained under normal circumstances will spread and early rapid detection and prevention is necessary. WHO reports that scrub typhus is one of the most common vector-borne diseases that can occur in humanitarian emergency settings.

Prognosis

The prognosis depends on what types of complications an individual patient experiences. Most patients usually recover well from epidemic typhus with treatment. However, older adults may have as much as a 60% death rate without treatment. Brill-Zinsser disease carries no threat of death. People usually recover uneventfully from endemic typhus, although the elderly, those with other medical problems, or people mistakenly treated with sulfa drugs may have a 1% death rate from the illness. Scrub typhus responds well to appropriate treatment, but untreated patients have a death rate of about 7%.

The relatively high death rate from untreated typhus is one reason there is some concern that its causative organisms might be used in the future as agents of **bioterrorism**.

QUESTIONS TO ASK YOUR DOCTOR

- Should I be worried about contracting typhus from fleas or lice?
- How dangerous is my form of typhus?
- Is typhus contagious before symptoms appear?
- What symptoms should I watch for with regards to typhus?
- If I was exposed to someone with typhus, can I give it to others?
- What types of tests do I need?
- Are treatments available to help me recover from typhus?
- How long will a full recovery take?
- When can I return to my daily routine?
- What are the possible causes for my symptoms?
- Am I at risk of any long-term complications?

Prevention

Prevention for each of these forms of typhus includes avoidance of the insects that carry the causative bacteria. Other preventive measures include good hygiene and the use of insect repellents.

Resources

BOOKS

Beers, Mark H., Robert S. Porter, and Thomas V. Jones, eds. *The Merck Manual of Diagnosis and Therapy*, 18th ed. Whitehouse Station, NJ: Merck Research Laboratories, 2006.

Bynum, William, and Helen Bynum, eds. *Great Discoveries in Medicine*. New York: Thames & Hudson, 2011.

Sartre, Jean-Paul. *Typhus*. London: Seagull Books, 2010.

Shannon, Joyce Brennfleck. ed. *Contagious Diseases Sourcebook: Basic Consumer Health Information about Diseases Spread from Person to Person*. Detroit: Omnigraphics, 2010.

Wilder-Smith, Annelies, Eli Schwartz, and Marc Shaw, eds. *Travel Medicine: Tales Behind the Science*. Amsterdam: Elsevier, 2007.

WEBSITES

David, Patrick. "Typhus." MedicineNet.com. http://www.medicinenet.com/typhus/article.htm (accessed October 13, 2012).

"Typhus." Medline Plus. (March 18, 2011). http://www.nlm.nih.gov/medlineplus/ency/article/001363.htm (accessed October 13, 2012).

"Typhus." World Health Organization. May 1997. http://www.who.int/mediacentre/factsheets/fs162/en/index.html (accessed October 13, 2012).

"Typhus Fever (Louse-Borne Typhus)." International Association for Medical Assistance to Travellers. http://www.iamat.org/disease_details.cfm?id=15 (accessed October 13, 2012).

ORGANIZATIONS

Centers for Disease Control and Prevention, 1600 Clifton Rd., Atlanta, GA 30333, (800) 232-4636, cdcinfo@cdc.gov, http://www.cdc.gov/.

National Institute of Allergy and Infectious Diseases, 1301 Pennsylvania Ave., NW, Ste. 800, Washington, D.C. 20004, (202) 785-3355, Fax: (202) 452-1805, http://www.niaid.nih.gov.

World Health Organization, Avenue Appia 20, Geneva, Switzerland 1211 27, 41 22 791-2111, Fax: 41 22 791-3111, http://www.who.int/en.

Rosalyn Carson-DeWitt, MD
Rebecca J. Frey, PhD
William A. Atkins, BB, BS, MBA

U

Ultraviolet radiation

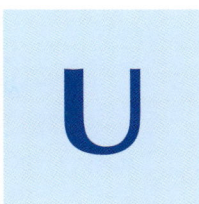

Definition

Ultraviolet (UV) **radiation** is invisible electromagnetic radiation with wavelengths that are shorter than the visible light spectrum and longer than x rays.

Description

Ultraviolet radiation comes primarily from sunlight. Very small amounts are emitted from black lights, bug zappers, specialized lamps and some medical and scientific equipment. The UV radiation spectrum ranges from wavelengths of 400 nanometers (nm) to 10 nm. The shorter the wavelength, the higher the energy and the greater the potential to damage the body. Three types of UV radiation are of primary concern to human health: ultraviolet A (UV-A, 320–400 nm), ultraviolet B (UV-B, 280–320 nm) and ultraviolet C (UV-C, 280–100 nm).

About 10% of radiation emitted by the sun is in the UV range. Another 40% is visible light, and 50% is infrared light that we perceive as heat. **Ozone**, a gas in Earth's atmosphere, blocks all but about 3% of the UV radiation from the sun. However, it blocks some wavelengths more effectively than others.

UV-A has the longest wavelength and the least amount of energy. It pass easily through Earth's atmosphere, and about 95% of what the sun emits reaches Earth. A great deal of UV-A radiation also passes through ordinary window glass. UV-B has a shorter wavelength and more energy. Its energy allows it to react with some ozone molecules. When the ozone molecules break apart, they absorb the UV-B energy, so only some of the UV-B radiation reaches the earth. UV-C has a shorter wavelength and more energy than UV-B. All the UV-C radiation reacts with ozone in the atmosphere. Its energy is absorbed by the ozone molecules as they split apart and no UV-C radiation from the sun reaches the surface of the earth. A small amount of UV-C radiation is generated through industrial activities such as welding. UV-C can be hazardous. Workers who may be exposed to man-produced UV-C must wear protective clothing.

Effects on public health

Exposure to UV radiation is both helpful and harmful. The body makes a form of vitamin D when the skin is exposed to sunlight, and more specifically to UV-B. Vitamin D is a fat-soluble steroid compound that the body needs to remain healthy. Its main role is to regulate amount of calcium circulating in the blood. Calcium is a mineral acquired through diet. Vitamin D helps regulate the absorption of calcium from the small intestine. Too little vitamin D can cause weak, brittle, deformed bones. UV-B at a wavelength of around 310 nm also is used to treat psoriasis, eczema, vitiligo, and other skin conditions. In addition, UV radiation can safely be used to sterilize food, water, and in laboratories and hospitals to kill or break down the DNA of undesirable microorganisms.

However, exposure to UV-B, either from sunlight or a tanning bed, may cause sunburn, basal and squamous cell **skin cancer** or malignant **melanoma**. UV-B directly damages DNA, the genetic material, thus causing mutations. UV-A penetrates the skin and does not cause sunburn. Because of its lower energy level, it does not directly damage DNA. Nevertheless, it contributes to the development of skin cancer, especially potentially fatal melanoma, by stimulating chemical reactions that release free radicals. In April 2011, the International Agency for Research on Cancer of the **World Health Organization** classified all ultraviolet radiation as a carcinogen in humans.

Both UV-A and UV-B damage collagen. Damage to the elastic cartilage found in skin accelerates aging and the formation of wrinkles. In addition, welders exposed to UV-B light may develop cataracts or sustain other damage to the eye.

KEY TERMS

Cataract—Cloudiness of the eye's natural lens.

Deoxyribonucleic acid (DNA)—The genetic material in cells that holds the inherited instructions for growth, development, and cellular functioning.

Free radical—A molecule with an unpaired electron that has a strong tendency to react with other molecules in DNA (genetic material), proteins, and lipids (fats), resulting in damage to cells. Free radicals are neutralized by antioxidants.

Melanoma—A malignant tumor of skin cells that produce dark pigment. It is the leading cause of skin cancer deaths.

Mutation—A permanent change in the genetic material that may alter a trait or characteristic of an individual, or manifest as disease and can be transmitted to offspring.

Psoriasis—A common recurring skin disease that is marked by dry, scaly, and silvery patches of skin that appear in a variety of sizes and locations on the body.

Vitiligo—A condition where the skin loses pigment and develops irregular white patches.

QUESTIONS TO ASK YOUR DOCTOR

- Is there a particular kind of sunscreen you recommend?
- What are the symptoms of skin cancer?
- Are tanning beds safe?
- Is it safe to tan if I do not burn?

Prevention

Individuals, especially those with fair skin, must avoid excessive exposure to the sun. Sunscreens contain substances that block UV-B. The degree of blocking power is indicated by the SPF number. The higher the number, the greater the protection against UV-B radiation. Some sunscreens contain compounds such as titanium dioxide, zinc oxide, and avobenzone that block UV-A. Europe and Japan have rating systems in place to allow consumers to determine the degree of protection against UV-A each sunscreen offers. **Food and Drug Administration** (FDA) regulates labeling of sunscreen in the United States. A rating system for UV-A is under consideration. However, some sunscreen products in the United States already indicate if they protect against both UV-B and UV-A.

Prevention must also occur on a global level. The ozone layer of Earth's atmosphere provides protection from ultraviolet radiation, but this protective layer has been depleted largely due to the reactions of chlorofluorocarbons (CFCs) and other ozone-depleting substances in the upper atmosphere. By 2010, there was evidence that adherence to the Montreal Protocol on Substances that Deplete the Ozone Layer and other international agreements might allow substantial ozone layer recovery by 2060. However, although the use of ozone-depleting compounds has declined due to bans on these substances, as of 2008, measurements reported by the National Oceanic and Atmospheric Administration (NOAA) indicated that the Antarctic ozone hole hit its maximum in 2006. The situation remains under study because other factors also contribute to the size of the cyclic Antarctic ozone hole.

Resources

BOOKS

Stille, Darlene. *Invisible Exposure: The Science of Ultraviolet Rays*. Mankato, MN: Compass Point Books, 2010.

WEBSITES

Allen, Jeannie. "Radiation—How It Affects Life on Earth." NASA. http://earthobservatory.nasa.gov/Features/UVB (accessed October 24, 2012).

Environmental Protection Agency. "UV Radiaton." http://www.epa.gov/sunwise/doc/uvradiation.html (accessed October 24, 2012).

World Health Organization. "Ultraviolet Radiation and Health." http://www.who.int/uv/uv_and_health/en/index.html (accessed October 23, 2012).

ORGANIZATIONS

American Academy of Dermatology, PO Box 4014, Schaumburg, IL 60168-4014, (866) 503 7546, Fax: (847) 240 1859, MRC@aad.org, http://www.aad.org.

Environmental Protection Agency, Ariel Rios Bldg., 1200 Pennsylvania Ave. NW, Washington, DC 20460, (202) 272-0167; TTY (202) 272-0165, http://www.epa.gov.

World Health Organization, Avenue Appia 20, 1211 Geneva 27, Switzerland, 2241 791 21 11, Fax: 2241 791 31 11, info@who.int, http://www.who.int.

Tish Davidson, AM

UNICEF

Definition

UNICEF stands for the United Nations Children's Fund (formerly known as the United Nations International Children's Emergency Fund). UNICEF is an agency of the United Nations (UN) that administers programs to aid and improve education and child and maternal health in developing countries. UNICEF employs 11,000 staff in 191 countries and territories. Eighty-eight per cent of the organization's staff are located in the field. There are eight regional offices and country offices worldwide, as well as a research center in Florence, a supply operation in Copenhagen and offices in Tokyo and Brussels. UNICEF headquarters are in New York, New York. As an operating agency of the United Nations, UNICEF is headed by an executive director, who is appointed by the Secretary General of the UN in consultation of its thirty-six-member executive board. Board members are elected by the Economic and Social Council of the UN.

Description

Origins

After World War II, European children were facing **famine** and disease. The United Nations International Children's Emergency Fund (UNICEF) was created as a temporary agency on December 11, 1946 by the United Nations (UN) to provide food, clothing, shelter, and health care to the affected children. In 1954 UNICEF became a permanent part of the UN and its mandate to aid children was extended indefinitely. Its name was shortened from United Nations International Children's Emergency Fund to the United Nations Children's Fund, although it is still known by its original acronym.

One of the first campaigns UNICEF undertook with its continued mandate was to work to eradicate infectious diseases that could be prevented or for which there was an effective treatment and that were widespread in many parts of the world. These diseases included **malaria**, yaws, **tuberculosis**, **typhus**, trachoma, and leprosy. UNICEF furnished medical equipment and supplies to countries, and the **World Health Organization** (WHO) provided technical support. In 1961, UNICEF broadened its focus from child health issues and began to address the needs of the "whole child," thus beginning an additional focus on education, including teacher training and classroom equipment in developing countries.

In 1965, nineteen years after it was founded, UNICEF, which had developed a global partnership involving governments, private and non-governmental organizations, and citizens, was awarded the Nobel Peace Prize for "the promotion of brotherhood among nations" and for emerging on the world stage as a "a peace-factor of great importance."

In 1978, WHO and UNICEF co-sponsored a conference that resulted in the Declaration of Alma-Ata on Primary Health Care (PHC). PHC involved a redefinition of health care for the poor and for rural communities by providing care "for the people and by the people" through training and employment of lay workers to provide care at the local level, with referrals to secondary and tertiary facilities as necessary.

The UN General Assembly designated 1979 as the Year of the Child (IYC), and UNICEF served as the IYC secretariat. This role provided an opportunity for UNICEF to expand its programs to many countries.

In 1982, UNICEF initiated a drive to save the lives of millions of children each year by focusing on four simple, low-cost techniques:

- growth monitoring, which is the process of following the growth rate of a child in comparison to a standard in order to assess growth adequacy and identify faltering at early stages. Assessing growth allows remediation of growth faltering before the child reaches the status of under-nutrition or identifies illnesses that may benefit from treatment;
- oral rehydration therapy to save the lives of infants with severe diarrhea;
- breastfeeding, for breastfeeding of infants under two years of age has the greatest potential impact on child survival of all preventive interventions, with the potential to prevent 1.4 million deaths in children under five in the developing world. Breastfed children have at least six times greater chance of survival in the early months than non-breastfed children, and reduces deaths from acute respiratory infection and diarrhea, two major child killers, as well as from other infectious diseases;
- immunization, which is a proven tool for controlling and even eradicating infectious diseases.

The Convention on the Rights of the Child, held in 1989, was the first legally binding international instrument to incorporate the full range of human rights, including civil, cultural, economic, political and social rights, for children. World leaders recognized that children under 18 years old had human rights as adults do, and often needed special care and protection that adults do not. The Convention defined the basic human rights that children everywhere have: to survive; to develop to the fullest; to be protected from harmful influences, abuse and exploitation; and to participate fully in family, cultural and social life. The four core principles of the Convention are non-discrimination; devotion to the best interests of the child; the right to life, survival and development; and respect for the views of the child. The Convention protects children's rights by setting standards in health care, education; and legal, civil and social services.

UNICEF organized the World Summit for Children in 1990, which brought more than seventy heads of state and representatives of more than eighty UN member states to New York for a two-day meeting. It produced a declaration, a plan of action, and a set of goals for children's health, nutrition and education to be achieved by the year 2000, most of which were in the realm of public health. UNICEF followed up the summit with individual national plans of action to reach the goals. UNICEF also developed programs concerning child labor and land mines.

In 2000, UNICEF, along with developing country and donor governments, WHO, the World Bank, vaccine industries in both industrialized and developing countries, research and technical agencies, the Bill & Melinda Gates Foundation, and other private philanthropists, formed the GAVI Alliance. This Alliance is a public-private global health partnership committed to saving children's lives and protecting people's health by increasing access to immunization in developing countries. By the end of the 1990s, nearly 30 million children born every year in developing countries were not fully immunized. In response to this statistic, the GAVI Alliance was started in 2000 with a $ 750 million commitment from the Bill & Melinda Gates Foundation. During GAVI's first decade, 288 million children were immunized against life-threatening diseases such as **diphtheria**, tetanus, **whooping cough**, hepatitis B, Haemophilus influenzae type b (Hib), and **yellow fever**. In 2010 WHO estimated that five million future deaths have been prevented by the efforts of the GAVI Alliance.

In 2002 a Session of the UN General Assembly was convened to review progress since the World Summit for Children in 1990 and to re-commit to children's rights. It was the first such Session devoted exclusively to children and the first to include them as official delegates.

Funding

UNICEF is funded entirely by voluntary contributions from governments, foundations, UN agencies, international financial institutions, individuals and businesses. In addition to regular contributions, many governments also make special contributions for specific purposes, especially during emergencies. UNICEF also sells cards, gifts, and other products to provide funds for its programs.

Another UNICEF funding source is "Trick or Treat for UNICEF". This activity began in 1950 when a group of Philadelphia school children went door-to-door collecting money in decorated milk cartons in order to help struggling children being served by UNICEF. They raised $17 that first year, but since then, the practice, now using orange collection boxes, has spread to other parts of the United States, Canada (since 1955), and Hong Kong, China (since 2001), as well as other locations around the world. Millions of dollars are raised each year that is used by UNICEF to provide medicine, better nutrition, clean water, education, emergency relief, and other aid to children. In addition to trick or treating, the children participate in educational programs concerning poverty, diseases, and armed conflicts that affect children throughout the world and learn how they can help improve the world. Since the program started over 60 years ago, U.S. children ("kids helping kids") have collected almost $160 million by going door-to-door and by holding fundraisers with schools or other groups.

UNICEF uses its resources for the poorest and most marginalized children because this aid often determines their chances of being educated, healthy, nourished and protected from harm. In 2011, UNICEF's cut headquarters management costs without cutting programs and field staff in order to realize greater results for children, Total expenditures in 2011 was $3,819 million, with spending on program was $3,472 million. Over half of program expenditures went to UNICEF's efforts to ensure that young children survive and develop; 57 per cent went to sub-Saharan Africa, which has the majority of the least developed countries.

The National Committees are an essential part of UNICEF's global organization and a unique feature of UNICEF. Currently there are 36 National Committees in the world, each established as an independent local non-governmental organization. The National Committees raise funds from the private sector, promote children's rights and provide worldwide visibility for children threatened by poverty, disasters, armed conflict, abuse and exploitation. About one-third of UNICEF's annual income is raised as a result of the National Committees' efforts.

Research

The UNICEF Innocenti Research Centre (IRC) in Florence, Italy was established in 1988 for conducting studies and developing knowledge on emerging issues affecting children. IRC collaborates with its host institution in Florence, the Istituto degli Innocenti, which is an organization established in the 15th century as a facility for the care and protection of abandoned children. Core funding for the IRC is provided by the Government of Italy. Financial support for specific projects is also provided by other governments, international institutions, and private sources, including UNICEF National Committees.

The goals of the IRC are to improve international understanding of the issues relating to children's rights, to promote economic policies that advance the cause of children, and to help facilitate implementation of the Convention on the Rights of the Child. To accomplish these goals, the IRC uses these approaches:

- evidence-based analysis, drawing on quantitative and qualitative information, the application of appropriate methodologies, and the development of recommendations concerning child well-being and the realization of children's rights;
- partnerships with a wide range of research and policy institutions and development groups, within and beyond the United Nations system;
- communication and leveraging of research findings and recommendations to support policy dialogue and development and advocacy initiatives;

The Centre produces a wide range of publications, often in multiple languages, that contribute to the global discussion on children's issues and include a wide range of opinions.

Purpose

To accomplish the purpose of UNICEF, the organization focuses on five areas concerning education and child and maternal health.

Child survival and development

UNICEF along with governments, national and international agencies, communities, and individuals, work to end preventable child deaths by supporting effective and life-saving actions at each phase in a child's life, from prenatal care in a mother's pregnancy to effective and affordable health care through childhood and into adulthood. Existing high-impact, low-cost interventions such as vaccines, antibiotics, micronutrient supplementation, insecticide-treated bed nets, improved breastfeeding practices, and safe hygiene practices have saved millions of lives. In 2010, 7.6 million children died before reaching their fifth birthday, which is an improvement from 1990, when more than 12 million children died under the age of five.

Proper nutrition is especially important to provide every child with a good start in life. UNICEF since it was founded concentrated on nutrition programs. One in four, or 143 million under-five children in the developing world are still underweight and only 38 per cent of children less than six months of age are exclusively breastfed. Specific UNICEF programs include infant and young child feeding, micronutrient deficiencies, nutrition security during emergencies, and nutrition and HIV/AIDS.

By 1977, **smallpox** had been eradicated from the world through the widespread and targeted use of the smallpox vaccine, which had been developed in 1792. In 1974, based on the success of smallpox eradication, WHO established the Expanded Programme on Immunization (EPI), for less than five per cent of the world's children were immunized during their first year of life against six life-threatening diseases: **polio**, diphtheria, tuberculosis, pertussis (whooping cough), **measles** and tetanus. During the 1980s, UNICEF worked with WHO to achieve Universal Childhood Immunization of the vaccines against the six diseases, with the aim of immunizing 80 percent of all children by 1990. By 2010, a record 109 million children were vaccinated and global immunization rates were at 85 percent. The present goal is to have 90 percent of all children vaccinated. In coordination with the GAVI Alliance, UNICEF provides vaccines to 58 percent of the world's children.

In the last 20 years many new vaccines have been developed and provided by the GAVI Alliance to developing countries. These vaccines include those against Hepatitis B and Haemophilus influenzae type b (Hib) and the pneumococcal conjugate vaccine (PCV) and rotavirus vaccine (RV). Polio and maternal neonatal tetanus have almost been eradicated, and measles deaths were reduced by 78% between 2000 and 2008. While health care teams are providing immunizations, they can also deliver other preventive services, such as vitamin A supplements, deworming medications, and insecticide-treated mosquito nets.

UNICEF also advocates for the protection of the rights of children with disabilities. One billion people have a disability, with at least 1 in 10 being children and 80 percent living in developing countries. As an example of UNICEF's involvement, UNICEF provides programs that give children with disabilities the opportunity to participate in sport activities. Participation in sport, recreation and play empowers children with disabilities and teaches them key life skills. It can help build more inclusive societies by raising awareness about the contributions children with disabilities can make in their communities.

UNICEF works with WHO and other groups to introduce Life Skills Education to children around the world. Life skills"are defined as psychosocial abilities for adaptive and positive behavior that enable individuals to deal effectively with the demands and challenges of everyday life. They are loosely grouped into three broad categories of skills: cognitive skills for analyzing and using information, personal skills for developing personal agency and managing oneself, and inter-personal skills for communicating and interacting effective- with others.

The School-in-a-Box is part of UNICEF's standard response in emergencies and used in many back-to-school operations around the world. The kit contains supplies and materials for a teacher and 40 students. The purpose of the kit is to ensure the continuation of children's education during the first 72 hours of an emergency. The Early Childhood Development Kit was created to aid younger children during conflict or emergencies. The Kit provides young children access to play, stimulation and early learning opportunities and permits them to achieve a sense of normalcy. The Kit contains materials to help caregivers create a safe learning environment for up to 50 young children ages 0-6. Contents include puzzles and games, counting circle and boxes to stack and sort, board books and puppets for storytelling, art supplies, and hygience supplies.

UNICEF initiated the "Days of Tranquillity", whereby ceasefires are arranged during war times so that children can be reached with lifesaving healthcare.

UNICEF works in more than 90 countries around the world to improve water supplies and **sanitation** facilities in schools and communities and to promote safe hygiene practices. In emergencies UNICEF provides relief to communities and nations with disrupted water supplies and disease. According to the WHO/UNICEF Joint Monitoring Programme for Water Supply and Sanitation, 37 percent of the developing world's population (2.5 billion people) lack improved sanitation facilities, and over 780 million people still use unsafe drinking water sources.

Basic education and gender equality

UNICEF works to ensure that all children, regardless of gender, ethnicity, socioeconomic background or circumstances, receive their right to a quality education. UNICEF supports programs and initiatives that focus on the world's most excluded and vulnerable children, including girls, the disabled, ethnic minorities, the rural and urban poor, victims of conflict and natural disasters and children affected by HIV and **AIDS**.

UNICEF provides opportunities for governments, communities and parents to gain the capacities and skills they need to fulfill their obligations for children, which include ensuring the right of all children to free, compulsory quality, child-friendly schooling, even during a humanitarian crisis, in the recovery period after a crisis, or in unstable situations.

Early childhood development programs sponsored by UNICEF that focus on the most significant developmental period of life, have been shown to lead to higher levels of primary school enrollment and educational performance, which in turn positively affect employment opportunities later in life. Children who start school late and lack the necessary skills to be able to learn constructively are more likely to fall behind or drop out completely, often perpetuating a cycle of poverty.

HIV/AIDS and children

UNICEF works to ensure that children, young people, and women have access to information regarding prevention, care, and treatment of HIV/AIDS, and that they have continuing access to programs such as those that provide preventative measures, antiviral and antibiotic treatments, nutrition support, psychosocial support and counseling, infant care for HIV-positive mothers, and peer support groups. Special focus is given to preventing mother-to-child transmission of HIV, providing pediatric treatment, preventing infection among adolescents and young people, and protecting and supporting children affected by HIV and AIDS.

Child protection

Millions of children worldwide from all socio-economic backgrounds, and across all ages, religions and cultures suffer violence, exploitation and abuse. Some children are particularly vulnerable because of gender, race, ethnic origin or socio-economic status. Higher levels of vulnerability are also often associated with children with disabilities, orphans, and indigenous and ethnic minorities. Other risks for children are associated with living and working on the streets, those living in institutions and detention and living in communities where inequality, unemployment and poverty are concentrated. Natural disasters and armed conflict may expose children to additional risks. violence, exploitation and abuse can affect the child's physical and mental health in the short and longer term, impairing their ability to learn and socialize, and impacting their transition to adulthood with adverse consequences later in life. UNICEF and its partners work to the strengthen all components of child protection systems, including human resources, finances, laws, standards, governance, monitoring and services.

In addition, in the last ten years, UNICEF has investigated social norms that result in violence, exploitation and abuse and has promoted change in a number of countries. To promote positive norms to bring about an end to harmful practices, UNICEF uses advocacy and awareness-raising and supports discussions and educational programs at community and national levels. This process, with its focus on community values and human rights, and when combined with legislation, policies, regulations and services, can lead to positive and lasting change, such as the abandonment of female genital mutilation/cutting, decrease in child marriage, and domestic violence.

Policy advocacy and partnerships

Policy analysis is another focus of UNICEF's work with governments, lawmakers, the media, society, and international organizations on behalf of children and women. By analyzing economic, social and legal policies, the circumstances and forces that affect the well-being of children and women in specific countries can be better understood and improved. UNICEF uses the standards outlined in the Convention on the Rights of the Child to conduct their analyses of specific policies. Analyses are shared with UNICEF'S partners so that programs and polices for the protection of children's rights can be developed and implemented.

Public health role and response

With its focus on the needs and rights of the child, UNICEF uses as much as 80 percent of its funds to programs that can be classified under the broad umbrella of public health. Working in partnership with governments as well as health-related organizations, especially WHO, UNICEF is active in programs ranging from immunization and oral rehydration campaigns to water and sanitation projects, and from the fight against acute respiratory infections to the elimination of polio and micronutrient deficiencies.

The world's population is at increased risk of recurring influenza pandemics as well as other newly emerging infectious diseases because of global changes in both animal and human population densities and ecological changes. UNICEF works with its partners to support national preparedness to respond to disease outbreaks and other emergencies as well as focuses on communication methods that can be used to mobilize communities and to inform individuals of how to protect themselves from infections.

UNICEF partners with public personalities, including those in the performing arts or athletics, to generate public support for public health issues. Goodwill ambassadors provide support in reaching specific audiences. In the last two decades of the twentieth century, UNICEF, with its activist leadership, helped shape the agenda of international health, especially for children and mothers.

> **KEY TERMS**
>
> **Oral rehydration therapy**—Oral administration of a solution of electrolytes and carbohydrates in the treatment of diarrhea-related dehydration.
>
> **Social norms**—Laws (not considered to be formal) that govern a society's behaviors, that is, the rules that a group uses for appropriate and inappropriate values, beliefs, attitudes and behaviors. These rules may be explicit or implicit and result in social control. Failure to abide by the rules can result in severe punishments, the most feared of which is exclusion from the group. What is considered "normal" is relative to the location of the culture in which the social interaction is taking place. Norms in every culture create conformity that allows for people to become socialized to the culture in which they live.
>
> **United Nations**—An international organization whose purpose is to facilitate cooperation in international law, international security, economic development, social progress, human rights, and achievement of world peace. The UN was founded in 1945 after World War II to replace the League of Nations, to stop wars between countries, and to provide a platform for dialogue. It contains multiple subsidiary organizations to carry out its missions.

Resources

BOOKS

Connolly, Sean. *UNICEF*. Collingwood ON: Saunders Book Co., 2011.

Jolly, Richard. *UNICEF (United Nations Children's Fund)*.London, UK: Routledge, 2013.

UNICEF. *The State of the World's Children 2012: Children in an Urban World.*. New York, NY: UNICEF, 2012.

UNICEF. *Committing to Child Survival: A Promise Renewed Progress Report 2012*. New York, NY: UNICEF, 2012.

UNICEF. *Humanitarian Action for Children 2012.* New York, NY: UNICEF, 2012.

ORGANIZATIONS

UNICEF, 3 United Nations Plaza, New York, NY, USA 10017, (212) 686-5522, Fax: (212) 887-7465, http://www.unicef-irc.org/.

UNICEF Innocenti Research Centre, Piazza SS. Annunziata, 12 50122, Florence, Italy, 39 055 20330, Fax: 39 055 2033220, http://www.unicef-irc.org/.

Judith L. Sims

U.S. Department of Health and Human Services

Definition

Established in 1979, the U.S. Department of Health and Human Services (HHS) is a cabinet-level department responsible for the welfare, safety, and health of United States citizens.

Purpose

HHS is comprised of several different programs. administers drug safety standards, prevents epidemics, and offers assistance to those who are economically disadvantaged.

Description

The **Public Health Service**, a division of HHS, helps state and city governments with health problems. The service studies ways of controlling infectious diseases, works to immunize children, and operates quarantine programs.

HHS also operates the Centers for Disease Control (CDC), where most of the nation's health problems are studied. These include occupational health and safety, the dangers of cigarette **smoking**, and childhood injuries, as well as **communicable diseases** and the epidemic of urban violence. In addition to investigating these problems, the CDC is charged with making policy suggestions on their management. HHS also administers the Social Security and Medicare programs, as well as the Head Start Program.

The **Food and Drug Administration** (FDA) is another agency of HHS. It is charged with responding to new drug research by drug development companies and approving new drugs for use in the United States.

Results

New lead-content standards for paint and other consumer items grew out of CDC studies. The agency conducts energy related epidemiological research for the U.S. Department of Energy, including studies on **radiation exposure**. Through the CDC, the HHS runs the National Center for Health Statistics, an **AIDS** Hotline, an international disaster relief team, and programs to monitor infectious disease epidemics worldwide.

Along with the U.S. Department of Agriculture, the FDA is responsible for maintaining the safety of the nation's food and drug supply. HHS also administers the **Agency for Toxic Substances and Disease Registry**, which carries out the health-related responsibilities of the Superfund legislation.

Resources

WEBSITES

"Department of Health and Human Services." USA.gov. August 8, 2012. http://www.usa.gov/Agencies/Federal/Executive/HHS.shtml (accessed August 11, 2012).

ORGANIZATIONS

U.S. Department of Health and Human Services, 200 Independence Ave., SW, Washington, DC 20201, (202) 619-0257, (877) 696-6775, http://www.hhs.gov.

Linda Rehkopf
Stacey Chamberlin

V

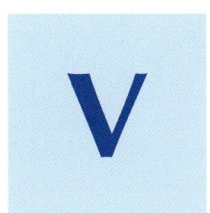

Vaccination

Definition

Vaccination, also called immunization, is the administration of a weakened (attenuated) or killed microorganism to stimulate immune system defenses against that organism. Upon future exposure to the pathogen, the immune system responds rapidly and prevents the development of disease.

Purpose

Vaccinations are among the most effective public health interventions. Vaccination has changed the course of human history, putting an end to plagues of infectious diseases that once wiped out large segments of the population. Vaccination has led to the worldwide eradication of **smallpox** and the near-eradication of poliomyelitis. In many parts of the world, vaccination has nearly eliminated diseases such as **measles**, **mumps**, rubella, and chickenpox (varicella), which were once considered to be a normal part of childhood, but sometimes led to debilitating or fatal complications. Vaccination has also drastically reduced the incidence of diseases such as **tuberculosis**, **whooping cough** (pertussis), rabies, **diphtheria**, **typhoid fever**, tetanus, and **plague**. More recent vaccines have decreased the incidence of hepatitis B infections that can lead to liver cancer and **human papilloma virus** (HPV) infections that can lead to cervical cancer. Vaccines are now available against more than 20 infectious diseases.

In the United States and other developed countries, children are routinely vaccinated against more than 12 diseases. In general, they must have at least some of these vaccinations before they can attend school. As a result, these diseases are now at their lowest levels in human history. Once most people in a population have been vaccinated against an infectious disease, it can no longer spread through the population. This is known as herd immunity, and provides protection against the disease, even for those who have not been vaccinated.

Description

Vaccines are produced from weakened or killed bacteria or **viruses**. Vaccination stimulates the body's immune system to respond to antigens or markers on the pathogen by producing proteins called antibodies that are specific for those antigens. Vaccines usually stimulate the cellular immune system as well. Later, if vaccinated people are exposed to the infectious microorganism, they already have antibodies to destroy it, thereby preventing the development of disease. This process of establishing specific immunity through vaccination is known as immunization.

It has been recognized for hundreds, if not thousands, of years that people who survived an infectious disease were very unlikely to contract that disease a second time. Traditional healers used intentional infections to try to protect people from devastating diseases. During the eighteenth century, smallpox was responsible for 60 million deaths worldwide—killing 45,000 people annually in the British Isles alone. Early in that century, Lady Mary Wortley Montagu observed the practice of variolation in Turkey. Every autumn, old women would collect pus from the victim of a mild smallpox attack and inject it into the veins of susceptible children. After a short illness, the children recovered and were thereafter immune to smallpox. Montagu popularized variolation among the British gentry. However, treatment with live virus sometimes resulted in disease transmission or death. Dr. Edward Jenner, adopting a related method used by some English farmers, developed the first vaccination against smallpox using the exudate from cowpox, a closely related cattle disease that does not cause human illness.

Vaccinations differ for different diseases. Some vaccinations, such as the rabies vaccine first developed

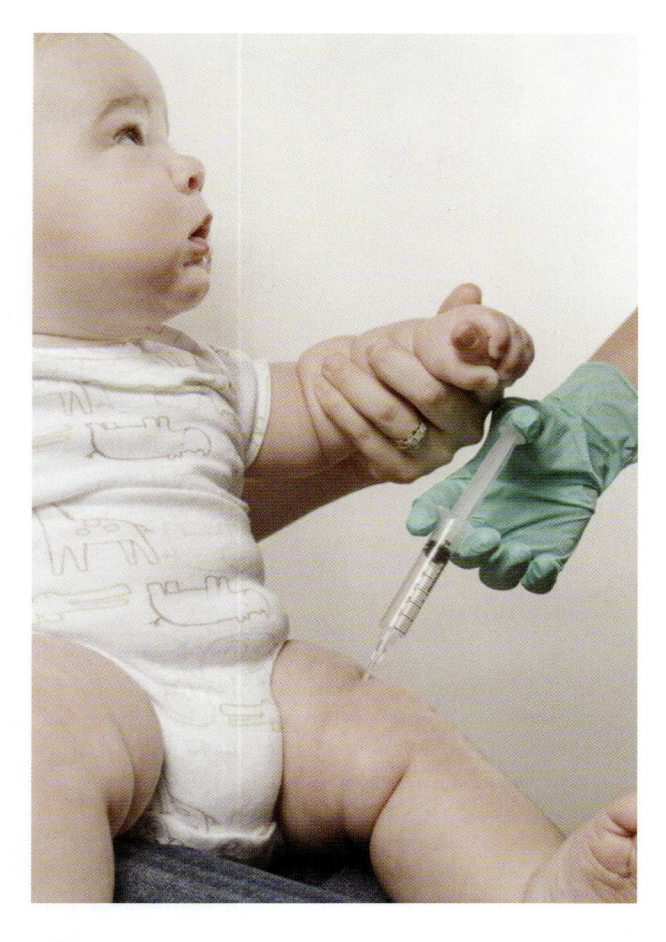

A baby receiving a vaccine injection. *(CDC/Amanda Mills)*

by Louis Pasteur and Emile Roux in 1885, are administered only when a person is likely to have been exposed to the pathogen or is at specific risk. Other vaccinations are given to travelers going to countries where certain diseases, such as typhoid or **yellow fever**, are common or **endemic**. Influenza vaccines are developed annually, based on the viral strains that are expected to be prevalent that year. Although annual flu shots were previously recommended only for specific groups who were particularly susceptible to complications—such as young children, the elderly, and people with compromised immune systems—they are now recommended for everyone. Attempts are also made to vaccinate almost everyone against certain other diseases, such as diphtheria, tetanus, **polio**, and measles. Some vaccinations are required only once, whereas as others require a series of vaccinations or must be repeated after a certain number of years. Most vaccines are given as injections, but a few are given by mouth (oral) or as a nasal spray. Some vaccinations are combined in one injection, such as the measles-mumps-rubella (MMR) or diphtheria-tetanus-pertussis (DTaP) combinations.

Recommended vaccinations

Because vaccinations are most effective when administered at certain ages, children in the United States and other developed countries are routinely vaccinated according to specific immunization schedules:

- hepatitis B (HepB) at birth, at 1–2 months of age, and again at 6–18 months
- rotavirus (RV) at 2, 4, and 6 months
- diphtheria, tetanus, and pertussis (DTaP) at 2, 4, 6, and 15–18 months and 4–6 and 11–12 years
- *Haemophilus influenzae* type b (Hib; a major cause of spinal meningitis) at 2, 4, 6, and 12–15 months
- pneumococcus (bacterial pneumonia, PCV) at 2, 4, 6, and 12–15 months and older children with certain medical conditions
- inactivated polio (IPV) at 2, 4, 6–18 months and 4–6 years
- influenza annually beginning at 6 months
- combination measles, mumps, and rubella or German measles (MMR) and varicella or the MMRV combination at 12–15 months and 4–6 years
- hepatitis A (HepA) at 12–23 months and 6–18 months later and older children with medical conditions that put them at risk
- human papillomavirus (HPV)—three doses at 11–12 years (before becoming sexually active)
- meningococcal conjugate vaccine (meningococcal meningitis, MCV) at age 11 or 12 and a booster at age 16

Since most vaccinations have only become available in recent decades, older adults are presumed to be immune to most common infectious diseases through previous exposure. For example, adults born before 1957 do not need measles vaccinations, because they have lived through several years of measles epidemics, and 95–97% are immune to measles. Recommendations for adult vaccinations include:

- influenza annually
- tetanus, diphtheria, pertussis (Tdap), with a Td booster shot every ten years
- varicella, two doses
- one or two doses of MMR before age 55
- zoster (shingles) at age 60 or older

Other available vaccinations protect against:

- anthrax
- cholera
- Japanese encephalitis
- plague

ALBERT BRUCE SABIN (1906–1993)

Albert Bruce Sabin was born on August 26, 1906, in Bialystok, Russia, to Jacob and Tillie Sabin. To escape extreme poverty, the Sabins immigrated to the United States and settled in Paterson, New Jersey. Following his graduation from high school in 1923, Sabin was able to attend dentistry school at New York University due to his uncle's generous financing. However, after reading Paul deKruif's *Microbe Hunters*, he became intrigued by virology and the idea of curing epidemic diseases. After two years of dentistry school, Sabin decided to switch to medicine, earning his M.D. in 1931. Sabin completed his residency and internship in the United States and then went to London to conduct research.

Sabin returned to the United States in 1935 to resume his research on polio at the Rockefeller Institute. In 1953, Jonas Salk announced that he had created a safe killed-virus polio vaccine, but soon after its introduction many people died. Sabin wanted to create a live-virus vaccine, which he believed would be safer. Sabin diluted three strains of the polio virus and tested these on himself, his family, and other volunteers. These live-virus vaccines (given orally) proved safe and effective and soon became the vaccine of choice worldwide. Sabin's published works include *Viruses and Cancer: A Public Lecture in Conversational Style* (1965), *Behavior of Chimpanzee-Avirulent Poliomyelitis Viruses in Experimentally Infected Human Volunteers* (1955), and *Recent Advances in Our Knowledge of Dengue and Sand Fly Fever* (1955). Sabin died of congestive heart failure on March 3, 1993.

- tuberculosis
- typhoid fever
- H1N1 or swine flu
- yellow fever

Recommended vaccination dosages depend on the type of vaccine and may be different for different patients and different ages. Some vaccines, such as MMR and MMRV, are not given during the first year, when babies are still protected by their mothers' antibodies that can destroy the vaccine. Most physicians follow recommended schedules, but there is some flexibility. For example, children are usually not vaccinated during an illness. An immunization record is used to keep track of children's vaccinations.

Some people—including healthcare workers, college students, cruise ship vacationers, and travelers to developing countries—may require additional vaccinations, some of which must be given as far as 12 weeks in advance. Women of childbearing age may also require additional vaccinations, since some infectious diseases are very dangerous if contracted during pregnancy, and some vaccines cannot be administered during pregnancy.

Precautions

Vaccines are not always 100% effective. To prevent outbreaks of disease, immunization programs depend on the participation of entire communities. The more people who are vaccinated, the lower everyone's risk of being exposed to a disease. People who are not immune through vaccination or prior exposure are safer when their family, friends, neighbors, and coworkers have been vaccinated.

Some vaccinations are not recommended for pregnant or breastfeeding women. Others may be given to pregnant women who are at especially high risk for a particular disease such as polio or to prevent medical problems in their babies. Women should avoid becoming pregnant within three months of vaccination against measles, mumps, or rubella, as these vaccines may harm the fetus. Certain vaccinations are not safe for infants.

Medical conditions, such as cancer or HIV/AIDS, can render vaccinations dangerous. Influenza vaccine may reactivate the rare Guillain-Barré syndrome or worsen illnesses that involve the lungs, such as **bronchitis** or pneumonia. Vaccines with fever as a side effect may trigger seizures in people with a history of fever-induced seizures.

Vaccines can cause allergic reactions in some people. People who have previously had an unusual reaction to a vaccine should inform their physician. Patients with allergies to:

- the antibiotics neomycin or polymyxin B should not have rubella, measles, mumps, or the combined MMR vaccines
- baker's yeast should not have the HepB vaccine
- antibiotics such as gentamicin, streptomycin, or other aminoglycosides should be aware that some influenza vaccines contain small amounts of these drugs
- chicken eggs or the fluids of chick embryos should not be used to produce influenza, measles, or mumps vaccines

KEY TERMS

Anthrax—An infectious bacterial disease of animals that can be passed to humans.

Antibodies—Proteins produced by specialized white blood cells after stimulation by a foreign substance (antigen), including a vaccine, that act against the antigen in an immune response.

Antigen—Any foreign substance, usually a protein, that stimulates the body's immune system to produce antibodies.

Attenuated—A vaccine made with live virus that has been modified so that it is no longer infective.

Autism—A variable developmental disorder that includes an impaired ability to communicate and form normal social relationships.

Booster shot—A supplementary vaccine dose.

Cellular immune system—Cell-mediated immunity; immune system cells that fight infection without specific antibodies against the disease-causing organism.

Cholera—A bacterial infection of the small intestine that spreads through feces-contaminated water and food and is often fatal in young children and the elderly; cholera vaccinations are essential in the overcrowded, unsanitary conditions of many refugee camps.

Cowpox—A mild disease in cows caused by a virus related to the smallpox virus.

Diphtheria—A serious, infectious disease caused by a toxin-producing bacterium.

DTap, TDap—Combination vaccines against diphtheria, tetanus, and pertussis; Td is a tetanus/diphtheria vaccine.

Endemic—Occurring naturally and consistently in a particular area.

Epidemic—An outbreak of disease where the number of cases exceeds the usual (endemic) or typical number of cases.

Hepatitis—Any of several viral diseases that affect the liver; vaccinations (HepA and HepB) are available against hepatitis A. B, and C.

Herd immunity—Disease protection for non-immune or unvaccinated individuals that is conferred by the prevailing immunity within a population due to widespread vaccination coverage.

Hib—A vaccine against *Haemophilus influenzae* type b, a major cause of spinal meningitis.

Human papillomavirus; HPV—A large family of viruses that cause warts and other growths on various parts of the body; the HPV vaccine is effective against sexually transmitted HPV strains that cause cervical cancer.

Immunization—The administration of a vaccine that stimulates the body to create antibodies to a specific disease (immunity) without causing symptoms of the disease.

Influenza—A disease caused by viruses that infect the respiratory tract.

Side effects

The most common vaccination side effects are minor pain, redness, or swelling at the site of the injection. Some people may develop a fever or rash. In rare cases, vaccines may cause severe allergic reactions. The Vaccine Adverse Event Reporting System (VAERS) is a national system for tracking side effects and adverse reactions to any vaccine licensed in the United States.

With the recent significant increases in the number of recommended childhood vaccinations, some parents have balked at having their children vaccinated. Although most vaccinations are required before children can enter school, all states make exceptions for children with specific medical conditions, and many states grant exemptions for children whose parents object for religious or other reasons. Although some early vaccines did cause various complications, vaccine development has taken advantage of advances in many fields, and rational vaccine design is a very sophisticated science. Purported links between childhood vaccinations and complications such as **autism** and seizures have been thoroughly disproven. Nevertheless, some consumers are genuinely concerned when pharmaceutical companies develop vaccines such as HPV and then aggressively market those vaccines and lobby state governments to require them for all children.

Interactions

Vaccines may interact with other medicines and medical treatments to alter the effects of the vaccine or the other medication or increase the risk of side effects.

Measles—An acute and highly contagious viral disease marked by distinct red spots followed by a rash; occurs primarily in children.

Meningitis—Inflammation of tissues that surround the brain and spinal cord; the meningococcal conjugate vaccine (MCV) protects against meningococcal meningitis.

MMR—A combination vaccine against measles, mumps, and rubella.

MMRV—A combination vaccine against measles, mumps, rubella, and varicella (chickenpox).

Mumps—An acute and highly contagious viral illness that usually occurs in childhood.

Pathogen—A disease-causing microorganism.

PCV—A vaccine against the pneumococcus that causes bacterial pneumonia.

Pertussis; whooping cough—An infectious bacterial disease, especially of children, that is on the increase due to under-vaccination.

Plague—A highly infectious and often fatal bacterial disease that is transmitted between humans and from rodents to humans by fleas.

Poliomyelitis; polio—An infectious viral disease that was very widespread, especially among children, before the introduction of polio vaccines in the 1950s; it has been eradicated in most of the world through vaccines such as inactivated polio vaccine (IPV).

Rabies—A rare but serious viral disease transmitted to humans by the bite of an infected animal.

Rotavirus (RV)—A genus of viruses, some of which are common causes of diarrhea and childhood death worldwide.

Rubella—German measles; a contagious viral disease that is milder than typical measles but is damaging to the fetus if it is contracted in early pregnancy.

Smallpox—A highly contagious viral disease that has been eradicated through worldwide vaccination.

Tetanus—An acute infectious disease caused by bacteria introduced into the body through a wound.

Tuberculosis—A chronic infectious bacterial disease of the respiratory system.

Typhoid fever—An infectious bacterial disease spread through poor sanitation.

Vaccine—A preparation of killed or attenuated-live bacteria or virus that is administered to stimulate immunity against that disease-causing organism.

Varicella; chickenpox—A childhood disease caused by a herpes virus that may be reactivated later in life to cause herpes zoster or shingles.

Variolation—The deliberate inoculation of an uninfected person with smallpox to protect against severe smallpox; widely used before the introduction of a vaccine.

Yellow fever—An infectious viral disease that is spread by mosquitoes and is most common in Central and South America and Central Africa.

For example, **radiation** therapy and cancer drugs may reduce the effectiveness of many vaccines or increase the chance of side effects.

Public health role and response

Vaccinations are a major—if not the major—public health concern worldwide. Vaccinations are essential for preventing or containing epidemics of infectious disease following natural and manmade disasters. Overcrowded refugee camps, where diseases such as **cholera** and measles can reach epidemic proportions, are a special focus for mass vaccinations.

Both the **Centers for Disease Control and Prevention** (CDC) and the **World Health Organization** (WHO) carefully track vaccination coverage throughout the world. Routine childhood vaccinations and mass immunization campaigns are primary public health strategies for both organizations, with the goals of reducing mortality from vaccination-preventable diseases and eventual worldwide eradication of those diseases. The WHO's fourth Millennium Development Goal is to reduce the mortality rate for children under five by two-thirds between 1990 and 2015. Measles vaccination coverage is an indicator of progress toward that goal, because it is considered an indicator of access to child health services. The Measles & Rubella (MR) Initiative is a joint effort of WHO, the CDC, **UNICEF**, the United Nations Foundation, and the American **Red Cross**. By the end of 2015, it aims to reduce global measles deaths by at least 95% from 2000 levels and to eliminate measles and rubella in at least five WHO regions by 2020. The MR Initiative works toward achieving and maintaining high vaccination

WHAT TO ASK YOUR DOCTOR

- Should I have my child vaccinated?
- What vaccinations does my child require?
- Who will keep track of my child's vaccinations?
- Are there any risks to childhood vaccinations?
- Will my child be fully protected against disease?

coverage, as well as providing disease surveillance, rapid response to outbreaks, and effective treatment.

Mass vaccination programs face a variety of obstacles around the world, ranging from lack of resources and healthcare infrastructures to cultural and political opposition. For example, in July of 2012, WHO doctors working for polio eradication in Pakistan were assassinated amid rumors that the polio vaccine was unsafe and an element in a plot to sterilize Muslim children. Pakistan, Afghanistan, and Nigeria are the three countries in which polio remains endemic, meaning that transmission of the polio virus has never been interrupted.

In the United States, falling vaccination rates are a major public health concern and have led to serious outbreaks of pertussis, and measles. Overall vaccination rates in some parts of the Pacific Northwest and a few other communities have fallen below 80%, well below the threshold needed for herd immunity. In some Oregon communities, more than 20% of children have religious exemptions from required vaccinations. Other parents delay vaccinations for their young children because of misinformed fears about the dangers of vaccines. Whereas in the developing world, poverty and poor healthcare infrastructure are common barriers to vaccination, in the United States, most low-income children receive the recommended vaccinations through the federal Vaccines for Children program, which provides free vaccinations for children without health insurance. In contrast, it tends to be wealthier, better-educated American parents who object to vaccinating their children. Under-vaccination has become so widespread that ScienceDebate.org named the issue of enforced vaccinations in the interests of public health and allowable circumstances for vaccination exemptions as one of the Top American Science Questions of the 2012 presidential campaign.

The development of new vaccines, especially for widespread infections such as **malaria** and HIV/AIDS, is also a major public health initiative. New vaccines for rare infectious diseases, such as **anthrax**, are being rapidly developed and tested for defense against potential **bioterrorism**.

Resources

BOOKS

Artenstein, Andrew W., ed. *Vaccines: A Biography*. New York: Springer, 2010.

Cochi, Stephen L., and Walter R. Dowdle. *Disease Eradication in the 21st Century: Implications for Global Health*. Cambridge, MA: MIT, 2011.

Merino, Noël. *Should Vaccinations be Mandatory?* Detroit: Greenhaven, 2010.

Offit, Paul A. *Deadly Choices: How the Anti-Vaccine Movement Threatens Us All*. New York: Basic Books, 2011.

Offit, Paul A., and Charlotte A. Moser. *Vaccines & Your Child: Separating Fact from Fiction*. New York: Columbia University, 2011.

Queijo, Jon. *Breakthrough: How the 10 Greatest Discoveries in Medicine Saved Millions and Changed Our View of the World*. Upper Saddle River, NJ: FT Press Science, 2010.

Sears, Robert. *The Vaccine Book: Making the Right Decision for Your Child*. New York: Little, Brown, 2011.

PERIODICALS

Diekema, Douglas S. "Improving Childhood Vaccination Rates." *New England Journal of Medicine* 366, no. 5 (February 2, 2012): 391–3.

Kim, Jane J. "The Role of Cost-Effectiveness in U.S. Vaccination Policy." *New England Journal of Medicine* 365, no. 19 (November 10, 2011): 1760–1.

Mascarelli, Amanda. "Vaccination Questions Answered." *Los Angeles Times* (August 8, 2011): E2.

Stein, Richard A. "Vaccination: A Public Health Intervention That Changed History & Is Changing With History." *American Biology Teacher* 73, no. 9 (November/December 2011): 513–19.

"The Value of HPV Vaccination." *Nature Medicine* 18, no. 1 (January 2012): 28–9.

WEBSITES

"Childhood Immunization." MedlinePlus. December 27, 2011. http://www.nlm.nih.gov/medlineplus/childhoodimmunization.html (accessed October 13, 2012).

"Immunization." MedlinePlus. June 15, 2012. http://www.nlm.nih.gov/medlineplus/immunization.html (accessed October 13, 2012).

"Immunization Schedules." Centers for Disease Control and Prevention. May 31, 2012. http://www.cdc.gov/vaccines/schedules/index.html (accessed October 13, 2012).

Reinberg, Steven. "Unvaccinated Kids Behind Largest U.S. Measles Outbreak in Years." *HealthDay*. October 11, 2011. http://health.usnews.com/health-news/family-health/childrens-health/articles/2011/10/20/unvaccinated-kids-behind-largest-us-measles-outbreak-in-years-study (accessed October 13, 2012).

"Vaccines & Immunizations." Centers for Disease Control and Prevention. January 4, 2010. http://www.cdc.gov/vaccines (accessed October 13, 2012.)

"Vaccines, Blood & Biologics: Vaccines." U.S. Food and Drug Administration. November 2, 2010. http://www.fda.gov/BiologicsBloodVaccines/Vaccines/default.htm (accessed October 13, 2012).

"Vaccine Safety." Centers for Disease Control and Prevention. October 26, 2010. http://www.cdc.gov/vaccinesafety/index.html (accessed October 13, 2012).

Wecker, Menachem. "Amid Rise in U.S. Measles Cases, High School Parents Divided on Vaccinations." *U.S. News & World Report*. May 15, 2012. http://www.usnews.com/education/high-schools/articles/2012/05/15/amid-rise-in-us-measles-cases-high-school-parents-divided-on-vaccinations (accessed October 13, 2012).

"Who & When: Infant & Young Child." Vaccines.gov. U.S. Department of Health and Human Services. http://www.vaccines.gov/who_and_when/infant/index.html (accessed October 13, 2012).

ORGANIZATIONS

American Academy of Pediatrics, 141 Northwest Point Blvd., Elk Grove Village, IL 60007-1098, (847) 434-4000, Fax: (847) 434-8000, info@healthychildren.org, http://www.healthychildren.org.

Centers for Disease Control and Prevention, 1600 Clifton Rd., Atlanta, GA 30333, (800) CDC-INFO (232-4636), cdcinfo@cdc.gov, http://www.cdc.gov.

National Institute of Allergy and Infectious Diseases Office of Communications and Government Relations, 6610 Rockledge Dr., MSC 6612, Bethesda, MD 20892-6612, (301) 496-5717, Fax: (301) 402-3573, (866) 284-4107, ocpostoffice@niaid.nih.gov, http://www.niaid.nih.gov.

National Network for Immunization Information, 301 University Blvd., Galveston, TX 77555-0351, (409) 772-3695, Fax: (409) 772-5208, dipineda@utmb.edu, http://www.immunizationinfo.org.

National Vaccine Program Office, Room 715-H, 200 Independence Ave., SW, Washington, DC 20201, (202) 690-5566, nvpo@hhs.gov, http://www.hhs.gov/nvpo.

World Health Organization, Avenue Appia 20, 1211 Geneva, Switzerland 27, 41 22 791 21 11, Fax: 41 22 791 31 11, info@who.int, http://www.who.int/en.

Larry I. Lutwick, MD
Monique Laberge, PhD
Margaret Alic, PhD

Variant Creutzfeldt-Jakob disease *see* **Creutzfeldt-Jakob disease**

Vector (mosquito) control

Definition

Control of disease-carrying mosquito vectors is the most effective method of preventing the transmission of some of the planet's most devastating diseases, including **malaria** and dengue.

Purpose

The purpose of vector control is to reduce illness and death from diseases such as malaria, dengue, and **West Nile virus** (WNV), which are transmitted to and among humans by mosquito bites. Controlling the transmission of these and other vector-borne diseases requires controlling or eliminating their vectors. It has been estimated that mosquitoes, especially those that transmit the malaria parasite, have been responsible for half of the deaths in human history.

Mosquitoes also transmit many other life-threatening infections, including **yellow fever**, chikungunya, lymphatic filariasis, Rift Valley fever, and several encephalitis **viruses**. With the exception of yellow fever, there are no vaccines for preventing these diseases, and malaria **parasites** quickly develop resistance to most antimalarial drugs. There are no medications for effectively treating dengue or WNV, so mosquito control is the only option. Furthermore, the mosquitoes that carry these diseases are expanding their ranges.

Description

Although various animals function as disease-carrying vectors, mosquitoes are the most important for human disease. Female mosquitoes of key species must consume vertebrate blood to provide nourishment for egg production. In the process, they can carry viral, bacterial, or parasitic disease-causing organisms between human and animal hosts.

Understanding the life cycles of disease agents and the habits of the mosquitoes that carry them is essential to vector control. Malaria is caused by five species of protozoan parasites of the genus *Plasmodium* that are transmitted from infected to uninfected people by *Anopheles* mosquitoes.

Dengue and yellow fever are viral infections carried by the *Aedes aegypti* mosquito. *A. aegypti* thrives in urban environments, breeding in manmade containers. Unlike other mosquitoes, it feeds in the daytime, in early morning and just before dusk. The female bites multiple people during each feeding period. *Aedes albopictus* or Asian tiger is a secondary dengue vector in Asia that, like *A. aegypti*, has spread to Europe and North America. *Aedes* mosquitoes are highly adaptive. They can survive temperatures below freezing by hibernating or sheltering in microhabitats, such as under houses where they are safe from aerial sprays. They can lie dormant in containers for months. The international trade in used tires, a prime breeding habitat, is a major factor in their expanding range. The mosquitoes also are resistant to many chemicals.

More than 130 bird species are infected with WNV. Mosquitoes that feed on the birds transmit the virus to humans. The birds and mosquitoes are attracted to the same pools of stagnant water that accumulate in droughts. Mosquitoes carrying WNV tend to feed at dusk and dawn.

Origins

A. aegypti probably arrived in the Western Hemisphere in water casks on slave ships from Africa, carrying yellow fever that caused a severe epidemic along the eastern seaboard in the eighteenth century. Although eradicated in North America in the mid-twentieth century, *A. aegypti* is back, this time carrying dengue.

One of the earliest large-scale vector-control campaigns occurred during the construction of the Panama Canal. In the French attempt to build the canal through mosquito-infested jungles, thousands of lives were lost to malaria and yellow fever. When the United States set out to construct the canal in the early twentieth century, thousands of workers and millions of dollars were invested in two years of vector control. In addition to identifying and isolating patients with malaria and yellow fever, swamps were drained, buildings were fumigated by burning sulfur or pyrethrum, and breeding areas were sprayed with oil and larvicides. Roads were paved and water systems replaced cisterns to eliminate stagnant water. Windows were covered with screens and beds with netting. The spread of mosquito-borne disease was nearly eliminated.

From the 1940s through the 1960s, massive vector-control programs using the pesticide DDT (dichlorodiphenyltrichloroethane) almost completely eradicated mosquito vectors in the United States and many other countries. However DDT, which persists in the environment, caused immense damage to wildlife—decimating bird populations around the world by weakening their eggshells—and threatened human health. Furthermore, DDT-resistant mosquito strains soon emerged. Rachel Carson's 1962 book *Silent Spring* brought the devastating consequences of DDT to the world's notice. DDT was banned in the United States in 1972, a major factor in the recovery of the bald eagle and many other North American birds. However, DDT is still used in many developing countries where mosquito infestations pose an even greater threat.

Treatment

Global mosquito control consumes tremendous financial resources, time, and labor, and can have significant environmental impacts. The choice of a control method depends on local circumstances—the magnitude of the disease burden, the ability to correctly apply interventions in a timely manner, and the likelihood that effective control can be sustained.

Insecticides

Insecticides may be used routinely or only during outbreaks of disease. They may be sprayed over large areas from the air, from trucks, or by hand on specific areas, structures, or outdoor water containers. Adulticiding is ground spraying of an insecticide fog to kill adult mosquitoes. Larviciding is the spraying of stagnant areas where mosquitoes lay their eggs and larvae develop. Many of the insecticides in use today are pyrethroids—synthetic chemicals that resemble the natural insecticides in chrysanthemums. Pyrethroids are deemed safe for humans—including infants, children, and the elderly—and for dogs, cats, and vegetables. New insecticides are continually being developed as mosquitoes develop resistance to those currently in use.

Insecticide-treated bed nets (ITNs) are one of the most effective means for controlling mosquitoes that bite people while they sleep. If used by an entire population, ITNs can reduce malaria transmission by 90%, malaria incidence by 50%, and child mortality by 18%. ITNs can reduce mortality from all causes by 20%. It has been estimated that for every 1,000 children protected with an ITN, five or six lives are saved each year. Pyrethroid-treated nets in malaria-endemic areas are a major component of the Roll Back Malaria initiative of the **World Health Organization** (WHO).

WHO recommends integrated vector management (IVM) that employs a range of methods based on scientific evidence and local circumstances. IVM requires collaboration between public and private sectors and healthcare workers, the involvement of local communities, good management practices, and rational use of insecticides. In addition to ITNs, IVM employs indoor residual spraying (IRS) to destroy malaria vectors in homes and sleeping areas, as well as larviciding and/or environmental management. Environmental management or modification prevents mosquitoes from accessing egg-laying habitats. It includes proper disposal of solid waste, removal of manmade habitats, draining areas where mosquitoes breed, filling in low-lying areas to prevent water from stagnating, and ongoing vector monitoring. These methods require more local technical expertise and are applicable to far fewer situations than ITNs and IRS.

Personal protection

Avoiding mosquito bites and mosquito-proofing homes, workplaces, and communities are effective methods of vector control.

- The U.S. Environmental Protection Agency (EPA) recommends using an insect repellant that contains N,N-diethyl-m-toluamide (DEET), picaridin, or oil of lemon eucalyptus on all exposed skin when outdoors for even a short time.
- Loose-fitting long sleeves, long pants, and socks should be worn outdoors whenever possible. Clothing can be sprayed with permethrin or another EPA-registered insect repellant. Permethrin cannot be applied directly to the skin, and no repellent should be sprayed on skin under clothing.
- People should remain indoors or take extra precautions during insect-feeding times, often between dusk and dawn.
- Standing water should be drained. Tires, flower pots, birdbaths, and clogged rain gutters are common breeding sites.
- Doors and windows should have well-fitting screens in good repair.
- In-home water storage containers should be emptied or covered and cleaned weekly.
- Grass should be kept mowed and bushes trimmed.
- Dead birds should be reported to public health officials, because they can be an indication that WNV is circulating between birds and mosquitoes.
- Insecticide-treated materials, coils, vaporizers, and ITNs can provide personal protection in mosquito-infested regions.

Biologic controls and genetic modification (GM)

In the early 2000s much research was being devoted to vector control by biological and GM methods. An example of biologic control is infection of *Anopheles* mosquitoes with *Wolbachia* bacteria that can decrease malaria parasite transmission. The bacteria are passed on to mosquito offspring, causing a self-sustaining infection.

The Grand Challenges in Global Health (an initiative of the Bill & Melinda Gates Foundation and the Foundation for the National Institutes of Health in the United States, the Canadian Institutes of Health Research, and the Wellcome Trust in the United Kingdom) support the development of genetic tools for controlling dengue transmission. For example, a group at the University of California-Irvine has engineered male *A. aegypti* mosquitoes that carry a gene that destroys the flight muscles of female offspring.

In the early 2000s, the British company Oxitec was at the forefront of GM vector control. It engineered *A. aegypti* that carry a lethal gene that is turned off by the antibiotic tetracycline. Released males pass on the gene to their offspring, which die as larvae without the antibiotic. Since *A. aegypti* fly only a few hundred feet during their lifetimes, the released males can be readily targeted to dengue-infected populations. The method is far cheaper than insecticide spraying and avoids poisoning the environment. Oxitec claims to have reduced *A. aegypti* populations by 80% in three months during field trials in Brazil, Malaysia, and the Cayman Islands. As of 2012, a Brazilian factory was producing four million of the GM mosquitoes every week.

Precautions

Pyrethroid sprays and other insecticides kill desirable insects, such as butterflies, dragonflies, and ladybugs, and essential insect pollinators including bees, although public health officials argue that aerial spraying at night reduces harm to honeybees and other beneficial insects. Pyrethroid sprays can also kill fish, birds, bats, and geckos that eat mosquitoes. Some insecticides may be harmful to humans, especially when they are sprayed from the air. Health officials recommend that children, pets, and those with respiratory problems remain indoors until aerial sprays have dried. Some physicians tell their chemically sensitive patients to leave areas of aerial spraying. Furthermore, vector control methods never eliminate every mosquito, so personal and household protection will continue to be mainstays of control.

GM vector control is very controversial, particularly since some GM vectors have been released in the wild in secret. There are many concerns about the introduction of new GM species. Critics have also argued that eradicating a mosquito species could have unintended consequences on ecosystems and the food chain. Some critics worry that wiping out *A. aegypti* could cause a takeover by the invasive dengue-carrying Asian tiger, which is very hard to control with insecticides. However, Oxitec claims to have already engineered mutant Asian tigers.

Complications

Many mosquito vector populations are resistant, not only to DDT, but also to other commonly used insecticides, including pyrethroids, and insecticide-resistance is

KEY TERMS

Adulticiding—Insecticide spraying to kill adult mosquitoes.

Aedes aegypti—A mosquito that transmits dengue and yellow fever worldwide.

Anopheles—A genus of mosquitoes that transmits the malaria parasite.

Asian tiger—*Aedes albopictus*; an invasive, dengue-transmitting mosquito that is resistant to most insecticides.

DDT—An insecticide widely used for mosquito control, but banned in the United States since 1972 because it accumulates in the environment and is toxic to birds and other vertebrates.

DEET—N,N-diethyl-m-toluamide; an insect and tick repellent.

Dengue—Infectious disease caused by RNA flaviviruses and transmitted by *Aedes* mosquitoes.

Genetic modification (GM)—Organisms that have been genetically modified in the laboratory, such as mosquitoes that destroy vector populations when released into the environment.

Indoor residual spraying (IRS)—The spraying of homes and sleeping areas with insecticides to control malaria-transmitting mosquitoes.

Insecticide-treated nets (ITNs)—Bed nets treated with pyrethroids to control malaria-transmitting mosquitoes.

Integrated vector management (IVM)—A vector control strategy that uses various methods depending on local conditions and circumstances.

Malaria—A disease caused by parasites of the genus *Plasmodium* that infect red blood cells and are transmitted from infected to uninfected people by bites of anopheline mosquitoes; the single largest cause of illness and death worldwide.

Permethrin—A common neurotoxic insecticide and insect repellent.

Picaridin—A mosquito repellent that is applied directly to the skin.

Pyrethroids—Synthetic insecticides that resemble pyrethrins from chrysanthemums.

West Nile virus (WNV)—A mosquito-transmitted flavivirus that can cause severe illness and whose geographical range is expanding rapidly.

---

spreading. As of 2012, WHO reported resistance to ITN and IRS insecticides in 64 countries.

A study of two African villages where every household used ITNs found that *Anopheles funestus* mosquitoes, one of the two primary African malaria vectors, were changing their habits. Instead of biting at 2–3 AM, they were biting around 5 AM, after the nets were put up. In one village, the number of outdoor mosquito bites had also increased significantly since the introduction of ITNs. Shifts from indoor night biting to early-morning and outside biting could undermine the effectiveness of ITNs.

Results

Some countries that had low transmission rates, such as Tunisia and the United Arab Emirates, have been able to eradicate malaria with vector control, strict monitoring, and aggressive malaria treatment. However, malaria is reemerging in most countries where the disease is **endemic**. In some parts of Africa, transmission rates are so high that even reducing mosquito bites by 99% would leave about ten infectious bites per person every year.

Public health role and response

Vector control is one of the four basic elements of WHO's global malaria control strategy. WHO also develops new insecticides and application technologies. In the United States, the **Centers for Disease Control and Prevention** (CDC) monitors and surveys for malaria and other vector-borne diseases. However, vector control is primarily the responsibility of local officials. Insecticide spraying of breeding areas remains the most cost-effective method of mosquito control. Cities and counties also conduct mosquito surveillance, and local authorities may be alerted to standing water, such as storm sewers, ditches, and abandoned properties that are potential breeding grounds.

In the summer 2012, there were hundreds of WNV infections and multiple deaths in Texas and Louisiana. Dallas, Texas, declared a state of emergency and aerial sprayed for the first time in 45 years. The spraying was controversial, not only because of risks to beneficial insects, animals, and humans, but because it killed only adult mosquitoes, leaving the larvae. The online social-action group, Change.org, petitioned to halt the spraying.

> **WHAT TO ASK YOUR DOCTOR**
>
> - Are there disease-carrying mosquitoes in our area?
> - Should I use insect repellent or take other personal measures to protect myself from mosquito bites?
> - How can I mosquito-proof my house?
> - What insecticides are safe to use?
> - Do we have mosquito control in our community?

In 2009, Key West, Florida experienced its first major outbreak of dengue since 1934. Despite blanket spraying with pesticides, the outbreak lasted for 15 months, sickening 93 people. By 2012, the Florida Keys Mosquito Control Board was awaiting approval from the U.S. **Food and Drug Administration** (FDA) to release Oxitec's GM mosquitoes to combat dengue. As a major tourist destination, the area spends more than $1 million a year on truck and helicopter spraying. Still, approximately 20% of Key West homes have dengue-infected mosquitoes, reaching as high as 40% or more in the summer rainy season.

Resources

BOOKS

Atkinson, Peter W. *Vector Biology, Ecology, and Control.* New York: Springer, 2010.

Becker, Norbert. *Mosquitoes and Their Control.* Heidelberg, Germany: Springer, 2010.

Perry, Alex. *Lifeblood: How to Change the World, One Dead Mosquito at a Time.* New York: Public Affairs, 2011.

PERIODICALS

Butler, Kiera. "Attack of the Mutant Mosquitoes." *Mother Jones* 37, no. 3 (May/June 2012): 66–67.

Gravitz, Lauren. "Vector Control: The Last Bite." *Nature* 484, no. 7395 (April 26, 2012): S26–S27.

Knickerbocker, Brad. "Dallas Launches Air War Against West Nile Mosquitoes. Is it Safe?" *Christian Science Monitor* (August 17, 2012): 10.

Maxmen, Amy. "Florida Abuzz Over Mosquito Plan." *Nature* 487, no. 7407 (July 19, 2012): 286.

Maxmen, Amy. "Malaria Surge Feared." *Nature* 485, no. 7398 (May 17, 2012): 293.

Petersen, Lyle R., and Marc Fischer. "Unpredictable and Difficult to Control—The Adolescence of West Nile Virus." *New England Journal of Medicine* 367, no. 14 (October 4, 2012): 1281–84.

Trivedi, Bijal P. "The Wipeout Gene." *Scientific American* 305, no. 5 (November 2011): 68–75.

WEBSITES

Ambizas, Emily M., and Alberto H. Ambizas. "West Nile Virus." *U.S. Pharmacist* 37, no. 8 (October 31, 2012): 31–4. http://www.medscape.com/viewarticle/772644_1 (accessed November 8, 2012).

"Fight the Bite! Avoid Mosquito Bites to Avoid Infection." West Nile Virus, Division of Vector-Borne Diseases, Centers for Disease Control and Prevention. August 30, 2012. http://www.cdc.gov/ncidod/dvbid/westnile/prevention_info.htm (accessed November 7, 2012).

Haskins, Michael. "Are Mutant Mosquitoes the Answer to Dengue Fever?" Reuters Health Information. July 25, 2012. http://www.medscape.com/viewarticle/768059 (accessed November 8, 2012).

Media Centre. "Dengue and Severe Dengue." World Health Organization. January 2012. http://www.who.int/entity/mediacentre/factsheets/fs117/en/index.html (accessed November 7, 2012).

"New Approaches for Fighting Emerging Diseases: Frequently Asked Questions." Genetic Strategies for Control of Dengue Virus Transmission. http://stopdengue.hs.uci.edu/FAQs.htm (accessed November 7, 2012).

Norton, Amy. "Facing Anti-Mosquito Nets, Mosquitoes Alter Habits." Reuters Health Information. September 21, 2012. http://www.medscape.com/viewarticle/771252 (accessed November 8, 2012).

Specter, Michael. "The Mosquito Solution: Can Genetic Modification Eliminate a Deadly Tropical Disease?" *New Yorker* 88, no. 20 (July 9–16, 2012). http://www.newyorker.com/reporting/2012/07/09/120709fa_fact_specter (accessed November 5, 2012).

"Vector Control of Malaria." World Health Organization. http://www.who.int/malaria/vector_control/en (accessed November 7, 2012).

ORGANIZATIONS

American Mosquito Control Association, 15000 Commerce Pkwy., Ste. C, Mount Laurel, NJ 08054, (856) 439-9222, Fax: (856) 439-0525, amca@mosquito.org, http://www.mosquito.org.

National Pesticide Information Center, Oregon State University, 333 Weniger Hall, Corvallis, OR 97331-6502, (800) 858-7378, npic@ace.orst.edu, http://npic.orst.edu.

U.S. Centers for Disease Control and Prevention, 1600 Clifton Rd., Atlanta, GA 30333, (800) CDC-INFO (232-4636), cdcinfor@cdc.gov, http://www.cdc.gov.

U.S. Environmental Protection Agency, 4601M, Ariel Rios Bldg., 1200 Pennsylvania Ave. NW, Washington, DC 20460, (202) 564-3750, ogwdw.web@epa.gov, http://www.epa.gov.

World Health Organization, Avenue Appia 20, 1211 Geneva, Switzerland 27, 41 22 791-2111, Fax: 41 22 791-3111, info@who.int, http://www.who.int/en.

Terry Watkins
Margaret Alic, PhD

Vegetation fire *see* **Wildfire**

Viral hemorrhagic fevers *see* **Hemorrhagic fevers**

Viruses

Definition

A virus is an infectious agent, often highly host-specific, consisting of genetic material surrounded by a protein coat.

Description

Viruses infect virtually every life form, including humans, animals, plants, fungi, and bacteria. So small that they cannot be seen by a light microscope, viruses range in size from about 30 nanometers (about 0.000001 in to about 450 nanometers (about 0.000014 in) and are between 100 to 20 times smaller than bacteria. As of 2011, the International Committee on Taxonomy of Viruses (ICTV) listed 2,475 species of viruses in 395 genera and 94 families. Many more viruses remain unclassified due to lack of information.

All standard viruses share a general structure of genetic material, or viral genome, and a protein coat, called a capsid. The viral genome is made of either deoxyribose nucleic acid (DNA), the genetic material found in plants and animals, or ribonucleic acid (RNA), a compound plant and animal cells use in protein synthesis. The protein capsid is made of repeating, often-identical subunits known as capsomeres. Viruses are not strictly free-living, as they cannot reproduce on their own. Instead, they use host cell machinery to make both the viral genome and capsids of the newly formed viruses, or virions.

The broad category of viruses also includes unusual infective agents that are missing one or more components of standard viruses. These unconventional viruses include viroids, which exist as circular RNA molecules that are not packaged, and prions, infective particles that contain protein and little or no nucleic acids.

Some viral infections can cause damage to the host cell, resulting in disease to the organism. Other viral infections appear to make the host cells divide uncontrollably, causing the development of cancer. However, many viral infections are asymptomatic and do not result in disease. There are no cures for viral infections, due in part to the difficulty of developing drugs that adversely affect only the virus and not the host. Accordingly, preventative measures such as vaccines play an important role in the treatment of viral diseases.

Function

The primary function of a virus is to infect host cells and create more viruses. The virus does this by taking over the host cell's protein and genetic material-making processes, forcing it to produce the new viruses. Exactly how viruses function in this manner is best understood by examining general viral structure, classification, and reproductive strategies.

Structure and classification

There are three basic structures for standard viral capsids: icosahedral, helical, and complex. Icosahedral capsids are 20-sided, made of triangular capsomere subunits. The points of the triangular subunits join at 12 vertices about the shape. Although exact structure varies from virus type to virus type, a common arrangement is five or six neighboring triangular subunits at each vertex. Some viruses show more than one capsomere arrangement within the capsid. An example of a virus having an icosahedral structure is adenovirus, the virus that can cause acute respiratory disease or viral pneumonia in humans.

The helical viruses have protein subunits that curve about a central axis running the length of the virus. The fanlike arrangement of protein forms a three-dimensional ribbon-shaped structure that covers the viral genome. Some of these capsid structures are stiff and rodlike, while other helical viruses are more flexible. The influenza virus is an example of a virus with a helical capsid structure.

The third type of virus capsid structure is called complex. Although the structure is regular from virus to virus of the same type, the symmetry is not patterned enough to be fully understood. For example, poxvirus, the virus that causes **smallpox** in humans, has a complex capsid structure of over 100 proteins.

The combination of the capsid and the viral genome is known as a nucleocapsid. Some nucleocapsids are infective in this form and are known as naked viruses. Others require a surrounding lipid membrane derived from the host cell to be infective. The membrane envelope can encompass one or more nucleocapsids and usually contains on its surface at least one viral protein in addition to the host cell components. Viruses of this type are called enveloped or coated viruses.

Viruses are classified according to structural characteristics such as whether the virus genome is made of DNA or RNA. Both of these nucleic acids can form ladder-like structures where each side of the ladder is known as a strand. Viruses are differentiated by whether the DNA or RNA is single or doubled-stranded. The type of capsid structure and whether the virus is naked or enveloped are also considered. A few viral classifications take into account differences in replication strategy.

Replication

The generalized replication cycle for standard viruses begins with the absorption of the virus by the host cell. Absorption involves an interaction between the viral particle and the potential host cell. This is often mediated by a viral protein that is recognized by a binding protein located on the surface of the host cell. Whether the host cell recognizes the viral protein often determines whether a particular cell can or cannot function as a host for a particular virus. For example, the hemagglutin protein of the influenza virus, a viral protein found within the lipid envelope of this coated virus, interacts with a receptor found on the surface of the epithelial cells that line the human respiratory tract.

The next step in the virus replication cycle is penetration and, if necessary, the uncoating of the virus in the host cell. With some coated viruses, the envelope membrane fuses directly with the host membrane, allowing movement of nucleocapsid into the cell's cytoplasm. Other coated viruses are brought into the cell using endosomes, small vesicles of cellular membrane that bud inwardly and are used to move materials into the cell. Due to the lower pH environment of the endosome, the virus coat can fuse with the endosomal membrane to gain access to the cell cytoplasm. Naked viruses are sometimes small enough to move without help through the host cellular membrane, while others use the endosome system.

Once inside the cell, the virus takes over the host cell's protein and nucleic acid production, directing it to produce viral proteins and genomes. For many viruses having a DNA genome, the viral nucleic acid is inserted or integrated directly into the host cell's own DNA, that make up the cell's chromosomes. RNA viruses tend to keep the genome independent from the host cell's genetic material. In either case, the host cell is fooled into using the viral genetic material as the instructions for the production of new infectious virions. In order to ensure that new virions will be formed, viruses often have mechanisms that speed up the protein formation of the host cell. Sometimes the mechanism will be specific for increased production of viral proteins, while others speed up all protein formation.

A special method of producing new virions is employed by retroviruses, such as the human immunodeficiency virus (HIV). These viruses carry their genomes as RNA, but upon entry into the host cell a viral enzyme known as reverse transcriptase converts the viral RNA into DNA, and that molecule is integrated into the host genome. The enzyme is called reverse transcriptase because generally genetic information moves from DNA to RNA copies rather than this reverse process. The integrated DNA is known as a provirus and will be replicated when the host cell divides, to be inherited by the two resulting daughter cells.

After production of the viral proteins and genomes by the host cellular machinery, the capsid is assembled around the genetic material and, for some viruses, a maturation step occurs that is necessary for infectivity. Finally, the new virions are released from the cell. Some coated viruses leave the cell by budding and do not cause the death of the host cell. The budding process is the process by which the virus acquires its lipid membrane envelope. Other viruses lyse, or break down, the host cell membrane. Lysis kills the host cell.

Because of the ability of viruses to carry genetic material into and out of a cell during the reproduction cycle, viruses can function as vectors in genetic engineering. This is done by inserting foreign genetic material into viral genomes and allowing the material to be integrated and expressed in bacteria and animal cells. Viral vectors are often the basis for gene therapies that in their simplest form attempt to cure genetic defects by providing non-mutated copies of a damaged gene to an organism.

Role in human health

Viruses that infect humans cause damage to the infected cells, resulting in outward symptoms seen as human disease. Human viruses gain entry into the body using various routes. Some viruses are transmitted through skin-to-skin contact, such as herpes simplex 1, the virus that causes cold sores. Others are transmitted through exposure to infected blood, the mode of transmission of the hepatitis B virus. Some of the most easily caught viruses, such as varicella-zoster, the virus that causes chicken pox, are transmitted through water droplets suspended in the air. The virus is transmitted when the droplets are breathed in and come in contact with the respiratory tract of the new host.

Gastrointestinal viruses are transmitted through exposure to waste products containing virus particles that has contaminated water or food, and enter the host's digestive tract through the mouth. Rotavirus, a cause of a diarrheal illness common in children, is transmitted in this manner. Sexually transmitted viruses move from host to host through sexual contact and enter the body most commonly by the genitourinary route. HIV and **human papilloma virus** (HPV) are examples of viruses that are sexually transmitted.

After gaining entry into the host, the response at a cellular level to the viral infection varies with the type of virus and the virulence of the strain. Thus, the response can vary from no apparent change, to detectable changes in the cell, known as cytopathic effects (CPE), to loss of growth control or malignancy. Virulence refers to the ability of a virus to cause disease in a host. Some viruses are highly virulent, causing disease with almost every infection. **Measles**, rabies, and influenza are virulent viruses. Other less virulent viruses, such as Epstein-Barr virus, which causes mononucleosis, only rarely result in disease symptoms.

Viral infections follow patterns that are specific to the virus. Some infections are localized, that is, restricted to a particular cell type or organ, while others are disseminated throughout the body. Disseminated infections are often propagated through the nervous system or the bloodstream. Infections can be acute, where the patient's immune system self-limits the disease and recovers, or chronic, where the infection continues for a long period of time.

Some viruses have the ability to cause an initial disease state upon infection and then establish a latent or dormant infective state. For example, herpes viruses cause blisters on the skin as a result of their lytic replication, but then establish a latent infection in nerve cells. Upon presentation of a stimulus such as exposure to the sun or stress the virus switches back to a lytic cycle, again producing blisters at the site of infection. In this way, the infection can persist for months or even years.

Several viruses, such as human papilloma viruses and Epstein-Barr virus, have been strongly associated with human cancers. The exact role of viruses in malignancy is not yet understood, as environmental and host genetic factors also seem to contribute to the development of tumors. However, it is highly probable that viruses are key triggers for a number of human cancers.

Another effect of viruses on human health is infection by zoonotic viruses, that is, viruses that can be transmitted from an animal host of another species to humans. Some of these viruses are transmitted through a blood-sucking insect intermediary, such as a mosquito, while others are transmitted directly from the infected animal to humans. Many of these viruses raise important public health concerns. An example of a mosquito-transmitted virus is the flavivirus that causes West Nile encephalitis in humans. A strain of hantavirus was discovered in 1993 that infects **rodents** and transmits directly to humans, causing a respiratory illness.

A few unconventional viruses cause human disease. The only know human viroid is the delta virus (hepatitis D) that requires co-infection with hepatitis B to be infective. The combined infection of hepatitis B and D causes more severe symptoms than B alone. An example of a human prion-mediated disease is Creutzfeldt-Jakob disease (CJD), which causes neurological symptoms and is fatal. Of significant concern is a possible variant of CJD reported in Great Britain that affects younger individuals. Although cause and effect has not been conclusively shown, there is now a strong suspicion that this disease results from eating beef contaminated with the prion that causes bovine spongiform encephalopathy, or mad cow disease.

Common diseases and disorders

Several hundred different viruses infect humans. The viruses that occur chiefly in humans can be categorized as respiratory, enteric, exanthematous, hepatitis, or persistent. The most common respiratory viruses include the rhinoviruses (the common cold) and the influenza viruses. Common enteric viruses include polioviruses (now rare because of vaccination), coxsachie viruses (herpangina), and epidemic gastroenteritis viruses such as rotaviruses. Rubeola (measles) and rubella (German measles) are two common exanthematous viruses.

Hepatitis viruses type A through E are known, with type A most often responsible for epidemics of the disease. Many of the persistent viruses are quite widespread and include cytomegalovirus (usually asymptomatic), Epstein-Barr virus (mononucleosis), herpes simplex virus (cold sores and genital herpes), human herpes virus type 6 (roseola), human papilloma virus (warts), and varicella-zoster virus (chicken pox and shingles).

Zoonotic viruses, that chiefly infect insects or animals, with humans as minor or accidental host, are generally rarer. The diseases caused by these viruses are limited to areas that can support the insect or animal host as well as humans. Rabies is the most widespread of these diseases. Flaviviruses (yellow and **dengue fever**), bunyaviruses (California encephalitis and hantavirus pulmonary syndrome), and filoviruses such as ebola (hemorrhagic fever) are other examples of zoonoitic viruses that cause human disease.

Human disease caused by nonconventional viruses is very rare. The most common is CJD, a prion-mediated disease that occurs in one in a million individuals. Hepatitis D is the only known human viroid, and it requires co-infection with hepatitis B. Other diseases caused by nonconventional viruses are kuru and

Gerstmann-Sträussler-Scheinker syndrome (GSS), both caused by prions.

Causes and symptoms

When challenged by a viral infection, the human body responds with both antibodies and cell-mediated responses to counteract the virus. Antibodies, produced by B lymphocytes, are specific for surface proteins of the virus. When acting as a target for antibodies, such viral proteins are known as antigens. The binding of the antibodies to the viruses can inactivate them or target them as foreign particles for destruction by other components of the immune system. Antibodies can also bind to viral proteins seen in the membrane of infected cells, directing their elimination by the immune system. Antibodies mediate the immunity to reinfection by the same virus. Unfortunately, many viruses have high rates of mutation that alter the surface antigens, rendering the host again susceptible to infection. This process is the reason that one cold does not make a person immune to all rhinoviruses, a virus with at least 95 different serotypes (a characteristic of a virus based on the antibodies that are produced against the surface antigens upon infection).

Non-specific cell-mediated responses are also important to the body's fight against viruses. The production of interferons and cytokines, in particular, is known to help control viral infections. However, the side effects of these molecules, including fever, malaise, fatigue and muscle pains, significantly contribute to the physical symptoms of viral infections.

Diagnosis

In general there are three methods of diagnosing viral disease in humans. Some viruses can be identified clinically, as the infection causes unmistakable outward signs. The blistery pox of the varicella-zoster or chicken pox virus is a good example of a clinically diagnosed viral disease. Viral diseases can also be diagnosed epidemiologically, through known exposure to certain viruses or virus-harboring hosts. However, many virus infections cannot be diagnosed definitively without diagnostic testing.

Diagnostic testing can involve direct detection, using electron microscopy, light microscopy of CPE seen in host cells, detection of viral antigen in patient samples, or detection of the viral genome using the polymerase chain reaction (PCR) test. Effective tests for some viral infections involve indirect detection, generally using cell culture systems to grow the virus *in vitro* (outside the organism). A final method of diagnosing viral illnesses is serological testing that

> **KEY TERMS**
>
> **Capsid**—The protein structure of a virus.
> **Capsomere**—The protein subunits of the capsid.
> **Endosome**—A membrane-mediated means of transporting materials from outside to inside the cell.
> **Genome**—The genetic material encoding the genes of an organism.
> **Nucleocapsid**—The combination of the capsid and viral genome.
> **Prion**—An unconventional virus that is made almost entirely of protein.
> **Reverse transcriptase**—A retroviral enzyme that produces DNA copies of genetic information encoded by RNA.
> **Virion**—A single infectious virus particle.
> **Viroid**—An unconventional virus that is made of uncoated RNA.
> **Zoonotic**—A type of virus that primarily infects an insect or animal, but can be transmitted to humans.

involves the detection of antibodies against the virus antigen in samples taken at presentation and during convalescence. A serious drawback to traditional serological testing is the amount of time needed to obtain the results. New techniques are being developed, however, that may speed serological tests and make them more useful.

Treatment

Most viral diseases have no cure, so treatment involves easing symptoms and allowing the body's immune system to eliminate the virus. Viruses are not affected by antibiotics, which target bacteria. However, a handful of anti-viral drugs have been developed and many more are in the developmental and drug trial stage. In general, the development of anti-viral drugs has been hampered by the parasitic relationship between viruses and their hosts. It has been difficult to find pharmacological means to kill the virus without harming the host. The speed of viral infection has also been a problem, as viral numbers are so high by the time the infection has symptoms, the drugs have little effect.

Amantadine and rimantiadine are two drugs that have been used successfully against influenza A. These drugs appear to inhibit the absorption of the influenza

> **QUESTIONS TO ASK YOUR DOCTOR**
>
> - Can you recommend a reliable source for current information on viral vaccines?
> - To which viral diseases are children in our geographic area most likely to be exposed?
> - Can you review with me the vaccination schedule recommended for very young children as protection against viral infections?
> - Are there any zoonotic disease about which we should be concerned in this region?

virus into the epithelial cells of the respiratory tract and, accordingly, are administered prior to infection as a prophylaxis.

Herpes simplex and varicella-zoster infections can be treated with acyclovir, valacyclovir, and famciclovir. Cytomegalovirus infection can be treated with ganciclovir, foscarnet, and cidofovir. All of these drugs are converted into a chemical that interferes with the production of the viral genome. As a viral enzyme produces the genome for these viruses, the chemical does not interfere with the production of genetic material for the host cell.

A number of drugs that inhibit reverse transcriptase have been developed for treatment of HIV. The best known of these is Zidovudine (AZT). The other major target for antiviral HIV drugs is the viral protease, an enzyme that cleaves both viral structural proteins and enzymes apart after formation by the host cell. Because the virus is noninfective if these cleavages do not occur, drugs inhibiting the protease action are effective antivirals. As advances in this field happen quickly, the International AIDS Society/USA Panel provides periodic recommendations as to what drugs given in what combinations have proven to be most effective inn the treatment of AIDS.

Finally, genetically engineered interferon has been used with some success against hepatitis B and C and human papillovirus. However, the severe side effects of this protein, in particular nausea and vomiting, have hampered its usefulness.

Prevention

The most effective method of treatment of viral diseases is prevention of the infection. Vaccines, where the immune system is exposed to non-infective viral antigens to allow the development of protective antibodies, have proven effective in controlling many viral illnesses. Vaccines are made of inactivated (killed) virus, attenuated (weakened) virus, or isolated viral proteins, that are known as subunit vaccines. Vaccines are available for the viruses that cause measles, **mumps**, rubella, poliomyelitis, rabies, hepatitis A and B, influenza, varicella-zoster (chicken pox) and **yellow fever**. Many other vaccines are in the developmental or clinical trial stages.

The greatest drawback to vaccines is the inability of the protection to counter the same virus that has altered its antigens through mutation. Thus, viruses that undergo rapid mutation are difficult to control using **vaccination**. One solution used for influenza is to create a new vaccine every season against the viruses that are predicted to be responsible for upcoming flu outbreaks. Although this is an imperfect system, influenza vaccination is instrumental in shortening epidemics and protecting the populations most at risk for complications, including the chronically ill, the elderly, and health care workers (primarily to prevent transmitting infection to those as risk).

A second preventative measure is the avoidance of infection by blocking transmission at the point of viral entry. This is done through the isolation of infected patients and avoiding contact with infected biological material such as lesions, blood, and airborne particles through the use of gloves, masks, and other barriers. Health care providers must practice careful hygiene of patients, including immediate removal of vomit or diarrhea, and thorough hand washing. These measures are taken equally to avoid patient-to-provider and provider-to-patient transmission of viruses. For zoonotic viruses, transmission can be reduced through pesticide control of the insect or animal reservoir of the disease.

Resources

BOOKS

Crawford, Dorothy H. *Viruses: A Very Short Introduction.* Oxford; New York: Oxford University Press, 2011.

Harper, David E. *Viruses: Biology, Applications, Control.* New York: Garland Science, 2012.

Sompayrac, Lauren. *How Pathogenic Viruses Think: Making Sense of Virology*, 2nd ed. Sudbury, MA: Jones and Bartlett, 2013.

WEBSITES

Freudenrich, *How Viruses Work*.http://science.howstuffworks.com/environmental/life/cellular-microscopic/virus-human.htm (accessed April 4, 2012).

Viral Infections. Medline Plus. http://www.nlm.nih.gov/medlineplus/viralinfections.html (accessed April 4, 2012).

Virus Structure. Molecular Expressions. http://micro.magnet.fsu.edu/cells/virus.html (accessed April 4, 2012).

Viruses.http://users.rcn.com/jkimball.ma.ultranet/BiologyPages/V/Viruses.html (accessed April 4, 2012).

What Is a Virus?.http://www.news-medical.net/health/What-is-a-Virus.aspx (accessed April 4, 2012).

Michelle L. Johnson, MS

VOC *see* **Volatile organic compound**

Volatile organic compound

Definition

The term volatile organic compound (VOC) refers to chemicals that are emitted as gases from certain solids or liquids.

Description

VOCs include hydrocarbons (excluding carbon dioxide, carbon monoxide, carbonic acid, metallic carbides or carbonates, and ammonium carbonate)—especially those considered as air pollutants—and usually include many other organic compounds found in air. In the presence of sunlight, hydrocarbons react with **ozone** (O_3), nitrogen oxides (NO_x), and other components of polluted air to form compounds that are hazardous to plants, animals, and humans. VOCs and nitrogen oxides, produced by motor vehicle exhaust, industrial emissions, gasoline vapors, and chemical solvents, react with sunlight to form ozone in the lower atmosphere, contributing to **climate change**. In 2008, VOCs ranked third behind carbon monoxide (CO) and nitrogen oxides and just above sulfur dioxide (SO_2) in annual pollutant emissions in the United States. Ozone, which is emitted indirectly from reactions of nitrogen oxides and VOCs, is one of the six common air pollutants regulated by the U.S. Environmental Protection Agency's (**EPA**) National Ambient Air Quality Standards (**NAAQS**).

Effects on public health

VOC concentrations (from paint, cleaning products, etc.) can be up to ten times higher indoors compared with outdoors and can affect **indoor air quality** (IAQ), leading to respiratory symptoms, liver and kidney problems, and central nervous system issues.

Resources

BOOKS

Anslyn, E.V. and D.A. Dougherty. *Modern Physical Organic Chemistry*. Herndon, VA: University Science Books, 2005.

Arms, Karen. *Environmental Science*. Orlando, FL: Holt, Rinehart & Winston, 2006.

Botkin, Daniel B. and Edward A. Keller. *Environmental Science: Earth as a Living Planet*. New York: John Wiley & Sons, 2004.

Pfafflin, J. R. *The Dictionary of Environmental Science and Engineering*. Routledge dictionaries. New York: Routledge, 2008.

Volcanic eruptions

Definition

A volcanic eruption is the sudden release of lava, tephra, and gasses from a volcanic vent or fissure.

Description

Many different types of volcanic eruptions are found around the world. The most common types of eruptions are:

- Hawaiian eruption. Named after the Kilauea volcano on the Big Island of Hawaii, during Hawaiian eruptions lava flows out of the volcano, most often from the central vent. The volcano may also throw lava hundreds of feet into the air for a few minutes to a few hours. The lava then collects and can flow for miles before cooling. Hawaiian eruptions are not considered a very destructive type of volcanic eruption.

- Strombolian eruption. Every few minutes bursts of fluid lava are sent into the air during a Strombolian eruption. Although the lava bursts can rise hundreds of meters high, this type of eruption is considered less dangerous than other types of volcanic eruptions. Strombolian eruptions are named after the Italian island of Stromboli.

- Vulcanian eruption. Vulcanian eruptions produce giant ash clouds that may occur repeatedly for days, weeks, or even years before stopping or developing into an even larger explosion. The name Vulcanian comes from the Italian island of Vulcano.

- Plinian eruption. This type of eruption is considered the most powerful and dangerous type of volcanic eruption. The released tephra and gases can rise over 35 miles (50 km) into the air and be blown hundreds of thousands of miles away from the eruption site, while pyroclastic flows of hot ash can engulf the surrounding landscape. Roman historian Pliny the Younger, described Plinian eruptions in 79AD and later they were named for him.

- Surtseyan eruption A Surtseyan eruption happens when an underwater volcano releases magma or lava into shallow water. These eruptions usually take place over a long period and are repetitive. The name comes from the volcanic island Surtsey, which was formed off the coast of Iceland from years of Surtseyan eruptions.

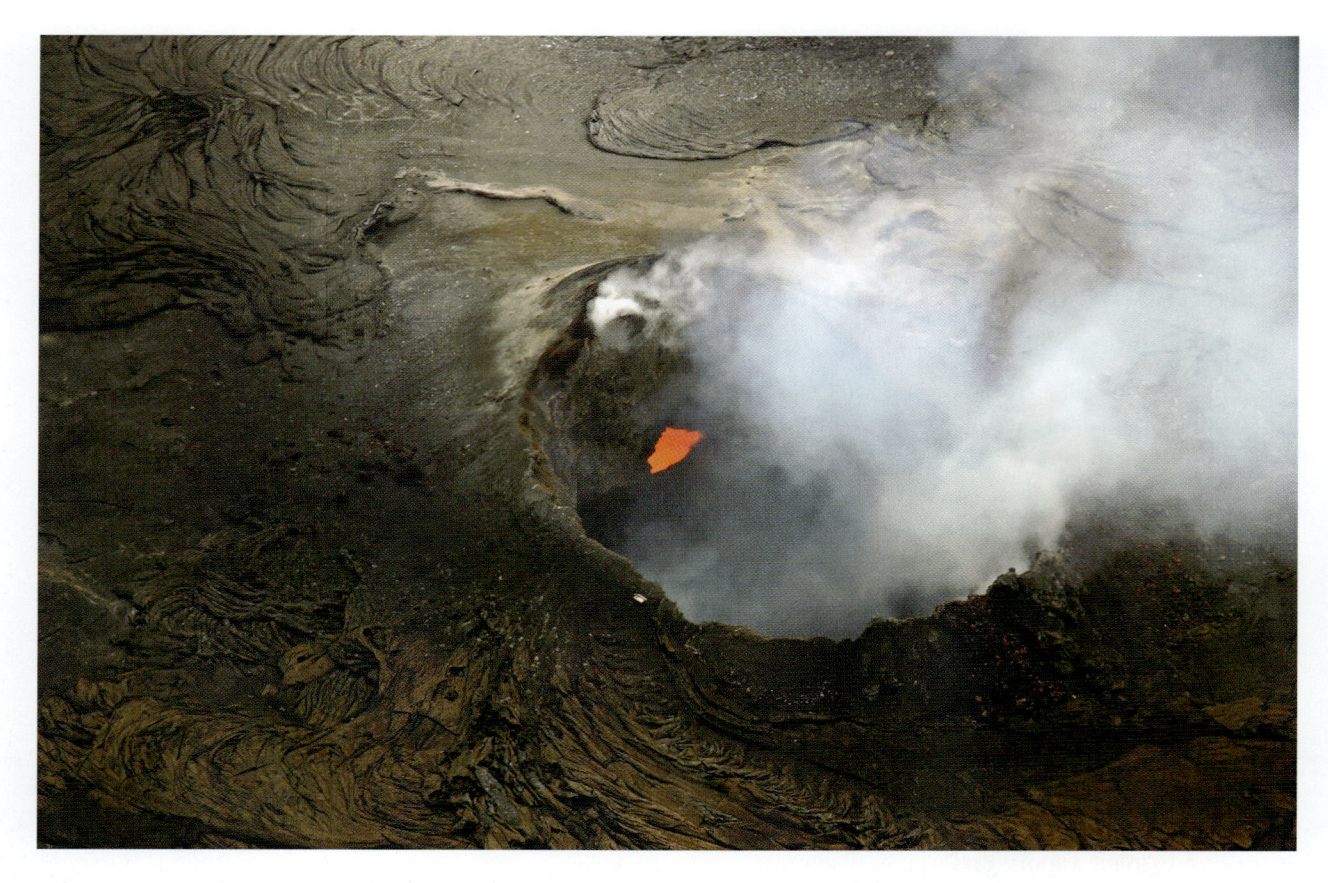

Pu'u'O'o Cone of Kilauea Volcano in Hawaii Volcanoes National Park on the Big Island of Hawaii. *(Bryan Busovicki/Shutterstock.com)*

These are only a few examples of the types of volcanic eruptions found around the world. Each eruption can vary in strength, time length, and amount of destruction done to the surrounding area. Additionally, what is released with an eruption can vary greatly, with different amounts of tephra, lava, and gases all possible.

Origins

Volcanoes form where Earth's plates move away from each other or collide, pushing one plate under the other. This action allows magma (melted mantle material) to flow out onto Earth's surface. Magma can also be released in the middle of a plate, if the magma is unusually hot and can rise to just under the plate's surface. This hot spot, which can be from 310–620 miles (500–1,000 km) wide, remains in one area as the plate continues to move above it, forming a line of volcanoes.

The heat of the magma causes solid rock to become liquid, building pressure and forcing the magma upwards. This melts more rock and adds to the amount of magma headed toward Earth's surface. The magma then collects in magma chambers below Earth's surface, where it stays until a crack opens or the pressure becomes great enough to force it out onto the surface of the earth. When this happens, magma becomes lava and it is said that the volcano is erupting. Depending on the type of volcanic eruption, the amount of lava, gas, and tephra (including ash, dust, lapilli, bombs, cinders, and blocks) released will vary.

Not all volcanic eruptions are devastating to the people around them. Volcanic eruptions on the ocean floor allow new crust to form, filling in gaps created by Earth's plates moving away from each other. Other eruptions may take place in sparsely populated or unpopulated areas or lead to the creation of new islands. Lava released from volcanic eruptions can also build on itself, developing larger volcanoes both under water and on Earth's surface.

Risk factors

Volcanoes can be found around the world; however, the most active volcanoes are in the Ring of Fire, an area around the Pacific Ocean where the most volcanic activity occurs. Because of the way volcanoes

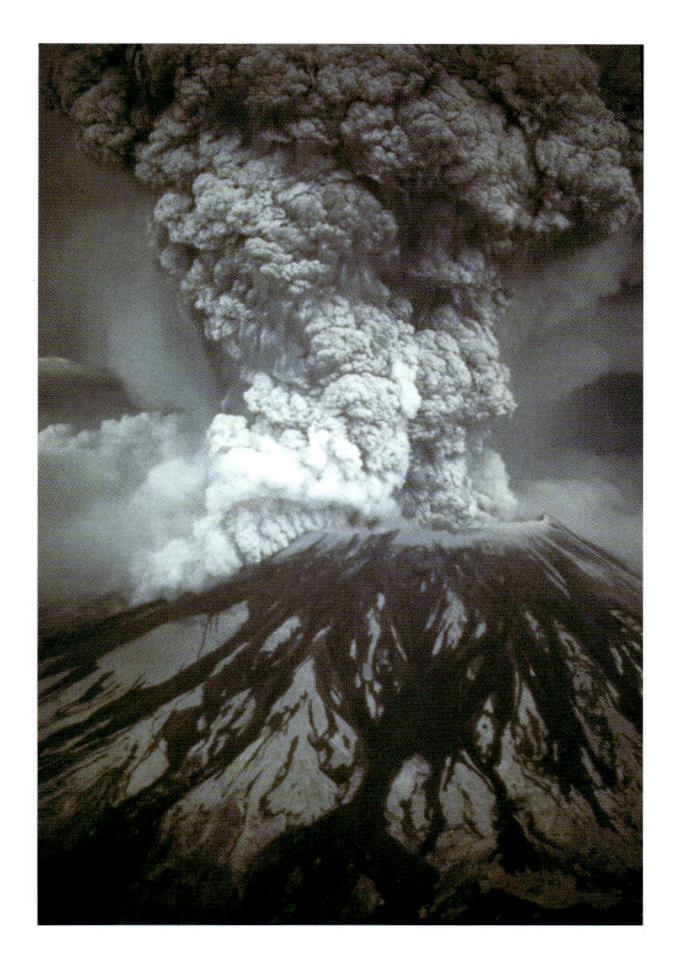

Mount St. Helens erupting. *(Courtesy of the USGS)*

are formed, the most common areas for volcanic eruptions are along tectonic plates that are either converging (coming together) or diverging (moving away from each other). Scientists and researchers monitor volcanic activity in order to try to predict when a volcanic eruption may occur. Signs of an upcoming eruption may develop months or weeks before the actual eruption. Other times, signs may lead to a false alarm and no eruption takes place. Monitoring volcanic activity allows for the development of early warning systems that can give people the chance to evacuate and prepare for a volcanic eruption.

Effects on public health

The material released during a volcanic eruption can pose a major health threat to people in the area. When breathed in, ash can cause difficulty breathing, especially for infants, the elderly, and those with respiratory problems such as **asthma**. Ash that contains silica can cause the respiratory disease **silicosis**. Additionally, ash can irritate and scratch the eyes.

KEY TERMS

Asthma—A disease in which the air passages of the lungs become inflamed and narrowed.

Lava—Also known as molten rock, lava is magma that has been exposed to the earth's surface through a volcano. Liquid lava can reach temperatures between 1,292 to 2,192°F (700 to 1,200°C). Lava forms rock when cooled.

Magma—An extremely hot fluid material found under Earth's crust. When magma hits the surface of the earth, it begins to cool and becomes lava.

Silicosis—A lung disease caused by inhaling silica dust. Silicosis is considered a type of occupational lung disease because it is most often found in people who are working in hard-rock mining, tunneling, quarrying, and other jobs that expose them to silica dust. Natural disasters, such as volcanoes, which cause a large amount of silica dust, can also cause silicosis.

Tephra—The general term for rock particles and fragments produced by a volcanic eruption.

The gases released by volcanoes often blow away very quickly, reducing their health threat. The pollution is sometimes called vog, or a volcanic fog. However, people exposed to a large amount of gas, or those who are in an area where the gas does not dissipate quickly, may have difficulty breathing or experience nose, throat, and eye irritation. Common volcanic gases include carbon dioxide, sulfur dioxide, hydrogen chloride, and hydrogen fluoride. People who are exposed to volcanic gases for a longer period may also experience headaches, swelling, dizziness, and suffocation. Suffocation because of volcanic gases is the most common cause of death from a volcanic eruption.

Other health threats from volcanic eruptions include burns, illness, injury, mudslides, floods, drinking water contamination, **wildfires**, and the spread of infectious diseases. Each volcanic eruption is unique and so are the health threats that go along with it.

Treatment

People who are in an area affected by a volcanic eruption should try to limit the amount of contact they have with ash and volcanic gases. This can be done by staying indoors or by using an air-purifying respirator. Injuries and burns should be seen by a physician as soon as possible. People who continue to experience headaches, dizziness, or respiratory problems after the initial eruption should also speak to a physician. For the most part, volcanic eruptions do not pose many long-term health threats if precaution is taken, such as not drinking water contaminated with ash and remaining indoors away from the ash and gases.

Public health role and response

Emergency response to a volcanic eruption may begin before the event has even taken place. An early warning system may be used to let citizens know that they need to evacuate from hazard zones and prepare for a potential eruption. People with disabilities or health problems may be evacuated with the help of support organizations or governmental groups. Bottled water and food, which can be stored and prepared without power, may be collected along with emergency supplies, such as first aid kits, flashlights, and air purifying respirators.

After the eruption, emergency personal may take a census of the population and search for people who need medical help. Refuge zones are set up in areas with cleaner air where affected citizens can receive water, food, and medical help. Transportation often is available to help people get to these refuge zones. Security in evacuated areas may also be set up in order to protect the property of those who have left the hazard zones.

Cleanup from a volcanic eruption can take anywhere from a few days to months depending on the amount of devastation. Ash may clog filters, destroy engines, and cause buildings to collapse because of the strain it puts on roofs. Drinking water may be contaminated and power may be out for an extended period. For these reasons, emergency response and refuge zone assistance usually continue well after the initial eruption has taken place.

Prognosis

Most people do not experience any long-lasting health effects after being in an area affected by a volcanic eruption. Symptoms should fade quickly once individuals reach an area where the air is free of volcanic gas and ash. Silicosis cannot currently be cured. Those individuals exposed to silica and diagnosed with the disease should work with their physician to alleviate symptoms and limit complications.

Prevention

Although volcanic eruptions cannot be prevented, current technology and careful preparation can reduce the health risks and destruction associated with volcanoes. The ability for scientists to monitor volcanic activity allows early warning systems to be used and people in high-risk zones are often able to evacuate before an eruption occurs. Additionally, having an emergency plan in place, along with extra food, water, and emergency supplies, such as a first aid kit and air purifying respirators, reduces the risk of injury and long-term negative health effects from ash and volcanic gases.

> **QUESTIONS TO ASK YOUR DOCTOR**
>
> - What types of medical supplies should I have in a volcanic eruption emergency kit?
> - What is the best way to treat a burn until I can get to a doctor?
> - How can I reduce the chance of ash and volcanic gases having long-term health effects on me and my family?

Resources

BOOKS

Kusky, Timothy. *Volcanoes: Eruptions and Other Volcanic Hazards.*. New York: Facts on File, 2008.

WEBSITES

Centers for Disease Control and Prevention. "Volcanoes." http://emergency.cdc.gov/disasters/volcanoes/index.asp (accessed October 9, 2012).

Federal Emergency Management Agency. "Volcanoes." http://www.ready.gov/volcanoes (accessed October 9, 2012).

How Stuff Works. "How Volcanoes Work." http://science.howstuffworks.com/nature/natural-disasters/volcano.htm(accessed October 9, 2012).

U.S. Geological Survey. "Current Alerts for U.S. Volcanoes." http://volcanoes.usgs.gov/activity/status.php (accessed October 9, 2012).

ORGANIZATIONS

Federal Emergency Management Agency (FEMA), PO Box 10055, Hyattsville, MD 20782, (202) 646 2500, (800) 621 3362, http://www.fema.gov.

International Union of Geodesy and Geophysics, Hertzstrasse 16, Karlsruhe, Germany 76187, 49(721) 6084-4494, Fax: 49(721) 711-73, secretariat@iugg.org, http://www.iugg.org.

World Organization of Volcano Observatories, 903 Koyukuk Dr., Fairbanks, AK 99775, (907) 474-1542, Fax: (907) 474-7290, wovo.iavcei@gmail.com, http://www.wovo.org.

Tish Davidson, AM

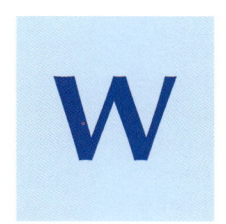

Water fluoridation

Definition

Water **fluoridation** is the public health practice of altering municipal water supplies to reflect an optimal range of fluoride in drinking water in order to combat dental caries (tooth decay).

Description

At the beginning of the twentieth century, dental caries were widespread and lead to serious tooth loss. In fact, having sound teeth was so important and such a rarity in the general population that the U.S. military made having a minimum of six opposing teeth a requirement during recruitment for WW I and II.

The first glimmer of an association between fluoride and oral health was observed by Dr. Frederick S. McKay in 1901. Noticing a brown stain on the teeth of his patients, Dr. McKay found that those who had these stains seemed to have fewer caries. In 1909, Dr. F.L. Robertson noticed mottling on the enamel (the hard outer surface) of children's teeth after the digging of a new well—source of the local drinking water. It wasn't until 1930 that the well water was analyzed, and high concentrations of fluoride were found. Fluoride, a naturally occurring fluorine ion, is found in soil, foods, and water.

The brown staining and mottling were characteristic of fluorosis, an abnormal condition caused by excessive exposure to fluoride while a child's teeth are forming under the gums. It affects the formation of tooth enamel and can vary from very mild to severe. Very mild fluorosis is manifested as tiny, white spots on 25% of a tooth's surface. Mild fluorosis covers 26–50%, and moderate fluorosis compromises all of a tooth's surface. It is most often characterized by brown discoloration of the tooth. Severe fluorosis involves pitting of the enamel and more serious brown staining. Approximately 94% of dental fluorosis today ranges from very mild to mild.

Extensive studies of national water supplies have been conducted. It has been found that dental caries were fewer in cities with more fluoride in the community water supply. A 1945 field study was conducted in four pairs of cities to determine whether a low level of fluoride (between 1.0 ppm and 1.2 ppm) could prevent dental caries. The result was a 50–70 reduction in the number of dental caries in communities with fluoridated water; only 10% of the people had mild fluorosis.

In 1962, another study found an optimal fluoride level of 0.7 parts per million (ppm) to 1.2 ppm (warm climates, where water consumption is higher, vs. cooler climates, respectively). This fluoride level range was determined to combat dental caries and pose only a slight risk of mild fluorosis.

Water fluoridation was rapidly adopted in major U.S. cities. About 46% of all public water supplies, however, remain non-fluoridated. Still, there has been a drastic reduction in the incidence of dental caries among children. In 2000, about half of all American children aged five to 17 years had never had a cavity in their permanent teeth. Adults also have experienced a 20–40 reduction in dental caries on enamel surfaces, as well as on exposed root caries—a condition peculiar to persons with gingival recession. Some of the earlier studies from the 1980s showed little difference in the reduction rates of dental caries between fluoridated communities and non-fluoridated communities. This may be due to improved dental hygiene, and the use of other fluoride products like fluoridated toothpaste and mouth rinses.

Effects on public health

Adding fluoride to drinking water has always been controversial. Though fluoride appears naturally in many water supplies, its purposeful introduction into community water supplies has brought claims of causing cancer, heart disease, Down Syndrome, osteoporosis, acquired immunedeficiency syndrome (**AIDS**), low intelligence, Alzheimer's disease, nephritis, cirrhosis, intracranial lesions, allergic reactions, and hip fractures. There has been no credible evidence to link fluoride to these diseases.

Early geographic studies in the 1980s reported a correlation between water fluoridation and bone fractures. However, an October 2000 study of women in four U.S. communities who had a continuous 20-year exposure to fluoride in drinking water found that fluoride was not a factor in increased spinal and hip fractures. In fact, these women exhibited greater bone density in the large bones like the femur, the hip, and the lumbar spine, with a slight decrease in hip and spine fractures. There was, however, a slight increase in the incidence of wrist fractures.

Though claims of increased medical risk when drinking fluoridated water still exist, opponents are finding other issues with platforms from which to fight fluoridation (for example, the fact the individuals do not get to decide whether to fluoridate their own personal drinking water) and whether dental caries are a serious public health problem anymore. These opponents cite studies from the mid-1980s that showed only an 18% difference in dental caries among children living in communities with and without fluoridated water. They claim, and rightly so, that this difference is due to widespread use of fluoridated toothpaste. However, increased use of bottled water, and processed foods that may contain fluoridated water, may also be contributing factors.

Water fluoridation provides inexpensive prevention for at-risk populations in every community. Despite Medicaid benefits that cover dental treatment, poor children often have less access than higher income families to dentists and fluoridated dental hygiene products. Children in non-fluoridated communities seek dental treatment in hospital emergency rooms more often than children in fluoridated communities; this increases costs for their dental treatment. The consumption of fluoridated water can reduce these expenses.

Adding fluoride to drinking water is the most cost-effective method for preventing dental caries. The average costs of fluoridation is around $0.50 per person annually, with some communities paying out only $0.12 per person. Smaller areas with fewer than 10,000 people, however, have costs that can run between $3 and $5 a year per person. Still, the cost of fluoridation for a single person over his or her lifetime can be less than the cost of one filling.

> ## KEY TERMS
>
> **Dental caries**—Tooth decay.
>
> **Enamel**—The hard, calcified outer surface of a tooth; the hardest known substance in the human body.
>
> **Fluoride**—A fluorine ion used to treat water or apply directly to tooth surfaces to prevent dental caries.
>
> **Fluorosis**—Fluorosis is an abnormal condition caused by excessive exposure to fluoride while a child's teeth are forming under the gums. It affects the formation of tooth enamel and can be very mild (a few white spots on a tooth) to severe (etching, pitting, and brown discoloration).

Fluoridation has been found to be effective for all citizens within a community regardless of socioeconomic status, and it has been proven safe for every person to use. Fluoridated water has a topical benefit. It provides ambient fluoride, which promotes remineralization of teeth to all ages and populations who consume the treated water. The latest concern, however, centers on over-fluoridation. There are many more ways to ingest fluoride than just in drinking water. Fluoride is added to prepared foods and bottled drinks. Carbonated drinks, juices, and some bottled waters have fluoride in varying amounts. Often, the fluoride in these products is not revealed on the label. Foods high in fluoride are fish with bones, tea, poultry products, cereals, or infant formula, which is made with fluoridated water. Dental products such as mouth rinses, toothpaste, and fluoride supplements all have added fluoride. Some pediatricians prescribe fluoride supplements without determining the fluoride content of the water a child drinks or assessing the amount of fluoride exposure the child has in his or her environment. Parents need to take a proactive role in learning the contents of their children's prescriptions.

It is of most concern when children ingest large amounts of fluoride, not because of known health risks related to fluoride, but because of the added potential of having fluorosis in children's permanent teeth. Young children under six years of age often use too much fluoride toothpaste and consistently swallow it. This alone has been the biggest cause of excess fluoride ingestion. For that reason, fluoride products should be kept out of the reach of children. Parents should supervise children who are under six years of age as they brush their teeth, ensuring that only a peasized drop of toothpaste is used, and directing them not to swallow toothpaste. Children under six should not use fluoridated mouth rinses.

Public health role and response

Water fluoridation has been recognized by more than 90 professional health organizations in the world as the most effective dental caries preventive in the 20th century. Dentists, dental hygienists, pediatricians, nurses, dietitians, and professionals from the United States Centers for Disease Control have endorsed the benefits of fluoridated water. Unfortunately, about half of the population of the United States lives in areas that do not have fluoridated water. Healthcare professionals need to be aggressive in their efforts to bring fluoride to these areas. Careful monitoring of fluoride present in all environments, and an assessment of the client's fluoride history, need to be carried out by local pediatricians and dentists before fluoride supplements are prescribed. Nurses and other professionals need to take a role in educating parents about fluoride dental products and foods containing fluoride, as well as proper fluoride consumption by children under the age of six.

Resources

BOOKS

Griffen, A.K., ed. *Pediatric Oral Health*. Philadelphia: Saunders, 2000.

PERIODICALS

Heilman, J.R., Kiritsy, M.C., Levy, S.M., and J.S. Wefel. "Assessing Fluoride Levels of Carbonated Soft Drinks." *Journal of the American Dental Association* 130, no. 11 (November 1999): 1593-1600.

Phipps, K.R., Orwoll, E.S., Mason, J.D., and J.A. Cauley. "Community Water Fluoridation, Bone Mineral Density, and Fractures: prospective study of effects in older women." *British Medical Journal* 321, no. 7265 (October 7, 2000):860.

Warren, J.J., Kanellis, M.J., and S.M. Levy. "Fluorosis of the Primary Dentitian: What Does it Mean for Permanent Teeth?" *Journal of the American Dental Association* 130, no. 3 (March 1999):347.

ORGANIZATIONS

American Academy of Pediatrics. 141 Northwest Point Boulevard, Elk Grove Village, IL 60007-1098. (847) 434-4000. http://www.aap.org.

American Dental Association. 211 East Chicago Ave., Chicago, IL 60611. (800)947-4746, (312)440-2500. http://www.ada.org.

Centers for Disease Control and Prevention. 4770 Buford Highway, NE, Atlanta, GA 30341. (770) 488-6054. http://www.cdc.gov/nohss.

National Association of Pediatric Nurse Associates & Practitioners. 1101 Kings Highway, N., Suite 206, Cherry Hill, NJ 08034-1912. http://www. napnap.org.

WEBSITES

"American Dental Association: Oral Health Topics: Fluoridation Facts: Safety Question 18." April 20, 2001. http://www.ada.org.

"American Dental Asscciation: Statement on Water Fluoridation Efficacy and Safety." April 20, 2001. http://www.ada.org.

Janie F. Franz

Water pollution

Definition

Water pollution is any physical, biological, or chemical change in **water quality** that adversely affects living organisms or makes water unsuitable for desired uses.

Description

Among the many environmental problems that offend and concern people, perhaps none is as powerful and dramatic as water pollution. Paradoxically, a change that adversely affects one organism may be advantageous to another. Nutrients that stimulate oxygen consumption by bacteria and other decomposers in a river or lake, for instance, may be lethal to fish but will stimulate a flourishing community of decomposers. There are natural sources of water contamination, such as poison springs, oil seeps, and sedimentation from erosion, but most discussions of water pollution focus on human-caused changes that affect water quality or usability.

Demographics

The most serious water pollutants affecting human health are pathogenic organisms. Altogether, at least 25 million deaths worldwide each year are blamed on these water-related diseases, including nearly two-thirds of the mortalities of children under five years old. The main source of these pathogens is untreated or improperly treated human wastes deposited into drinking water sources. In more developed countries, sewage treatment plants and other pollution control techniques have reduced or eliminated most of the worst sources of pathogens in inland surface waters. The United Nations estimates that 90 percent of the people in

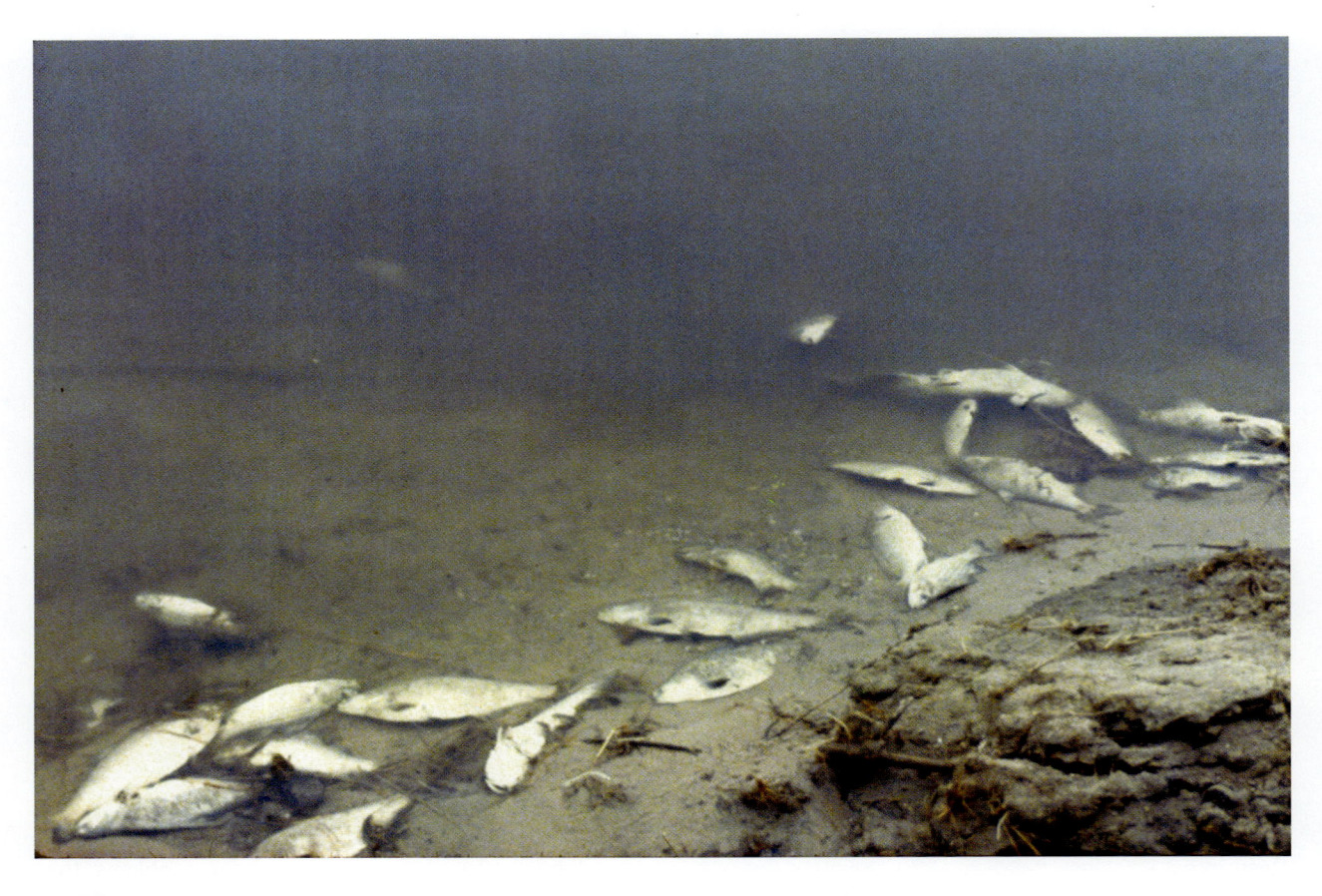

Fish killed by water pollution. (© U.S. Fish & Wildlife Service.)

high-income countries have adequate sewage disposal, and 95 percent have clean drinking water.

For developing countries, the situation is quite different. The United Nations estimates that three-fourths of the population in less-developed countries have inadequate **sanitation**, and that less than half have access to clean drinking water. Conditions are generally worse in remote, rural areas where sewer systems and waste water treatment are ineffective or nonexistent, and purified water is either unavailable or too expensive to obtain. In the thirty-three poorest countries, 60 percent of the urban population have access to clean drinking water but only 20 percent of people living in rural areas do.

A lack of pollution control is reflected in surface and groundwater quality in countries that lack the resources or political will to enforce pollution control. In Poland, for example, 95 percent of all surface water is unfit to drink. The Vistula River, which winds through the country's most heavily industrialized region, is so badly polluted that more than half the river is utterly devoid of life and unsuited even for industrial use. In Russia, the lower Volga River is reported to be on the brink of disaster due to the 300 million tons (272.2 million metric tons) of solid waste and 5 trillion gallons (20 trillion liters) of liquid effluent dumped into it annually.

The least developed countries of South America, Africa, and Asia have even worse water quality. Sewage treatment is either totally lacking or woefully inadequate. Low technological capabilities and little money for pollution control are made even worse by burgeoning populations, rapid urbanization, and the shift of heavy industry from developed countries where pollution, labor and other laws are strict to less developed countries where regulations are more lenient.

In Malaysia, 42 of 50 major rivers are reported to be ecological disasters as a result of contamination and flooding. Residues from palm oil and rubber manufacturing, along with heavy erosion from logging of tropical rain forests, have destroyed all higher forms of life in most of these rivers. In the Philippines, domestic sewage makes up 60%–70% of the total volume of Manila's Pasig River. Thousands of people use the river not only for bathing and washing clothes, but also as their source of drinking and cooking water. Only 63 percent of groundwater resources in China can be used for drinking water due to high pollution levels rendering them unsuitable for human consumption. As of 2005, wastewater treatment in China was estimated at or below 20%; however, the government now requires wastewater treatment facilities in all Chinese cities, which will raise the percentage of treated water to 45-60 percent. Approximately 75 percent of lakes in China are reported to be seriously polluted.

Pollution control standards and regulations usually distinguish between point and nonpoint pollution sources. Factories, power plants, sewage treatment plants, underground coal mines, and oil wells are classified as point sources because they discharge pollution from specific locations, such as drainpipes, ditches, or sewer outfalls. These sources are discrete and identifiable, so they are relatively easy to monitor and regulate. It is generally possible to divert effluent from the waste streams of these sources and treat it before it enters the environment. In contrast, nonpoint sources of water pollution are scattered or diffused, having no specific location where they discharge into a particular body of water. Nonpoint sources include runoff from farm fields, golf courses, lawns and gardens, construction sites, logging areas, roads, streets, and parking lots. Multiple origins and scattered locations make this pollution more difficult to monitor, regulate, and treat than point sources.

Desert soils often contain high salt concentrations that can be mobilized by irrigation and concentrated by evaporation, reaching levels that are toxic for plants and animals. Salt levels in the San Joaquin River in central California rose about 50 percent from 1930 to 1970 as a result of agricultural runoff. Salinity levels in the Colorado River and surrounding farm fields had become so high that millions of acres of previously valuable cropland was abandoned. The United States constructed a huge desalination plant at Yuma, Arizona, to reduce salinity in the river. In northern states, millions of tons of sodium chloride (NaCl) and calcium chloride ($CaCl_2$) are used to melt road ice in the winter. The corrosive damage to highways and automobiles and the toxic effects on vegetation are enormous. Leaching of road salts into surface waters has a similarly devastating effect on aquatic ecosystems.

Acids are released by mining and as by-products of industrial processes, such as leather tanning, metal smelting and plating, petroleum distillation, and organic chemical synthesis. Coal mining is an especially important source of acid water pollution. Sulfides (S^{2-}) in coal are solubilized to make sulfuric acid. Thousands of miles of streams in the United States have been poisoned by acids and metals, some so severely that they are essentially lifeless.

Effects on public health

Thousands of different natural and synthetic organic chemicals are used in the chemical industry to make pesticides, plastics, pharmaceuticals, pigments, and other products that we use in everyday life. Many of these chemicals are highly toxic. Exposure to very low concentrations can cause birth defects, genetic disorders, cancer, and can affect reproductive development. Some synthetic chemicals are resistant to degradation, allowing them to persist in the environment for many years. Contamination of surface waters and groundwater by these chemicals is a serious threat to human health.

Costs to society

Hundreds of millions of tons of hazardous organic wastes are thought to be stored in dumps, landfills, lagoons, and underground tanks in the United States. Many, perhaps most, of these sites are leaking toxic chemicals into surface waters or groundwater or both. The **Environmental Protection Agency (EPA)** estimates that about 26,000 **hazardous waste** sites will require cleanup because they pose an imminent threat to public health, mostly through water pollution.

In addition to pollution from natural sources and industrial runoff, the possible intentional pollution of water supplies and resources is a recognized vulnerability and an area of concern for scientists and security specialists.

Although the oceans are vast, unmistakable signs of human abuse can be seen even in the most remote places. Garbage and human wastes from coastal cities are dumped into the ocean. Silt, fertilizers, and pesticides from farm fields smothered coral reefs, coastal spawning beds, and result in eutrophication (excess nutrient deposition into bodies of water altering water quality) of estuaries. Every year millions of tons of plastic litter and discarded fishing nets entangle aquatic organisms, dooming them to a slow death. Generally coastal areas, where the highest concentrations of sea life are found and human activities take place, are most critically affected. Solid wastes and toxic substances derived from discarded computers and other types of electronics (e-waste) are also a growing concerns.

Effects on the environment

The amount of oxygen dissolved in water is a good indicator of water quality and of the kinds of life it will support. Water with an oxygen content above eight parts per million (ppm) will support game fish and other desirable forms of aquatic life. Water with less than two ppm oxygen will support only worms, bacteria, fungi, and other decomposers. Oxygen is added to water by diffusion from the air, especially when turbulence and mixing rates are high, and by photosynthesis of green plants, algae, and cyanobacteria. Oxygen is removed from water by respiration and chemical processes that consume oxygen. As water temperature increases, the amount of dissolved oxygen decreases. Global **climate change** is resulting in a warming of the Earth that could affect water quality and the health of aquatic ecosystems and organisms.

Public health role and response

The Federal Water Pollution Control Act was passed in 1972 to "restore and maintain the physical, chemical, and biological integrity of the nation's waters by preventing point and nonpoint pollution sources, providing assistance to publicly owned treatment works for the improvement of wastewater treatment, and maintaining the integrity of wetlands." This act is more commonly referred to as the **Clean Water Act** (CWA) and regulates both direct and indirect discharges of the 126 priority pollutants, conventional pollutants (e.g., total suspended soils, oils), and non-conventional pollutants, which are any pollutants not included in the two former categories. The National Pollutant Discharge Elimination System (NPDES) regulates direct (or point source) discharges of pollutants. A permit must be obtained to discharge pollutants into navigable waters after review of analytical data provided by the applicant detailing the pollutant content of the effluent (treated water).

In spite of the enormous bad news about water quality, some encouraging pollution control stories are emerging. One of the most outstanding examples is the Thames River in London. With the Industrial Revolution, the Thames became little more than an open sewer, full of toxic waste products from domestic and industrial sewers. In the l950s, however, England undertook a massive cleanup of the Thames. More than $250 million in public funds plus millions more from industry were spent to curb pollution. By the early l980s, the river was showing remarkable signs of rejuvenation. Oxygen levels had rebounded and some 95 species of fish had returned, including the pollution-sensitive salmon, which had not been seen in London for three hundred years. With a little effort, care, and concern for the environment, similar improvements can develop elsewhere.

Resources

BOOKS

Brinkman, Stephen, and Nicole M. K. Vieira. *Water Pollution Studies*. Federal aid in fish and wildlife restoration job progress report. Fort Collins, CO: Colorado Division of Wildlife, Fish Research Section, 2008.

Economy, Elizabeth. *The River Runs Black: The Environmental Challenge to China's Future*. Ithaca, NY: Cornell University Press, 2004.

Morris, Robert D. *The Blue Death: Disease, Disaster, and the Water We Drink*. New York: HarperCollins Publishers, 2007.

Strange, Cordelia. *Water Pollution & Health* (Health and the Environment). New York: AlphaHouse, 2009.

Thomas, Sarah V., and Claudia Copeland. *Water Pollution Issues and Developments*. New York: Nova Science, 2008.

Tripathi, A. K., and S. N. Pandey. *Water Pollution*. New Delhi: APH, 2009.

WEBSITES

Environmental Protection Agency. "Water: Water Pollution." http://www.epa.gov/ebtpages/watewaterpollution.html (accessed October 25, 2012).

Environmental Protection Agency. "Water: Water Pollution: Community Involvement." http://www.epa.gov/ebtpages/watewaterpollutioncommunityinvolvement.html (accessed October 25, 2012).

World Business Council for Sustainable Development. "Water: Fact and Trends." WBCSD, August 2005. http://www.unwater.org/downloads/Water_facts_and_trends.pdf (accessed October 25, 2012).

ORGANIZATIONS

Environmental Protection Agency, 1200 Pennsylvania Ave. NW, Washington, DC 20460, (202) 272-0167, http://water.epa.gov.

William P. Cunningham
Alison C. Heimer, MA

Water quality

Definition

Water quality refers to how suitable water is for its intended use, often for drinking. A wide range of water characteristics, including biological, chemical, and physical descriptions of water clarity or contamination can be used to help determine water quality.

Description

The quality of water is critical to health. Around the world, there are many places where access to enough quality water is a challenge for people and communities. Water that is not properly managed can cause diseases related to drinking, **sanitation** problems, or microorganisms harbored in the water. Most urban areas, especially in developed countries, have safe drinking water supplies and systems in place to properly process and store sewage. Cities also ensure that water from precipitation is properly managed to that it doesn't affect drinking or sanitation water supplies, cause damage to structures or crops, or stand and stagnate so that it can harbor microorganisms.

In many ways, the effects of poor-quality water on the spread of disease in communities formed the basis of public health. In mid-nineteenth century England, John Snow traced a **cholera** outbreak in London's East End to a single pump that was supplying water contaminated with human waste. He was able to halt the disease by removing the handle from the pump so people stopped using it. Until that time, people did not understand how cholera was spread, and they suspected other methods, such as transmission through air. His work was followed by that of Edwin Chadwick, who wrote *Report on an Inquiry into the Sanitary Condition of the Labouring Population of Great Britain,* which argued that problems such as inadequate waste disposal, overcrowding, poverty, and other issues in society were causing disease and the high economic burden of disease.

Water quality assessment usually involves the examination of a lake, river, bay, aquifer, or other water body for characteristics that are mandated by municipal, state, and/or federal legislation. The most important of these attributes are pollutants that deplete the oxygen content of the water or cause disease, nutrients that stimulate excessive plant growth, synthetic organic and inorganic chemicals, mineral substances, sediments, radioactive substances, and temperature.

After the 1950s, routine tests for water quality have evaluated temperature, turbidity, color, odor, total solids after evaporation, hardness (pH), and concentrations of carbon dioxide, iron, nitrogen, chloride, active chlorine, microorganisms, coliform bacteria, and amorphous matter. More parameters were added in later decades, in response to growing public concern over water quality: these included algal growth, chemical oxygen demand, and the presence of hydrocarbons, metals, and other toxic substances.

Water quality is evaluated through a set of samples taken at different depths of water (a water column), if the watercourse is sufficiently deep, or at selected sites in shallower watercourses. Because quality conditions change continually, each set of samples reflects the conditions at the time of sampling. Over time, samples collected from the same site can provide an indication of the temporal quality of the particular watercourse, which can be used to reveal conditions when water quality deteriorates (e.g., runoff following excessive rainfall).

To ensure that quality measurements are consistent at different times and locations, standards are legally set for various water uses and contaminant levels. As well, the testing protocols are standardized, allowing comparison of results obtained from different testing facilities, and permitting the auditing of testing laboratories to ensure that the tests are being done in a valid fashion. Two general types of standards are used around the globe to measure water quality. Water quality-based standards ensure that a water body is clean enough for its expected uses, which can include fishing, swimming, industrial use, or drinking. Technology-based standards are set for wastewater entering a water body so that overall water conditions remain acceptable. In the United States, the **Environmental Protection Agency (EPA)** is responsible for developing **water quality standards** and criteria for surface, ground, and marine waters.

Water quality standards are based upon criteria that designate acceptable levels of specific pollutants, water clarity, or oxygen content. Acceptable levels of these criteria are typically measured in parts per million (ppm) of each contaminant or nutrient. These measurements allow scientists to assess whether or not a body of water meets the prescribed water quality standards. If standards are not met, then local governing bodies or industries must develop and implement cleanup strategies that target specific criteria.

Risk factors

Both point and nonpoint sources of pollution affect water quality. Point sources are discrete locations that discharge pollutants, mainly industrial outflow pipes or sewage treatment plants. Nonpoint sources are more diffuse and include storm runoff and runoff from farming, logging, construction, and other land use activities.

In the United States, more than 50 percent of the population relies on underground sources for drinking water. Because groundwater receives an enormous range of agricultural, industrial, and urban pollutants, groundwater quality is a growing concern. Preventing groundwater pollution is especially important because remedial action in an aquifer is expensive and technologically difficult. Major sources of groundwater pollution include nitrate contamination from septic systems, nitrate from fertilizers added to agricultural land, organic pollutants from leaking fuel tanks and other storage containers, and an array of contaminants leached from landfills.

In rivers, the most extensive causes of water quality impairment are usually siltation, nutrient concentration (nitrogen and phosphorus), fecal coliform bacteria, and low dissolved oxygen levels caused by high organic content (e.g., sewage, grass clippings, pasture and feedlot runoff). Agricultural runoff, including pesticides, fertilizers, and sediments, is the largest source of river pollution, followed by municipal sewage discharge. Estuaries, rich ecosystems of mixed salt and fresh water where rivers enter a sea or ocean, often have serious water quality problems. Estuarine contaminants are usually the same as those in rivers—high organic content and low oxygen, disease-causing pathogens, organic chemicals, and municipal sewage discharge.

In most lakes, water quality is affected primarily by nitrogen and phosphorus loading, siltation and low dissolved oxygen. Like rivers, lakes suffer from agricultural runoff, habitat modification, storm runoff, and municipal sewage effluent. Lakes especially suffer from eutrophication (the excessive growth of aquatic algae and other plants) caused by high levels of nutrients. This burst of growth, also called an **algal bloom**, feeds on concentrated nutrients. Thick mats of algae and other aquatic plants clog water systems, increase turbidity, and suffocate aquatic animals so that an entire ecosystem is disrupted.

Effects on public health

Water quality degradation affects the stability of aquatic ecosystems as well as human health. Much is still unknown about the effects of specific pollutants on ecosystem health. However, fish and other aquatic organisms exposed to elevated levels of pollutants may have lowered reproduction and growth rates, diseases, and, in severe cases, high death rates.

Common diseases and disorders

Contaminated drinking water can cause a number of short-term and long-term health problems, and the number of possible contaminants, such as chemicals and minerals, is lengthy. Several waterborne substances can cause illness if people drink water containing them. Some of the most common diseases are:

- Giardiasis, a severe diarrhea from the giardia parasite
- Shigellosis, an infectious bacterial disease that can cause fever, stomach cramps, and bloody diarrhea
- Norovirus, spread in water and other ways, causing stomach swelling, severe cramping, and nausea
- Hepatitis A, a virus that causes inflammation of the liver
- Cryptosporidiosis, a disease caused by a parasite that is tolerant to chlorine and affects people and animals
- High levels of the metal copper, causing vomiting and nausea. Very high levels can cause severe disease or death

Drinking water quality is not the only cause of disease, however. The bacteria *Legionella* is natural in ground and sea water. Under certain conditions, it can transmit from water to air. Systems such as faucets, showerheads, cooling towers, and nebulizers can help transmit the bacteria from water to air. Human inhalation of contaminated aerosols leads to infection and Legionnaire's disease. Some diseases are spread by people washing their hands in water or are water-related diseases. An example is **malaria**, which can be spread by mosquitoes that breed in standing water.

Further, pollution of water can be a public health hazard that causes numerous problems later on. For example, if wastewater is dumped into the rivers or lakes and is not treated properly, the polluted water affects aquatic populations and can make fish unsafe to eat. If quantities of certain nutrients, such as nitrogen, become too high in water used to irrigate crops, the water can damage the crops. Too much nitrogen also kills algae, which in turn affects the water body's ecosystem.

Costs to society

In the United States, public water systems supply nearly 90 percent of drinking water to residents, or about 286 million Americans. The **EPA** regulates the private and public entities that run the systems. The **Centers for Disease Control and Prevention** (CDC) estimates that up to 15 percent of Americans get their drinking water from private wells, which neither the EPA nor any federal agency regulates. Globally, safe community drinking water is more problematic. Diarrheal disease accounts for about 4 percent of all disease and could kill nearly 1.8 million people a year, according to the **World Health Organization**. WHO estimates that 88 percent of the diarrheal disease is caused by unsafe water supplies, poor sanitation, and insufficient hygiene.

The CDC estimates that the costs of the three most common waterborne diseases, **cryptosporidiosis**, **giardiasis**, and Legionnaire's disease, are more than

$500 million a year in hospitalizations and other medical care.

Public health role and response

Public health officials monitor diseases that might be caused by drinking or exposure to bacteria or other substances in water. Hospitals and healthcare providers should report waterborne diseases to public health departments for this reason. They usually have policies and procedures in place to work with local hospitals, community agencies, and government entities to help curb disease spread. Public health professionals first try to prevent disease by educating people, ensuring adequate and safe water supplies through setting standards and practices, and by advocating for change when necessary.

In the United States and many other countries, national water quality criteria have been developed for most conventional, toxic, and nonconventional pollutants. Conventional pollutants include suspended solids, biochemical oxygen demand (BOD), pH (acidity or alkalinity), presence and/or quantity of fecal coliform bacteria, oil, and grease. Toxic priority pollutants include metals and organic chemicals. Nonconventional pollutants are any other contaminants that harm humans or marine resources and require regulation.

Drinking water must meet especially high standards to be safe for human consumption, and its quality is strictly monitored in most developed countries, including the United States. Most governments have a legal responsibility to maintain acceptable drinking water quality. Indeed, in the United States, the **Clean Water Act** was conceived based on the belief that clean water was a national necessity.

Until 1974, efforts to maintain acceptable levels of drinking water quality in the United States were limited to preventing the spread of contagious diseases. The **Safe Drinking Water Act** of 1974 expanded the government's regulatory role to cover all substances that may adversely affect human health or a water body's odor or appearance. This act established national regulations for acceptable levels of various contaminants.

Even ocean waters, with their massive volume of water, are vulnerable. One example began on April 20, 2010, when the Deepwater Horizon oil drilling platform exploded and sank in the Gulf of Mexico, triggering the rupture of a deep water oil pipeline. Estimates were that up to 60,000 barrels of oil (2,500,000 US gallons) per day flowed into the Gulf before the rupture was capped on July 15. Some beaches were soiled and wildlife affected. But as of July 2010, the ultimate environmental fate of the massive amount of oil that remained underwater was unknown. Fears were that the oil would be pushed ashore during a tropical storm or hurricane, which could be disastrous for the coastline of the Gulf states.

Resources

BOOKS

American Water Works Association and James Edzwald. *Water Quality & Treatment: A Handbook on Drinking Water* (Water Resources and Environmental Engineering Series). New York: McGraw-Hill, 2011.

Chapra, Steven C. *Surface Water-Quality Modeling*. Long Grove, IL: Waveland Press, 2008.

Craig, Robin Kundis. *The Clean Water Act and the Constitution*. Washington, DC: Environmental Law Institute, 2009.

Virgil, Kenneth M. *Clean Water: An Introduction to Water Quality and Pollution Control*. Corvallis: Oregon State University Press, 2003.

WEBSITES

Centers for Disease Control and Prevention. "Water-related Emergencies and Outbreaks: Outbreak Response Resources." http://www.cdc.gov/healthywater/emergency/ (accessed October 13, 2012).

Centers for Disease Control and Prevention. "Water Quality." http://www.cdc.gov/healthyplaces/healthtopics/water.htm (accessed October 14, 2012).

Eisenberg, Joseph N. S., Jamie Bartram, and Paul R. Hunter. "A Public Health Perspective for Establishing Water-related Guidelines and Standards." WHO. http://www.who.int/water_sanitation_health/dwq/iwachap11.pdf(accessed October 13, 2012).

United States Geological Service. "Nitrogen and Water." http://ga.water.usgs.gov/edu/nitrogen.html (accessed October 14, 2012).

ORGANIZATIONS

Environmental Protection Agency, 1200 Pennsylvania Ave. NW, Washington, DC 20460, (202) 272-0167, http://water.epa.gov.

Marci L. Bortman
Teresa G. Odle

Water quality standards

Definition

Water quality standards refer to mandated conditions that drinking and recreational water must achieve to be judged acceptable for use.

Purpose

Water quality standards set the conditions that drinking and recreational water must meet in order to be deemed acceptable for use. Failure to meet the various water quality standards for organic chemicals, inorganic chemicals, and biological material, including bacteria, **viruses**, and protozoa, by different municipal, state, and federal government authorities, can trigger actions designed to restore water quality.

In the United States, the legislative process is used to establish standards for stream water quality by taking into account the use and value of a stream for public water supplies, propagation of fish and wildlife, recreational purposes, as well as agricultural, industrial, and other legitimate uses. The goals of water quality standards are to protect public health and the environment and to maintain a standard of water quality consistent with its designated uses.

Description

To establish water quality standards for a water body, officials (a) determine the designated beneficial water use; (b) adopt suitable water quality criteria to protect and maintain that use; and (c) develop a plan for implementing and enforcing the water quality criteria.

Water quality is evaluated based on how well the designated uses are supported. In the United States, the **Federal Water Act** of 1972 and following amendments, together known as the **Clean Water Act**, require that, whenever possible, water quality standards should ensure the protection and propagation of fish, shellfish, and wildlife and should provide for recreation. States have primary responsibility for designating stream segment uses, so stream uses may vary from state to state. However, stream use as designated by one state must not result in the violation of another state's use of the same stream.

The 1987 amendments to the Clean Water Act required states to identify water not meeting its standards due to nonpoint source pollution (i.e., addition of pollutants from a wider geographical area, such as runoff from a field), identify general and specific nonpoint sources causing the problems, and develop management plans for the control of the these sources. The Clean Water Act also charged the federal government with the responsibility of setting standards for water quality and enforcing those standards. Until the implementation of the act, this responsibility rested with the individual states, which were free to enacted different standards.

> ### KEY TERMS
>
> **Contaminant**—A type of unwanted microparticle or organism. In water, a contaminant may reduce clarity, quality, or be a health hazard.
>
> **Protozoa organisms**—Single-celled organisms that have animal-like behavior. Certain protozoa are harmful to humans and are found in water, making it important that water is treated and filtered before drinking.
>
> **Virus**—A tiny particle that can cause infections by duplicating itself inside a cell using the cell's own software. Antibiotics are ineffective against viruses, though antiviral drugs exist for some viruses.

Before the passage of the Clean Water Act, **water pollution** control efforts were considered successful if they achieved water quality standards. Water quality standards were retained as part of the overall strategy to control water pollution. However, rather than using water quality standards as the highest goal for determining water quality, state and federal authorities now consider water quality control standards to be the lowest acceptable level of water quality. In addition, point sources of pollution (i.e., addition of a contaminant at a single site, such as a pipeline) may be subject to more stringent requirements.

Origins

The development of water quality standards was first mandated in the United States by the Water Quality Act of 1965. Under this legislation, states had to develop water quality standards and water quality goals. By the early 1970s, these standards and goals had been adopted by all U.S. states. With the advancement of technology and scientific information, states have updated their standards over time. Legally enforceable legislation was also expanded by requirements in the Federal Water Pollution Control Act of 1972, with amendments in 1977 and 1987 (collectively referred to as the Clean Water Act).

Other nations also focus on water quality standards; however, each nations' standards vary. For example, whereas the United States has drinking water quality regulations, Canada only has drinking water quality guidelines, meaning they are not enforceable by law. The **World Health Organization** (WHO) also has drinking water quality guidelines. The European Union has both a drinking water directive and a water framework directive, which covers all

> **QUESTIONS TO ASK YOUR DOCTOR**
>
> - How can I protect myself in countries with low water-quality standards?
> - Where can I find information about the water quality in water sources near me?
> - Does my personal well water need to meet federal water quality standards?

bodies of water. It is the responsibility of each country in the European Union to make sure that the regulations are implemented. Water quality standards are still a major problem in developing countries.

Results

The focus on protecting and improving water quality has made drastic changes to water quality around the world. In the United States, the Environmental Protect Agency (**EPA**) requires that 99.9% of viruses and protozoan organisms are removed before the water can be considered safe for human consumption. Water used for recreation must also pass strict standards. The EPA also requires that water to be consumed by humans be monitored for over 90 contaminants. This is much stricter than in Canada, which recommends checking for fewer than 70 contaminants, or the European Union, which requires that water be checked for 48 contaminants. Although these regulations and guidelines vary by country, all work to keep citizens healthy through protecting and improving both recreational and drinking water.

Resources

BOOKS

American Water Works Association and James Edzwald. *Water Quality & Treatment: A Handbook on Drinking Water* (Water Resources and Environmental Engineering Series). New York: McGraw-Hill, 2011.

Chapra, Steven C. *Surface Water-Quality Modeling.* Long Grove, IL: Waveland Press, 2008.

Craig, Robin Kundis. *The Clean Water Act and the Constitution.* Washington, DC: Environmental Law Institute, 2009.

Virgil, Kenneth M. *Clean Water: An Introduction to Water Quality and Pollution Control.* Corvallis: Oregon State University Press, 2003.

WEBSITES

United Nations Department of Economic and Social Affairs. "Water Quality." http://www.un.org/water forlifedecade/quality.shtml (accessed October 18, 2012).

United Nations Environment Programmes. "Clearing the Waters: A Focus on Water Quality Solutions." http://www.unep.org/PDF/Clearing_the_Waters.pdf (accessed October 18, 2012).

United States Environmental Protection Agency. "Water Quality Criteria." http://water.epa.gov/scitech/swguidance/standards/criteria/index.cfm (accessed October 18, 2012).

United States Environmental Protection Agency. "Water Quality Standards History." http://water.epa.gov/scitech/swguidance/standards/history.cfm (accessed October 18, 2012)

United States Environmental Protection Agency. "What Are Water Quality Standards?" http://water.epa.gov/scitech/swguidance/standards/about_index.cfm (accessed October 18, 2012).

ORGANIZATIONS

Centers for Disease Control and Prevention (CDC), 1600 Clifton Rd., Atlanta, GA 30333, (404) 639-3534, (800) CDC-INFO (800-232-4636); TTY: (888) 232-6348, inquiry@cdc.gov, http://www.cdc.gov.

Environmental Protection Agency, 1200 Pennsylvania Ave., NW, Washington. DC 20460, (202) 272-0167; (202) 272-0165, http://water.epa.gov.

National Institute of Environmental Health Science, PO Box 12233, MD K3-16, Research Triangle Park, NC 27709, (919) 541-1919, Fax: (919) 541-4395, http://www.niehs.nih.gov.

Water Quality Association, 4151 Naperville Rd., Lisle, IL 60532, (630) 505-0160, Fax: (630) 505-9637, http://www.wqa.org.

Judith L. Sims
Tish Davidson, AM

Waterborne illness

Definition

Waterborne illness is a disease or condition caused by a pathogenic organism or toxic chemical that is directly spread via water. Waterborne illnesses are sometimes categorized as either potable (drinking) water illnesses or a recreational water illnesses (RWIs).

Description

Waterborne illness is most often contracted from drinking or swallowing water contaminated with a pathogen (a parasite, bacterium, or virus) or a chemical. Many waterborne disease-causing agents can also cause **foodborne illness**. Some waterborne illnesses can be contracted by inhaling mist from contaminated water or through contact of contaminated water with the skin or mucus membranes. In contrast, water-related illnesses are due to secondary effects, such as a lack of water for hygiene, poor **sanitation**, or water-breeding insects that spread disease.

Most waterborne illness results from swallowing water contaminated with animal or human feces. However, recreational water illnesses (RWIs) from swimming pools, hot tubs, fountains, springs, streams, rivers, ponds, lakes, and oceans are also a serious concern. RWIs can be contracted while swimming, boating, or participating in other water or shoreline activities.

Water systems in the United States have been chlorinated since the early twentieth century. This has eliminated life-threatening illnesses such as **cholera** and typhoid. However, these waterborne illnesses are **endemic** to much of the developing world. Even in developed countries, travelers to wilderness areas can be at risk for waterborne illness, especially **giardiasis** caused by the *Giardia* parasite.

Groundwater supplies occasionally become contaminated with sewage from wastewater treatment plants and septic tanks and with animal waste from concentrated animal feeding operations (CAFOs) and manure-augmented fields. In addition to livestock and agricultural operations, industrial and other business, residential, recreation, and transportation activities can contaminate drinking and recreational waters with pathogens and chemicals. Heavy rains and natural disasters increase the risk of contamination. The 2010 Pakistani floods led to millions of cases of waterborne illness, and a cholera epidemic followed in the wake of the 2010 Haitian earthquake. Even normal rainfall or snowmelt can wash human and animal waste into groundwater, streams, rivers, and lakes. **Climate change** is projected to affect rainfall patterns in ways that may increase the rates of waterborne illness. Hydraulic fracturing ("fracking") for natural gas and oil extraction appears to be an emerging source of groundwater contamination.

Waterborne illnesses occasionally occur even with water systems that meet current regulations and standards. Furthermore, water-purification technologies are sometimes inadequate for dealing with emerging waterborne pathogens and chemicals. Water is usually tested for safety by measuring the number of fecal coliform bacteria such as ***Escherichia coli***, which are found in human and animal intestines. The presence of *E. coli* is a strong indication of recent contamination with sewage or animal waste that may harbor various disease-causing organisms.

Demographics

Worldwide, more than one billion people are at risk for waterborne illness due to lack of access to clean water for drinking, cooking, and washing. An estimated 200 million people are infected with *Giardia* annually. An estimated 1.5 million people—mostly children—die of waterborne illness every year.

Even though 94% of Americans are on community water systems, there are an estimated 19.5 million cases of waterborne illness annually in the United States. It has been estimated that as many as 300,000 Americans are infected with waterborne pathogens in hospital facilities, and about 250 out of every 10,000 Americans contract giardiasis from public drinking water every year.

Of the approximately 53,000 community water systems and 100,000 other public drinking-water systems in the United States, just 8% serve 81% of all Americans. These systems vary greatly in technology and quality. There are more groundwater than surface-water systems, but more Americans get their drinking water from surface sources. Every year, there are an estimated:

- 26 million infections and 13 million illnesses in populations served by municipal surface-water systems
- 10.7 million infections and 5.4 million illnesses in populations with community groundwater systems
- 2.2 million infections and 1.1 million illnesses in populations with noncommunity groundwater systems

Causes and symptoms

Nearly one-half of all waterborne illnesses in the United States are caused by unidentified agents. Approximately one-fourth are caused by bacteria, an estimated 18% by **parasites**, about 10% by **viruses**, and about 5% by chemical contamination.

Bacteria

Many different bacteria can cause waterborne illness. Cholera is caused by *Vibrio cholerae*, which thrives in unsanitary water. It is endemic in many parts of the world and is associated with natural and human disasters and with contaminated ballast water dumped from ships near shore.

Most of the hundreds of *E. coli* strains that live in the intestines of healthy humans and animals are harmless. However, some enterovirulent *E. coli* (EEC) strains can cause waterborne illness. Strain 0157:H7, a Shiga toxin-producing *E. coli* (STEC), is most often identified in North America. It causes severe, usually bloody, diarrhea and abdominal cramps. Symptoms usually appear within two–four days after ingestion, but sometimes not for as long as eight days. In 2–7% of infections, especially in young children and the elderly, 0157:H7 causes a life-threatening type of kidney failure, called hemolytic uremic syndrome (HUS), in which red blood cells are destroyed.

Other waterborne-illness-causing bacteria include:

- *Pseudomonas* that has been associated with inadequately treated hot tubs
- *Legionella* that causes Legionnaires' disease and has been associated with hospital-acquired infections and even retail store whirlpool spa displays
- *Salmonella* spp., widespread intestinal bacteria including *S. typhi* that causes typhoid fever
- *Shigella*, a family of bacteria responsible for nearly a half-million diarrheal illnesses annually
- *Campylobacter* spp. that live in the intestines of healthy birds and are the most commonly identified cause of diarrheal illness worldwide and the second most common cause of bacterial diarrhea in the United States

Parasites

Cryptosporidiosis, or "crypto", caused by the one-celled (protozoan) parasite *Cryptosporidium parvum*, is now recognized as one of the most common waterborne illnesses, contaminating drinking and recreational waters in the United States and around the world. The parasite lives in the intestines of infected people and herd animals, including cows, sheep, goats, deer, and elk. Infective crypto oocysts are shed in human and animal feces. These oocysts have a tough outer shell and can survive for long periods in the environment. They can survive for days even in properly chlorinated pools and sometimes pass through water-filtration systems. The most common symptom of crypto is watery diarrhea, beginning two to ten days after ingestion of the oocysts and lasting for one to two weeks. Other symptoms of intestinal cryptosporidiosis include stomach cramps, upset stomach, and slight fever, although many infected people have no symptoms. Crypto can also cause tracheal or pulmonary illnesses. Young children, pregnant women, and anyone with a weakened immune system are at risk for serious illness from crypto infection.

Like crypto, *Giardia duodenalis* or *G. intestinalis* (formerly called *G. lamblia*) is a one-celled parasite in human and animal intestines. It is associated with contaminated drinking water worldwide. International travelers and hikers and campers drinking untreated water are at particular risk. Symptoms, if present, include diarrhea, abdominal cramps, gas, and nausea, generally appearing one–two weeks after ingestion of *Giardia* cysts.

Other common waterborne parasites include:

- the ameba *Entamoeba histolytica*, found in drinking water contaminated with fecal matter and causing amebiasis or amebic dysentary
- the Guinea worm *Dracunculus medinensis* that is transmitted when people with open Guinea worm wounds contaminate wells or ponds that are used for drinking water
- *Schistosoma* spp., parasitic worms carried by snails and birds that bore into humans in contaminated freshwater, causing schistosomiasis

Viruses

Hepatitis A is one of the most frequently reported waterborne viruses. It causes fever, nausea, and diarrhea. Other waterborne viral pathogens include:

- noroviruses, major sources of foodborne illness that can also contaminate water
- adenoviruses, a virus family that can cause a range of illnesses, especially diarrheal and respiratory infections
- reoviruses that cause a range of illnesses
- poliovirus that causes poliomyelitis

Chemicals

There are a large number of chemicals that can pollute drinking water and cause illness. These include pesticides, fertilizers, industrial solvents, and petroleum products. Chemical contamination occurs primarily through water run-off and cross-connections between waterways. There are also some naturally occurring waterborne toxins that can cause illness.

Diagnosis

Waterborne illness often goes undiagnosed. Specific symptoms and the length of time between exposure to suspect water and symptom appearance may suggest the culprit. However, unless the illness is associated with a known outbreak of waterborne illness, laboratory tests may be necessary. These usually involve microscopic examination of stool samples for parasites, culturing stool samples for bacteria, or testing stool samples for genetic markers of a specific virus. Diagnosis of a waterborne illness from a naturally occurring or manmade chemical may require extensive blood tests. Blood and urine tests may also be required to determine the extent of dehydration and electrolyte imbalances from diarrhea and vomiting.

KEY TERMS

Amebic dysentery; amebiasis—A common waterborne illness caused by the protozoan ameba *Entamoeba histolytica* and characterized by severe diarrhea, abdominal pain, and erosion of the intestinal wall.

Chlorination—Water treatment with chlorine or chlorine compounds to kill or inactivate disease-causing organisms.

Cholera—Severe waterborne diarrheal disease caused by the bacterium *Vibrio cholerae*.

Coliform—Gram-negative, rod-shaped bacteria, such as *Escherichia coli*, that are normally present in the human intestine and that are measured to monitor drinking water for contamination.

Cryptosporidiosis; crypto—A waterborne illness caused by the one-celled parasite *Cryptosporidium parvum*.

Dehydration—The abnormal depletion of body fluids, as from vomiting and diarrhea.

Electrolytes—Ions—such as sodium, potassium, calcium, magnesium, chloride, phosphate, bicarbonate, and sulfate—that are dissolved in bodily fluids and regulate or affect most metabolic processes.

Endemic—Restricted or peculiar to a specific locale or region; especially a disease that is prevalent only in a particular population.

Giardiasis—A waterborne illness caused by a widespread flagellate protozoan of the genus *Giardia*, usually characterized by diarrhea.

Halogenation—Water treatment with chlorine or bromine to kill or inactivate disease-causing organisms.

Hemolytic uremic syndrome (HUS)—Kidney failure, usually in infants and young children, that can be caused by waterborne illness, especially *Escherichia coli* strain O157:H7 and related bacteria.

Oocyst—A thick-walled spore that is the infective stage of certain waterborne illnesses, such as cryptosporidiosis.

Parasite—An organism that survives by living with, on, or in another organism, usually to the detriment of the host.

Pathogen—A causative agent of disease, such as a bacterium, virus, or parasite.

Potable—Water or other liquid that is suitable for drinking.

Recreational water illness (RWI)—An illness contracted by swallowing or contacting recreational waters during activities such as swimming and boating, and including pools, hot tubs, lakes, rivers, and oceans.

Shiga toxin-producing *E. coli* (STEC)—Shiga toxin-producing strains of the common, normally harmless, intestinal bacterium *Escherichia coli*, such as strain O157:H7.

Typhoid fever—A waterborne illness caused by the bacterium *Salmonella typhi*.

Treatment

The immediate treatment for waterborne illness is to prevent or reverse dehydration by replacing fluids and electrolytes lost through vomiting and diarrhea. Worldwide, dehydration is the biggest killer of children under age five. The loss of 10–15% of body fluids is very serious and the loss of 20% is fatal. Small sips of over-the-counter (OTC) oral rehydration solutions should be given to young children as soon as vomiting and diarrhea begin. International travelers suffering from diarrhea should be careful to drink only boiled or bottled water. Severe dehydration may require hospitalization and intravenous fluids. Antidiarrheal medications may slow the elimination of toxins and pathogens and delay recovery. Antibiotics are not usually required for waterborne bacterial illnesses. With *E. coli* infections, some antibiotics can lead to kidney complications. HUS caused by *E. coli* O157:H7 is life-threatening and is usually treated in an intensive-care unit. Blood transfusions and kidney dialysis are often required.

Prognosis

Most waterborne illnesses are mild and resolve quickly as the body's immune system kicks in. For example, crypto usually resolves within three or four days without medical intervention, although symptoms may last up to two weeks, even in otherwise healthy people. In people with weakened immune systems, crypto can be a serious, long-lasting, and even fatal illness. Giardiasis can last for two to six weeks in otherwise healthy individuals, and chronic infections have been known to last for months or years, accompanied by dehydration and severe weight loss.

> **WHAT TO ASK YOUR DOCTOR**
>
> - How do I know if my drinking water is safe?
> - Will using a water filter or bottled water protect me from waterborne illness?
> - How can I protect myself and my children from recreational water illnesses?
> - Does waterborne illness require medical attention?
> - How do I report a waterborne illness

Most people recover from *E. coli* O157:H7 infection within five–ten days without specific treatment. However, children under age five, the elderly, and immunocompromised patients are at risk for severe illness. Hemolytic uremic syndrome (HUS) is the most common cause of acute kidney failure in children and is fatal in 3–5% of cases. Certain other waterborne bacterial illnesses can also have chronic complications.

Waterborne chemical illnesses are more likely than pathogen-associated illnesses to have serious long-term complications. Pesticides and other chemical contaminants can cause liver damage, kidney failure, and nervous system complications.

Prevention

To a large extent, prevention of waterborne illness is the responsibility of public officials. Water-distribution and recreational-water systems require proper maintenance and disinfection, with no water stagnation, biofilm development, or dead ends. Public water systems are required by law to send out annual water-quality reports and to notify consumers if the water becomes unsafe. Public water systems are generally treated with chlorine, ultraviolet light, or **ozone** to kill or inactivate *E. coli* and other bacteria. About 89% of community water systems in the United States meet all health-based standards.

Obtaining drinking water only from treated municipal water systems that are safe from source contamination is the best protection against waterborne illness. Boiling water for one minute or halogenation with chlorine or bromine kills most waterborne bacteria. Hot water systems should be kept at or above 122°F (50°C), with hot water tanks set at 160–171°F (71–77°C), to protect against *Legionella*. Hepatitis A virus can be resistant to **chlorination** and the presence of fecal matter may protect it from the effects of chlorine.

Water from private wells should be tested for *E. coli* and total coliforms. Wells that test positive should be disinfected and tested regularly. All water for consumption should be boiled until tests are negative. Most in-home water filters do not protect against *E. coli* and other bacteria. Filtration to remove *Cryptosporidium* requires a pore size no larger than one micron or reverse-osmosis filtration. When hiking, camping, or traveling to countries where the water supply is questionable, all drinking water should be boiled for one minute or only bottled beverages should be consumed.

Preventing RWIs involves:

- avoiding recreational waters when suffering from diarrhea
- keeping recreational water out of one's mouth
- proper hand washing after using the toilet or changing diapers
- showering with soap and washing children thoroughly before swimming
- taking children for frequent toilet breaks
- changing diapers in a bathroom or diaper-changing area away from swimming areas
- using a molluscicide to eliminate snails or treating birds with anti-helmetic drugs to eliminate parasitic worms

Resources

BOOKS

Chandra, Amit, and Matthew Dacso. *Tarascon Global Health Pocketbook*. Sudbury, MA: Jones and Bartlett, 2011.

PERIODICALS

Kozicki, Zigmond A., et al. "Waterborne Pathogens: A Public Health Risk in U.S. Hospitals." *American Water Works Association* 104, no. 1 (January 2012): 52–56.

WEBSITES

Center for Food Safety and Applied Nutrition. "Bad Bug Book—Foodborne Pathogenic Microorganisms and Natural Toxins." U.S. Food and Drug Administration. March 3, 2011. http://www.fda.gov/Food/FoodSafety/FoodborneIllness/FoodborneIllnessFoodbornePathogensNaturalToxins/BadBugBook/default.htm (accessed February 8, 2012).

Centers for Disease Control and Prevention. "Parasites: Water." http://www.cdc.gov/parasites/water.html (accessed February 8, 2012).

Centers for Disease Control and Prevention. "Water-Related Diseases, Contaminants, & Injuries." http://www.cdc.gov/healthywater/disease (accessed February 8, 2012).

U.S. Environmental Protection Agency. "Basic Information about E. coli 0157:H7 in Drinking Water." Water: Basic Information about Regulated Drinking Water

Contaminants. http://water.epa.gov/drink/contaminants/basicin formation/ecoli.cfm (accessed February 8, 2012).

ORGANIZATIONS
Centers for Disease Control and Prevention, 1600 Clifton Rd., Atlanta, GA 30333, (800) 232-4636, cdcinfor@cdc.gov, http://www.cdc.gov.
Environmental Protection Agency, 1200 Pennsylvania Ave. NW, Washington, DC 20460, (202) 272-0167, http://water.epa.gov.

Margaret Alic, PhD

West Nile virus

Definition

West Nile virus is a mosquito-borne virus that causes viral illnesses of varying seriousness, ranging from no symptoms or mild flu-like symptoms to encephalitis or **meningitis**.

Demographics

In the United States, the **Centers for Disease Control and Prevention** (CDC) monitors and records human WNV infections. In 2011, 714 cases and 43 deaths due to WNV were reported in the United States. In that year, only Maine, Alaska, and Hawaii were free of the virus, although South Carolina, New Hampshire, Washington, and Oregon reported no human cases. In those states the virus only detected only in animals. As of 2012, the virus was found from Canada to Venezuela and in Africa, Europe, the Middle East, North America and West Asia.

Among those with severe illness due to West Nile virus, fatality rates range from 3% to 15% with the highest rates are among the elderly. Less than 1% of people who become infected with West Nile virus develop severe illness. According to the **World Health Organization** (WHO), about 80% of people who are infected do not show any symptoms of the disease at all. Others have mild flu-like symptoms.

Description

The primary hosts of West Nile virus (WNV) are birds, in which the virus numbers multiply before being transmitted by mosquitoes to the next victim. Over 140 species of birds can be infected with WNV. Besides birds, the virus can infect other vertebrates, including humans and horses.

WNV is a flavivirus that belongs to the Japanese encephalitis serocomplex, which includes St. Louis encephalitis, Murray Valley encephalitis, and Kunjin virus. Infections occur generally between late summer and early fall in temperate areas, and throughout the year in southern climates. Although typical manifestation of WNV is asymptomatic, the virus can cross the blood-brain barrier and cause severe illness and paralysis.

WNV was originally isolated in a feverish woman living in the West Nile District of Uganda during 1937. The virus was ecologically characterized in Egypt during the 1950s and later linked to severe human meningoencephalitis in elderly patients during a 1957 outbreak in Israel. Since 1937, subsequent outbreaks of WNV have been reported in Africa, Asia, Australia, Oceania, Western Europe, and the Middle East.

In the summer of 1999, WNV was first reported in the New York City area and then spread rapidly across the entire continent. It is suspected that the transport of infected birds or the international travel of infected humans from Israel and/or Tunisia may have imported the disease into North America. After its arrival in the New Work area, the virus spread rapidly across the United States, as well as north into Canada and south into Mexico. In 2002, a severe outbreak of WNV in the United States killed 284 people and caused 2,944 cases of severe brain damage. This was the worst outbreak in the United States to date.

Life cycle and Transmission

Like most flaviviruses, the WNV is maintained in a natural host-vector-host cycle, where the primary vector is the mosquito. The zoonotic cycle begins with a reservoir host, which is most commonly of avian origin. When a mosquito feeds on the infected bird, the virus is passed to the insect along with the blood meal. The virus then multiplies rapidly within the mosquito's body and salivary glands over the next few days. When the insect feeds on another animal or human, the virus can be transmitted through the bite and cause serious illness.

Most mosquitoes can become infected with the WNV. However, female mosquitoes of the *Culex pipiens* species are of particular concern, as they live in suburban and urban areas, can survive through the winter, prefer to feed on birds, and frequently bite humans. The *C. pipiens*, also known as the house mosquito, is also the most common vector for WNV transmission. *Culex restuan*, *Culex quinquefasciatus*, *Aedes Albopictus*, and *Aedes Vexans* are also common carriers of the WNV.

Common food sources for mosquitoes, birds represent the primary WNV reservoir species. A continent-wide study published in 2007 suggests that WNV has severely affected bird populations associated with human habitats in North America. Many in the scientific community believe that the rapid spread of WNV in North America may be due in part to the migratory nature of birds. Infected birds carry the virus with them as they travel in summer and winter, thus acting as reservoirs in their new nesting sites. Across the world, outbreaks occur most commonly along the main migration routes of migratory birds.

Most vertebrates, such as alligators, bats, chipmunks, skunks, squirrels, and rabbits, can also be infected with WNV. Horses, in particular, are commonly infected with WNV. Like humans, the majority of horses suffer either no or mild symptoms, but severe illness and death can and does occur. There are relatively few cases of dogs and cats becoming infected with WNV. Animals of all species exhibiting fever, weakness, poor coordination, spasms, seizures, and/or personality changes may be infected with WNV.

Risk factors

There is no evidence of WNV transmission from person-to-person through touch, kissing, or other contact. However, there is evidence of WNV transplacental (mother-to-child) transmission, as well as viral transmission through breastfeeding. As such, pregnant mothers should be aware of the presence of WNV in their area and take appropriate precautions. The transmission of WNV has also occurred in blood transfusions and organ transplants although the current blood supply is now tested for the presence of the WNV. People that are immunocompromised (from disease or chemotherapy, for example) and people aged 50 and older represent the highest risk group for serious WNV infection.

Causes and symptoms

The exact mechanism of WNV–caused illnesses remains unclear. However, it is suspected that the virus enters the host's blood stream and multiples. The incubation period for WNV after infection typical ranges between 3 to 14 days. WNV can then develop to the point where it crosses the blood-brain barrier, which separates the blood from the central nervous system. When this occurs, the virus can infect the brain, spinal cord, and other vital systems, creating a potentially deadly inflammatory response.

Most infected persons will exhibit a series of mild flu-like symptoms, also known as West Nile Fever. These mild symptoms can persist for 3–6 days, and occasionally for weeks. They include:

- eye pain
- fever
- headache
- loss of appetite
- lymphadenopathy (abnormal enlargement of the lymph nodes)
- malaise (nonspecific bodily discomfort)
- myalgia (nonspecific muscular pain/tenderness)
- nausea
- rash (on the neck, torso, and limbs)
- vomiting

In rare cases, approximately 1 in 150 cases (0.7%), WNV can cross the blood-brain barrier and develop into a severe neuroinvasive disease. Immunocompromised individuals and those over age 50 years are at an increased risk for developing more severe syndromes; a 20-fold increase in incidence among older patients has been reported. Symptoms indicating the possible presence of severe West Nile-related syndromes include:

- severe headache
- high fever
- acute muscle weakness
- neck stiffness
- convulsions and tremors
- disorientation and stupor
- paralysis
- coma

People exposed to WNV infection, especially the immunocompromised and elderly, should contact their health provider immediately if they develop a severe headache accompanied by high fever.

Typically, severe WNV syndromes manifest as one of three syndromes: West Nile encephalitis (inflammation of the brain); West Nile meningitis (inflammation of the meninges of the brain and spinal cord); or West Nile meningoencephalitis (inflammation of both the brain and the meninges). These three syndromes can cause severe brain damage and death. The majority of deaths result from complications attributable to West Nile meningoencephalitis. Additionally, severe WNV disease can cause acute vision loss due to inflammatory disorders of the eye, such as chorioretinitis, optic neuritis, retinal vasculitis, uveitis, and vitritis. Less frequently, the patient can exhibit acute flaccid paralysis, similar to poliomyelitis (**polio**) or Guillain-Barré syndrome, caused by inflammation of the spinal cord and/or damage to the peripheral nerves. In some severe cases, this acute flaccid paralysis can disrupt muscles that control breathing and result in respiratory failure.

Diagnosis

A proper diagnosis of WNV infection depends heavily upon clinical presentation, laboratory testing, and patient history. Patients with a known susceptibility to WNV (the elderly and immunocompromised) who exhibit symptoms during the late spring to early fall, or at any time in warmer climates, should be tested for WNV and other arboviral infections. Additionally, healthcare providers should remain aware of the local presence of WNV activity, such as reports of recent animal and/or human cases. Similarity of symptoms and serological cross-reactivity of WNV and other flaviviruses, may lead to confusion and an incorrect diagnosis. Healthcare providers must use thorough laboratory testing to differentiate WNV antibodies from those of other arboviruses.

Symptomatic WNV infection can be classified as either non–neuroinvasive or neuroinvasive, with each being identified according to certain criteria.

Non-neuroinvasive

The majority of WNV infections are asymptomatic. In approximately 20% of WNV cases, clinically recognizable symptoms can manifest. However, to be clinically classified as non-neuroinvasive West Nile disease, the following must be true:

- no neuroinvasive symptomology
- presence of fever without other recognizable cause
- four-fold or greater increase in serum antibody titer
- virus isolated from and or demonstrated in blood, tissue, cerebrospinal fluid (CSF), or other bodily fluid
- virus-specific immunoglobulin M (IgM antibodies demonstrated in CSF through antibody-capture methods

Neuroinvasive

In rare cases (0.7%) of West Nile disease, the virus crosses the blood-brain barrier and manifests in severe and life-threatening symptoms. Clinical confirmation of neuroinvasive of neuroinvasive disease requires the presence of a fever and at least one of the following:

- acutely altered mental status, such as disorientation, stupor, or coma
- acute central or peripheral neurological difficulties, such as paralysis, nerve palsy, sensory deficits, and abnormal muscle function
- an increased white blood cell concentration in the CSF coupled with symptoms of meningitis, such as severe headache and neck pain

---

KEY TERMS

Blood-brain barrier—An arrangement of cells within the blood vessels of the brain that prevents the passage of toxic substances, including infectious agents, from the blood and into the brain. It also makes it difficult for certain medications to pass into brain tissue.

Flavivirus—An arbovirus that can cause potentially serious diseases, such as dengue, yellow fever, Japanese encephalitis, and West Nile fever.

Guillain-Barré—A disorder in which the body's immune system attacks part of the peripheral nervous system. Weakness, tingling, and abnormal sensations in the arms and upper body can progress until the muscles become totally disabled and the patient is effectively paralyzed.

Meninges—A series of membranous layers of connective tissue that protect the central nervous system (brain and spinal cord). Damage or infection to the meninges, such as in meningitis, can cause serious neurological damage and even death.

Zoonotic diseases—Diseases caused by infectious agents that can be transmitted between (or are shared by) animals and humans. This can include transmission through the bite of an insect, such as a mosquito.

Treatment

As of 2012, there are no treatment modalities for WNV infection. Antibiotics are ineffective against WNV as they are against all **viruses**. Instead, supportive care is used to treat the varying symptoms and syndromes associated with the various West Nile diseases. Although milder symptoms can be treated at home, severe symptoms can require hospitalization. Treatment of severe symptoms may require the use of intravenous infusions, airway and respiratory management and support, and use of preventive measures against secondary infection.

In severe cases of flaccid paralysis, physical therapy and occupational therapy may be used to help restore some muscle function.

Prognosis

The majority of WNV infections are asymptomatic. West Nile fever offers an excellent prognosis associated with quick recovery and no long-term side effects. The majority of symptoms resolve within a few days or weeks.

> ## QUESTIONS TO ASK YOUR DOCTOR
>
> - Have any WNV cases been reported in this area recently?
> - I am going to travel abroad to areas where WNV is common. What precautions should I take?
> - I know that horses often are infected with WNV. Does being around horses increase my chance of infection?
> - My child handled a dead bird. Does that increase his chances of developing WNV?

The prognosis is not as positive for patients experiencing the more severe syndromes attributable to WNV infection. Symptoms of West Nile encephalitis, West Nile meningitis, and West Nile meningoencephalitis can last for several weeks, as well as cause severe and permanent neurological damage. Inflammation can interfere with the brain and central nervous system and result in death, especially among the elderly population. Patients may suffer prolonged muscle weakness and loss of motor control. Long-term rehabilitation is typically required and a full recovery is not assured. If the muscles used for breathing are affected, death from respiratory failure may result.

Public health role and response

The CDC requires that state and local public health offices report cases of WNV. These cases are tracked and updated weekly on the CDC website. When a major outbreak occurs, public service announcements are made reminding individuals of preventative measure. Internationally WHO also monitors outbreaks of WNV.

Local municipalities are responsible for mosquito abatement programs, which help control various mosquito-borne diseases including WNV. These programs usually involve widespread aerial spraying of insecticide. Often there is opposition to insecticide spraying by individuals concerned with exposure to chemicals. Mosquito abatement programs try to balance the need for disease control and the desire of residents to remain pesticide-free.

Prevention

Although there is a vaccine used for horses and exotic birds in zoos, there is no WNV vaccine for humans at the current time. Several pharmaceutical companies, however, have WNV vaccines in development.

Prevention techniques of WNV typically coincide with avoidance measures against mosquito bites, the primary source of the virus. These include the use of insect repellant (with 5–20% DEET) on exposed body parts, wearing loose-fitting clothes over the limbs and torso while outdoors, using mosquito coils and/or citronella candles outdoors, and limiting outdoor activities during peak biting periods and/or in areas with high mosquito density. While camping outdoors, knockdown spray or bed netting with pyrethrum is suggested. Mosquito eradication programs have been instituted in most major cities.

The *C. pipiens* mosquito is the primary vector of WNV transmission and also commonly lives and feeds in urban areas. Special precautions should be taken to reduce exposure to these potentially infected insects. Screen doors and enclosed porches can help keep mosquitoes from coming into the house. It should be noted that studies have shown that mosquito control devices such as "bug zappers" and CO2-baited traps do not significantly reduce the risk of being bitten.

Removing potential mosquito breeding areas from near the home and from the neighborhood can further reduce the risk of bites. Any container which can collect half an inch of standing water can become a potential breeding site in as little as five days. Old tires, empty plant pots, and empty trashcans should be removed, while water sources like ponds or birdbaths should be cleaned regularly. Standing water on any property should be drained, such as from clogged eaves. Swimming pools and hot tubs should be properly covered and chlorinated to prevent mosquitoes breeding in them.

Resources

BOOKS

Oldstone, Michael B. A. *Viruses, Plagues, and History: Past, Present, and Future.* Oxford, UK; New York: Oxford University Press, 2010.

Sfakianos, Jeffrey and Alan Hecht. *West Nile Virus*, 2nd ed. New York: Chelsea House, 2009.

Wiwanitkit, Viroj *Focus on Arbovirus Infections.* Hauppauge NY: Nova Science Publishers, 2009.

WEBSITES

West Nile Virus: Fight the Bite. Centers for Disease Control and Prevention (CDC). June 19, 2012. http://www.cdc.gov/ncidod/dvbid/westnile/index.html (accessed June 27, 2012).

Salinas, Jess D. West Nile Virus. Medscape.com January 18, 2012. http://emedicine.medscape.com/article/312210-overview (accessed June 27, 2012).

West Nile Virus. MedlinePlus June 11, 2012. http://www.nlm.nih.gov/medlineplus/westnilevirus.html (accessed June 27, 2102).

West Nile Virus. World Health Organization (WHO) July 2011. http://www.who.int/mediacentre/factsheets/fs354/en/index.html (accessed June 27, 2102).

ORGANIZATIONS

National Institute of Allergy and Infectious Diseases Office of Communications and Government Relations, 6610 Rockledge Drive, MSC 6612, Bethesda, MD 20892-6612, (301) 496-5717, (866) 284-4107 or TDD: (800)877-8339 (for hearing impaired), Fax: (301) 402-3573, http://www3.niaid.nih.gov.

United States Centers for Disease Control and Prevention (CDC), 1600 Clifton Road, Atlanta, GA 30333, (404) 639-3534, 800-CDC-INFO (800-232-4636). TTY: (888) 232-6348, inquiry@cdc.gov, http://www.cdc.gov.

World Health Organization, Avenue Appia 20, 1211 Geneva 27, Switzerland, +22 41 791 21 11, Fax: +22 41 791 31 11, info@who.int, http://www.who.int.

Monique Laberge, PhD
Tish Davidson, AM

Whooping cough

Definition

Whooping cough, also known as pertussis, is a highly contagious disease that causes spasms (paroxysms) of uncontrollable coughing, followed by a sharp, high-pitched intake of air that creates the characteristic "whoop" of the disease's name.

Demographics

Pertussis was once one of the most deadly of all infectious childhood diseases in the United States and most other parts of the world. In 1923, 9,269 deaths from the disease were recorded in the United States, the largest number ever. In the period between 1934 and 1943, an average of more than 200,000 new cases of pertussis were being reported annually in the United States, with an average of just over 4,000 deaths per year from the disease. Since the 1940s, the rate of morbidity and mortality from the disease has continued to decrease to very low levels. In 1950, the U.S. **Centers for Disease Control and Prevention** (CDC) reported 120,718 new cases of pertussis in the United States, a number that gradually fell to 14,809 in 1960, 4,249 in 1970, and 1,730 in 1980. Since that time, the number of new cases of pertussis remained at less than 10,000 per year until 2003, when the rate began to climb, to a high of 25,616 new cases in 2005. It fell again to a total of 16,858 new cases in 2009. The cause for this resurgence of the disease in the twenty-first century is not known for certain, although some experts believe that doubts about the safety of pertussis vaccines may be partially responsible for fewer children being vaccinated and, hence, at greater risk for the disease.

Pertussis occurs equally in males and females. Whites make up the large majority at over 85% of cases diagnosed. People under the age of 20 years make up over 75% of cases, most of these being reported in children under the age of one or between the ages of 10 and 19. Because the whooping cough **vaccination** does not provide lifelong immunity and immunity is no longer evident after 12 years, people must be revaccinated in order to be protected.

Description

Whooping cough is caused by a bacterium called *Bordatella pertussis*. *B. pertussis* causes its most severe symptoms by attaching itself to cells in the respiratory tract that have cilia. Cilia are small, hair-like projections that beat continuously, and serve to constantly sweep the respiratory tract clean of such debris as mucus, bacteria, **viruses**, and dead cells. When *B. pertussis* interferes with this normal janitorial function, mucus and cellular debris accumulate and cause constant irritation to the respiratory tract, triggering coughing and increasing further mucus production.

Whooping cough is a disease that exists throughout the world. While people of any age can contract whooping cough, children under the age of two are at the highest risk for the disease and for serious complications and death. Apparently, exposure to *B. pertussis* bacteria earlier in life gives a person some immunity against infection with it later on. Subsequent infections resemble the common cold.

Causes and symptoms

Whooping cough has four somewhat overlapping stages: incubation, the catarrhal stage, the paroxysmal stage, and the convalescent stage.

An individual usually acquires *B. pertussis* by inhaling droplets infected with the bacteria coughed into the air by someone with the infection. Incubation is the symptomless period of 7 to 14 days after breathing in the *B. pertussis* bacteria, and during which the bacteria multiply and penetrate the lining tissues of the entire respiratory tract.

The catarrhal stage is often mistaken for an exceedingly heavy cold. The patient has teary eyes, sneezing, fatigue, a poor appetite, and an extremely runny nose (rhinorrhea). This stage lasts about 10 to 14 days.

The paroxysmal stage, lasting two to four weeks, begins with the development of the characteristic whooping cough. Spasms of uncontrollable coughing, the "whooping" sound of the sharp inspiration of air, and vomiting are all hallmarks of this stage. The whoop is believed to occur due to inflammation and mucus, which narrow the breathing tubes, causing the patient to struggle to get air into his or her lungs; the effort results in intense exhaustion. The paroxysms (spasms) can be induced by activity, feeding, crying, or even overhearing someone else cough.

The mucus produced during the paroxysmal stage is thicker and more difficult to clear than the more watery mucus of the catarrhal stage, and the patient becomes increasingly exhausted attempting to clear the respiratory tract through coughing. Severely ill children may have great difficulty maintaining the normal level of oxygen in their system and may appear somewhat blue (cyanotic) after a paroxysm of coughing, due to the low oxygen content of their blood. Such children may experience swelling and degeneration of the brain (encephalopathy), which is believed to be caused both by lack of oxygen to the brain during paroxysms and by bleeding into the brain caused by increased pressure during coughing. Seizures may result from decreased oxygen to the brain. Some children have such greatly increased abdominal pressure during coughing that hernias result. (Hernias are the abnormal protrusion of a loop of intestine through a weak area of muscle.) Another complicating factor during this phase is the development of pneumonia from infection with another bacterial agent; the bacteria take hold due to the patient's already-weakened condition.

If the patient survives the paroxysmal stage, recovery occurs gradually during the convalescent stage, usually taking about three to four weeks. However, spasms of coughing may continue to occur over a period of months, especially when a patient contracts a cold or other respiratory infection.

Diagnosis

Examination

Diagnosis based just on the patient's symptoms is not particularly accurate, as the catarrhal stage may appear to be a heavy cold, a case of influenza, or a simple **bronchitis**. Other viruses and **tuberculosis** infections can cause symptoms similar to those found during the paroxysmal stage. The presence of a pertussis-like cough along with an

> **KEY TERMS**
>
> **Bordatella pertussis**—A bacterium that causes whooping cough by attaching itself to cells in the respiratory tract.
>
> **Cilia**—Tiny, hair-like projections from a cell. In the respiratory tract, cilia beat constantly in order to move mucus and debris up and out of the respiratory tree, in order to protect the lung from infection or irritation by foreign bodies.
>
> **Encephalopathy**—Swelling and degeneration of the brain.
>
> **Lymphocytes**—A type of white blood cell.
>
> **Nasopharynx**—The breathing tube continuous with the nose.
>
> **Rhinorrhea**—A name for the common cold.

increase of certain specific white blood cells (lymphocytes) is suggestive of whooping cough. However, cough can occur from other pertussis-like viruses.

Tests

The most accurate method of diagnosis is to culture (grow on a laboratory plate) the organisms obtained from swabbing mucus out of the nasopharynx (the breathing tube continuous with the nose). *B. pertussis* can then be identified by examining the culture under a microscope.

Treatment

Drugs

Treatment with the antibiotic erythromycin is helpful only at very early stages of whooping cough, during incubation and early in the catarrhal stage. After the cilia and the cells bearing those cilia are damaged, the process cannot be reversed. Such a patient will experience the full progression of whooping cough symptoms; symptoms only improve when the old, damaged lining cells of the respiratory tract are replaced over time with new, healthy, cilia-bearing cells. However, treatment with erythromycin is still recommended to decrease the likelihood of *B. pertussis* spreading. In fact, all members of the household where a patient with whooping cough lives should be treated with erythromycin to prevent the spread of *B. pertussis* throughout the community.

Home remedies

The only other treatment is supportive and involves careful monitoring of fluids to prevent dehydration; rest in a quiet, dark room to decrease paroxysms; and suctioning of mucus. Patients should be hospitalized if at risk for complication, such as infants from birth to six months of age.

Prognosis

Just under 1% of all cases of whooping cough cause death. Children who die of whooping cough usually have one or more of the following three conditions present:

- severe pneumonia, perhaps with accompanying encephalopathy
- extreme weight loss, weakness, and metabolic abnormalities due to persistent vomiting during paroxysms of coughing
- other pre-existing conditions, so that the patient is already in a relatively weak, vulnerable state (such conditions may include low birth weight, poor nutrition, infection with the measles virus, presence of other respiratory or gastrointestinal infections or diseases)

Prevention

The mainstay of prevention lies in programs similar to the mass immunization program in the United States, which begins immunization inoculations when infants are two months old. The pertussis vaccine, most often given as one immunization together with **diphtheria** and tetanus (DTP or DTaP), has greatly reduced the incidence of whooping cough.

There has been some concern about serious neurologic side effects from the vaccine itself. This concern has led many parents in England, Japan, and Sweden to avoid immunizing their children, which in turn has led to major epidemics of disease in those countries. However, several carefully constructed research studies have disproved the idea that the pertussis vaccine is the cause of neurologic damage. Furthermore, a newer formulation of the pertussis vaccine is available. Unlike the old whole cell pertussis vaccine, which is composed of the entire bacterial cell that has been deactivated (and therefore unable to cause infection), the newer acellular pertussis vaccine does not use a whole cell of the bacteria. Instead, it is made up of between two and five chemical components of the *B. pertussis* bacterium. The acellular pertussis vaccine appears to greatly reduce the risk of unpleasant reactions to the vaccine, including high fever and discomfort following vaccination.

Resources

BOOKS

Kitta, Andrea. *Vaccinations and Public Concern in History: Legend, Rumor, and Risk Perception*. New York: Routledge, 2012.

Long, Sarah S. *Principles and Practice of Pediatric Infectious Disease*. Edinburgh: Churchill Livingstone, 2012.

Stratton, Kathleen R., ed. *Adverse Effects of Vaccines: Evidence and Causality*. Washington, DC: National Academies Press, 2012.

Wertheim, Heiman F.L., Peter Horby, and John P. Woodall. *Atlas of Human Infectious Diseases*. Hoboken, NJ: John Wiley & Sons, 2012.

PERIODICALS

Bugenske, E., et al. "Middle School Vaccination Requirements and Adolescent Vaccination Coverage." *Pediatrics* 129, 6. (2012): 1056–63.

Clark, Thomas A., Nancy E. Messonnier, and Stephen C. Hadler. "Pertussis Control: Time for Something New?." *Trends in Microbiology* 20, 5. (2012): 211–13.

Girard, D.Z. "Recommended or Mandatory Pertussis Vaccination Policy in Developed Countries: Does the Choice Matter?" *Public Health* 126, 2. (2012): 129–34.

Libster, R., and K.M. Edwards. "How Can We Best Prevent Pertussis in Infants?" *Clinical Infectious Diseases* 54, 1. (2012): 85–87.

WEBSITES

Bocka, Joseph J. "Pertussis." Medscape Reference. http://emedicine.medscape.com/article/967268-overview. Accessed on November 2, 2012.

"DTaP Immunization (Vaccine)." Medline Plus. http://www.nlm.nih.gov/medlineplus/ency/article/002021.htm. Accessed on November 2, 2012.

"Pertussis (Whooping Cough) Vaccination." Centers for Disease Control and Prevention. http://www.cdc.gov/vaccines/vpd-vac/pertussis/default.htm. Accessed on November 2, 2012.

"Whooping Cough." Medline Plus. http://www.nlm.nih.gov/medlineplus/whoopingcough.html. Accessed on November 2, 2012.

ORGANIZATIONS

American Academy of Family Physicians, P.O. Box 11210, Shawnee Mission, KS 66207, (913) 906–6000, (800) 274-2237, Fax: (913) 906–6075, http://familydoctor.org/familydoctor/en/about/contact-us.html, http://familydoctor.org.

American Academy of Pediatrics, 141 Northwest Point Blvd., Elk Grove Village, IL 60007–1098, (847) 434–4000, Fax: (847) 434–8000, http://www2.aap.org/visit/contact.htm, http://www.aap.org.

Centers for Disease Control and Prevention (CDC), 1600 Clifton Rd., Atlanta, GA 30333, (404) 639–3534, (800) CDC–INFO (800–232–4636). TTY: (888) 232–6348, inquiry@cdc.gov, http://www.cdc.gov.

National Institute of Allergy and Infectious Diseases Office of Communications and Government Relations, 6610 Rockledge Dr., MSC 6612, Bethesda, MD 20892-6612, (301) 496–5717, (866) 284–4107, or TDD: (800) 877–8339 (for hearing impaired), Fax: (301) 402-3573, ocpostoffice@niaid.nih.gov, http://www3.niaid.nih.gov.

World Health Organization, Avenue Appia 20, 1211 Geneva 27, Switzerland, +22 41 791 21 11, Fax: +22 41 791 31 11, info@who.int, http://www.who.int.

Rosalyn Carson-DeWitt, MD
Tish Davidson, AM
Paul Checchia, MD

Wildfires

Definition

A wildfire is a quick-spreading, uncontrolled fire in the countryside or a wilderness area.

Demographics

Wildfires are a serious threat throughout the world. One very bad wildfires took place in February 2009, in the Australian state of Victoria. On February 7, over 400 small fires were reported, which resulted in destroying over 820,000 acres, killing 173 people, and injuring at least 414 more. Another deadly wildfire took place in Russia during the summer 2010. Over 280,000 acres burned in Western Russia killing at least 60 people. In September 2012, Russia experienced another giant wildfire in Siberia that burned over 74 million acres of land. Earlier that same year, 16 wildfires blazed simultaneously in the western United States. On average, over 5 million acres of land is burned due to wildfire each year in the United States alone. Although these fires can replenish soil nutrients and give space for new plants to grow, they also cause millions of dollars of damage and put thousands of lives at risk.

Description

Few natural forces match fire for its range of impact on the human consciousness, with a roaring forest fire at

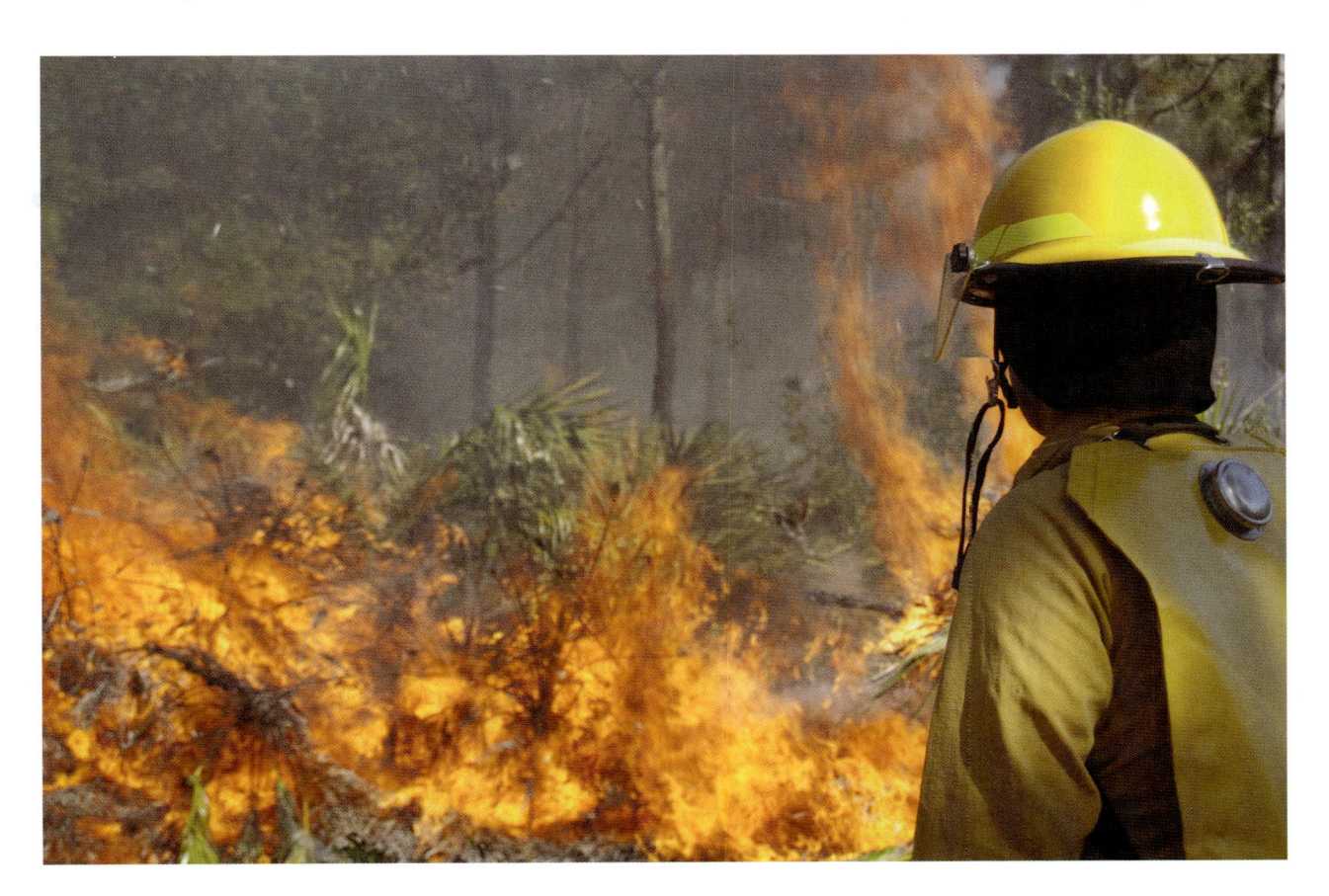

A firefighter watches a blazing wildfire (© iStockphoto.com/Jeremy Sterk.)

INDONESIAN FOREST FIRES (1997–1998)

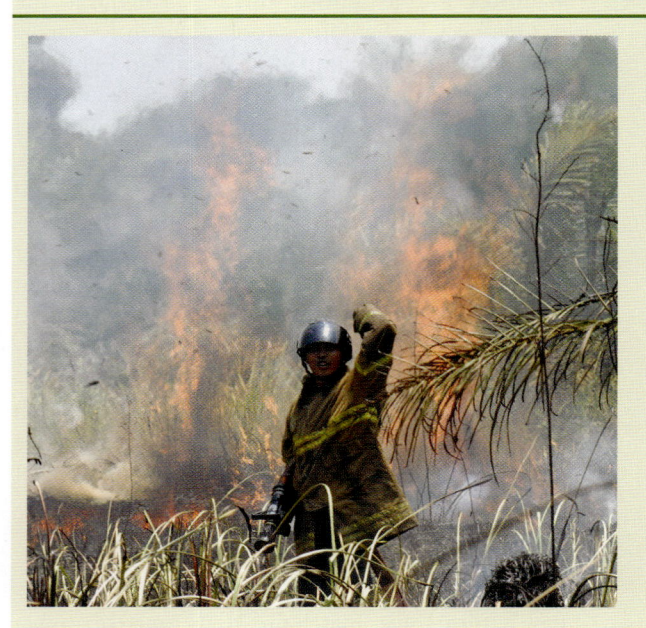

To prepare the Indonesian forestland for the upcoming planting season, farmers use fire to burn specific forest areas. Unfortunately, the droughts of 1997 and 1998 caused extremely dry conditions. Fires spread quickly, destroying approximately 8,000 square miles of Indonesian forest. The smoke and haze spread to other counties, affecting 75 million people. The poor air quality resulted in severe health problems, including asthma, emphysema, bronchitis, and death.

The fires did not only affect humans. The wildlife suffered from loss of habitat and health issues. Creatures, such as orangutans, were in a disorientated state due to the noxious smoke, and aquatic life lost their clear waters.

The dire effects of these forest fires did nothing to quell future fires. Farmers continue to set fires every year. In 2002, the Association of Southeast Asian Nations (ASEAN) countries signed the "ASEAN Agreement on Transboundary Haze Pollution", in an attempt to control the burning. However, Indonesia has not ratified this agreement.

A fire fighter battles a blaze in the sub-district of Ilir Barat outside Palembang city, South Sumatra on September 3, 2006. (© STRINGERINDONESIAReutersCorbis.)

---

one extreme and a warming and comforting campfire or cooking flame at the other. Along with earth, water, and air, fire is one of the original "elements" once thought to comprise the universe, and it frightened and fascinated people long before the beginning of modern civilization. In nature, fire both destroys and renews. A wildfire is a fire that spreads quickly in the wilderness. Depending on what type of vegetation is burned, wildfire may also be called bush fire, brushfire, forest fire, desert fire, grass fire, or vegetation fire.

Fire is an oxidation process that rapidly transforms the potential energy stored in chemical bonds of organic compounds into the kinetic energy forms of heat and light. Like the much slower oxidation process of decomposition, fire destroys organic matter, creating a myriad of gases and ions and liberating much of the carbon and hydrogen as carbon dioxide and water. A large portion of the remaining organic matter is converted to ash, which may go up in the smoke, blow or wash away after the fire, or, like the humus created by decomposition, be incorporated into the soil.

Risk factors

Wildfires take place on every continent except Antarctica. Wildfires are especially common in Australia, Southeast Asia, and Southern Africa. In the United States, all 50 states have experienced wildfires; however, most fires take place in the West where conditions are optimal for wildfires to start.

Areas in the most danger of wildfire have long dry summers or suffer from **drought** conditions. These areas have dried out vegetation that can catch fire easily.

Wildfires can start in many ways. Sometimes there is a natural cause that starts a wildfire, for example, a lightning strike. Nevertheless, four out of five wildfires are started by humans. Sometimes this is by accident, such as a dropped cigarette butt or uncontrolled campfire. Other times, wildfires are started deliberately by an arsonist. With the right conditions, a tiny spark can cause hundreds of thousands of acres of wilderness to burn. Once a fire starts in a dry area, it moves quickly and is hard to control, moving at speeds up to 14 miles per hour (22 km/h).

Effects on public health

Beyond destroying land and homes, wildfires also pose a serious risk to people. Smoke caused by wildfire can worsen chronic heart and lung diseases and cause

KEY TERMS

Anxiety—Worry or tension in response to real or imagined stress, danger, or dreaded situations. Physical reactions, such as fast pulse, sweating, trembling, fatigue, and weakness may accompany anxiety.

Asthma—A disease in which the air passages of the lungs become inflamed and narrowed.

Depression—A mental condition in which a person feels extremely sad and loses interest in life. A person with depression may also have sleep problems and loss of appetite and may have trouble concentrating and carrying out everyday activities. Severe depression may instigate a suicide attempt.

Phobia—An intense, abnormal, or illogical fear of something specific, such as heights or open spaces.

healthy people to become sick. Smoke is especially dangerous for the young, the elderly, and people suffering from a chronic respiratory illness such as cystic **fibrosis** or **asthma**. Being in a smoky area can cause coughing, irritation to the eyes and sinuses, a scratchy throat, headaches, a runny nose, chest pains, and difficulty breathing. Burns or injuries that happen while trying to fight the wildfire or evacuate the area also are common health problems associated with wildfires. Those who do not evacuate in time may become trapped and die of smoke inhalation. Depression, **post-traumatic stress disorder**, anxiety, and phobia have been seen in people who are directly or indirectly affected by wildfires.

Treatment

Typically, once a person is away from a wildfire and has clean, smoke-free air to breathe, symptoms fade quickly. People who continue to experience symptoms or have a chronic disease or a history of heart or lung disease should speak to their doctor about possible complications. Burns and serious smoke inhalation or other injuries sustained should be treated by a healthcare professional right away. People showing signs of depression, phobia, anxiety, or post-traumatic stress disorder should also speak to their healthcare professional about treatment possibilities.

Public health role and response

Although fire is vital to the long-term health and sustainability of many ecosystems, wildfires cause numerous human deaths and destroy millions of dollars of property each year. Controlling these destructive fires means fighting them aggressively. Fire fighters can be exposed to furfural (an organic compound created when wheat, sawdust, and other materials burn) produced in the combustion process. Fire suppression efforts are based on the fact that any fire requires three factors: heat, fuel, and oxygen. Together, these make up the three parts of the "fire triangle" known to all fire fighters. The strategy in all fire fighting is to extinguish the blaze by breaking one part of this triangle. An entire science has developed around fire behavior and the effects of changing weather, topography, and fuels on that behavior. Common responses to wildfire include sending in firefighters on the ground or dropping fire retardants and water by planes, helicopters, and unmanned aerial vehicles.

Prognosis

Many people do not experience any long-lasting effects after being in or close to a wildfire area. Most symptoms fade quickly once people are back in clean and smoke-free air. However, long-term exposure to smoke can cause serious problems. It is estimated that 339,000 deaths each year are caused by exposure to wildfire smoke. Firefighters also experience health problems due to breathing in smoke and chemicals repeatedly.

Prevention

The first step to preventing wildfires is education. Educating the public about how to prevent fires, such as extinguishing campfires completely and not dropping lit cigarette butts, can make a major impact on the number of wildfires that occur each year. Mascots, such as the U.S. Forest Service's Smokey the Bear, are used to teach children and adults the importance to preventing wildfires. Other prevention methods include controlled burns, clearing trees or dried brush, and developing fuel-free fire lines between homes and wilderness.

Resources

BOOKS

Silverstein, Alvin, et al. *Wildfires: The Science Behind Raging Infernos.* Berkeley Heights, NJ: Enslow, 2009.

WEBSITES

Bonsor, Kevin. "How Wildfires Work." http://science.howstuffworks.com/nature/natural-disasters/wildfire.htm (accessed September 26, 2012).

Centers for Disease Control and Prevention. "Wildfires." http://www.bt.cdc.gov/disasters/wildfires (accessed September 26, 2012).

QUESTIONS TO ASK YOUR DOCTOR

- How can I protect myself from smoke during a wildfire?
- Are my anxiety and nightmares normal after experiencing a wildfire?
- How long does it typically take for a burn to heal?

Federal Emergency Management Agency. "Wildfires." www.ready.gov/wildfires (accessed September 26, 2012).
National Geographic. "Wildfires." http://environment.nationalgeographic.com/environment/natural-disasters/wildfires (accessed September 26, 2012).

ORGANIZATIONS

Federal Emergency Management Agency (FEMA), PO Box 10055, Hyattsville, MD 20782, (202) 646-2500, (800) 621-3362, http://www.fema.gov.
International Association of Wildland Fires, 1418 Washburn St., Missoula, MT 59801, (406) 531-8264, (888) 440-4293, iawf@iawfonline.org, http://www.iawfonline.org.
National Wildfire Suppression Association, PO Box 330, Lyons, OR 97358, (877) 676-6972, Fax: (866) 854-8186, http://www.nwsa.us.

Tish Davidson, AM

Wool-sorter's disease *see* **Anthrax**

World Health Organization

Definition

The World Health Organization (WHO) is the health authority within the United Nations (UN). The UN is an international organization concerned with coordinating efforts to make the world safer for future generations.

Purpose

WHO is charged by the UN with coordinating and directing global health issues. In this role, WHO leads research in countries around the world concerning public health problems, diseases, and treatments. The research can involve monitoring and improving health trends. WHO also suggests or sets policies regarding health and disease prevention, along with becoming involved in global matters that can prevent disease or improve health. WHO also provides resources and technical support to countries around the world. The philosophy of the organization is that health is a shared responsibility, as is access to health care.

WHO has set an agenda aimed at improving public health that included the following:

- Promote health development, and specifically prevent and treat chronic diseases by ensuring care is not denied and by addressing neglected tropical diseases.
- Foster health security by continuing to strengthen revised health regulations and helping all people and communities defend against disease outbreaks.
- Strengthen health systems to help reduce poverty by supporting financing, staffing, and technology in areas that need it.
- Harness research and information to provide evidence needed to set and monitor health priorities.
- Enhance partnerships to gain collaboration of private partners to best establish and reach goals in countries.
- Improve performance of WHO by being more effective and efficient.

Demographics

The UN has 193 member states, and these countries plus two associate members belong to WHO. A meeting of countries is held every year in Geneva, Switzerland, to set organization policy and budget. Every five years, the countries appoint a new director-general. WHO has an executive board with 34 members that the entire health assembly elects. It also has six regional committees that focus on health matters specific to their regions of the world.

WHO is not strictly a volunteer assembly, however. The organization employs more than 8,000 public health professionals in its Geneva headquarters, six regional offices, and 147 country offices. These include physicians, epidemiologists, scientists, and administrators. More than 85 of WHO's countries have dedicated HIV/AIDS staff. Less than one-third of the WHO budget is based on assessed contributions from member states; the rest is based on voluntary contributions, primarily from member states. The money helps WHO address problems around the world; the organization estimates that up to 2 billion people face health threats every day.

Description

WHO has several core functions. One is to provide global leadership on critical health matters and partner to take joint action when necessary to address those matters. WHO also engages in research and in helping to ensure important research is conducted and that the results are published. WHO sets various standards and promotes and monitors them to help improve health and provides technical support to communities or regions to help them create change. The organization emphasizes policies that are ethical and based on evidence and monitors and assesses health trends.

Origins

The United Nations was founded in 1945 following World War II. The 51 founding nations were committed to maintaining peace and security around the world, along with improving relations, social progress, and human rights. The first meeting of the nations' diplomats was held in San Francisco, and the discussion included developing a global health organization. By 1948, WHO had accepted responsibility for a system called the International Classification of Diseases, which had begun in the 1850s under a different name. The standard was used to help classify causes of death then to classify diseases and other health problems for doctors and epidemiologists.

Top priorities in the early years of WHO were **malaria**, women's and children's health, **tuberculosis**, venereal disease, nutrition, and **sanitation**. Many of these priorities still exist today, and other diseases, such as HIV/AIDS, have been added as priorities. Some, such as **smallpox**, have been eradicated or at least controlled. In 1974, the organization began bringing vaccinations to children around the world.

Results

In addition to tackling specific diseases and outbreaks and responding to disasters, WHO global and regional teams work strategically ahead of and during **disease outbreaks**. International Health Regulations provide rules that countries must follow when disease outbreaks occur to prevent diseases from spreading globally. By 1988, WHO had virtually eradicated **polio** by working with partnering organizations and volunteers to immunize children. Global treaties or strategies have been adopted to address the major health risk factors of tobacco and obesity. Most impressively, deaths of children younger than age five in all regions of the world were reduced from 12 million in 1990 to 6.9 million in 2011.

WHO remains the global source for public health information. In September 2012, the organization alerted doctors around the world of a new virus related to **severe acute respiratory syndrome (SARS)** that behaved differently than in the past. WHO also serves as an important marker for keeping industries and governments as consistent as possible in actions that affect public health. For example, the organization added diesel fuel to a list of carcinogens that included **asbestos**, cigarette smoke, and **radiation**. Each year on April 7, WHO marks the anniversary of its 1948 founding with a World Health Day that focuses on a different health initiative. In 2011, the focus was resistance to antibiotics, and in 2012, it was aging and health.

Research and general acceptance

The goals of WHO are large, and yet the organization continues to serve as the global repository for public health data and policies. WHO statistics often are cited by clinicians, public health professionals, and policymakers. The organization publishes data on its millennium development goals, disease-specific information, country-specific statistics, and world statistics. Though there are criticisms from time to time, such as 2010 calls from some critics that WHO overstated the H1N1 influenza **pandemic**, the organization largely serves as a trusted resource, particularly to countries with the most limited resources of their own.

Resources

WEBSITES

Alphonso, Caroline. "WHO Fights Back Over Criticism That It Exaggerated H1N1 Threat." The Globe and Mail. http://www.theglobeandmail.com/life/health-and-fitness/health/conditions/who-fights-back-over-criticism-that-it-exaggerated-h1n1-threat/article1207764/ (accessed October 6, 2012).

World Health Organization. "About WHO." http://www.who.int/about/en/ (accessed October 6, 2012).

World Health Organization. "Working for Health: An Introduction to the World Health Organization." http://www.who.int/about/brochure_en.pdf (accessed October 6, 2012).

ORGANIZATIONS

World Health Organization, Avenue Appia 20, 1211 Geneva 27, Switzerland, 41 22 (791) 2111, Fax: 41 22 (791) 3111, publications@who.int, www.who.int/en.

Teresa G. Odle

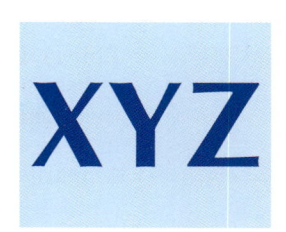

Yellow fever

Definition

Yellow fever, also known as sylvatic fever and viral hemorrhagic fever or VHF, is a severe infectious disease caused by a type of virus called a flavivirus. This flavivirus can cause outbreaks of epidemic proportions throughout Africa and tropical America. It is **endemic** in 33 countries in Africa and 11 countries in South America.

Description

The first written evidence of a yellow fever epidemic occurred in the Yucatan (Mexico) in 1648. Since that time, much has been learned about the transmission patterns of this illness. It is thought that the disease originated in Africa and spread to the Americas in the seventeenth and eighteenth centuries through trading ships. The flavivirus that causes yellow fever was first identified in West Africa, in 1928, and the first vaccine (17D) to fight against the disease was produced by South African-born American microbiologist Max Theiler (1899–1972) at the Rockefeller Institute in New York City in 1937. Based on work from American pathologist and physician Ernest Goodpasture (1886–1960), Theiler used chicken eggs to culture the virus. He won a Nobel Prize in 1951 for his work. Over 400 million doses of vaccine 17D have been used throughout the years.

Many common illnesses in the United States (including the common cold, many viral causes of diarrhea, and influenza) are spread by direct passage of the causative virus between human beings. Yellow fever, however, cannot be passed directly from one infected human to another. Instead, the virus responsible for yellow fever requires an intermediate vector. A vector is an organism that can carry a particular disease-causing agent (such as a virus or bacteria) without actually developing the disease. In the case of yellow fever, a mosquito is the vector that carries the virus from one host to another.

A host is an animal that can be infected with a particular disease. The hosts of yellow fever include both humans and monkeys. The cycle of yellow fever transmission begins when a tree-hole breeding mosquito bites an infected monkey. This mosquito acquires the virus and can pass the virus to any number of other monkeys that it may bite. This form of yellow fever is known as sylvatic yellow fever, and usually affects humans only incidentally. When an infected mosquito bites a human, the human may acquire the virus. In the case of South American yellow fever, the infected human may return to the city, where an urban mosquito (*Aedes aegypti*) serves as a viral vector, spreading the infection rapidly by biting humans. This form of the disease is known as urban yellow fever or epidemic yellow fever.

Yellow fever epidemics also may occur after flooding caused by **earthquakes** and other natural disasters. They result from a combination of new habitats available for the vectors of the disease and changes in human behavior (spending more time outdoors and neglecting **sanitation** precautions).

Cases of yellow fever are uncommon in the United States and Canada, as of 2012. The last reported case of a U.S. citizen dying of yellow fever concerned a man who contracted yellow fever after visiting Venezuela in 1999. The man had not been vaccinated against yellow fever. The last epidemic in the United States occurred in New Orleans, Louisiana, in 1905.

Risk factors

The major risk factor for contracting yellow fever is residing in or traveling to an area where mosquitoes carry the virus. These areas include South America and sub-Saharan Africa. To provide protection from yellow fever, a **vaccination** is recommended for anyone traveling to affected areas at least 10 to 14 days before the departure date.

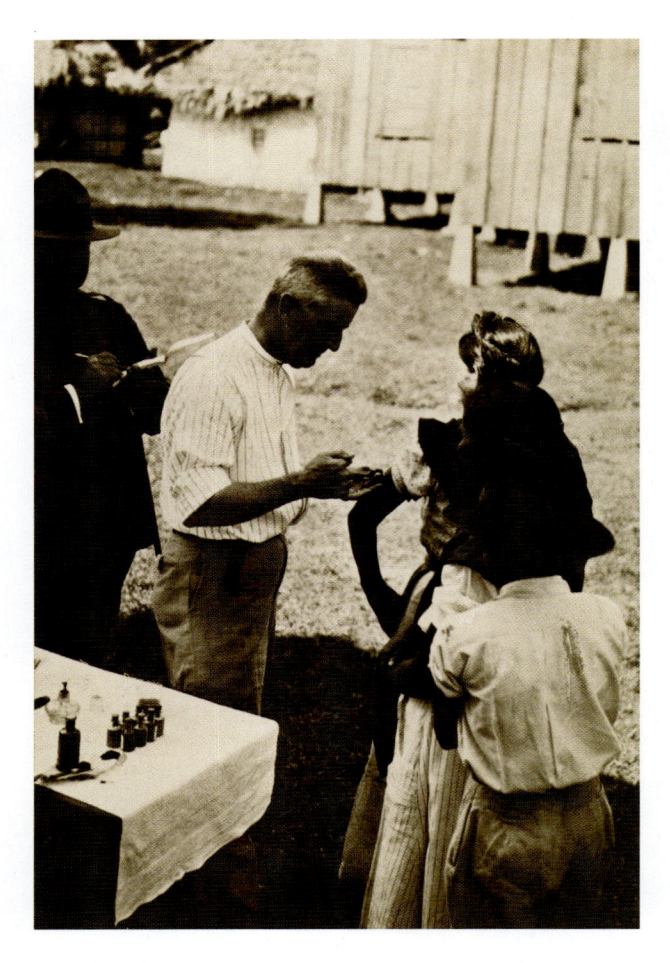

A Rockefeller scientist administers anti-yellow-fever vaccine. (© National Geographic Image Collection / Alamy)

Demographics

Anyone can get yellow fever; however, older people are more at risk than younger ones. Yellow fever is found most commonly in men between the ages of 15 and 45 years who work outdoors and live in fever-endemic areas. Race has not been shown to be a factor in contraction or transmission. Between 1970 and 2002, only nine cases of yellow fever were reported in travelers from the United States and Europe. All cases were found in unimmunized travelers who had visited South America or Africa. Seven of the cases were fatal.

According to the **World Health Organization** (WHO), as of 2011, about 200,000 cases of yellow fever occur annually around the world (mostly in tropical endemic areas of Africa and the Americas), with approximately 30,000 deaths caused by the disease. Thirty-three countries are at risk of yellow fever in Africa and in the Americas; several Caribbean islands and nine South American countries (including Bolivia, Brazil, Columbia, Ecuador, and Peru) are also at risk. Up to 50% of severely affected persons without treatment die from yellow fever. The number of yellow fever cases has increased over the past several decades primarily due to fewer people becoming immune to it and fewer immunizations, along with environmental factors such as urbanization, deforestation, global **climate change**, and population movements into areas more prone to the virus. The vaccine for yellow fever protects humans for 30 to 35 years. About 95% of people vaccinated are immune to the disease within one week of the vaccination.

Causes and symptoms

Once a mosquito passes the yellow fever virus to a human, the chance of disease developing ranges from 5–20%. Infection may be fought off by the host's immune system or may be so mild that it is never identified.

In human hosts who develop the disease yellow fever, there are five distinct stages through which the infection evolves. These have been termed the periods of incubation, invasion, remission, intoxication, and convalescence.

Yellow fever's incubation period (the amount of time between the introduction of the virus into the host and the development of symptoms) is three to six days. During this time, there are generally no symptoms identifiable to the host.

The period of invasion lasts two to five days, and begins with an abrupt onset of symptoms, including fever and chills, intense headache and lower backache, muscle aches, nausea, and extreme exhaustion. The patient's tongue shows a characteristic white, furry coating in the center, surrounded by a swollen, reddened margin. While most other infections that cause a high fever also cause an increased heart rate, yellow fever results in an unusual finding, called Faget's sign. This is the simultaneous occurrence of a high fever with a slowed heart rate. Throughout the period of invasion, there are live **viruses** circulating in the patient's bloodstream. Therefore, a mosquito can bite an ill patient, acquire the virus, and continue passing it on to others.

The next phase is the period of remission. The fever falls, and symptoms decrease in severity for several hours to several days. In some patients, this signals the end of the disease; in other patients, this is the calm before the storm.

The period of intoxication represents the most severe and potentially fatal phase of the illness. During this time, lasting three to nine days, a type of degeneration of the internal organs (specifically the kidneys,

WILBUR AUGUSTUS SAWYER (1879–1951)

Wilbur Augustus Sawyer was born in Appleton, Wisconsin, on August 7, 1879, to Minnie Edmea (Birge) and Wesley Caleb Sawyer. The Sawyers moved to Oshkosh, Wisconsin, and finally to Stockton, California in 1888. Sawyer spent two years at the University of California and then entered Harvard College where he earned his A.B. degree in 1902. In 1906, Sawyer graduated from Harvard Medical School and began a private practice, which lasted until he started his internship at Massachusetts General Hospital. Sawyer returned to California in 1908 in order to obtain a position at the University of California as a medical examiner. He then worked with the California State Board of Health from 1910 until 1918. In 1911, Sawyer married Margaret Henderson. The couple had three children.

Sawyer's first publication (1913) dealt with his research into poliomyelitis. His discovery, in 1915, that examination of an individual's stool could lead to detection of the disease was later regarded as very significant. In 1918 and 1919, Sawyer worked to control venereal disease while employed by the Army Medical Corps. In 1926 and 1927, while director of the West African Yellow Fever Commission, Sawyer succeeded in isolating the yellow fever virus. He ultimately returned to the United States, where he and Wray Lloyd devised an immunization against yellow fever (1931).

In 1944, Sawyer became director of health for the United Nations Relief and Rehabilitation Administration, a position he held for three years. He retired to Berkeley, California, where he died on November 12, 1951. The company he built with his brother still thrives today.

---

liver, and heart) occurs. This fatty degeneration results in what is considered the classic triad of yellow fever symptoms: jaundice, black vomit, and the dumping of protein into the urine. Jaundice causes the whites of the patient's eyes and the patient's skin to take on a distinctive yellow color. This is due to liver damage, and the accumulation of a substance called bilirubin, which is normally processed by a healthy liver. The liver damage also results in a tendency toward bleeding; the patient's vomit appears black due to the presence of blood. Protein, which is normally kept out of the urine by healthy, intact kidneys, appears in the urine due to disruption of the kidney's healthy functioning.

Patients who survive the period of intoxication enter into a relatively short period of convalescence. They recover with no long-term effects related to the yellow fever infection. Surviving an infection with the yellow fever virus results in lifelong immunity against repeated infection by the virus.

The course of yellow fever is complicated in some patients by secondary bacterial infections.

Diagnosis

Diagnosis for yellow fever includes examination, testing, and procedures.

Examination

A diagnosis of yellow fever may be suspected during a physical examination when the classic triad of symptoms are present. These include:

- a sudden onset of fever, chills, intense headaches and lower backaches, muscle aches, nausea, and exhaustion
- Faget's sign—simultaneous occurrence of a high fever and decreased heart rate
- a white furry coating in the center of the tongue surround by a swollen, red margin

Tests

Diagnosis of yellow fever depends on the examination of blood by various techniques in order to demonstrate either yellow fever viral antigens (the part of the virus that stimulates the patient's immune system to respond) or specific antibodies (specific cells produced by the patient's immune system that are directed against the yellow fever virus). The most rapid method of diagnosis, as of 2012, was capture enzyme immunoassay.

Procedures

Typically, the only procedure required for diagnosis is a blood draw so that the blood can be evaluated for signs of yellow fever.

Treatment

Treatment for yellow fever includes traditional approaches, along with the use of drugs.

The only treatments for yellow fever are given to relieve its symptoms. Fevers and pain should be relieved with acetaminophen, not aspirin or ibuprofen, both of which could increase the already-present risk of bleeding. Dehydration (due to fluid loss, both from fever and bleeding) needs to be carefully avoided. This can be accomplished by increasing fluids. The risk of bleeding into the stomach can be decreased through the administration of antacids and other medications. Hemorrhage (heavy bleeding) may require blood transfusions. Kidney failure may require dialysis (a process that allows the work of the kidneys in clearing the blood of potentially toxic substances to be taken over by a machine, outside of the body).

Drugs

There are no antiviral treatments available as of 2012 to combat the yellow fever virus. Nonclinical research has yielded limited results.

Researchers have found that ribavirin (Virazole, Rebetol), a drug that is given by mouth to treat hepatitis C, is successful in reducing mortality from yellow fever in hamsters, but only if given within 120 hours of infection. Another drug, Interferon-alpha has also been found to reduce mortality in monkeys with yellow fever but only when administered within 24 hours of infection.

Public health role and response

The World Health Organization (WHO) recommends routine childhood vaccination to prevent yellow fever in endemic countries where epidemics are possible. Quick detection of yellow fever and fast response of governments through emergency vaccination campaigns are important in controlling outbreaks. WHO recommends that at-risk countries maintain at least one national laboratory where blood tests for yellow fever can be performed.

The organization Secretariat for the International Coordinating Group (ICG) for Yellow Fever Vaccine Provision provides an emergency stockpile of yellow fever vaccines whenever outbreaks occur in any country of the world. WHO also leads the Yellow Fever Initiative (YFI), which is a preventive vaccination effort for at-risk countries, especially 12 participating African countries where the disease is most likely to occur. The YFI recommends "including yellow fever vaccines in routine infant immunizations (starting at age 9 months), implementing mass vaccination campaigns in high-risk areas for people in all age groups aged 9 months and older, and maintaining surveillance and outbreak response capacity."

Prognosis

Five to ten percent of all diagnosed cases of yellow fever are fatal. Jaundice occurring during a yellow fever

---

KEY TERMS

Antibody—A protein normally produced by the immune system to fight infection or rid the body of foreign material. The material that stimulates the production of antibodies is called an antigen. Specific antibodies are produced in response to each different antigen and can only inactivate that particular antigen.

Antigen—Any foreign substance, usually a protein, that stimulates the body's immune system to produce antibodies.

Bilirubin—A reddish-yellow bile pigment made by the liver.

Dialysis—The cleansing of the blood through use of a special machine that filters the blood. The process is performed when the kidneys are unable to filter blood properly.

Epidemic—A situation in which the number of cases of a particular disease exceeds the endemic or average number of cases. Infections of such diseases often spread through a population of people in a relatively short period of time.

Faget's sign—The simultaneous occurrence of a high fever with a slowed heart rate.

Flavivirus—The species to which the virus that causes yellow fever belongs.

Hemorrhage—Abnormal and obsessive bleeding.

Host—The organism (such as a monkey or human) in which another organism (such as a virus or bacteria) is living.

Jaundice—The yellowing of the skin and whites of the eyes caused by an increased level of bilirubin in the blood.

Sylvatic—Pertaining to or living in the woods or forested areas. The form of yellow fever transmitted by mosquitoes to rainforest monkeys is called sylvatic yellow fever.

Vector—A carrier organism (such as a fly or mosquito) that serves to deliver a virus (or other agent of infection) to a host.

---

infection is an extremely grave predictor; 20–50% of these patients die of the infection. Death may occur due to massive bleeding (hemorrhage), often following a lapse into a comatose (unconscious) state.

Prevention

A very safe and very effective yellow fever vaccine exists. The Arilvax vaccine is made from a live

> **QUESTIONS TO ASK YOUR DOCTOR**
>
> - Should I be worried about contracting yellow fever?
> - Should I receive a yellow fever vaccination?
> - What symptoms should I watch for with regards to yellow fever?
> - What are my treatment options and the risks associated with treatment?
> - How long will I be taking medication for yellow fever? What are the potential side effects of my medication?
> - Does my yellow fever medication interact with my medicines or supplements?
> - When can I resume my normal activities? When can I return to work?
> - What can I do to reduce my risk for having yellow fever again?
> - How often will I need to follow-up with my doctor?
> - What community support and other resources are available to help me?

attenuated (weakened) form of the yellow fever virus, strain 17D. In the United States, the vaccine is given only at Yellow Fever Vaccination Centers authorized by the U.S. **Public Health Service**. About 95% of vaccine recipients acquire long-term immunity to the yellow fever virus. Careful measures to decrease mosquito populations in both urban areas and jungle areas where humans are working, along with programs to vaccinate all people living in such areas, are necessary to avoid massive yellow fever outbreaks.

Individuals planning to travel in countries where yellow fever is endemic may obtain up-to-date information on yellow fever vaccination from the U.S. **Centers for Disease Control and Prevention** (CDC).

Resources

BOOKS

Crosby, Molly Caldwell. *The American Plague: The Untold Story of Yellow Fever, the Epidemic That Shaped Our History*. New York: Berkley Books, 2006.

Shannon, Joyce Brennfleck, editor. *Contagious Diseases Sourcebook: Basic Consumer Health Information about Diseases Spread from Person to Person*. Detroit: Omnigraphics, 2010.

Shmaefsky, Brian R. *Yellow Fever*. New York: Chelsea House, 2010.

Wilder-Smith, Annelies, Eli Schwartz, and Marc Shaw, editors. *Travel Medicine: Tales Behind the Science*. Amsterdam: Elsevier, 2007.

WEBSITES

Busowski, Mary T. *Yellow Fever*. Medscape Reference. (September 15, 2011). http://emedicine.medscape.com/article/232244-overview (accessed October 9, 2012).

Country List: Yellow Fever Vaccination Requirements and Recommendations; and Malaria Situation. World Health Organization. http://www.who.int/ith/ITH2010countrylist.pdf (accessed October 9, 2012).

Dugdale, David, and Jatin M. Vyas. *Yellow Fever*. Medline Plus. (December 6, 2011). http://www.nlm.nih.gov/medlineplus/ency/article/001365.htm (accessed October 9, 2012).

Yellow Fever. Fact Sheet No. 100. World Health Organization. (January 2011). http://www.who.int/mediacentre/factsheets/fs100/en/ (accessed October 9, 2012).

Yellow Fever. Mayo Clinic. (August 27, 2011). http://www.mayoclinic.com/health/yellow-fever/DS01011 (accessed October 9, 2012).

Yellow Fever Vaccine. Medline Plus. (July 15, 2011). http://www.nlm.nih.gov/medlineplus/druginfo/meds/a607030.html (accessed October 9, 2012).

ORGANIZATIONS

Centers for Disease Control and Prevention, 1600 Clifton Rd., Atlanta, GA 30333, (800) 232-4636, cdcinfo@cdc.gov, http://www.cdc.gov.

National Institute of Allergy and Infectious Diseases, 6610 Rockledge Dr., MSC 6612, Bethesda, MD 20892, (301) 496-5717, (866) 284-4107, Fax: (301) 402-3573, http://www.niaid.nih.gov.

World Health Organization, Avenue Appia 20, Geneva, Switzerland 1211 27, 41 22 791-2111, Fax: 41 22 791-3111, http://www.who.int/en/.

Rosalyn Carson-DeWitt, MD
Paul Checchia, MD
William A. Atkins, BB, BS, MBA

Yokkaichi asthma

Definition

Yokkaichi **asthma** was a major health crisis that occurred in the city of Yokkaichi in Mie Prefecture, Japan, between 1960 and 1972. Known as one of the "Four Big Pollution Diseases of Japan", it was caused by the burning of crude oil and from petrochemical processing facilities and refineries, which released huge amounts of sulfur oxide and other pollutants into the atmosphere. Such pollution caused serious

smog, which resulted in numerous respiratory-related problems to many local residents.

Description

Nowhere is the connection between industrial development and environmental and human health deterioration more graphically demonstrated than at Yokkaichi, Japan. An international port located on the Ise Bay, Yokkaichi was a major textile center by 1897. The shipping business shifted to nearby Nagoya in 1907, and Yokkaichi filled in its coastal lowlands in a successful bid to attract modern industries, especially chemical processing, steel production, and oil and gasoline refining.

Spurred by both the World War II (1939–1945) demand and the postwar recovery effort, several more petrochemical companies were added through the 1950s, creating an oil refinery complex called the Yokkaichi Kombinato. In 1959 it began 24-hour operations, and the sparkle of hundreds of electric lights became known as the "million-dollar night view." Although citizens took pride in the growing industrial complex, their enthusiasm waned when **air pollution** and **noise pollution** created human health problems. As early as 1953, the central government sent a research group to try to discover the cause, but no action was taken. Instead, the petrochemical complex was expanded.

Demographics

The construction of the Daichi Petrochemical Complex was begun in 1955 as a way for Japan to start converting from coal to petroleum as its primary source of fossil fuel. The city of Yokkaichi was selected as the site of the new complex. A second petrochemical production complex was constructed north of Yokkaichi in 1960 in order to increase capacity for petrochemicals. For even larger capacity, a third complex became operational in 1972.

Causes and symptoms

In the early 1960s, residents of Yokkaichi began to complain of respiratory problems. For instance, increased incidence of chronic obstructive pulmonary disease (COPD) and bronchial asthma were especially noticeable at this time. The cause of the disease was air pollution from sulfur oxide. It became known as Yokkaichi Asthma (Yokkaichi Zensoku, in Japanese). As citizens began to complain about breathing difficulties, scientists documented a high correlation between airborne sulfur dioxide concentrations and bronchial asthma in schoolchildren and chronic **bronchitis** in individuals over the age of 40. Despite this knowledge, a second industrial complex was opened in 1963. In the Isozu district of Yokkaichi, the average concentration of sulfur dioxide was eight times that of unaffected districts. Taller smokestacks spread pollution over a wider area but did not resolve the problem; increased production also added to the volume discharged. Despite resistance, a third industrial complex was added in 1973, one of the largest petroleum refining and ethylene-producing facilities in Japan.

As the petrochemical industries continued to expand, local citizens' quality of life deteriorated. In the early years, heavy smoke was emitted by coal combustion, and parents worried about the exposure of schoolchildren whose playground was close to the emissions source. Switching from coal to oil in the 1960s seemed to be an improvement, but the now-invisible stack gases still contained large quantities of

---

KEY TERMS

Bronchial asthma—A respiratory disorder characterized by chronic inflammation of the airways.

Carbon monoxide—With the chemical formula CO (where C stands for carbon, and O for oxygen), a colorless, odorless, and tasteless gas that is toxic to humans in higher than normal concentrations.

Chronic obstructive pulmonary disease (COPD)—Also known by such names as chronic obstructive airway disease (COAD) and chronic obstructive respiratory disease (CORD), a respiratory disorder that causes both chronic bronchitis and emphysema.

Chronic bronchitis—A respiratory disorder that causes chronic inflammation of the bronchi within the lungs.

Flue-gas de sulfurization—Technologies used to remove sulfur dioxide from exhaust flue gases of fossil-fuel power plants and other such processes.

Fossil fuels—Any type of fuel, such as coal, natural gas, peat, and petroleum, derived from the decomposed remains of prehistoric plants and animals.

Pulmonary emphysema—A progressive respiratory disorder that causes shortness of breath.

Sulfur dioxide—With the chemical formula SO_2 (where S stands for sulfur, and O for oxygen), a toxic gas with a strong, irritating smell; in nature it is released from spewing volcanoes and it is also released by human-producing industrial processes.

sulfur oxides, and more people developed respiratory diseases. By 1960, fish from the local waterways had developed such a bad taste that they were unable to be sold, and fishermen demanded compensation for their lost livelihood. By 1961, 48% of children under the age of six years, 30% of people over 60, and 19% of those in their twenties had respiratory abnormalities. In 1964, a pollution-free room was established in the local hospital where victims could take refuge and breathe freely.

Even so, two desperate people committed suicide in 1966, and 12 Yokkaichi residents who had been trying to resolve the problem by negotiation finally filed a damage suit against the Shiohama Kombinato in 1967. In 1972, the judge awarded the plaintiffs $286,000 in damages to be paid jointly by the six companies. This was the first case in which a group of Japanese companies was forced to pay damages, making other kombinatos vulnerable to similar suits.

Diagnosis

Medical professionals diagnosed the problems of the citizens of Yokkaichi as being primarily chronic obstructive pulmonary disease, chronic bronchitis, pulmonary **emphysema**, and bronchial asthma. The problems were diagnosed based on clinical signs and symptoms and laboratory findings such as arterial blood oxygen tension, chest x ray, and lung function.

Treatment

In 2008, Japanese researchers Peng Guo, Kazuhito Yokoyama, Masami Suenaga, and Hirotaka Kida published the paper "Mortality and Life Expectancy of Yokkaichi Asthma Patients, Japan: Late Effects of Air Pollution in 1960–70s," in the journal *Environmental Health*. The authors stated that laws were implemented to provide financial support to victims of Yokkaichi asthma. The petrochemical companies paid medical expenses based on the following requirements:

- diseases, such as bronchial asthma, chronic bronchitis, pulmonary emphysema, and their complication, occurred in the polluted areas and were confirmed epidemiologically
- in specific areas, where prevalence of the specific diseases increased
- During a specific period, stated as three years of residence in the specific area

Public health role and response

In 1960, officials of Yokkaichi organized a committee to measure the pollution in the city. Three years later, the Japanese national government sent researchers to assess the situation. In 1965, the city established a medical aid program for its citizens. Two years later, several local citizens brought legal action against the petrochemical companies. Because of successful litigation by the Yokkaichi victims, the Japanese government enacted a basic antipollution law in 1967. Two years later, the Law Concerning Special Measures for the Relief of Pollution-Related Patients was enacted. It applied to chronic bronchitis and bronchial-asthma victims from Yokkaichi but also from Kawasaki and Osaka. In addition, national air-pollution standards were strengthened to require that oil refineries adhere to air pollution abatement policies.

> ## QUESTIONS TO ASK YOUR DOCTOR
> - Am I susceptible to respiratory problems?
> - How can air pollution be harmful to me?
> - What are the risks associated air pollution?
> - Should I be concerned if I live near a petrochemical plant?

Prognosis

The Japanese researchers Peng Guo and colleagues found in 2008 that the mortality rates for COPD and asthma for local residents were significantly higher than in the whole population of Mie Prefecture. In addition, they found that for all ages of residents, except for men between the ages of 80 and 84 years, their life expectancy was significantly reduced when compared to the entire population of Mie Prefecture. Even though pollution levels decreased substantially by the end of 1970s and no new cases had been reported since 1988, the Japanese researchers concluded that "Mortality and life expectancy were adversely affected in patients from Yokkaichi-city, despite the fact that the air pollution problem has been already solved."

Prevention

Eventually, flue-gas de sulfurization technologies were implemented and, by 1975, the annual mean sulfur dioxide levels had decreased by a factor of three, below the target level of 0.017 parts per million (ppm). The prevalence of respiratory diseases on the Yokkaichi was also reduced. In 1973, the Law Concerning Compensation for Pollution-Related Health Damages and Other Measures aided sufferers of chronic bronchitis and bronchial asthma from the other affected areas of Japan, especially Tokyo. By December 1991, 97,276 victims throughout Japan, including 809 from Yokkaichi, were eligible for compensation. Since that time, residents near heavily industrialized areas in China and Mexico City have experienced similar increases in sulfur oxide-related respiratory illnesses.

Resources

BOOKS

Ayres, Jon, Robert Maynard, and Roy Richards. *Air Pollution and Health.* London: Imperial College, 2006.
Phalen, Robert F., and Robert N. Phalen. *Introduction to Air Pollution Science: A Public Health Perspective.* Burlington, MA: Jones & Bartlett Learning, 2013.
Yu, Ming-Ho, Humio Tsunoda, and Masashi Tsunoda. *Environmental Toxicology: Biological and Health Effects of Pollutants.* Boca Raton, FL: CRC Press, 2012.

PERIODICALS

Guo, P., K. Yokoyama, M. Suenaga, and H. Kida. "Mortality and Life Expectancy of Yokkaichi Asthma Patients, Japan: Late Effects of Air Pollution in 1960–70s." *Environmental Health: A Global Access Science Source* 7 (2008): 8.

WEBSITES

Academia.edu. "Public health Experts on Yokkaichi Asthma." http://u-tokyo.academia.edu/TomohisaSumida/Papers/1267153/Public_health_experts_on_Yokkaichi_asthma (accessed September 21, 2012).
Environmental Protection Agency. "Air Pollutants." http://www.epa.gov/oar/airpollutants.html (accessed September 10, 2012).
Environmental Protection Agency. "Air Quality and Public Health." http://www.epa.gov/oia/air/pollution.htm (accessed September 10, 2012).
Environmental Protection Agency. "Particulate Matter (PM)." http://www.epa.gov/pm/health.html (accessed September 21, 2012).
Nolen, Janice. "5 Steps to Clean Up Air Pollution." Scientific American. http://www.scientificamerican.com/article.cfm?id=5-steps-to-clean-up (accessed September 10, 2012).
World Health Organization. "Chronic Respiratory Diseases." http://www.who.int/respiratory/en/ (accessed September 21, 2012).

ORGANIZATIONS

American Lung Association, 1301 Pennsylvania Ave. NW, Ste. 800, Washington, DC 20004, (202) 785-3355, Fax: (202) 452-1805, (800) 621-8335, http://www.lung.org.
American Medical Association, 515 N. State St., Chicago, IL 60654, (800) 621-8335, http://www.ama-assn.org.
Environmental Defense Fund, 1875 Connecticut Ave. NW, Ste. 600., Washington, D.C. 20009, (800) 684-3322, http://www.edf.org/.
Environmental Protection Agency, 1200 Pennsylvania Ave. NW, Ariel Rios Bldg., Washington, DC 20460, (202) 272-0167, http://www.epa.gov.
Global Alliance Against Chronic Respiratory Diseases, World Health Organization, 20 Avenue Appia, Geneva, Switzerland 1211 27, gard@who.int, http://www.who.int/gard/en.
World Health Organization, Avenue Appia 20, Geneva, Switzerland 1211 27, 41 22 791-2111, Fax: 41 22 791-3111, cdcinfo@cdc.gov, http://www.who.int/en.

Frank M. D'Itri
William A. Atkins, BB, BS, MBA

Zero population growth

Definition

Zero population growth (also called the replacement level of fertility) refers to stabilization of a population at its current level.

Description

A population growth rate of zero means that a population remains stable over time, with no net change in numbers of entities within the population (i.e., birthrate is in balance with death rate). In more developed countries (MDC), where infant mortality rates are low, a fertility rate of about 2.2 children per couple results in zero population growth. This rate is slightly more than two because the extra fraction includes infant deaths, infertile couples, and couples that choose not to have children. In less developed countries (LDC), the replacement level of fertility is often as high as six children per couple.

Zero population growth, as a term, lends its name to a national, nonprofit organization founded in 1968 by Paul R. Ehrlich, which works to achieve a sustainable balance between population, resources, and the environment worldwide.

ORGANIZATIONS

Zero Population Growth, 1400 16th Street NW, Suite 320, Washington, DC 20036

Zoonoses

Definition

Zoonoses, also called zoonotic diseases, refers to diseases or infections that can be naturally passed (transmitted) from vertebrate animals, whether wild or domesticated, to humans, and vice-versa. According to the **World Health Organization** (WHO), over 250 distinct zoonoses have been medically described.

Description

Bacteria, fungi, **parasites**, **viruses**, and other disease-causing organisms cause zoonosis. The following are examples of zoonosis caused by:

- bacteria: leptospirosis (scientific name *Leptopiras spp*) that is transmitted by direct contact with an infected animal or indirect contact with urine-infected food, soil, or water
- fungi: aspergillosis (*Aspergillus fumigatus*) that is transmitted by the inhalation of fungal spores
- parasites: raccoon roundworm (*Baylisascaris procyonis*) that is transmitted by the ingestion of eggs
- viruses: rabies (no scientific name) that is transmitted by a bite wound

In the twenty-first century, zoonoses continue to be significant public health threats around the world, affecting hundreds of thousands of people annually especially in developing countries. However, most zoonoses can be prevented.

Many modern diseases are known to have started as zoonotic diseases when humans first began to record history. Biblical references to a **plague** are thought to have been caused by bacterial zoonosis transmitted from fleas to humans. The Plague of Athens, in 430 BC is thought to have been caused by one of the bacteria in the family Rickettsiae. History continues to hold the secret as to when many diseases were first transported from other animals to humans. Medical science is quite confident, however, that many long-known diseases such as influenza (flu), **smallpox**, and **measles** had their beginnings as zoonotic diseases. In addition, even though with much less certainty, the common cold may have first been a problem in other animals before becoming a problem for humans. Other diseases that were virtually unknown within humans in the twenty century, such as **West Nile virus**, are causing serious problems with people in the twenty-first century.

Although many diseases are species specific, meaning that they can only occur in one animal species, many other diseases can be spread between different animal species. These are infectious diseases caused by bacteria, viruses, or other disease-causing organisms that can live as well in humans as in other animals.

There are different methods of transmission for different diseases. In some cases, zoonotic diseases are transferred by direct contact with infected animals, much as being near an infected human can cause the spread of an infectious disease. Other diseases are spread by drinking water that contains the eggs of parasites. The eggs enter the water supply from the feces of infected animals. Others are spread by eating the flesh of infected animals. Tapeworms are spread this way. Insect vectors spread other diseases. An insect, such as a flea or tick, feeds on an infected animal, and then feeds on a human. In the process, the insect transfers the infecting organism.

The **Centers for Disease Control and Prevention** (CDC), headquartered in Atlanta, Georgia, has said that most emerging diseases around the world are zoonotic. The director of the CDC has stated that 11 of the last 12 emerging infections in the world with serious health consequences have probably arisen from animal "1"s. Wild animal trade occurs across countries and many people take in wild animals as domestic pets. However, many pet shops and food markets are not properly testing for diseases and parasites that can cause harm to humans and other animals.

Some zoonotic diseases are well known, such as plague (rats) and **Lyme disease** (deer ticks). Others are not as well known. For example, elephants may develop **tuberculosis** and spread it to humans.

Risk factors

According to the WHO, the largest risk for the transmission of zoonotic disease "occurs at the human-animal interface through direct or indirect human exposure to animals, their products, and/or their environments." WHO adds, "More than 60% of the newly identified infectious agents that have affected people over the past few decades have been caused by pathogens originating from animals or animal products. Seventy percent of these zoonotic infections originate from wildlife."

Many zoonoses continue to occur in several developing countries of the world. These continue to be transmitted to humans through bites from infected mammals (rabies), food (such as **brucellosis** and tuberculosis), and insects (Rift Valley Fever), along with environmental contamination (echinococcosis/hydatidosis).

Demographics

Human health has been adversely effected by zoonoses. One particular major outbreak involved the Nipah virus and **severe acute respiratory syndrome**

(SARS) coronavirus (CoV). Such outbreaks are becoming more complex due to changing circumstances.

A 2010 paper "Public Health Threat of New, Reemerging, and Neglected Zoonoses in the Industrialized World" in the CDC publication *Emerging Infectious Diseases* discusses how zoonoses are changing in the face of these changing circumstances:

- Changes in agriculture, such as containment of large numbers of animals or close proximity of several different species can promote the spread of disease between animals
- Increased movement of people, animals, and products across the globe allows introduction of disease and disease carriers to more populations despite measures to control spread of disease
- Movement of people into natural habitats for housing or tourism puts them in circumstances where they may be exposed to new types of zoonoses
- Changes in climate may promote opportunity for mutation or variation of pathogens as well as the vectors they use to spread disease

Common diseases and disorders

The following is a partial list of animals and the diseases that they may carry. Not all animal carriers are listed, nor are all the diseases that the various species may carry:

- Bats are important rabies carriers and also carry other viral diseases that can affect humans.
- Cats may carry the causative organisms for plague, anthrax, cowpox, tapeworm, and many bacterial infections.
- Dogs may carry plague, tapeworm, rabies, Rocky Mountain Spotted Fever, and Lyme disease.
- Horses may carry anthrax, rabies, and *Salmonella* infections.
- Cattle may carry the organisms that cause anthrax, European tick-borne encephalitis, rabies, tapeworm, *Salmonella* infections, and many bacterial and viral diseases.
- Pigs are best known for carrying tapeworm, but may also carry a large number of other infections including anthrax, influenza, and rabies.
- Sheep and goats may carry rabies, European tick-borne encephalitis, *Salmonella* infections, and many bacterial and viral diseases.
- Rabbits may carry plague and Q-Fever.
- Birds may carry *Campylobacteriosis, Chlamydia psittaci, Pasteurella multocida, Histoplasma capsulatum, Salmonellosis*, and others.

KEY TERMS

Anthrax—A disease of warm blooded animals, particularly cattle and sheep, transmissible to humans. The disease causes severe skin and lung damage.

Bovine spongiform encephalopathy—Also known as Mad Cow disease, a progressive, fatal disease of the nervous system of domestic animals that is transmitted by eating infected food.

Lyme disease—An acute disease that is usually marked by skin rash, fever, fatigue, and chills. Left untreated, it may cause heart and nervous system damage.

Q-Fever—A disease marked by high fever, chills, and muscle pain. It is seen in North America, Europe, and parts of Africa. It may be spread by drinking raw milk or by tick bites.

Zoonotic—A disease that can be spread from animals to humans.

Causes and symptoms

Zoonotic diseases may be spread in different ways. Tapeworms can often spread to humans when people eat the infected meat of cattle and swine. Other diseases are transferred by insect vectors, often blood-feeding insects that carry the cause of the disease from one animal to another.

Diagnosis

Diagnosis of the disease is made by identifying the infecting organism. Each disease has established symptoms and tests. Identifying the carrier may be easy or may be more difficult when the cause is a common infection. For example, tapeworms are usually species specific. Cattle, pigs, and fish all carry different species of tapeworms, although all can be transmitted to humans who eat undercooked meat containing live tapeworm eggs. Once the tapeworm has been identified, it is easy to tell from which species the tapeworm came.

Other zoonotic infections may be more difficult to identify. Sometimes the infection is common among both humans and animals, and it is impossible to tell the difference. Snakes may carry the bacteria *Escherichia coli* and *Proteus vulgaris*, but since these bacteria are already common among humans, it would be difficult to trace infections back to snakes.

Increased trade between nations and changes in animal habitats has introduced new zoonotic diseases.

These may be found in animals transported from one nation to another, bringing with them new diseases. In some cases, changes in the environment lead to changes in the migratory habits of animal species, bringing new infections.

Treatment

The treatment of zoonotic infections depends on the specific disease. Many are treated with prescription drugs such as antibiotics. For instance, Lyme disease is caused by the bacterium *Borrelia burgdorferi*. The bacterium gets inside a tick from infected deer, mice, or other animals. The tick can then attach itself onto the skin of a human. The infected tick feeds on a person's blood, which then infects the human. Lyme disease is treated with antibiotics.

Public health role and response

The Global Early Warning System for Major Animal Diseases, including Zoonoses (GLEWS) is an early warning system for outbreaks of animal diseases. The World Health Organization (WHO), the Food and Agricultural Organization of the United Nations (FAO), and the World Organization for Animal Health (OIE) created GLEWS. It is used to help alert the international community in the prevention and control of threats from animal diseases, including zoonoses.

Prognosis

The prognosis for zoonoses is dependent on the particular organism; however, for the most part, the prognosis for fully recovering from such a disease is good if treatment is promptly given with appropriate medicine.

Prevention

Prevention of zoonotic infections may take different forms, depending on the nature of the carrier and the infection.

Some zoonotic infections can be avoided by immunizing the animals that carry the disease. Pets and other domestic animals should have rabies vaccinations, and wild animals are immunized with an oral vaccine that is encased in suitable bait. In some places, the bait is dropped by airplane over the range of the potential rabies carrier. When the animals eat the bait, they also ingest the oral vaccine, thereby protecting them from rabies and reducing the risk of spread of the disease. This method has been used to protect foxes, coyotes, and other wild animals.

> **QUESTIONS TO ASK YOUR DOCTOR**
>
> - Should I be worried about zoonotic disease?
> - What are the possible causes for my symptoms?
> - What symptoms should I be watching for with regards to this zoonotic disease?
> - If I was exposed to someone with a zoonotic disease, can I give it to others?
> - What types of tests do I need?
> - Are treatments available to help me recover from zoonotic disease? What are the risks associated with treatment?
> - How long will a full recovery take?
> - When can I return to my daily routine?
> - Am I at risk of any long-term complications?

Zoonotic diseases that are passed by eating the meat of infected animals can often be prevented by proper cooking of the infected meat. Tapeworm infestations can be prevented by cooking, and *Salmonella* infections from chickens and eggs can be prevented by ensuring that both the meat and the eggs are fully cooked.

For other zoonotic diseases, programs are in place to eliminate the host, or the vector, that spreads the disease. Plague is prevented by elimination of rats—a common "1" of the infection—and of fleas that carry the disease from rats to humans. Efforts around the world to control bovine spongiform encephalitis, better known as Mad Cow disease, have focused on the destruction of infected cattle to prevent spread of the disease. Regulations on the makeup of the cattle feed to ensure safety and prevent the disease have helped curb its spread.

Other means of prevention simply rely on care. People living in areas where Lyme disease is common are warned to take precautions against the bite of the deer tick, which transfers the disease. These precautions include not walking in tall grass, not walking bare legged, and wearing light-colored clothing so that the presence of the dark ticks can be readily seen.

Resources

BOOKS

Link, Kurt. *Understanding New, Resurgent, and Resistant Diseases: How Man and Globalization Create and Spread Illness.* Westport, CT: Praeger, 2007.

Palmer, S. R., et al., eds. *Oxford Textbook of Zoonoses: Biology, Clinical Practice, and Public Health Control.* Oxford: Oxford University Press, 2011.

Shannon, Joyce Brennfleck, ed. *Contagious Diseases "1"book: Basic Consumer Health Information about Diseases Spread from Person to Person.* Detroit: Omnigraphics, 2010.

Wilder-Smith, Annelies, Eli Schwartz, and Marc Shaw, eds. *Travel Medicine: Tales Behind the Science.* Amsterdam: Elsevier, 2007.

PERIODICALS

Cutler, Sally J., Anthony R. Fooks, and Wim H.M. van der Poel. "Public Health Threat of New, Reemerging, and Neglected Zoonoses in the Industrialized World." *Emerging Infectious Diseases* 16, no. 1 (January 2010): DOI 10.3201/eid1601.081467.

WEBSITES

Outbreak Alerts: Global Early Warning System for Major Animal Diseases, including Zoonoses (GLEWS). World Health Organization. http://www.who.int/zoonoses/outbreaks/en/ (accessed July 6, 2012).

Zoonoses. World Health Organization. http://www.who.int/foodsafety/zoonoses/en/ (accessed October 13, 2012).

Zoonoses and Veterinary Public Health (VPH). World Health Organization. http://www.who.int/zoonoses/en/ (accessed October 13, 2012).

ORGANIZATIONS

Centers for Disease Control and Prevention, 1600 Clifton Rd., Atlanta, GA 30333, (800) 232-4636, cdcinfo@cdc.gov, http://www.cdc.gov/.

National Institute of Allergy and Infectious Diseases, 1301 Pennsylvania Ave., NW, Ste. 800, Washington, DC 20004, (202) 785-3355, Fax: (202) 452-1805, http://www.niaid.nih.gov.

World Health Organization, Avenue Appia 20, Geneva, Switzerland 1211 27, 41 22 791-2111, Fax: 41 22 791-3111, http://www.who.int/en/.

Samuel D. Uretsky, PharmD
Teresa G. Odle
William A. Atkins, BB, BS, MBA

ORGANIZATIONS

The following is an alphabetical compilation of relevant organizations listed in the *Resources* sections of the main body entries. Although the list is comprehensive, it is by no means exhaustive. It is a starting point for gathering further information. E-mail addresses and web addresses listed were provided by the associations; Gale, Cengage Learning is not responsible for the accuracy of the addresses or the contents of the websites.

A

Academy of Nutrition and Dietetics
120 South Riverside Plaza, Ste. 2000
Chicago, IL 60606-6995
Phone: (312) 899-0040
Toll free: (800) 877-1600
E-mail: amacmunn@eatright.org
Website: http://www.eatright.org

Agency for Toxic Substances and Disease Registry (ATSDR)
4770 Buford Hwy. NE
Atlanta, GA 30341
Toll free: (800) 232-4636; TTY: (888) 232-6348
E-mail: cdcinfo@cdc.gov
Website: http://www.atsdr.cdc.gov/

Agency for Toxic Substances and Disease Registry (ATSDR)Division of Toxicology and Environmental Medicine
4770 Buford Hwy NE
Atlanta, GA 30341
Toll free: (800) CDC-INFO
E-mail: cdcinfo@cdc.gov
Website: http://www.atsdr.cdc.gov/

Agricultural Research Service
Jamie L. Whitten Bldg. 1400 Independence Avenue SW
Washington, DC 20250
Phone: (301) 504-1637
Website: http://www.ars.usda.gov

AIDS.GOV
200 Independence Ave. SW, Rm 443H
Washington, DC 20201
Toll free: (800) 448-0440
E-mail: contact aids.gov.
Website: http://www.aids.gov

Allergy and Asthma Foundation of America
8201 Corporate Dr., Ste. 1000
Landover, MD 20785
Toll free: (800) 727-8462
E-mail: Info@aafa.org
Website: http://www.aafa.org

Allergy and Asthma Network: Mothers of Asthmatics (AANMA)
2751 Prosperity Ave., Ste. 150
Fairfax, VA 22031
Toll free: (800) 878-4403
Fax: (703) 573-7794
Website: http://www.aanma.org

Alliance for the Prudent Use of Antibiotics (APUA)
200 Harrison Ave. Posner 3 (Business)
Boston, MA 02111
Phone: (617) 636-0966
Fax: (617) 636-0458
E-mail: apua@tufts.edu
Website: http://www.tufts.edu/med/apua/

America's Clean Water Foundation
750 First St. NE, Ste. 1030
Washington, DC 20002
Phone: (202) 898-0908
Fax: (202) 898-0977
E-mail: webmasteracwf@acwf.org
Website: http://agripollute.nstl.gov.cn/MirrorResources/6492/index.html

American Academy of Allergy Asthma and Immunology (AAAAI)
555 East Wells St., Ste. 1100
Milwaukee, WI 53202-3823
Phone: (414) 272-6071
E-mail: info@aaaai.org
Website: http://www.aaaai.org

American Academy of Dermatology
PO Box 4014
Schaumburg, IL 60168-4014
Toll free: (866) 503 7546
Fax: (847) 240 1859
E-mail: MRC@aad.org
Website: http://www.aad.org

American Academy of Environmental Medicine
6505 E Central Ave. No. 296
Wichita, KS 67206
Phone: (316) 684-5500
Website: http://www.aaemonline.org

American Academy of Family Physicians
P.O. Box 11210
Shawnee Mission, KS 66207
Phone: (913) 906–6000
Toll free: (800) 274-2237
Fax: (913) 906–6075
E-mail: http://familydoctor.org/familydoctor/en/about/contact-us.html
Website: http://familydoctor.org

American Academy of Pediatrics (AAP)
141 Northwest Point Blvd.
Elk Grove Village, IL 60007-1098
Phone: (847) 434-4000
Fax: (847) 424-8000
E-mail: kidsdocs@aap.org
Website: http://www.aap.org

American Association of Poison Control Centers
3201 New Mexico Ave., Ste. 330
Washington, DC 20016
Toll free: (800) 222-1222
Website: http://www.aapcc.org

American Associations of Poison Control Centers
515 King St., Ste. 510
Alexandria, VA 22314
Phone: (703) 894-1858
Fax: (703) 683-2812
Website: http:// info@aapcc.org

American Biological Safety Association
1200 Allanson Rd.
Mundelein, IL 60060
Phone: (847) 949-1517
Toll free: (866) 425-1385
Fax: (847) 566-4580
E-mail: info@absa.org
Website: http://www.absa.org

American Board of Industrial Hygiene
6015 W St. Joseph, Ste. 102
Lansing, MI 48917
Phone: (517) 321-2638
Fax: (517) 321-4624
Website: http://www.abih.org

American Burn Association
311 S Wacker Dr. Ste. 4150
Chicago, IL 60606
Phone: (312) 642-9260
Fax: (312) 642-9130
E-mail: info@ameriburn.org
Website: http://www.ameriburn.org

American Cancer Society
250 Williams St. NW
Atlanta, GA 30303
Toll free: (800) 227-2345
Website: http://www.cancer.org

American College of Allergy Asthma and Immunology
85 West Algonquin Rd. Ste. 550
Arlington Heights, IL 60005
Phone: (847) 427-1200
E-mail: mail@acaai.org
Website: http://www.acaai.org

American College of Emergency Physicians (ACEP)
1125 Executive Cir.
Irving, TX 75038-2522
Phone: (972) 550-0911
Toll free: (800) 798-1822
Fax: (972) 580-2816
Website: http://www.acep.org

American College of Hyperbaric Medicine
6737 W. Washington St., Ste. 3265
West Allis, WI 53214
Phone: (414) 918-9300
Fax: (414) 918-9301
E-mail: admin@achm.org
Website: http://www.achm.org

American College of Medical Toxicology (ACMT)
10645 N. Tatum Blvd., Ste. 200-111
Phoenix, AZ 85028
Phone: (623) 533-6340
Fax: (623) 533-6520
E-mail: info@acmt.net
Website: http://www.acmt.net/

American College of Nutrition
300 S. Duncan Ave., Ste. 225
Clearwater, FL 33755
Phone: (727) 446-6086
Fax: (727) 446-6202
E-mail: office@AmericanCollegeofNutrition.org
Website: http://www.americancollegeofnutrition.org

American College of Sports Medicine
401 West Michigan St.
Indianapolis, IN 46206-3233
Phone: (317) 637-9200
Fax: (317) 634-7817
Website: http://www.acsm.org

American College of Toxicology (ACTOX)
9650 Rockville Pike #3408
Bethesda, MD 20814
Phone: (301) 634-7840
Fax: (301) 634-7852
Website: http://www.actox.org/Home/tabid/726/Default.aspx

American Contact Dermatitis Society
2323 North State St., #30
Bunnell, FL 32110
Phone: (386) 437-4405
Fax: (386) 437-4427
E-mail: info@contactderm.org
Website: http://www.contactderm.org

American Council on Science and Health
1995 Broadway, Ste. 202
New York, NY 10023
Phone: (212) 362-7044
Toll free: (866) 905-2694
Fax: (212) 362-4919
E-mail: acsh@acsh.org
Website: http://www.acsh.org

American Industrial Hygiene Association
3141 Fairview Park Dr., Ste. 777
Falls Church, VA 22042
Phone: (703) 849-8888
Fax: (703) 207-3561
E-mail: infonet@aiha.org
Website: http://www.aiha.org

American Kidney Fund
11921 Rockville Pike, Ste. 300
Rockville, MD 20852
Toll free: (800) 638-8299
Website: http://www.kidneyfund.org

American Legion
700 N Pennsylvania St.
Indianapolis, IN 46206
Toll free: (800) 433-3318
Website: http://www.legion.org

American Lung Association
1301 Pennsylvania Ave. NW, Ste. 800
Washington, DC 20004
Phone: (202) 785-3355
Toll free: (800) LUNGUSA (586-4872)
Fax: (202) 202 452 1805
Website: http://www.lungusa.org

American Lyme Disease Foundation
P. O. Box 466
Lyme, CT 06371
E-mail: inquire@adlf.com
Website: http://www.aldf.com

American Medical Association
515 N State St.
Chicago, IL 60654
Toll free: (800) 621-8335
Website: http://www.ama-assn.org

American Mosquito Control Association
15000 Commerce Pkwy., Ste. C
Mount Laurel, NJ 08054
Phone: (856) 439-9222
Fax: (856) 439-0525
E-mail: amca@mosquito.org
Website: http://www.mosquito.org

American Physical Therapy Association
1111 North Fairfax St.
Alexandria, VA 22314-1488
Phone: (703) 684-APTA (2782). TDD: (703) 683-6748
Toll free: (800) 999-APTA (2782)
Fax: (703) 683-6748
Website: http://www.apta.org

American Psychiatric Association
1000 Wilson Blvd., Ste. 1825
Arlington, VA 22209-3901
Phone: (703) 907-7300
Toll free: (888) 357-7924
E-mail: apa@psych.org
Website: http://www.psych.org

American Public Health Association (APHA)
800 I St. NW
Washington, DC 20001-3710
Phone: (202) 777-APHA
Fax: (202) 777-2534
Website: http://apha.org/

American Red Cross
2025 E St.
Washington, DC 20006
Phone: (202) 303-4498
Toll free: (800) 733-2767
Website: http://www.redcross.org

American Social Health Association (ASHA)
PO Box 13827
Research Triangle Park, NC 27709
Phone: (919) 361-8400
Toll free: (800) 227-8922
Fax: (919) 361-8425
Website: http://www.ashastd.org/index.cfm

American Society for Nutrition
9650 Rockville Pike
Bethesda, MD 20814
Phone: (301) 634-7050
Fax: (301) 634-7894
Website: http://www.nutrition.org

American Society of Clinical Oncology
2318 Mill Rd., Ste. 800
Alexandria, VA 22314
Phone: (571) 483-1300
Website: http://www.asco.org

American Society of Plastic Surgeons
444 E Algonquin Rd.
Arlington Heights, IL 60005
Phone: (847) 228-9900
Website: http://www.plasticsurgery.org

American Thoracic Society
25 Broadway 18th Fl.
New York, NY 10004
Phone: (212) 315-8600
Fax: (212) 315-6498
E-mail: atsinfo@thoracic.org
Website: http://www.thoracic.org/

Organizations

American Veterinary Medical Association (AVMA)
1931 North Meacham Rd., Ste. 100
Schaumburg, IL 60173-4360
Phone: (847) 925-8070
Fax: (847) 925-1329
E-mail: avmainfo@avma.org
Website: http://www.avma.org

Anxiety Disorders Association of America
8701 Georgia Ave., Ste. 412
Silver Spring, MD 20910
Phone: (240) 485-1001
Website: http://www.adaa.org

APEC Emerging Infections Network
1107 NE 45th St., Ste. 400
Seattle, WA 98195
E-mail: apecein@u.washington.edu
Website: http://depts.washington.edu

Asthma and Allergy Foundation of America
1233 20th Street NW, Ste. 402
Washington, DC 20036
Toll free: (800) 7-ASTHMA or (800) 727-8462
E-mail: info@aafa.org
Website: http://www.aafa.org

Autism Research Institute/Autism Resource Center
4182 Adams Ave.
San Diego, CA 92116
Phone: English: (866) 366-3361; Spanish: (877) 644-1184 ext. 5
Fax: (619) 563-6840
Website: http://www.autism.com

Autism Society of America
4340 East-West Hwy., Ste. 350
Bethesda, MD
Phone: (301) 657-0881
Toll free: (800) 3-AUTISM [(800) 328-8476]
Website: http://www.autismsource.org

Autism Speaks
1 East 33rd St., 4th Floor
New York, NY 10016
Phone: (212) 252-8584
Fax: (212) 252-8676
E-mail: contactus@autismspeaks.org
Website: http://www.autismspeaks.org

B

Beryllium Network Brayton Purcell LLP
222 Rush Landing Rd.
Novato, CA 94948
Phone: (415) 898-1555
Website: http://www.chronicberylliumdisease.com

Better Hearing Institute
1444 I St. NW, Ste. 700
Washington, DC 20005
Phone: (202) 449-1100
Fax: (202) 216-9646
E-mail: mail@betterhearing.org
Website: http://www.betterhearing.org

Bill & Melinda Gates Foundation
500 Fifth Ave. N
Seattle, WA 98102
Phone: (206) 709-3100
E-mail: info@gatesfoundation.org
Website: http://www.gatesfoundation.org

C

CARE International Secretariat
Chemin de Balexert 7–9
Chatelaine, 1219 France
Phone: 41 22 795 10 20
Fax: 41 22 795 10 29
Toll free: (800) 521-CARE (2273)
Website: http://www.care-international.org

Center for Environmental Research and Children's Health (University of California at Berkeley)
1995 University Ave., Ste. 265
Berkeley, CA 94720-7392
Phone: (510) 643-9598
Fax: (510) 642-9083
E-mail: cerch@berkeley.edu
Website: http://cerch.org

Center for Food Safety
660 Pennsylvania Ave. SE, Ste. 302
Washington, DC 20003
Phone: (202) 547-9359
Fax: (202) 547-9429
E-mail: office@centerforfoodsafety.org
Website: http://www.centerforfoodsafety.org

Center for Food Safety and Applied Nutrition (CFSAN) U.S. Food and Drug Administration
5100 Paint Branch Pkwy.
College Park, MD 20740
Toll free: (888) SAFEFOOD (723-3366)
E-mail: consumer@fda.gov
Website: http://www.fda.gov/Food/default.htm

Center for the Study of Bioterrorism and Emergency Infections-Saint Louis University
3545 Lafayette, Ste. 300
St. Louis, MO 63104
Website: http://bioterrorism.slu.edu

Centers for Disease Control and Prevention (CDC)
1600 Clifton Rd.
Atlanta, GA 30333
Phone: (404) 639-3534
Toll free: (800) 232-4636; TTY: (888) 232-6348
E-mail: inquiry@cdc.gov
Website: http://www.cdc.gov

Centers for Disease Control and Prevention Public Inquiries/MASO
Mailstop F07 1600 Clifton Rd.
Atlanta, GA 30333
Toll free: (800) 311-3435
Website: http://www.cdc.gov

Centers for Disease Control and Prevention—Bioterrorism Preparedness & Response Program (CDC)
1600 Clifton Rd.
Atlanta, GA 30333
Phone: (404) 639-3534
Toll free: (888) 246-2675
E-mail: cdcresponse@ashastd.org
Website: http://www.bt.cdc.gov

Centers for Disease Control Malaria Hotline
Phone: (770) 332-4555

Centers for Disease Control Travelers Hotline
Phone: (770) 332-4559

Charity Navigator
139 Harristown Rd., Ste. 201
Glen Rock, NJ 07452
Phone: (201) 818-1288
Fax: (201) 818-4694
E-mail: info@charitynavigator.org
Website: http://www.charitynavigator.org

Chartered Institute of Environmental Health
Chadwick Court 15 Hatfields
London, SE1 8DJ United Kingdom
Phone: +44(0)20 7928 6006
Fax: +44(0)20 7827 5862
E-mail: https://forms.cieh.org/ciehorg/forms/ciehform.aspx?ekfrm=154
Website: http://www.cieh.org/

Chemical Safety and Hazard Investigation Board (CSB)
2175 K St. NW
Washington, DC 20037
Phone: (202) 261-7600
Fax: (202) 261-7650
E-mail: http://www.csb.gov/service/contact.aspx
Website: http://www.csb.gov/

Chicago Electrical Trauma Research Institute
4047 W 40th St.
Chicago, IL 80532
Phone: (773) 904-0347
Toll free: (800) 516-8709
E-mail: info@cetri.org
Website: http://www.cetri.org/

Children & Nature Network
7 Avenida Vista Grande B-7, no. 502
Santa Fe, NM 87508
E-mail: info@childrenandnature.org
Website: http://www.cnaturenet.org

CJD Aware!
2527 South Carrollton Ave.
New Orleans, LA 70118-3013
Phone: (504) 861-4627
E-mail: info@cjdaware.com
Website: http://www.cjdaware.com

Consumer Product Safety Commission
4330 East West Hwy.
Bethesda, MD 20814
Phone: (301) 504-7923
Website: http://www.cpsc.gov/

Convention on Biological Diversity
413 Saint-Jacques St., Ste. 800
Montreal, H2Y 1N9 Quebec Canada
Phone: (514) 288-2220
Fax: (514) 288-6588
E-mail: bch@cbd.int
Website: http://bch.cbd.int

Creutzfeldt-Jakob Disease Foundation
3632 W Market St.
Akron, OH 44333
Toll free: (800) 659-1991
E-mail: help@cjdfoundation.org
Website: http://www.cjdfoundation.org

D

Department of Agriculture
1400 Independence Ave. SW
Washington, DC 20250
Phone: (202) 720-2791
Website: http://www.usda.gov/wps/portal/usdahome

Divers Alert Network
6 W, Colony Place
Durham, NC 27705
Phone: (919) 684-2948
Fax: (919) 490-6630
Toll free: (800) 446-2671
Website: http://www.diversalertnetwork.org

E

Earth Day Network
1616 P St. NW, Ste. 340
Washington, DC 20036
Phone: (202) 518-0044
E-mail: buchanan@earthday.org
Website: http://www.earthday.org

Environmental Defense Fund
1875 Connecticut Ave. NW, Ste. 600
Washington, DC 20009
Toll free: (800) 684-3322
Website: http://www.edf.org/

Environmental Protection Agency (EPA)
Ariel Rios Bldg., 1200 Pennsylvania Ave. NW
Washington, DC 20460
Phone: (202) 272-0167; TTY (202) 272-0165
Website: http://www.epa.gov

Environmental Research Foundation
PO Box 160
New Brunswick, NJ 08908
Phone: (732) 828-9995
E-mail: erf@rachel.org
Website: http://www.rachel.org

European Bioinformatics Institute
Wellcome Trust Genome Campus Hinxton
Cambridge, CB10 1SD United Kingdom
Phone: 44 (0)1223 494 444
Fax: 44 (0)1223 494 468
Website: http://www.ebi.ac.uk

European Commission Directorate General for Health and Consumers
B-1049 Brussels, Belgium
Phone: 011 32(2) 299-11-11
Website: http://ec.europa.eu/dgs/health_consumer/index_en.htm

European Food Safety Authority
Via Carlo Magno 1A
Parma, 43126 Italy
Phone: +39 0521 036111
Fax: +39 0521 036110
Website: http://www.efsa.europa.eu

Exxon Valdez Oil Spill Trustee Council
4230 University Dr., Ste. 230
Anchorage, AK 99508-4650
Phone: (907) 278-8012
Fax: (907) 276-7178
Toll free: (800) 478-7745
Website: http://www.evostc.state.ak.us

F

Federal Communications Commission
445 12th St. SW
Washington, DC 20554
Phone: (202) 418-1440
Fax: (866) 418-0232
Toll free: (888) CALL FCC (225-5322)
E-mail: fccinfo@fcc.gov
Website: http://www.fcc.gov

Federal Emergency Management Agency (FEMA)
PO Box 10055
Hyattsville, MD 20782
Phone: (202) 646-2500
Toll free: (800) 621-3362
Website: http://www.fema.gov

Federal Emergency Management Agency U.S. Department of Homeland Security
500 C St. SW
Washington, DC 20472
Phone: (206) 646-2500
Toll free: (800) 621-FEMA (3362)
Website: http://www.fema.gov

Food Allergy and Anaphylaxis Network (FAAN)
11781 Lee Jackson Hwy., Ste. 160
Fairfax, VA 22033
Toll free: (800) 929-4040
Fax: (703) 691-2713
E-mail: faan@foodallergy.org
Website: http://www.foodallergy.org

Food and Agriculture Organization of the United Nations (FAO Headquarters)
Viale delle Terme di Caracalla
Rome, 00153 Italy
Phone: 39 06 570 53625
Fax: 39 06 5705 3699
E-mail: AGN-Director@fao.org (Nutrition and Consumer Protection)
Website: http://www.fao.org

Food and Drug Administration (FDA)
10903 New Hampshire Ave.
Silver Spring, MD 20993
Toll free: (888) INFO-FDA (463-6332)
Website: http://www.fda.gov/default.htm

Food and Nutrition Information Center National Agricultural Library
10301 Baltimore Ave., Rm. 105
Beltsville, MD 20705
Phone: (301) 504-5414
Fax: (301) 504-6409
E-mail: fnic@ars.usda.gov
Website: http://fnic.nal.usda.gov

Food Safety and Inspection Service (FSIS) U.S. Department of Agriculture (USDA)
1400 Independence Ave. SW
Washington, DC 20250-3700
Toll free: (888) 674-6854 (USDA Meat and Poultry Consumer Hotline)
E-mail: MPHotline.fsis@usda.gov
Website: http://www.fsis.usda.gov

Food Standards Agency
Aviation House 125 Kingsway
London, WC2B 6NH United Kingdom
Website: http://www.food.gov.uk

G

Gay Men's Health Crisis (GMHC)
Tisch Bldg., 446 West 33rd St.
New York, NY 10001-2601
Phone: (212) 367-1000
Website: http://www.gmhc.org

Global Alliance Against Chronic Respiratory Diseases World Health Organization
20 Avenue Appia
Geneva, 1211 27 Switzerland
E-mail: gard@who.int
Website: http://www.who.int/gard/en

Global Fund to Fight AIDS Tuberculosis and Malaria
Geneva Secretariat Chemin de Blandonnet 8 1214 Vernier
Geneva Switzerland
Phone: 41 58 791-1700
Fax: 41 58 791-1701
E-mail: info@theglobalfund.org
Website: http://www.theglobalfund.org/en

H

Health Physics Society
1313 Dolley Madison Blvd., Ste. 402
McLean, VA 22101
Phone: (703) 790-1745
Fax: (703) 790-2672
E-mail: hps@burkinc.com
Website: http://www.hps.org

Human Factors and Ergonomics Society
PO Box 1369
Santa Monica, CA 90406-1369
Phone: (310) 394-1811
Fax: (310) 394-2410
E-mail: info@hfes.org
Website: http://www.hfes.org

I

Immunization Action Coalition
1573 Selby Ave., Ste. 234
St. Paul, MN 55104
Phone: (651) 647-9009
Fax: (651) 647-9131
E-mail: admin@immunize.org
Website: http://www.immunize.org

Infectious Diseases Society of America (IDSA)
1300 Wilson Blvd., Ste. 300
Arlington, VA 22209
Phone: (703) 299-0200
Fax: (703) 299-0204
E-mail: info@idsociety.org
Website: http://www.idsociety.org

Institute for Altitude Medicine
PO Box 1229
Telluride, CO 81435
Phone: (970) 728-6767
E-mail: info@altitudemedicine.org
Website: http://www.altitudemedicine.org

Institute of Food Technologies
525 W. Van Buren, Ste. 1000
Chicago, IL 60607
Phone: (312) 782-8424
Fax: (312) 792-8348
E-mail: info@ift.org
Website: http://www.ift.org

International Agency for Research on Cancer
150 Cours Albert Thomas CEDEX 08
Lyons, 69372 France
Phone: 33 0 4 72 73 8485
Fax: 33 0 4 72 73 8575
Website: http://www.iarc.fr

International AIDS Society (IAS)
Ave. Louis Casaï 71 P. O. Box 28
Geneva, CH - 1216 Cointrin Switzerland
Phone: +41-(0)22-7 100 800
Fax: +41-0)22-7 100 899
E-mail: info@iasociety.org
Website: http://www.iasociety.org

International Association of Wildland Fires
1418 Washburn St.
Missoula, MT 59801
Phone: (406) 531-8264
Toll free: (888) 440-4293
E-mail: iawf@iawfonline.org
Website: http://www.iawfonline.org

International Atomic Energy Agency (IAEA)
Vienna International Center PO Box 100
Vienna, A-1400 Austria
Phone: +4312600-0
Fax: +4312600-7
E-mail: Official.Mail@iaea.org
Website: http://www.iaea.org

International Atomic Energy Agency
1 United Nations Plaza, Rm DC-1-1155
New York, NY 10017
Phone: (212) 963-6010
Fax: (917) 367-4046
E-mail: iaeany@un.org
Website: http://www.iaea.org

International Centre for Genetic Engineering and Biotechnology Biosafety
Padriciano 99
Trieste, 34149 Italy
Phone: 39(040) 3757320
Fax: 39(040) 226555
E-mail: biosafe@icgeb.org
Website: http://www.icgeb.org

International Committee of the Red Cross
19 Avenue de la Paix
Geneva, 1202 Switzerland
Phone: 41 22 734 60 01
Fax: 41 22 733 20 57
E-mail: webmaster@icrc.org
Website: http://www.icrc.org

International Council for the Control of Iodine Deficiency Disorders
PO Box 51030 375 des Epinettes
Ottawa, K1E 3E0 Ontario Canada
Website: http://www.iccidd.org

International Federation of Red Cross and Red Crescent Societies
PO Box 372
Geneva, 1211 Switzerland
Phone: 41 22 730 42 22
Fax: 41 22 733 03 95
Website: http://www.ifrc.org

International Food Information Council Foundation
1100 Connecticut Ave. NW, Ste. 430
Washington, DC 20036

Phone: (202) 296-6540
E-mail: info@foodinsight.org
Website: http://www.foodinsight.org

International Leptospirosis Society
Faculty of Medicine Nursing and Health Sciences Monash University
Victoria 3800 Australia
Phone: +61 3 9905 4301
Fax: +61 3 9905 4302
E-mail: enquiries@med.monash.edu.au
Website: http://www.med.monash.edu.au/microbiology/staff/adler/ils.html

International Manganese Institute
17 rue Duphot
Paris, France
Phone: +33(0) 145 63 06 34
Fax: +33(0) 1 42 89 42 92
Website: http://www.manganese.org

International Occupational Hygiene Association
5/6 Melbourne Business Court Pride Park
Derby, DE24 8LZ United Kingdom
Phone: +44(332) 298 101
Fax: +44(332) 298 099
E-mail: admin@ioha.net
Website: http://www.ioha.net

International Rescue Committee
122 E 42nd St.
New York, NY 10168-1289
Phone: (212) 551-3000
Fax: (212) 551-3179
Website: http://www.rescue.org

International Society for Traumatic Stress Studies
111 Deer Lake Rd., Ste. 100
Deerfield, IL 60015
Phone: (847) 480-9028
Fax: (847) 480-9282
Website: http://www.istss.org

International Society of Explosives Engineers (ISEE)
30325 Bainbridge Rd.
Cleveland, OH 44139
Phone: (440) 349-4400
Fax: (440) 349-3788
Website: http://www.isee.org

International Society of Exposure Science Secretariat
c/o JSI Research and Training Institute
44 Farnsworth St.
Boston, MA 02201
Phone: (617) 482-9485
Fax: (617) 482-0617
Website: http://isesweb.org

International Solid Waste Association
Auerspergstrasse 15 Top 41
Vienna, 1080 Austria
Phone: 43 1(253) 6001
Fax: 43 1(253) 6001 99
E-mail: iswa@iswa.org
Website: http://www.iswa.org

International Union for Conservation of Nature
Rue Mauverney 28
Gland, 1196 Switzerland
Phone: 41(999) 0000
Fax: 41(999) 0002
Website: http://www.iucn.org

International Union of Geodesy and Geophysics
Hertzstrasse 16
Karlsruhe, 76187 Germany
Phone: 49(721) 6084-4494
Fax: 49(721) 711-73
E-mail: secretariat@iugg.org
Website: http://www.iugg.org

L

Leukemia and Lymphoma Society
1311 Mamaroneck Ave., Ste. 310
White Plains, NY 10605
Phone: (914) 949-5213
Website: http://www.lls.org

Lyme Disease Network of NJ.
43 Winton Road
East Brunswick, NJ 08816
Website: http://www.lymenet.org

M

March of Dimes Foundation
1275 Mamaroneck Ave.
White Plains, NY 10605
Phone: (914)997-4488
E-mail: askus@marchofdimes.com
Website: http://www.marchofdimes.com

Mine Safety and Health Administration
4015 Wilson Blvd.
Arlington, VA 22203
Toll free: (877) 778-6055
E-mail: MSHAhelpdesk@dol.gov
Website: http://www.msha.gov

N

National Agriculture Center U.S. Environmental Protection Agency
901 N 5th St.
Kansas City, KS 66101
Toll free: (888) 663-2155
Fax: (913) 551-7270
E-mail: agcenter@epa.gov
Website: http://www.epa.gov/agriculture/agctr.html

National Agriculture Compliance Assistance Center U.S. Environmental Protection Agency
901 North 5th St.
Kansas City, KS 66101
Toll free: (888) 663-2155
Fax: (913) 551-7270
E-mail: agcenter@epa.gov
Website: http://www.epa.gov/agriculture

National Alliance on Mental Illness
3803 N. Fairfax Dr., Ste. 100
Arlington, VA 22203
Phone: (703) 524-7600
Fax: (703) 524-9094
Toll free: (800) 950-6264
Website: http://www.nami.org

National Cancer Institute (NCI)
6116 Executive Blvd., Ste. 300
Bethesda, MD 20892-8322
Toll free: (800) 422-6237
E-mail: http://www.cancer.gov/global/contact/email-us
Website: http://www.cancer.gov

National Center for Biotechnology Information
8600 Rockville Pike
Bethesda, MD 20894
Phone: (301) 496-2475
Website: http://www.ncbi.nlm.nih.gov

National Center for Emerging and Zoonotic Infectious Diseases Centers for Disease Control and Prevention
1600 Clifton Rd.
Atlanta, GA 30333
Toll free: (800) 232-4635
E-mail: cdcinfo@cdc.gov
Website: http://www.cdc.gov/ncezid/

National Center for Posttraumatic Stress Disorder
810 Vermont Ave. NW
Washington, DC 20420
Website: http://www.ptsd.va.gov

National Children's Leukemia Foundation
7316 Ave. U
Brooklyn, NY 11234
Phone: (800) 448-4673
Website: http://www.leukemiafoundation.org

National Coalition for Cancer Survivorship
1010 Wayne Ave., Ste. 770
Silver Spring, MD 20910
Toll free: (877) 622-7937
Website: http://www.canceradvocacy.org/

National Comprehensive Cancer Network
275 Commerce Dr., Ste. 300
Fort Washington, PA 19034
Phone: (215) 690-0300
Website: http://www.nccn.org

National Digestive Diseases Information Clearinghouse (NDDIC)
2 Information Way
Bethesda, MD 20892-3570
Toll free: (800) 891-5389; TTY (866) 569-1162
Fax: (703) 738-4929
E-mail: info@niddk.nih.gov
Website: http://digestive.niddk.nih.gov

National Earthquake Information Center
PO Box 25046 DFC MS 967
Denver, CO 80225
Phone: (303) 273-8500
Fax: (303) 273-8450
E-mail: sedas@neis.cr.usgs.gov
Website: http://www.neic.usgs.gov

National Environmental Education Foundation
4301 Connecticut Ave., Ste. 160
Washington, DC 20008
Phone: (202) 833-2933
Fax: (202) 261-6464
Website: http://www.outdoorfoundation.org

National Foundation for Infectious Diseases
4733 Bethesda Ave., Ste. 750
Bethesda, MD 20814
Phone: (301) 656-0003
Fax: (301) 907-0878
Toll free: (800) 232-4636
Website: http://www.nfid.org

National Health Information Center. Office of Disease Prevention and Health Promotion. U.S. Department of Health and Human Services
P. O. Box 1133
Washington, DC 20013-1133
Phone: (847) 434-4000
Website: http://www.health.gov/nhic/

National Hearing Conservation Association
3030 W 81st Ave.
Westminster, CO 80031
Phone: (303) 224-9022
Fax: (303) 458-0002
E-mail: nhcaoffice@hearingconservation.org
Website: http://www.hearingconservation.org

National Heart Lung and Blood Institute
PO Box 30105
Bethesda, MD 20824-0105
Phone: (301) 592-8573
Fax: (240) 629-3246
E-mail: nhlbiinfo@nhlbi.nih.gov
Website: http://www.nhlbi.nih.gov

National Human Genome Research Institute Communications and Public Liaison Branch National Institutes of Health
Building 31, Room 4B09
31 Center Drive MSC 2152 9000 Rockville Pike
Bethesda, MD 20892-2152
Phone: (301) 402-0911
Fax: (301) 402-2218
Website: http://www.genome.gov

National Hurricane Center
11691 SW 17th St.
Miami, FL 33165

Phone: (305) 229-4404
E-mail: NHC.Public.Affairs@noaa.gov
Website: http://www.nhc.noaa.gov

National Institute for Occupational Safety and Health Centers for Disease Control and Prevention
1600 Clifton Rd.
Atlanta, GA 30333
Toll free: (800) 232-4636
E-mail: cdcinfo@cdc.gov
Website: http://www.cdc.gov/niosh/

National Institute for Occupational Safety and Health Education and Information Division
4676 Columbia Pkwy.
Cincinnati, OH 45226
Toll free: (800) 232-4636
Fax: (513) 533-8347
E-mail: cdcinfo@cdc.gov
Website: http://www.cdc.gov/niosh

National Institute of Allergy and Infectious Diseases Office of Communications and Government Relations
6610 Rockledge Dr. MSC 6612
Bethesda, MD 20892-6612
Phone: (301) 496-5717
Toll free: (866) 284-4107 or TDD: (800)877-8339 (for hearing impaired)
Fax: (301) 402-3573
Website: http://www3.niaid.nih.gov

National Institute of Allergy and Infectious Diseases
1301 Pennsylvania Ave. NW, Ste. 800
Washington, DC 20004
Phone: (202) 785-3355
Fax: (202) 452-1805
Website: http://www.niaid.nih.gov

National Institute of Arthritis and Musculoskeletal and Skin Diseases (NIAMS)Information Clearinghouse
1 AMS Circle
Bethesda, MD 20892-3675
Phone: (301) 495-4484
Toll free: (877) 22-NIAMS (226-4267); TTY: (301) 565«2966
E-mail: NIAMSinfo@mail.nih.gov
Website: http://www.niams.nih.gov

National Institute of Child Health and Human Development (NICHD)
PO Box 3006
Rockville, MD 20847
Toll free: (800) 370-2943
Fax: (866) 760-5947
E-mail: NICHDInformationResourceCenter@mail.nih.gov
Website: http://www.nichd.nih.gov

National Institute of Diabetes and Digestive and Kidney Diseases
Office of Communications & Public Liaison NIDDK NIH
Building 31 Rm. 9A06 31 Center Dr. MSC 2560
Bethesda, MD 20892-2560
Phone: (301) 496-3583
Website: http://www2.niddk.nih.gov

National Institute of Environmental Health Sciences (NIEHS)
P.O. Box 12233 MD K3-16
Research Triangle Park, NC 27709-2233
Phone: (919) 541-3345
Fax: (919) 541-4395
Website: http://www.niehs.nih.gov/

National Institute of Mental Health
6001 Executive Blvd., Rm. 8184 MSC 9663
Bethesda, MD 20892-9663
Phone: (301) 443-4513
Fax: (301) 443-4279
Toll free: (866) 615-6464
E-mail: nimhinfo@nih.gov
Website: http://www.nimh.nih.gov

National Institute of Neurological Disorders and Stroke
P.O. Box 5801
Bethesda, MD 20824
Phone: (301) 496-5751
Toll free: (800) 352-9424
Website: http://www.ninds.nih.gov/

National Institute on Drug Abuse
6001 Executive Blvd., Rm 5213
Bethesda, MD 20892-9561
Phone: (301) 443-1124; en espanole (240) 221-4007
E-mail: information@nida.nih.gov
Website: http://drugabuse.gov/nidahome.html

National Institutes of Health
9000 Rockville Pike
Bethesda, MD 20892
Phone: (301) 496-4000
E-mail: NIHinfo@od.nih.gov
Website: http://www.nih.gov

National Kidney Disease Education Program
3 Kidney Information Way
Bethesda, MD 20892
Toll free: (866) 4-KIDNEY (454-3639)
Fax: (301) 402-8182
E-mail: nkdep@info.niddk.nih.gov
Website: http://www.nkdep.nih.gov

National Kidney Foundation
30 East 33rd St.
New York, NY 10016
Phone: (212) 889-2210
Toll free: (800) 622-9010
Fax: (212) 689-9261
Website: http://www.kidney.org

National Meningitis Association
PO Box 725165
Atlanta, GA 31139
Phone: (866) FONE-NMA (366-3662)
Fax: (877) 703-6096
Website: http://www.nmaus.org

National Necrotizing Fasciitis Foundation
2731 Porter SW
Grand Rapids, MI 49509

E-mail: nnfffeb@aol.com
Website: http://www.nnff.org

National Network for Immunization Information
301 University Blvd.
Galveston, TX 77555-0350
Phone: (409) 772-0199
Fax: (409) 772-5208
E-mail: nnii@i4ph.org
Website: http://www.immunizationinfo.org

National Oceanic and Atmospheric Administration
1401 Constitution Ave. NW, Rm. 5128
Washington, DC 20230
Website: http://www.noaa.gov

National Office for Marine Biotoxins and Harmful Algal Blooms Woods Hole Oceanographic Institution
Biology Dept. MS No. 32
Woods Hole, MA 02543
Phone: (508) 289-2252
Fax: (508) 457-2180
E-mail: jkleindinst@whoi.edu
Website: http://www.redtide.whoi.edu/hab

National Park Conservation Association
777 6th St. NW, Ste. 700
Washington, DC 20001
Phone: (202) 223-6722
Toll free: (800) NAT-PARK (628-7275)
Fax: (202) 454-3333
E-mail: npca@npca.org
Website: http://www.npca.org

National Park Foundation
1201 Eye St. NW, Ste. 550B
Washington, DC 20005
Phone: (202) 354-6460
Fax: (202) 371-2066
E-mail: ask-npf@nationalparks.org
Website: http://www.nationalparks.org

National Pesticide Information Center
Oregon State University, 333 Weniger Hall
Corvallis, OR 97331-6502
Toll free: (800) 858-7378
E-mail: npic@ace.orst.edu
Website: http://npic.orst.edu

National Safety Council
1121 Spring Lake Dr.
Itasca, IL 60143-3201
Phone: (630) 285-1121
Toll free: (800) 621-7615
E-mail: info@cetri.org
Website: http://www.nsc.org/Pages/Home.aspx

National Solid Waste Management Association
4301 Connecticut Ave. NW, Ste. 300
Washington, DC 20008
Phone: (202) 244-4700
Toll free: (800) 424-2869
Fax: (202) 966-4824
Website: http://www.environmentalistseveryday.org

National Toxicology Program (NTP)
P.O. Box 12233 MD K2-05
Research Triangle Park, NC 27709
Phone: (919) 541-3419
Website: http://ntp.niehs.nih.gov/

National Vaccine Program Office. U.S. Dep. of Health & Human Services
200 Independence Ave. SW, Rm. 715-H
Washington, DC 20201
Phone: (202) 690-5566
E-mail: nvpo@hhs.gov
Website: http://www.hhs.gov/nvpo

National Wildfire Suppression Association
PO Box 330
Lyons, OR 97358
Toll free: (877) 676-6972
Fax: (866) 854-8186
Website: http://www.nwsa.us

National Wildlife Federation
PO Box 1583
Merrifield, VA 22116-1583
Phone: (703) 438-6000
Toll free: (800) 822-9919
Website: http://www.nwf.org

O

Occupational Safety and Health Organization U.S. Department of Labor
200 Constitution Ave. NW
Washington, DC 20210
Toll free: (800) 321-6742
Website: http://www.osha.gov

Office of Cancer Clinical Proteomics Research Center for Strategic Scientific Initiatives Office of the Director National Cancer Institute
31 Center Dr. MS 2580
Bethesda, MD 20892-2580
Phone: (301) 451-8883
E-mail: cancer.proteomics@mail.nih.gov
Website: http://proteomics.cancer.gov

Office of the Special Assistant for Gulf War Illnesses
Force Health Protection & Readiness Policy & Programs
Four Skyline Place 5113 Leesburg Pike, Ste. 901
Falls Church, VA 22041
Toll free: (800) 497-6261
Website: http://www.gulflink.osd.mil

Oncology Nursing Society
125 Enterprise Dr.
Pittsburgh, PA 25275
Phone: (866) 257-4667
Website: http://www.ons.org

Outdoor Foundation
1776 Massachusetts Ave. NW, Ste. 450
Washington, DC 20036

Phone: (202) 271-3252
E-mail: info@outdoorfoundation.org
Website: http://www.outdoorfoundation.org

Oxfam America
226 Causeway St. 5th Fl.
Boston, MA 02114-2206
Phone: (617) 482-121
Fax: (617) 728-2594
Toll free: (800) 77-OXFAM (776-9326)
Website: http://www.oxfamamerica.org

Oxfam International Secretariat
266 Banbury Rd. Ste. 20
Oxford, OX2 7DL United Kingdom
Phone: 44 865 339 100
Fax: 44 865 339 101
Website: http://www.oxfam.org

P

Pan American Health Organization
525 23rd St. NW
Washington, DC 20037
Phone: (202) 974-3000
Fax: (202) 974-3663
Website: http://www.paho.org

Partnership for Food Safety Education
2345 Crystal Dr., Ste. 800
Arlington, VA 22202
Phone: (202) 220-0651
Fax: (202) 220-0873
E-mail: info@fightbac.org
Website: http://www.fightbac.org

Pesticide Action Network North America
1611 Telegraph Ave., Ste. 1200
Oakland, CA 94612
Phone: (510) 788-9020
Website: http://www.panna.org

Pulmonary Fibrosis Association
811 W Evergreen Ave., Ste. 303
Chicago, IL 60642-2642
Toll free: (888) 733-6741
E-mail: info@pulmonaryfibrosis.org
Website: http://www.pulmonaryfibrosis.org

R

Rachel Carson Council
PO Box 10779
Silver Spring, MD 20914
Phone: (301) 593-7507
E-mail: rccouncil@aol.com
Website: http://www.rachelcarsoncouncil.org

S

Save the Children (United Kingdom)
1 St. John's Lane
London, EC1M 4AR United Kingdom
Phone: 44 20 7012 6400
E-mail: supporter.care@savethechildren.org.uk
Website: http://www.savethechildren.org.uk

Save the Children (United States)
54 Wilton Rd.
Westport, CT 06880
Phone: (203) 221-4030
Toll free: (800) 728-3843
E-mail: twebster@savechildren.org
Website: http://www.savethechildren.org

Sierra Club Canada
412-1 Nicholas St.
Ottawa, K1N 7B7 Ontario Canada
Phone: (613) 241-4611
Toll free: (888) 810-4204
Website: http://www.sierraclub.ca

Sierra Club
85 Second St. 2nd Fl.
San Francisco, CA 94105
Phone: (415) 977-5500
Fax: (415) 977-5797
E-mail: information@sierraclub.org
Website: http://www.sierraclub.org

Skin Cancer Foundation
149 Madison Ave., Ste. 901
New York, NY 10016
Phone: (212) 725-5176
E-mail: http://www.skincancer.org/contact-us
Website: http://www.skincancer.org

Society of Environmental Toxicology and Chemistry (Asia/ Pacific/Latin and North America)
229 South Baylen St., 2nd Fl.
Pensacola, FL 32502
Phone: (850) 469-1500
Fax: (850) 469-9778
E-mail: setac@setac.org
Website: http://www.setac.org

Society of Forensic Toxicologists (SOFT)
One MacDonald Center
1 N. MacDonald St., Ste. 15
Mesa, AZ 85201
Toll free: (888) 866-SOFT (7638)
E-mail: office@soft-tox.org
Website: http://soft-tox.org/

STOP Foodborne Illness
3759 N Ravenswood, Ste. 224
Chicago, IL 60613
Phone: (773) 269-6555
Fax: (773) 883-3098
Toll free: (800) 350-STOP
Website: http://www.stopfoodborneillness.org

Superfund TRI EPCRA RMP & Oil Information Center
Ariel Rios Bldg., 1200 Pennsylvania Ave. NW
Washington, DC 20460
Phone: (703) 412-9810
Toll free: (800) 424-9346
Website: http://www.epa.gov/superfund

T

Tennessee Valley Authority
400 W Summit Hill Dr.
Knoxville, TN 37902-1499
Phone: (865) 632-2101

Texas Department of Health Bioterrorism Preparedness Program (TDH)
1100 W 49th St.
Austin, TX 78756
Phone: (512) 458-7676
Toll free: (800) 705-8868
Website: http://www.tdh.state.tx.us/bioterrorism/default.htm

The National Law Center on Homelessness and Poverty
1411 K Street NW, Ste. 1400
Washington, DC 20005
Phone: (202) 638-2535
Toll free: (202) 628-2737
Website: http://www.nlchp.org/

The National Lead Information Center
422 S. Clinton Ave.
Rochester, NY 14620
Toll free: (800) 424-5323
Fax: (585) 232-3111
Website: http://www.epa.gov/lead/pubs/nlic.htm

The Nature Conservancy
4245 North Fairfax Dr., Ste. 100
Arlington, VA 22203-1606
Phone: (703) 841-5300
Toll free: (800) 628-6860
E-mail: member@tnc.org
Website: http://www.nature.org

U

United States Centers for Disease Control and Prevention (CDC)
1600 Clifton Rd.
Atlanta, GA 30333
Phone: (404) 639-3534
Toll free: (800) CDC-INFO (232-4636)
E-mail: cdcinfo@cdc.gov
Website: http://www.cdc.gov

United States Department of Agriculture
1400 Independence Ave. SW, Rm. 1180
Washington, DC 20250
Phone: (202) 720-2791
Website: http://www.usda.gov

United States Department of Health and Human Services
200 Independence Ave. SW
Washington, DC 20201
Phone: (202) 619-0257
Toll free: (877) 696-6775
Website: http://www.hhs.gov

United States Department of Labor Occupational Safety & Health Administration–Room N3641
200 Constitution Ave.
Washington, DC 20210
Toll free: (800) 321-OSHA (6742)
Website: http://www.osha.gov

United States Department of Veterans Affairs
810 Vermont Ave. NW
Washington, DC 20420
Toll free: (877) 222-8387
Website: http://www.publichealth.va.gov

United States Environmental Protection Agency (EPA)
4601M Ariel Rios Bldg., 1200 Pennsylvania Ave. NW
Washington, DC 20460
Phone: (202) 272-0167; TTY (202) 272-0165
Website: http://www.epa.gov

United States National Park Service
1849 C St. NW
Washington, DC 20240
Phone: (202) 208-3818
Website: http://www.nps.gov

Undersea and Hyperbaric Medical Society
21 W Colony Place, Ste. 280
Durham, NC 27705
Phone: (919) 490-5140
Fax: (919) 490-5149
Toll free: (877) 533-UHMS (8467)
E-mail: uhms@uhms@org

United Nations Environment Programme
United Nations Avenue Gigiri
PO Box 30552 00100
Nairobi, Kenya Africa
Phone: 254(20) 76-1234
Fax: 254(20) 76-448990
E-mail: unepinfo@unep.org
Website: http://www.unep.org

United Nations Environment Programme Global Environment Facility
UNEP-GEF Biosafety Unit DEPI UNEP
Nairobi, Kenya Africa
Phone: 254(20) 7624066
E-mail: unepgef@unep.org
Website: http://www.unep.org/biosafety

United Nations Foundation
1800 Massachusetts Ave. NW, Ste. 400
Washington, DC 20036
Phone: (202) 887-9040
Fax: (202) 887-9021
E-mail: inquiries@un.org
Website: http://www.unfoundation.org

UNICEF Headquarters
2 United Nations Plaza
New York, NY 10017
Phone: (212) 326-7000
Fax: (212) 887-7465
Website: http://www.unicef.org

UNICEF Innocenti Research Centre
Piazza SS. Annunziata 12 50122
Florence, Italy
Phone: 39 055 20330
Fax: 39 055 2033220
Website: http://www.unicef-irc.org/

United States Centers for Disease Control and Prevention (CDC)
1600 Clifton Rd.
Atlanta, GA 30333
Phone: (404) 639-3534
Toll free: (800) CDC-INFO (800-232-4636); TTY: (888) 232-6348
E-mail: inquiry@cdc.gov
Website: http://www.cdc.gov

United States Consumer Products Safety Commission
4330 East West Highway
Bethesda, MD 20814
Phone: (301) 504-7923; TTY(301) 595-7054
Toll free: (800) 638-2772
Fax: Fax (301) 504-0124 and (301) 504-0025
Website: http://www.cpsc.gov

United States Department of Agriculture (USDA)
1400 Independence Ave. SW
Washington, DC 20250
Phone: (202) 720-2791
Toll free: (800) 232-4636
E-mail: cdcinfo@cdc.gov
Website: http://www.usda.gov

United States Department of Labor Occupational Safety & Health Administration (OSHA)
200 Constitution Ave.
Washington, DC 20210
Toll free: (800) 321-OSHA (6742); TTY: 1-877-889-5627
Website: http://www.osha.gov

United States Environmental Protection Agency (EPA)
Ariel Rios Building, 1200 Pennsylvania Avenue N.W.
Washington, DC 20460
Phone: (202) 272-0167; TTY (202) 272-0165
Website: http://www.epa.gov

United States Food and Drug Administration (FDA)
10903 New Hampshire Ave.
Silver Spring, MD 20993-0002
Toll free: (888) INFO-FDA (463-6332)
Website: http://www.fda.gov

W

Water Environment Federation
601 Wythe St.
Alexandria, VA 22314-1994
Fax: (703) 684-2492
Toll free: (800) 666-0206
Website: http://www.wef.org

Water Quality Association
4151 Naperville Rd.
Lisle, IL 60532
Phone: (630) 505-0160
Fax: (630) 505-9637
Website: http://www.wqa.org

World Food Program
Via C.G.Viola 68 Parco dei Medici
Rome, 00148 Italy
Phone: 39 06 65131
Fax: 39 06 6590632
Website: http://www.wfp.org

World Health Organization (WHO)
Avenue Appia 20
1211 Geneva 27 Switzerland
Phone: +2241 791 21 11
Fax: +2241 791 31 11
E-mail: info@who.int
Website: http://www.who.int

World Health Organization Europe
Scherfigsvej 8 DK-2100
Copenhagen, Denmark
Phone: 45391-1717
E-mail: infohcp@euro.who.int
Website: http://www.euro.who.int/en/home

World Organization of Volcano Observatories
903 Koyukuk Dr.
Fairbanks, AK 99775
Phone: (907) 474-1542
Fax: (907) 474-7290
E-mail: wovo.iavcei@gmail.com
Website: http://www.wovo.org

Z

Zero Population Growth
1400 16th Street NW, Ste. 320
Washington, DC 20036

GLOSSARY

The glossary is an alphabetical compilation of terms and definitions listed in the *Key Terms* sections of the main body entries. Although the list is comprehensive, it is by no means exhaustive.

A

ABJECT POVERTY. The most extreme poverty which occurs when individuals cannot meet their basic needs for food, water, shelter, sanitation, and health care. The World Health Organization defines abject poverty as living on less than US $1.25 a day.

ABLATIVE. Also known as ablation and referring to the surgical removal of lesions associated with HPV.

ABSCESS. An accumulation of pus caused by localized infection in tissues or organs. *L. monocytogenes* can cause abscesses in many organs, including the brain, spleen, and liver.

ACARACIDE. A pesticide used to kill or disable arachnids.

ACETYLCHOLINE. A chemical called a neurotransmitter that functions to excite nerve cells.

ACETYLCHOLINESTERASE. An enzyme that breaks down acetylcholine.

ACQUIRED IMMUNE DEFICIENCY SYNDROME (AIDS). HIV infection that has led to certain opportunistic infections, cancers, or a CD4+ T-lymphocyte (helper cell) blood cell count lower than 200/mL.

ACUTE. Short in duration. Often used to mean both short and severe when used to describe a disease or symptom.

ACUTE RETROVIRAL SYNDROME (ARS). A syndrome that develops in about 30% of HIV patients within a few weeks of infection. ARS is characterized by nausea, vomiting, fever, headache, general tiredness, and muscle cramps.

ACUTE WATER DIARRHEA (AWD). Acute diarrhea and vomiting from consuming contaminated water, especially common in children in refugee camps and disaster areas.

ADJUVANT THERAPY. Therapy administered to patients who are at risk of having microscopic untreated disease present but have no manifestations.

ADULTICIDING. Insecticide spraying to kill adult mosquitoes.

AEDES AEGYPTI. A mosquito that transmits dengue and yellow fever worldwide.

AEROBIC BACTERIA. Bacteria that require oxygen to live and grow.

AIDS DEMENTIA COMPLEX. A type of brain dysfunction caused by HIV infection that causes difficulty thinking, confusion, and loss of muscular coordination.

ALBUMIN. A protein in the blood; albumin in the urine is an indication of kidney disease.

ALLERGEN. A foreign substance, such as mites in house dust or animal dander which, when inhaled, causes the airways to narrow and produces symptoms of asthma.

ALLERGIC RHINITIS. Inflammation of the mucous membranes of the nose and eyes in response to an allergen; hay fever, for example, is seasonal allergic rhinitis.

ALLERGY. extra sensitivity of the body to certain substances, such as pollens, foods, molds, or microorganisms, that produces an immune responses and that results in symptoms such as sneezing, itching, and skin rashes.

ALOPECIA. Loss of hair.

ALPHA PARTICLE. A positively charged particle emitted during radioactive decay. It contains two protons and two and is the same as the nucleus of the helium atom.

ALTERNARIA. A group of fungi known as major plant pathogens and as common allergens in humans.

They grow indoors and can cause hay fever or extra sensitive reactions that can lead to asthma. They can also cause infections in persons who are immunocompromised.

ALTERNATING CURRENT (AC). An electric current in which the flow of the electric charge periodically reverses direction. AC is the form in which electricity is usually delivered to homes. The usual household wall outlet (120 volts, or V) provides a current with 120 reversals of the direction of flow occurring each second and is termed 60-cycle alternating current.

ALVEOLI. The small air sacs located at the ends of the breathing tubes of the lung, where oxygen normally passes from inhaled air through the membranes into the capillaries and the bloodstream.

ALZHEIMER'S DISEASE. An incurable disease of older individuals that results in the destruction of nerve cells in the brain and causes gradual loss of mental and physical functions.

AMBIENT. Relating to surrounding conditions.

AMEBIC COLITIS. Inflammation of the colon caused by the ameba *Entamoeba histolytica*.

AMEBIC DYSENTERY. A common waterborne illness caused by the protozoan ameba *Entamoeba histolytica* and characterized by severe diarrhea, abdominal pain, and erosion of the intestinal wall. Also known as amebiasis.

AMENDMENT. A change or addition to a legal document.

AMPERAGE. A measurement of the amount of electric charge passing a given point per unit time. One ampere represents about 6.241×10^{18} electrons passing a given point in a wire in one second of time.

AMYOTROPHIC LATERAL SCLEROSIS (ALS). Also called Lou Gehrig's disease, a disease that causes degeneration of the nerves that control muscle movement. Eventually breathing muscles become paralyzed and the individual dies.

ANAEROBIC BACTERIA. Bacteria that require the absence of oxygen to live and grow.

ANAPHYLAXIS. Also called anaphylactic shock; a severe allergic reaction characterized by airway constriction, tissue swelling, and lowered blood pressure.

ANDROGENS. Male sex hormones.

ANEMIA. A condition in which there are too few red blood cells, too many abnormal red blood cells or too little iron-containing hemoglobin for normal oxygen transport in the body.

ANGIOTENSIN-CONVERTING ENZYME (ACE) INHIBITORS. Medications for lowering blood pressure and treating heart, blood vessel, and kidney diseases.

ANGIOTENSIN-II RECEPTOR BLOCKERS (ARBS). Medications for lowering blood pressure and treating heart, blood vessel, and kidney diseases.

ANHYDROUS AMMONIA. Ammonia gas that lacks water.

ANOPHELES. A genus of mosquitoes that transmits the malaria parasite.

ANTHELMINTHIC (ALSO SPELLED ANTHELMINTIC). A type of drug or herbal preparation given to destroy parasitic worms or expel them from the body.

ANTHRAX. A disease of warm blooded animals, particularly cattle and sheep, transmissible to humans. The disease causes severe skin and lung damage. It has also been used as a bioweapon.

ANTIBIOTIC. A medication that is designed to kill or weaken bacteria.

ANTIBODY. A protein normally produced by the immune system to fight infection or rid the body of foreign material. The material that stimulates the production of antibodies is called an antigen. Specific antibodies are produced in response to each different antigen and can only inactivate that particular antigen.

ANTIDEPRESSANTS. A type of medication that is used to treat depression; it is also sometimes used to treat autism.

ANTIDOTE. A substance that combats the effects of a poison or toxin.

ANTIGEN. Any foreign substance, usually a protein, that stimulates the body's immune system to produce antibodies.

ANTIHISTAMINE. A medication that blocks or counteracts the action of histamine; used to alleviate respiratory symptoms such as runny nose, watering eyes, and sneezing.

ANTIMICROBIAL. A general term for any drug that is effective against disease organisms, including bacteria, viruses, fungi, and parasites. Antibiotics, which are used to treat bacterial infections, are one type of antimicrobial.

ANTI-MOTILITY MEDICATIONS. Medications such as loperamide (Imodium), dephenoxylate (Lomotil), or medications containing codeine or narcotics that decrease the ability of the intestine to contract. This can worsen the condition of a patient with dysentery or colitis.

ANTIOXIDANT. A molecule that prevents oxidation. In the body antioxidants attach to other molecules called free radicals and prevent the free radicals from causing damage to cell walls, DNA, and other parts of the cell. Vitamin E, vitamin C, and beta carotene are common antioxidants.

ANTITOXIN. An antibody that neutralizes a toxin.

ANXIETY. Worry or tension in response to real or imagined stress, danger, or dreaded situations. Physical reactions, such as fast pulse, sweating, trembling, fatigue, and weakness may accompany anxiety.

ARC FLASH. A type of electrical explosion resulting from electrical breakdown of the gases in air, which normally does not conduct electricity. Arc flashes can occur when there is sufficient voltage in an electrical system and a path to the ground or to lower voltage.

AROMATIC HYDROCARBON. An organic compound that contains at least one benzene ring.

ARRHYTHMIA. Abnormal heart rhythm.

ARTEMINISININS. A family of antimalarial products derived from an ancient Chinese herbal remedy. Two of the most popular varieties are artemether and artesunate, used mainly in Southeast Asia in combination with mefloquine.

ASBESTOS. Asbestos is the commercial name, not a mineralogical term, given to a variety of six naturally occurring fibrous minerals that have been mined for wide use because of their heat resistance and chemical resistance properties. These minerals possess high tensile strength, flexibility, resistance to chemical and thermal degradation, and electrical resistance. These minerals have been used for decades in more than 3,000 types of commercial products, such as insulation and fireproofing materials, automotive brakes, textile products, and cement and wallboard materials. Asbestos has been classified as a known human carcinogen by the U.S. Department of Health and Human Services, the EPA, and the International Agency for Research on Cancer.

ASCITES. Abnormal accumulation of fluid in the abdomen, making the abdomen appear distended.

ASEPTIC MENINGITIS. A term for meningitis not caused by bacteria.

ASEPTIC. Sterile; containing no microorganisms, especially no bacteria.

ASIAN TIGER. *Aedes albopictus*—an invasive, dengue-transmitting mosquito that is resistant to most insecticides.

ASPERGER SYNDROME. Children who have autistic behavior but no problems with language and no clinically significant cognitive delay.

ASPERGILLUS. A group of several hundred mold species found in various climates worldwide, some of which are important medically and commercially while others cause infection in humans and other animals.

ASTHMA. A disease in which the air passages of the lungs become inflamed and narrowed.

ASYMPTOMATIC. Showing no symptoms of a disease even though the person may be infected by the organism that causes the disease.

ATAXIA. Lack of coordination.

ATOPY. A state that makes persons more likely to develop allergic reactions of any type, including the inflammation and airway narrowing typical of asthma.

ATTENTION DEFICIT/HYPERACTIVITY DISORDER (ADHD). Conditions characterized by age-inappropriate attention span, hyperactivity, and impulsive behavior.

ATTENUATED. A vaccine made with live virus that has been modified so that it is no longer infective.

AUTISM. A variable developmental disorder that includes an impaired ability to communicate and form normal social relationships.

AUTOIMMUNE DISEASE. A disease that develops when the immune system attacks normal cells or organs.

AUTOSOMAL DOMINANT INHERITANCE. A pattern of inheritance in which a trait will be expressed if the gene is inherited from either parent.

B

B CELL. A type of lymphocyte. B lymphocytes (B cells) produce antibodies to help the body fight infection.

BABESIOSIS. A disease caused by protozoa of the genus *Babesia* characterized by a malaria-like fever, anemia, vomiting, muscle pain, and enlargement of the spleen. Babesiosis, like Lyme disease, is carried by a tick.

BACILLUS. A rod-shaped bacterium.

BACILLUS CALMETTE-GUÉRIN (BCG). A vaccine made from a weakened bacillus similar to the tubercle bacillus that may help prevent serious pulmonary TB and its complications.

BACKGROUND RADIATION. The radiation in the natural environment, including cosmic rays and radiation from the naturally radioactive elements, both outside and inside the bodies of humans and animals. The usually quoted average individual exposure from background radiation is 300 millirem per year.

BACTEREMIA. The presence of bacteria in the bloodstream.

BACTERIA. Single-celled organisms without nuclei, some of which are infectious.

BACTERICIDAL. A state that prevents growth of bacteria.

BACTERIOPHAGE. A type of virus that can be used to treat bacterial infections. Bacteriophages (or simply phages) work by injecting their own genetic material into bacteria and forcing the bacteria to produce new virus particles rather than a new generation of bacteria.

BACTERIOSTATIC. A substance that kills bacteria.

BACTERIUM. A single-celled microorganism, which does not possess any distinct nuclei or complex cell structures, that is responsible for many diseases.

BELL'S PALSY. Facial paralysis or weakness with a sudden onset, caused by swelling or inflammation of the seventh cranial nerve, which controls the facial muscles. Disseminated Lyme disease sometimes causes Bell's palsy.

BENIGN. Harmless, not disease causing. Most often, benign is used to mean not malignant or noncancerous.

BENZODIAZEPINES. A class of drugs that have a hypnotic and sedative action, used mainly as tranquilizers to control symptoms of anxiety.

BERYLLIUM (BE). A steel-grey, metallic element used in the aerospace and nuclear industries and in a variety of manufacturing processes.

BERYLLIUM LYMPHOCYTE PROLIFERATION TEST (BELPT). A blood test for measuring the reaction of the body's immune system to beryllium; used as a screening test for beryllium sensitivity and berylliosis.

BERYLLIUM SENSITIZATION (BES). An allergic or hypersensitivity reaction to beryllium that can lead to berylliosis.

BETA BLOCKERS. Drugs used to treat high blood pressure (hypertension) that limit the activity of epinephrine, a hormone that increases blood pressure.

BETA PARTICLE. High-energy electrons (negatively charged) or positrons (positively charged) emitted during radioactive decay. They are a form of ionizing radiation.

BILIRUBIN. A reddish-yellow bile pigment made by the liver.

BIOACCUMULATION. The concentration of a substance, such as a chemical, in living organisms.

BIOFUELS. Liquid fuels from biomass, especially ethanol made from corn or sugarcane, and biodiesel from vegetable oils and animal fats.

BIOHAZARDOUS. Describes biological agents or conditions and materials that pose potential hazards or harms to people and the environment.

BIOMARKER. A biological indicator, such as a metabolite in the blood, of an event or condition such as exposure to a toxin.

BIOPSY. The surgical removal and microscopic examination of living tissue for diagnostic purposes.

BIOSENSOR. A device for detecting a target substance, usually incorporating a biological component such as an enzyme.

BIOSTATISTICS. The branch of statistics that focuses on the collection and analysis of biological and medical data.

BIOTERRORISM. The intentional use of pathogens to cause illness in population groups or to cause fear of such harm.

BIOTYPE. A variant strain of a bacterial species with distinctive physiological characteristics.

BISPHENOL A (BPA). An organic compound that is one of the most widely produced chemicals. Its use in many plastic containers has been questioned since it has potentially harmful health effects.

BLASTING CAP. A small tube filled with a small amount of a primary explosive.

BLIGHT. Any cause of impairment, destruction, ruin, or frustration; the state or result of being blighted or deteriorated, dilapidated or decaying.

BLOOD-BRAIN BARRIER. An arrangement of cells within the blood vessels of the brain that prevents the passage of toxic substances, including infectious agents, from the blood and into the brain. It also makes it difficult for certain medications to pass into brain tissue.

BONE MARROW. Spongy material that fills the inner cavities of the bones. The progenitors of all the blood cells are produced in this bone marrow.

BOOSTER SHOT. A supplementary vaccine dose.

BORDATELLA PERTUSSIS. A bacterium that causes whooping cough by attaching itself to cells in the respiratory tract.

BOTULISM. A life-threatening paralytic illness from food contaminated with botulinum toxin from the bacterium *Clostridium botulinum*.

BOVINE SPONGIFORM ENCEPHALOPATHY. Also known as Mad Cow disease, a progressive, fatal disease of the nervous system of domestic animals that is transmitted by eating infected food.

BRAIN STEM. The posterior portion of the brain that connects directly to the spinal cord. It regulates breathing, heart function, and the sleep-wake cycle as well as maintaining consciousness.

BRAINSTEM. The stalk of the brain that connects the two cerebral hemispheres to the spinal cord.

BRONCHIAL ASTHMA. A respiratory disorder characterized by chronic inflammation of the airways.

BRONCHITIS. A respiratory disorder caused by a viral or bacterial infection. Bronchitis is characterized by inflamed bronchi, excessive mucus production, and coughing.

BRONCHOALVEOLAR LAVAGE (BAL). A procedure for washing cells from the lungs to test for berylliosis.

BRONCHODILATOR. A drug that causes the expansion of the bronchial air passages.

BRONCHOSCOPY SCAN. The examination of the air passages through a flexible or rigid tube inserted into the nostril (or mouth). Sometimes cells are collected by washing the lungs with a small amount of fluid.

BRONCHOSCOPY. A procedure in which a fiber optic instrument called a bronchoscope is inserted in the airways allowing the physician to inspect the linings of the airways.

BRUCELLA. Bacteria of the genus *Brucella* that can cause brucellosis in wild and domestic animals and humans.

BUBOES. Smooth, oval, reddened, and very painful swellings in the armpits, groin, or neck that occur as a result of infection with the plague.

BUSHMEAT. The meat of wild animals killed for subsistence or sale throughout the tropics, especially in Central and West Africa.

BUTTON BATTERIES. Tiny, round batteries containing mercuric chloride that power items such as watches, hearing aids, calculators, cameras, and penlights.

C

CACHEXIA. Severe malnutrition involving muscle wasting and organ damage.

CALDERA. Volcanic crater.

CALICIVIRUS. A member of the Caliciviridae family of viruses that includes noroviruses.

CALORIC TESTING. Flushing warm and cold water into the ear to stimulate the labyrinth and cause vertigo and nystagmus if all the nerve pathways are intact.

CAMPYLOBACTER. A genus of bacteria that is found in almost all raw poultry and that can contaminate food and cause illness.

CAP AND TRADE. Part of environmental policy that uses a mandatory cap on emissions while providing flexibility on how to comply with the rules.

CAPSID. The protein structure of a virus.

CAPSOMERE. The protein subunits of the capsid.

CARBON MONOXIDE. With the chemical formula CO (where C stands for carbon, and O for oxygen), a colorless, odorless, and tasteless gas that is toxic to humans in higher than normal concentrations.

CARBOXYHEMOGLOBIN (COHB). Hemoglobin that is bound to carbon monoxide instead of oxygen.

CARCINOGEN. An agent that is known to cause cancer.

CARPAL TUNNEL SYNDROME. A condition in the wrist and forearm caused by repetitive tasks. The median nerve in the wrist is compressed, or entrapped, by swelling. The person experiences pain, numbness, and some loss of use.

CARRIER. A person who has a particular disease agent present within his or her body, and can pass this agent on to others, but who displays no symptoms of infection.

CARRIER STATE. The continued presence of an organism (bacteria, virus, or parasite) in the body that does not cause symptoms but is able to be transmitted and infect other persons.

CATARACT. Clouding of the lens of the eye or its capsule (surrounding membrane).

CD4. A type of protein molecule in human blood. The HIV virus infects cells with CD4 surface proteins and, as a result, depletes the number of T cells, B cells, natural killer cells, and monocytes in the patient's blood.

CELLULAR IMMUNE SYSTEM. Cell-mediated immunity; immune system cells that fight infection without specific antibodies against the disease-causing organism.

CENTRAL NERVOUS SYSTEM. Consists of the brain and spinal cord and integrates and processes information.

CEPHALOSPORINS. A class of beta-lactam antibiotics originally derived from the fungus *Acrimonium*, which was previously called *Cephalosporium*.

CERCARIAE. The free-living form of the schistosome worm that has a tail, swims, and has suckers on its head for penetration into a host.

CEREBRAL. Pertaining to the brain.

CEREBRAL PALSY. Brain damage before, during, or just after birth that results in lack of muscle coordination and problems with speech.

CEREBROSPINAL FLUID. A clear fluid that fills the hollow cavity inside the brain and spinal cord. The cerebrospinal fluid has several functions, including providing a cushion for the brain against shock or impact, and removing waste products from the brain.

CERVICAL CANCER. Cancer of the entrance to the womb (uterus). The cervix is the lower, narrow part of the uterus (womb).

CERVICAL CANCER SCREENING. Use of the Papanicolaou (Pap) smear test to detect cervical cancer in the early curable stage.

CERVICAL INTRA-EPITHELIAL NEOPLASIA (CIN). A precancerous condition in which a group of cells grow abnormally on the cervix but do not extend into the deeper layers of this tissue.

CERVID. The term for hoofed, even-toed animals that usually are horned (at least the males). Typically, this includes deer, elk, moose, and reindeer.

CERVIX. The narrow neck or outlet of the uterus.

CHELATING. A chemical term denoting a compound that has a central metallic ion attached via covalent bonds to two or more nonmetallic atoms in the same molecule.

CHELATION. The process by which a molecule encircles and binds to a metal and removes it from tissue.

CHELATION THERAPY. A treatment used for many types of heavy metal poisonings in which edetate calcium disodium is administered intravenously. The drug attracts molecules of the heavy metal and binds with them in such a way that they can be eliminated in urine.

CHELATORS. Various compounds that bind to metals such as mercury.

CHEMOTHERAPY. Treatment with anticancer drugs.

CHLORACNE. A skin rash that resembles acne, which is caused by repeated contact with chlorinated hydrocarbons.

CHLORINATION. Water treatment with chlorine or chlorine compounds to kill or inactivate disease-causing organisms.

CHLOROQUINE. An antimalarial drug that began being used in the 1940s and stopped being used after evidence of quinine resistance appeared in the 1960s. In the early 2000s, it was considered ineffective against falciparum malaria almost everywhere. However, because it is inexpensive, it continued to be still the antimalarial drug most widely in Africa. Native individuals with partial immunity may have better results with chloroquine than travelers with no previous exposure.

CHOLERA. An infection of the small intestine caused by a type of bacterium. The disease is spread by drinking water or eating seafood or other foods that have been contaminated with the feces of infected people. It occurs most often in parts of Asia, Africa, Latin America, India, and the Middle East. Symptoms include watery diarrhea and exhaustion. Cholera is often fatal to young children and the elderly.

CHRONIC BERYLLIUM DISEASE (CBD). Berylliosis; chronic, progressive lung damage caused by exposure to beryllium.

CHRONIC BRONCHITIS. A respiratory disorder that causes chronic inflammation of the bronchi within the lungs.

CHRONIC OBSTRUCTIVE PULMONARY DISEASE (COPD). Chronic obstructive pulmonary disease (COPD) is a progressive disease that makes it hard to breathe. COPD can cause coughing that produces large amounts of mucus, wheezing, shortness of breath, chest tightness, and other symptoms. Cigarette smoking is the leading cause of COPD. Most people who have COPD smoke or used to smoke. Long-term exposure to other lung irritants, such as air pollution, chemical fumes, or dust, also may contribute to COPD.

CHRONIC. A disease or condition characterized by slow onset over a long period of time.

CILIA. Tiny, hair-like projections from a cell. In the respiratory tract, cilia beat constantly in order to move mucus and debris up and out of the respiratory tree, in order to protect the lung from infection or irritation by foreign bodies.

CLADDING. The thin-walled metal tube that forms the outer jacket of a nuclear fuel rod. It prevents the corrosion of the fuel by the coolant and the release of fission products in the coolants. Aluminum, stainless steel and zirconium alloys are common cladding materials.

CLADOSPORIUM. A group of fungi that includes some of the most common indoor and outdoor molds. Their spores are wind-dispersed and are often extremely abundant in outdoor airs. They can grow on surfaces when moisture is present. The airborne spores are significant allergens and in large amounts they can severely affect asthmatics and people with respiratory diseases. Prolonged exposure may weaken the immune system.

CLASS ACTION SETTLEMENT. A form of lawsuit in which a large group of people collectively bring a claim to court and/or in which a class of defendants is being sued.

CLEAN WATER ACT (CWA). The U.S. environmental law that establishes the basic structure for regulating discharges of pollutants into the waters of the United States and for regulating quality standards for surface waters. The basis of the CWA was enacted in 1948 and was called the Federal Water Pollution Control Act, but the act was significantly reorganized and expanded in 1972. Clean Water Act became its common name with amendments in 1972.

CLIMATE CHANGE. The ongoing increase in average global temperatures due to the release of carbon dioxide and other greenhouse gases, primarily from the burning of fossil fuels for energy production.

CLOSTRIDIUM PERFRINGENS. A bacterium that is a common food contaminant.

COAGULATING FACTORS. Components within the blood that help form clots.

COGNITIVE-BEHAVIORAL THERAPY. A type of psychotherapy used to treat anxiety disorders (including PTSD) that emphasizes behavioral change as well as alteration of negative thought patterns.

COLIFORM. Gram-negative, rod-shaped bacteria, such as *Escherichia coli*, that are normally present in the human intestine and that are measured to monitor drinking water for contamination.

COLITIS. Inflammation of the colon or large intestine, usually causing diarrhea that may be bloody.

COLPOSCOPY. Procedure in which the cervix is examined using a special microscope.

COMPUTED TOMOGRAPHY (CT). A special x-ray technique that produces a cross sectional image of the organs inside the body.

CONCENTRATED ANIMAL FEEDING OPERATION (CAFO). An agricultural operation in which animals are raised in confined situations, with animals, feed, manure, urine, dead animals, and production operations concentrated in a small area.

CONDYLOMATA ACUMINATA (SINGULAR, CONDYLOMA ACUMINATUM). The medical term for infectious warts on the genitals caused by HPV.

CONGENITAL. existing at, and usually before, birth; referring to conditions that are present at birth, regardless of their causation.

CONJUGATION. The transfer of genetic material between two bacteria through cell-to-cell contact.

CONTACT DERMATITIS. Skin inflammation from contact with an allergen or other irritating substance.

CONTAINMENT. The gas-tight shell or other enclosure around a reactor to confine fission products that otherwise might be released to the atmosphere in the event of an accident.

CONTAMINANT. A type of unwanted microparticle or organism. In water, a contaminant may reduce clarity, quality, or be a health hazard.

CONVULSION. Also termed seizure; a sudden violent contraction of a group of muscles.

COOLANT. A substance circulated through a nuclear reactor to remove or transfer heat. The most commonly used coolant in the U.S. is water. Other coolants include air, carbon dioxide, and helium.

CORE. The central portion of a nuclear reactor containing the fuel elements, and control rods.

CORTICOSTEROID. A hormonal drug, such as cortisone or prednisone, used to treat inflammation.

CORTISOL. A hormone produced by the adrenal glands near the kidneys in response to stress.

COWPOX. A mild disease in cows caused by a virus related to the smallpox virus.

CREATININE. A protein produced by muscles and filtered out by the kidneys; high creatinine levels in the blood are indicators of kidney disease.

CREUTZFELDT-JAKOB DISEASE. A rare and progressive disease that targets certain brain tissue and causes early dementia and loss of muscle coordination.

CROHN'S DISEASE. A chronic inflammatory intestinal disease that can affect any part of the digestive tract but is most common in the lower part of the small intestine. Crohn's disease is genetic and often requires medical and surgical treatment.

CRYOTHERAPY. The use of liquid nitrogen or other forms of extreme cold to destroy tissue.

CRYPTOSPORIDIOSIS. A waterborne illness caused by the one-celled parasite *Cryptosporidium parvum*.

CULTURE. A laboratory system for growing bacteria for further study.

CUMULATIVE. Increasing in effects or quantity by successive additions.

CURETTAGE. The removal of tissue or growths by scraping with a curette.

CURIE. A unit of radioactivity abbreviated Ci that is equal to approximately 3.7 times 10^{10} decays per second.

CUTANEOUS. Located in the skin.

CYANOSIS. The appearance of a blue or purple coloration of the skin or mucous membranes due to the tissues near the skin surface being low on oxygen

CYBERATTACK. Attacks on computer systems, such as those that run power grids or nuclear power plants, and which could cause large-scale disasters.

CYST. A liquid-filled structure developing abnormally in the body.

D

DDT. An insecticide with the formal name dichlorodiphenyltrichloroethane and the chemical formula $C_{14}H_9Cl_5$, widely used for mosquito control, but banned in the United States since 1972 because it accumulates in the environment and is toxic to birds and other vertebrates.

DEBRIDEMENT. Surgical procedure in which dead or dying tissue is removed.

DECONTAMINATION. The reduction or removal of contaminating radioactive material from a structure, area, object, or person. Decontamination may be accomplished by (1) treating the surface to remove or decrease the contamination; (2) letting the material stand so that the radioactivity is decreased by natural decay; and (3) covering the contamination to shield the radiation emitted.

DEEPWATER HORIZON. A floating semi-submersible drilling unit, an ultra-deep water, column stabilized drilling rig owned by Transocean and built in Korea that sunk in 2010 in the Gulf of Mexico. The platform was 396 feet (121 m) long and 256 feet (78 m) wide and could operate in waters up to 8,000 feet (2,400 m) deep, to a maximum drill depth of 30,000 feet (9,100 m). A semi-submersible obtains its buoyancy from ballasted, watertight pontoons located below the ocean surface and wave action. The operating deck can be located high above the sea level due to the stability of the design, and therefore the operating deck is kept well away from the waves. Structural columns connect the pontoons and operating deck. With its hull structure submerged at a deep draft, the semi-submersible is less affected by wave loadings than a normal ship. With a small water-plane area, however, the semi-submersible is sensitive to load changes, and therefore must be carefully trimmed to maintain stability. Unlike a submarine or submersible, during normal operations, a semi-submersible vessel is never entirely underwater.

DEET. N,N-diethyl-m-toluamide; an insect and tick repellent.

DEFLAGRATION. The process by which a fuel burns at a rate somewhere ia few centimeters per second to about the speed of sound (343.2 meters per second).

DEHYDRATION. The abnormal depletion of body fluids, as from vomiting and diarrhea.

DELAYED HYPERSENSITIVITY REACTION. An allergic reaction mediated by T cells that occurs hours to days after exposure to an antigen such as beryllium.

DENGUE. Infectious disease caused by RNA flaviviruses and transmitted by *Aedes* mosquitoes.

DENTAL CARIES. Tooth decay.

DEOXYRIBONUCLEIC ACID (DNA). The genetic material in cells that holds the inherited instructions for growth, development, and cellular functioning.

DEPRESSION. A mental condition in which a person feels extremely sad and loses interest in life. A person with depression may also have sleep problems and loss of appetite and may have trouble concentrating and carrying out everyday activities. Severe depression may instigate a suicide attempt.

DERMATOLOGIST. A doctor who specializes in diseases and disorders of the skin.

DERMIS. The deepest layer of skin.

DETONATION. The process by which combustion occurs so rapidly in an explosive mixture that the shock wave generated travels at supersonic speeds (greater than 343.2 meters per second)

DETOXIFICATION. A structured program for removing stored toxins from the body.

DIABETES. Type 2 diabetes, the most common form, develops in obese adults and, increasingly, in children, and is characterized by high blood sugar (hyperglycemia); it can cause chronic kidney disease.

DIALYSIS. A form of treatment for patients with kidneys that do not function properly. The treatment removes toxic wastes from the body that are normally removed by the kidneys.

DIARRHEA. Abnormally frequent intestinal emptying with liquid stools.

DIAZINON. A member of the organophosphate family of pesticides. This chemical causes nerve and reproductive damage.

DICHLORODIPHENYLTRICHLOROETHANE (DDT). A synthetic organic compound first developed in 1874 and made popular in the 1940s for its use as an insecticide. DDT was banned by most developed countries in the 1970s, including by the United States in 1972. In 2006, the World Health Organization promoted the use of DDT indoors as a vector control in African countries.

DIETITIAN. A health care professional who specializes in individual or group nutritional planning, public education in nutrition, or research in food science. To be licensed as a registered dietitian (RD) in the United States, a person must complete a bachelor's degree in a nutrition-related field and pass a state licensing examination. Dietitians are also called nutritionists.

DIOXINS. Any of numerous by-products of various industrial processes, which are regarded as extremely toxic. These dioxins or dioxin-like compounds include polychlorinated dibenzo-p-dioxins (PCDDs), polychlorinated dibenzofurans (PCDFs), and polychlorinated biphenyls (PCBs).

DIPHTHERIA-TETANUS-PERTUSSIS (DTP). The standard preparation used to immunize children against diphtheria, tetanus, and whooping cough. A so-called "acellular pertussis" vaccine (aP) is usually used since its release in the mid-1990s in a combined vaccine known as DTaP.

DIPHTHERIA. A serious, infectious disease caused by a toxin-producing bacterium.

DIRECT CURRENT (DC). An electric current in which the electric charge moves in only one direction. It is the type of current produced by batteries and solar cells.

DIRTY BOMB. A radiological weapon that combines radioactive material and conventional explosives; in other words, a conventional bomb could be exploded near radioactive material causing the area to become contaminated with radioactive material.

DISPERSANT. A chemical that breaks up spilled oil into small particles that can be further scattered and broken down by water and wind, thus theoretically sparing oil damage to marine and coastal environments.

DISSEMINATED. Scattered or distributed throughout the body. Lyme disease that has progressed beyond the stage of localized EM is said to be disseminated.

DISSOCIATION. The splitting off of certain mental processes from conscious awareness. Many PTSD patients have dissociative symptoms.

DIURETIC. A substance that removes water from the body by increasing urine production

DNA PROBE. An agent that binds directly to a predefined sequence of nucleic acids.

DNA SEQUENCING. Determining the exact order of the bases A, T, G, and C in a length of DNA.

DOUBLE BURDEN OF DISEASE. The situation in which a country or region has to simultaneously address problems posed by both infectious and non-infectious (degenerative) diseases.

DTAP, TDAP. Combination vaccines against diphtheria, tetanus, and pertussis; Td is a tetanus/diphtheria vaccine.

DYSENTERY. A disease marked by frequent watery bowel movements, often with blood and mucus, and characterized by pain, urgency to have a bowel movement, fever, and dehydration.

DYSPLASTIC NEVUS SYNDROME. A familial syndrome characterized by the presence of multiple atypical appearing moles, often at a young age.

DYSPNEA. Difficult or labored breathing.

E

EARTHQUAKE. ground shaking caused by a sudden slip on a fault. Stresses in the earth's outer layer push the sides of the fault together. Stress builds up and the rocks slips suddenly, releasing energy in waves that travel through the earth's crust and cause the shaking that is felt during an earthquake.

ECOLOGY. The study of how organisms relate to one another and to their environment.

ECOSYSTEM. A biological community made up of interacting organisms and their environment.

ECOTHERAPY. Psychotherapy that uses nature-based methods for treating anxiety and depression.

EDEMA. Accumulation of excess fluid in the tissues of the body.

ELECTRODESICCATION. To make dry, dull, or lifeless with the use of electrical current.

ELECTROLYTE. Ions in the body that participate in metabolic reactions. The major human electrolytes are sodium ($Na+$), potassium ($K+$), calcium ($Ca\ 2+$), magnesium ($Mg2+$), chloride ($Cl-$), phosphate ($HPO4\ 2-$), bicarbonate ($HCO3-$), and sulfate ($SO4\ 2-$). Careful and regular monitoring of electrolytes and intravenous replacement of fluid and electrolytes are part of the acute care in many illnesses.

ELECTROMAGNETIC FIELD. An area containing both electric and magnetic components, also known as electromagnetic radiation. Areas with high levels of electromagnetic radiation can be a health threat to people.

ELECTROMAGNETIC FIELD RADIATION. Microwaves and radio waves.

ELECTROMAGNETIC RADIATION (EMR). A type of energy that is both absorbed and emitted by particles. Forms of EMR demonstrate wave-like movement as they travel through space and can be measured along the electromagnetic spectrum based on the frequency of wavelengths of emitted light or energy. Forms of EMR include radio radiation, infrared radiation, light on the visible spectrum, ultraviolet light, x rays and Gamma rays.

ELECTROMAGNETIC SPECTRUM. The range of all possible electromagnetic radiation.

ELEMENTAL MERCURY (HG). Metallic mercury; quicksilver; a heavy, silvery, poisonous metallic element that is a liquid at room temperature but vaporizes readily.

ELISA PROTOCOLS. ELISA is an acronym for "enzyme-linked immunosorbent assay." It is a highly sensitive technique for detecting and measuring antigens or antibodies in a solution.

ELONGATED MINERAL PARTICLES (EMPS). Substances with some of the same properties as asbestos that are used in various industrial processes.

EMACIATED. Extremely thin or wasted away physically.

EMERGENCY ALERT SYSTEM (EAS). A U.S. national public warning system that requires television and radio broadcasters to make emergency communications available to public officials.

EMERGENCY MANAGEMENT. An overall term for organization and management procedures for critical events that includes response to and recovery from emergencies as well as emergency preparedness.

EMPHYSEMA. A lung disease in which there is an abnormal accumulation of air in the tissues. Symptoms often include trouble breathing and a cough. Emphysema is frequently caused by long-term smoking.

EMPOWERMENT. The act of investing individuals with an understanding of their own potential and their own self-worth, while simultaneously providing them with the tools by which to achive their maximum personal potential.

ENAMEL. The hard, calcified outer surface of a tooth; the hardest known substance in the human body.

ENCEPHALITIS. Acute inflammation of brain tissue.

ENCEPHALOPATHY. Brain disorder characterized by memory impairment and other symptoms.

ENDANGERED SPECIES. A species vulnerable to extinction.

ENDEMIC. Restricted or peculiar to a specific locale or region; especially a disease that is prevalent only in a particular population.

ENDOCARDITIS. Inflammation of the endocardium, the inner layer of heart tissue.

ENDOCRINE DISRUPTOR. A chemical that interferes with the endocrine or hormone system, causing adverse developmental, neurological, reproductive, or immunological effects.

ENDOCRINE SYSTEM. A system of glands that secrete different types of hormones directly into the bloodstream for the purpose to regulate the body.

ENDOSOME. A membrane-mediated means of transporting materials from outside to inside the cell.

ENDOTOXIN. A poisonous substance in bacteria that is released when bacterial cells disintegrate.

END-STAGE LUNG DISEASE. The final stages of lung disease, when the lung can no longer keep the blood supplied with oxygen. End-stage lungs in pulmonary fibrosis have large air spaces separated by bands of inflammation and scarring.

END-STAGE RENAL DISEASE (ESRD). The final stage of kidney failure, with a complete or near-complete and irreversible loss of kidney function.

ENRICHMENT. The addition of vitamins and minerals to improve the nutritional content of a food.

ENTAMOEBA DISPAR. An ameba that appears identical to *Entamoeba histolytica*, but is much more common and does not cause illness.

ENTAMOEBA HISTOLYTICA. The ameba that causes amebiasis.

ENTEROTOXIGENIC E. COLI (ETEC). Strains of the normally harmless gut bacterium *Escherichia coli* that produce a toxin causing diarrhea and that are responsible for some cruise ship outbreaks of disease.

ENTEROTOXIN. A type of harmful protein released by bacteria and other disease agents that affects the tissues lining the intestines.

ENTEROVIRUSES. A family of viruses that normally live in the digestive tract and that can cause viral meningitis.

ENVIRONMENTAL IMPACT STATEMENT (EIS). A document required by the National Environmental Policy Act (NEPA) for certain actions "significantly affecting the quality of the human environment." An EIS, a tool for decision making, describes the positive and negative environmental effects of a proposed action and usually also lists one or more alternative actions that may be chosen instead of the action described in the EIS.

ENZYME. A protein that speeds up a chemical reaction but is not consumed during the process.

ENZYME-LINKED IMMUNOSORBENT ASSAY (ELISA). A laboratory technique used to detect specific antigens or antibodies. It can be used to diagnose giardiasis.

EOSINOPHIL. A type of white blood cell that increases in number in response to certain medical conditions, such as allergy or parasitic infection.

EPICENTER. In the case of earthquakes, epicenter in the case of earthquakes, the epicenter is directly above the point where the fault begins to rupture, and in most cases, it is the area of greatest damage.

EPIDEMIC. An outbreak of disease where the number of cases exceeds the usual (endemic) or typical number of cases.

EPIDEMIC PAROTITIS. The medical name for mumps.

EPIDEMIOLOGY. The study of the transmission and control of disease.

EPIDERMIS. The superficial layer of the skin.

EPIGENETIC. Modifications to DNA independent of the DNA sequence that affect gene expression.

EPINEPHRINE. A nervous system hormone stimulated by the nicotine in tobacco. It increases heart rate and may raise smokers' blood pressure.

EPITHELIAL. Of or relating to the epithelium, the layer of cells forming the epidermis of the skin and the surface layer of mucous membranes.

EPITHELIUM. The layer of cells covering the body's surface and lining the internal organs and various glands.

ERADICATE. To completely do away with something, eliminate it, end its existence.

ERYTHEMA MIGRANS (EM). A red skin rash that is one of the first signs of Lyme disease in about 75% of patients.

E. COLI. *Escherichia coli*; a bacterium that usually resides harmlessly in the lower intestine but can spread to cause infection elsewhere; also, some infectious strains produce a toxin that causes intestinal illness.

ESOPHAGUS. The muscular tube that leads from the back of the throat to the stomach. Coated with mucus and surrounded by muscles, it pushes food to the stomach by contraction.

ESSENTIAL MINERAL. A mineral required in one's diet for optimal health and functioning of the body. Examples of essential minerals include manganese, iron, and zinc.

ESTIMATED GLOMERULAR FILTRATION RATE (EGFR). A method for estimating kidney function from the level of creatinine in the blood serum.

ESTRADIOL. The most potent naturally occurring estrogen.

ESTROGEN. A steroid hormone produced primarily in the ovaries that is used for the development of female sexual characteristics.

EUTHYROID. Having the right amount of thyroxin stimulation.

EXANTHEM (PLURAL, EXANTHEMS OR EXANTHEMATA). A skin eruption regarded as a characteristic sign of such diseases as measles, German measles, and scarlet fever.

EXOBIOLOGY. The branch of science that focuses on the effects of outer space on organisms and the search for extraterrestrial life.

EXOTOXIN. A poisonous secretion produced by bacilli which is carried in the bloodstream to other parts of the body.

EXPOSOME. Lifetime exposure, both external and internal, to environmental factors, including pollution, radiation, chemicals, microorganisms, and food.

F

FAGET'S SIGN. The simultaneous occurrence of a high fever with a slowed heart rate.

FAMINE. A humanitarian crisis defined as the most severe stage of food insecurity.

FARMER'S LUNG. An allergic reaction to moldy hay, most often seen in farmers, that results in lung disease.

FASCIA, DEEP. A fibrous layer of tissue that envelopes muscles.

FASCIA, SUPERFICIAL. A fibrous layer of tissue that lies between the deepest layer of skin and the subcutaneous fat.

FEEDWATER. Water supplied to the steam generator that removes heat from the fuel rods by boiling and becoming steam. The steam then becomes the driving force for the turbine generator.

FERMENTATION. A reaction performed by yeast or bacteria to make alcohol.

FERTILITY. The ability to conceive children.

FETUS. An unborn vertebrate in which all structural features of the associated adult are recognizable.

FIBROSIS. A condition characterized by the presence of scar tissue or collagen proliferation in tissues to the extent that it replaces normal tissues.

FIRST RESPONDER. A generic term for the first medically trained responder to arrive at the scene of an emergency. First responders include police officers, firefighters, emergency medical technicians, and paramedics.

FLACCID. Weak, soft, or floppy.

FLAGELLUM. A tail-like projection extending from the cell walls of certain bacteria. Its name is the Latin word for whip.

FLASHBACK. A temporary reliving of a traumatic event.

FLAVIVIRUS. An arbovirus that can cause potentially serious diseases, such as dengue, yellow fever, Japanese encephalitis, and West Nile fever.

FLAVONOID. A food chemical that helps to limit oxidative damage to the body's cells, and protects against heart disease and cancer.

FLUE-GAS DE SULFURIZATION. Technologies used to remove sulfur dioxide from exhaust flue gases of fossil-fuel power plants and other such processes.

FLUORIDE. A fluorine ion used to treat water or apply directly to tooth surfaces to prevent dental caries.

FLUOROQUINOLONES. A class of synthetic broad-spectrum antibiotics that contain a fluorine atom in addition to the basic quinolone structure. They work by preventing the DNA in bacteria from unwinding and replicating.

FLUOROSIS. Fluorosis is an abnormal condition caused by excessive exposure to fluoride while a child's teeth are forming under the gums. It affects the formation of tooth enamel and can be very mild (a few white spots on a tooth) to severe (etching, pitting, and brown discoloration).

FLY ASH. One of the residues generated in combustion; in industrial settings, it refers to ash produced during combustion of coal.

FOOD SAFETY AND INSPECTION SERVICE (FSIS). The public health agency within the U.S. Department of Agriculture that is responsible for the safety of meat, poultry, and egg products.

FOOD SECURITY. Access for all people at all times to the food required to lead a healthy and active life.

FOODBORNE ILLNESS. A disease that is transmitted by eating or handling contaminated food.

FOOD-IRRADIATION METHODS. A process using radiant energy to kill microorganisms in food, to extend the amount of time in which food can be sold and eaten safely.

FORENSIC. Dealing with matters of interest to a court of law, whether criminal or civil proceedings.

FORTIFICATION. The addition of vitamins and minerals to improve the nutritional content of a food.

FOSSIL FUEL. Any type of fuel, such as coal, natural gas, peat, and petroleum, derived from the decomposed remains of prehistoric plants and animals.

FRACTIONAL DISTILLATION. A process by which petroleum is divided into its component parts by heating it in a tall tower.

FRAGILE X SYNDROME. A genetic condition related to the X chromosome that affects mental, physical and sensory development.

FREE RADICAL. A molecule with an unpaired electron that has a strong tendency to react with other molecules in DNA (genetic material), proteins, and lipids (fats), resulting in damage to cells.

FREQUENCY. The number of wavefronts that pass some given point in a designated period of time.

FROSTBITE BURN. Destruction of a specific area of skin and other body tissue due to direct contact with a certain chemical, such as chlorine or liquid nitrogen.

FULMINANT. Occurring or flaring up suddenly and with great severity. A potentially fatal complication of amebic dysentery is an inflammation of the colon known as fulminant colitis.

FUNGI. A group of organisms with a membrane-bound nucleus that derive their nourishment from dead or decaying organic matter. The group includes mushrooms, yeasts, mildew, and molds. They have rigid cell walls but lack chlorophyll.

FUNGICIDE. A substance that kills or slows the growth of fungi.

G

GANGRENE. Dead tissue.

GAS EMBOLISM. The presence of a gas bubble in the bloodstream that obstructs circulation.

GASTRIC LAVAGE. The act of emptying out the stomach via orogastric or nasogastric tube.

GASTROENTERITIS. An inflammation of the lining of the stomach and intestines, usually caused by a viral or bacterial infection.

GASTROINTESTINAL. Pertaining to the stomach and intestines.

GENE TRANSFER. The exchange of genetic material between bacteria during conjugation. It is a common mechanism for developing antimicrobial resistance.

GENES. Lengths of DNA that are the units of heredity passed from parent to offspring; genes contain the information for producing specific proteins or for RNAs that regulate gene expression.

GENETIC CLUSTER. A group of viral strains with very similar, yet distinct, nucleic acid sequences.

GENETIC MODIFICATION (GM). Organisms that have been genetically modified in the laboratory, such as mosquitoes that destroy vector populations when released into the environment.

GENETICALLY MODIFIED (GM OR GMO) FOODS. Food or ingredients derived from genetically modified organisms.

GENOGROUP. Related viruses within a genus; may be further subdivided into genetic clusters.

GENOME. The genetic material encoding the genes of an organism.

GENOMICS. The science of mapping genes and sequencing the DNA of an organism, collecting the results in a database, and analyzing and applying those results.

GENOTOXIC. Having the tendency to damage the DNA in a cell.

GIARDIA LAMBLIA. A type of protozoa with a whip-like tail that infects the human intestinal tract, causing giardiasis. The protozoa will not spread to other parts of the body.

GIARDIASIS. A waterborne illness caused by a widespread flagellate protozoan of the genus *Giardia*, usually characterized by diarrhea.

GLASNOST. In the former Soviet Union, the policy or practice of more open consultative government and wider dissemination of information, initiated by leader Mikhail Gorbachev from 1985.

GLUCOCORTICOSTEROIDS. Also called glucocorticoids, a class of steroid hormones that play important roles in metabolism and the immune system. Synthetic glucocorticosteroids are drugs given to control certain allergic and immune system disorders; they include cortisone, prednisone, aldosterone, and dexamethasone. These drugs suppress the immune response to infection; thus they can increase a person's risk of listeriosis.

GRAM-NEGATIVE. Refers to the property of many bacteria that causes them to not take up color with Gram's stain, a method which is used to identify bacteria. Gram-positive bacteria that take up the stain turn purple, while Gram-negative bacteria which do not take up the stain turn red.

GRAM'S STAIN. A dye staining technique used in laboratory tests to determine the presence and type of bacteria.

GRANULOMA. A small nodule that forms when immune system cells called macrophages gather to wall off foreign material in the body. Granulomas are a specialized type of inflammation that can occur many places in the body.

GRAY. Abbreviated Gy, a unit within the International System of Units (SI) that refers to absorbed radiation dose of ionizing radiation. One Gray is defined as the absorption of one joule of ionizing radiation by one kilogram of matter.

GREENHOUSE EFFECT. The overall warming of Earth's atmosphere as the result of atmospheric pollution by gases.

GREENHOUSE GAS. Any gas (such as carbon dioxide and ozone) that absorbs radiation and contributes to the warming of Earth's atmosphere by reflecting radiation from the surface of Earth.

GUILLAIN-BARRÉ SYNDROME. Progressive and usually reversible paralysis or weakness of multiple muscles usually starting in the lower extremities and often ascending to the muscles involved in respiration. The syndrome is due to inflammation and loss of the myelin covering of the nerve fibers, often associated with an acute infection.

H

HALOGENATION. Water treatment with chlorine or bromine to kill or inactivate disease-causing organisms.

HANTAVIRUS. A genus of viruses in the Bunyaviridae family that infect specific rodent species as their natural hosts and that can cause hemorrhagic fever with renal syndrome or hantavirus pulmonary syndrome in humans.

HAZARD. In the context of emergency preparedness, a general term for any agent, whether biological, chemical, mechanical, or other, that is likely to cause harm to humans or the environment in the absence of protective measures.

HAZARDOUS WASTE. Waste that is potentially harmful to public health or the environment, for example, paints, batteries, cleaners, and oil.

HEAT CRAMPS. The least severe sign of excessive exposure to heat and a warning sign or an impending heat disorder.

HEAT EXHAUSTION. A complex heat disorder resulting from exposure to a high index, restricted fluid intake, and/or failure of temperature regulation mechanisms of the body. It often affects athletes, firefighters, and construction workers.

HEATSTROKE. A life-threatening heat disorder caused by continued exposure to conditions that cause heat exhaustion. Heatstroke has a high potential for causing death, and immediate medical attention is critical.

HEAVY METAL. One of 23 chemical elements that has a specific gravity (a measure of density) at least five times that of water.

HELMINTHIASIS. Diseases caused by parasitic worms, including tapeworms, flukes, hookworm, *Ascaris*, and whipworm.

HEMATOTOXIC. Having a tendency to destroy blood cells.

HEMODIALYSIS. A method of mechanically cleansing the blood outside of the body, in order to remove various substances that would normally be cleared by the kidneys. Hemodialysis is used when an individual is in relative, or complete, kidney failure.

HEMOGLOBIN (HB). A molecule that normally binds to oxygen in order to carry it to the body's cells, where it is required for life.

HEMOGLOBIN A1C (A1C TEST). A test for determining the average blood sugar level for the previous two to three months.

HEMOLYTIC UREMIC SYNDROME (HUS). Kidney failure, usually in infants and young children, that can be caused by food contaminated with bacteria such as STEC or *Shigella*.

HEMORRHAGE. Bleeding that is massive, uncontrollable, and often life-threatening.

HEMORRHAGIC FEVER. Viral diseases that are transmitted to humans by insects or rodents and are characterized by the sudden onset of fever, bleeding from internal organs, and shock.

HEPATITIS. Any of several viral diseases that affect the liver; vaccinations (HepA and HepB) are available against hepatitis A. B, and C.

HERD IMMUNITY. Disease protection for non-immune or unvaccinated individuals that is conferred by the prevailing immunity within a population due to widespread vaccination coverage.

HIB. A vaccine against *Haemophilus influenzae* type b, a major cause of spinal meningitis.

HIGHLY ACTIVE ANTIRETROVIRAL THERAPY (HAART). An individualized combination of three or more antiretroviral drugs used to treat patients with HIV infection. It is sometimes called a drug cocktail.

HIGH-RISK HPV TYPE. A member of the HPV family of viruses that is associated with the development of cervical cancer and precancerous growths.

HISTOLOGY. The study of the structure of biological tissues at the microscopic level.

HORMONE. Any chemical secreted by the endocrine gland or some types of nerve cells, which regulates the function of a specific tissue or organ.

HORMONE THERAPY. Treatment of cancer by inhibiting the production of hormones such as testosterone and estrogen.

HOST. The organism (such as a monkey or human) in which another organism (such as a virus or bacteria) is living.

HUMAN GENOME PROJECT (HGP). An international project begun in 1990 and completed in 2003 that sequenced the three billion bases of DNA in the human genome.

HUMAN IMMUNODEFICIENCY VIRUS (HIV). The virus that causes AIDS, which is the most advanced stage of HIV infection. HIV is a retrovirus that occurs as two types: HIV-1 and HIV-2. Both types are transmitted through direct contact with HIV-infected body fluids, such as blood, semen, and genital secretions, or from an HIV-infected mother to her child during pregnancy, birth, or breastfeeding (through breast milk).

HUMAN PAPILLOMAVIRUS (HPV). A large family of viruses that cause warts and other growths on various parts of the body; the HPV vaccine is effective against sexually transmitted HPV strains that cause cervical cancer.

HYDROCARBONS. Any organic chemical compound containing hydrogen (H) and carbon (C).

HYPERACTIVITY. A state in which a person is abnormally active.

HYPERAROUSAL. A state of increased emotional tension and anxiety, often including jitteriness and being easily startled.

HYPERBARIC CHAMBER. A sealed compartment in which air pressure is gradually increased and then gradually decreased, allowing nitrogen bubbles to shrink and the nitrogen to safely diffuse out of body tissue.

HYPERBARIC OXYGEN THERAPY. A treatment in which the patient is placed in a chamber and breathes oxygen at higher-than-atmospheric pressure. This high-pressure oxygen stops bacteria from growing and, at high enough pressure, kills them.

HYPERSENSITIVITY. An excessive immune response to a foreign substance.

HYPERTENSION. High blood pressure, which can cause or be caused by chronic kidney disease.

HYPERTHYROID. Having too much thyroxin stimulation.

HYPERVIGILANCE. A condition of abnormally intense watchfulness or wariness. It is one of the most common symptoms of PTSD.

HYPOTHERMIA. Lower-than-normal body temperature.

HYPOTHYROID. Having too little thyroxin stimulation.

HYPOXEMIA. An abnormally low amount of oxygen in the blood, one of the major consequences of respiratory failure.

HYPOXIA. A deficiency in the amount of oxygen required for effective ventilation.

I

IATROGENIC. Caused by a medical procedure.

IMMUNE SYSTEM. The network of tissues and cells throughout the body that is responsible for ridding the body of any invaders, such as viruses, bacteria, and protozoa.

IMMUNIZATION. The administration of a vaccine that stimulates the body to create antibodies to a specific disease (immunity) without causing symptoms of the disease.

IMMUNOCOMPROMISED. A state in which the immune system is suppressed or not functioning properly.

IMMUNOGLOBULIN E. A class of antibodies produced in the lungs, skin, and mucous membranes that are responsible for allergic reactions.

IMMUNOGLOBULIN G (IGG). A group of antibodies against certain viral infections that circulate in the bloodstream. One type of IgG is specific against the mumps paramyxovirus.

IMMUNOSUPPRESSIVE THERAPY. Medical treatment in which the immune system is purposefully thwarted. Such treatment is necessary, for example, to prevent organ rejection in transplant cases.

IMMUNOTHERAPY. Treatment of cancer by stimulating the body's immune defense system.

IMMUNOTHERAPY. Therapy using biologic agents that either enhance or stimulate normal immune function.

INCISOR. A tooth at the front of the mouth adapted for biting and gnawing.

INCONTINENCE. The inability to control one's bowel movements.

INCUBATION. The time between exposure to an infectious agent, such as a virus or bacteria, and the appearance of symptoms of illness.

INDOOR RESIDUAL SPRAYING (IRS). The spraying of homes and sleeping areas with insecticides to control malaria-transmitting mosquitoes.

INFLAMMATION. The body's reaction to an irritant, characterized by the accumulation of immune cells, redness, and swelling.

INFLUENZA. A disease caused by viruses that infect the respiratory tract.

INFORMATION TECHNOLOGY (IT). The development, management, and use of computer-based data systems, such as bioinformatics.

INORGANIC MERCURY. Inorganic compounds such as mercuric oxide (HgO) and mercuric chloride ($HgCl_2$).

INSECTICIDE-TREATED NETS (ITNS). Bed nets treated with pyrethroids to control malaria-transmitting mosquitoes.

INSECTICIDES. Any substance used to kill insects.

INTEGRATED VECTOR MANAGEMENT (IVM). A vector control strategy that uses various methods depending on local conditions and circumstances.

INTEGUMENT. The skin.

INTESTINES. Also called the bowels and divided into the large and small intestine. They extend from the stomach to the anus, where waste products exit the body. The small intestine is about 20 ft (6.1 m) long and the large intestine, about 5 ft (1.5 m) long.

INTRAMUSCULARLY. A medication given by needle into a muscle.

INTRAVENOUS (IV). The process of giving a liquid through a vein.

IODINE-131. A radioactive material that, depending on its form, can be used in diagnosing or treating thyroid disease.

IONIZE. to transform a molecule or atom—a neutral particle—into an ion—a particle with a positive or negative charge.

IONIZING RADIATION. Electromagnetic radiation with enough energy to remove electrons from atoms, causing those atoms to become ionized or charged; high-frequency radiation including x rays and gamma rays.

IRRITANT CONTACT DERMATITIS. A type of skin disease that develops when the skin is repeatedly exposed over a long period to acids or alkaline materials that irritate the skin. Symptoms include red rashes, dry skin, and cuts.

ISOTOPE. An unstable form of an element that gives off radiation to become stable. Elements are characterized by the number of electrons around each atom. One electron's negative charge balances the positive charge of each proton in the nucleus. To keep all those positive charges in the nucleus from repelling each other (like the same poles of magnets), neutrons are added. Only certain numbers of neutrons work. Other numbers cannot hold the nucleus together, so it splits apart, giving off ionizing radiation. Sometimes one of the split products is not stable either, so another split takes place. The process is called radioactivity.

ITAI-ITAI DISEASE. The first reported cases of cadmium poisoning in the world, seen in Japan in about 1950. The name means "ouch-ouch" and conveys the sufferers' screams of pain. The disease causes bone and kidney defects. It was caused by cadmium pollution from mines.

J

JAPANESE SELF DEFENSE FORCES (JSDF). The military forces of Japan that were established after the end of the post-World War II Allied occupation of Japan. Since World War II, the JSDF have mostly been confined to the Japanese islands and not permitted to be deployed abroad. In recent years, however, they have been engaged in international peacekeeping operations.

JARISCH-HERXHEIMER REACTION. A rare reaction to the dead bacteria in the blood stream following antibiotic treatment.

JAUNDICE. The yellowing of the skin and whites of the eyes caused by an increased level of bilirubin in the blood.

K

KAPOSI'S SARCOMA. A cancer of the connective tissue that produces painless purplish red (in people with light skin) or brown (in people with dark skin) blotches on the skin. It is a major diagnostic marker of AIDS.

KOPLIK'S SPOTS. Tiny spots occurring inside the mouth, especially on the inside of the cheek. These spots consist of minuscule white dots (like grains of salt or sand) set onto a reddened bump. Unique to measles.

L

LA NIÑA. Unusually cold temperatures in the Equatorial Pacific that can contribute to drought in the Horn of Africa.

LATHYRISM. A disorder that affects humans and some domestic animals and results in degeneration of the nerves of the spinal cord. It is caused by eating legumes that contain the naturally occurring neurotoxin oxalyldiaminopropionic acid (ODAP).

LAVA. Also known as molten rock, lava is magma that has been exposed to the earth's surface through a volcano. Liquid lava can reach temperatures between 1,292–2,192°F (700–1,200°C). Lava forms rock when cooled.

LEAVENING. Yeast or other agents used for rising bread.

LEGIONELLOSIS. A disease caused by infection with a Legionella bacterium.

LESION. A patch of skin that has been infected or diseased.

LEVEE. A manmade embankment built to handle the overflow of water from a river.

LIPODYSTROPHY. The medical term for redistribution of body fat in response to HAART, insulin injections in diabetics, or rare hereditary disorders.

LISTERIOSIS. A usually mild foodborne illness caused by *Listeria monocytogenes*, which can be serious or fatal for fetuses, newborns, the elderly, and immunocompromised patients.

LIVER ABSCESS. An accumulation of pus in the liver that can occur if *Entamoeba histolytica* travels through the bloodstream to the liver.

LOEFFLER'S MEDIUM. A special substance used to grow diphtheria bacilli to confirm a diagnosis.

LOGARITHMIC. Pertaining to the logarithm of a number, which is the exponent by which another fixed value, the base, has to be raised to produce that number; for example, the logarithm of 100 to base 10 is 2, because 100 is 10 to the power 2.

LUMBAR PUNCTURE. A procedure in which the doctor inserts a small needle into the spinal cavity in the lower back to withdraw some spinal fluid for testing; also known as a spinal tap.

LUNG FUNCTION TESTS. Tests of how much air the lungs can move in and out, and how quickly and efficiently this can be done. Lung function tests are usually done by breathing into a device that measures air flow.

LYME DISEASE. An acute disease that is usually marked by skin rash, fever, fatigue, and chills. Left untreated, it may cause heart and nervous system damage.

LYMPH NODE. Small, bean-shaped mass of tissue scattered along the lymphatic system that act as filters and immune monitors, removing fluids, bacteria, or cancer cells that travel through the lymph system.

LYMPH NODE DISSECTION. Surgical removal of an anatomic group of lymph nodes.

LYMPHATIC. One of the three body fluids that is transparent and a slightly yellow liquid that is collected from the capillary walls into the tissues and circulates back to the blood supply.

LYMPHATIC VESSELS. Vessels that carry a fluid called lymph from the tissues to the bloodstream.

LYMPHEDEMA. Swelling of an extremity following surgical removal of the lymph nodes draining that extremity.

LYMPHOCYTES. A type of white blood cell.

LYMPHOMA. A cancerous tumor in the lymphatic system that is associated with a poor prognosis in AIDS patients.

M

MACROPHAGES. White blood cells whose job is to destroy invading microorganisms. *Listeria monocytogenes* avoids being killed and can multiply within the macrophage.

MADHYA PRADESH. State in central India. Its capital is Bhopal.

MAGMA. An extremely hot fluid material found under Earth's crust. When magma hits the surface of the earth, it begins to cool and becomes lava.

MAGNETIC RESONANCE IMAGING (MRI). An imaging technique that uses a large circular magnet and radio waves to generate signals from atoms in the body. These signals are used to construct images of internal structures.

MAJOR TRANQUILIZERS. The family of drugs that includes the psychotropic or neuroleptic drugs, sometimes used to help autistic people. They carry significant risk of side effects, including Parkinsonism and movement disorders, and should be prescribed with caution.

MALABSORPTION SYNDROME. A condition characterized by indigestion, bloating, diarrhea, loss of appetite, and weakness, caused by poor absorption of nutrients from food as a result of HIV infection itself, giardiasis or other opportunistic infections of the digestive tract, or certain surgical procedures involving the stomach or intestines.

MALARIA. A disease caused by parasites of the genus *Plasmodium* that infect red blood cells and are transmitted from infected to uninfected people by bites of anopheline mosquitoes; the single largest cause of illness and death worldwide.

MALIGNANT. A general term for cells and the tumors they form that can invade and destroy other tissues and organs.

MALIGNANT MESOTHELIOMA. Malignant mesothelioma is a rare form of cancer that develops from transformed cells originating in the mesothelium, the protective lining that covers many of the internal organs of the body. It is usually caused by exposure to asbestos. The most common anatomical site for the development of mesothelioma is the pleura (the outer lining of the lungs and internal chest wall), but it can also arise in the peritoneum (the lining of the abdominal cavity), and the pericardium (the sac that surrounds the heart), or the tunica vaginalis (a sac that surrounds the testis).

MALNUTRITION. Inadequate or unbalanced intake of nutrients that affects health.

MANTOUX TEST. Another name for the PPD test.

MATURATION. The process by which stem cells transform from immature cells without a specific function into a particular type of blood cell with defined functions.

MEASLES. An acute, highly contagious viral disease marked by distinct red spots followed by a rash; occurs primarily in children and is often epidemic in refugee camps.

MECHANICO-CHEMICAL. Relating to both mechanical and chemical processes.

MECONIUM. The first feces of a newborn. Meconium is the waste products accumulated in the bowel during fetal life.

MEDIA. Substance which contains all the nutrients necessary for bacteria to grow in a culture.

MEFLOQUINE. An antimalarial drug that was developed by the U.S. Army in the early 1980s. By the early 2000s, malaria resistance to this drug had become a problem in some parts of Asia (especially Thailand and Cambodia).

MELANOCYTE. Cells derived from the neural crest that are in the skin and produce the protein pigment melanin.

MELANOMA. A malignant tumor of skin cells that produce dark pigment. It is the leading cause of skin cancer deaths.

MENINGES. Outer covering of the spinal cord and brain. Infection is called meningitis, which can lead to damage to the brain or spinal cord and lead to death.

MENINGITIS. Inflammation of the meninges, the layers of membranes that cover and protect the brain and spinal cord.

MENINGOCOCCAL MENINGITIS. Highly contagious meningitis caused by the bacterium *Neisseria meningitidis*.

MERCURIC CHLORIDE; MERCURY(II) CHLORIDE; $HGCL_2$. A poisonous crystalline form of inorganic mercury that is used as a disinfectant and fungicide.

MERCURY POISONING. The exposure to the heavy metal mercury. Exposure to mercury can cause vomiting, diarrhea, shaking, kidney and respiratory problems, and brain damage.

METABOLOMICS. The study of all of the chemicals or metabolites involved in cellular processes.

METAMORPHISM. Changes in form to mineral assemblages and textures of rock, in this context, as a result of high pressures and temperatures that differ from the conditions the rock was formed under.

METASTASIS. The spread of cancer from one part of the body to another.

METHEMOGLOBINEMIA. A condition in which the oxygen-carrying capacity of the blood is impaired by an oxidizing agent.

METHICILLIN-RESISTANT *STAPHYLOCOCCUS AUREUS* (MRSA). A common healthcare-associated "staph" infection that is resistant to most common antibiotics.

METHYL ISOCYANATE (MIC). An organic compound is an intermediate chemical in the production of carbamate pesticides (such as carbaryl, carbofuran, methomyl, and aldicarb). Exposure symptoms include coughing; chest pain; Dyspnea; asthma; irritation of the eyes, nose and throat; and skin damage. Higher levels of exposure can result in pulmonary or lung edema, emphysema and hemorrhages, bronchial pneumonia, and death.

METHYLMERCURY. Any of various toxic compounds containing the organic grouping CH_3Hg. These compounds occur as industrial byproducts and pesticide residues, accumulate in fish and other organisms, especially those high on the food chain, and are rapidly absorbed through the human intestine to cause neurological disorders such as Minamata disease.

MICROBIOMICS. The study of microbes and their interactions in an ecosystem, such as the human gut, often based on their genomic sequences or metagenomics.

MICROORGANISM. An organism that can be seen only through a microscope. Microorganisms include bacteria, protozoa, algae, and fungi.

MILIARY TUBERCULOSIS. The form of TB in which the bacillus spreads through all body tissues and organs, producing many thousands of tiny tubercular lesions. It is often fatal unless promptly treated.

MINIMATA DISEASE. Sometimes referred to as Chisso-Minamata disease, it is a neurological syndrome caused by mercury poisoning.

MIRACIDIUM. The form of the schistosome worm that infects freshwater snails.

MITIGATION. A general term for attempts to prevent disasters or reduce their impact.

MMR VACCINE. The standard measles, mumps, and rubella (MMR) vaccine that is given to prevent measles, mumps and rubella (German measles). The MMR vaccine is now given in two dosages. The first should be given at 12-15 months of age. The second vaccination should be given at 4-6 years. There are some exceptions depending on a person's health condition.

MMRV VACCINE. A combination vaccine against measles, mumps, rubella, and varicella (chickenpox).

MONONUCLEAR PHAGOCYTE. A type of cell of the human immune system that ingests bacteria, viruses, and other foreign matter, thus removing potentially harmful substances from the bloodstream. These substances are usually then digested within the phagocyte.

MOTOR NEURON. A type of cell in the central nervous system that controls the movement of muscles either directly or indirectly.

MOUSSE OIL. Crude oil that has emulsified or weathered, mixed with dispersants, water, and marine material to form a spongy, light brown, mousse-like material.

MUMPS. An acute and highly contagious viral illness that usually occurs in childhood.

MUNICIPAL. Relating to a town or city.

MUSCULOSKELETAL DISORDER. Injuries or disorders of the muscles, nerves, joints, tendons, cartilage, or spinal discs.

MUTAGENIC. Having a tendency to produce mutations in an organism.

MUTATE. A make a permanent change in the genetic material that may alter a trait or characteristic of an individual or manifest as disease and can be transmitted to offspring.

MUTATION. A permanent change in the genetic material that may alter a trait or characteristic of an individual, or manifest as disease and can be transmitted to offspring.

MYCOBACTERIA. A group of bacteria that includes *Mycobacterium tuberculosis*, the bacterium that causes tuberculosis, and other forms that cause related illnesses.

MYOCARDITIS. Inflammation of the heart tissue.

MYOPIA. Nearsightedness.

N

N-95 RESPIRATOR. most common of the types of particulate filtering face piece respirators. It filters at least 95 percent of airborne particles but is not resistant to oil.

NASOPHARYNX. The breathing tube continuous with the nose.

NATIONAL DISASTER MEDICAL SYSTEM (NDMS). A federally coordinated system that augments the U.S. medical response capability. The overall purpose of the NDMS is to supplement an integrated National medical response capability for assisting State and local authorities in dealing with the medical impacts of major peacetime disasters and to provide support to the military and the Department of Veterans Affairs medical systems in caring for casualties evacuated back to the U.S. from overseas armed conventional conflicts.

NATIONAL ENVIRONMENTAL POLICY ACT OF 1969 (NEPA). The environmental law that established a national policy promoting the enhancement of the environment and also established the President's Council on Environmental Quality. The purpose of NEPA is to ensure that environmental factors are weighted equally when compared to other factors in the decision making process undertaken by federal agencies.

NATIONAL OCEANIC AND ATMOSPHERIC ADMINISTRATION (NOAA) WEATHER RADIO (NWR). A nationwide network of radio stations that broadcast continuous weather information to special receivers.

NATURAL SELECTION. The process by which certain biological traits become either more or less common in the population of a given species as a result of the different rates of reproduction of individuals bearing those traits.

NAVIGABLE WATERS. Waters that provide a channel for commerce and transportation of people and goods. Under U.S. law, bodies of water are defined according to their use. Navigable waters are used for business or transportation. The federal government has jurisdiction over navigable waters rather than states or municipalities. The federal government can determine how the waters are used, by whom, and under what conditions, and also has the power to alter the waters, such as by dredging or building dams. Generally a state or private property owner who is inconvenienced by such work has no remedy against the federal government unless state or private property itself is taken; if such property is taken, the laws of Eminent Domain would apply, which may lead to compensation for the landowner.

NEBULIZER. A device that delivers a regulated flow of medication into the airways; patients often use them at home to take bronchodilator drugs.

NECROSIS. Abnormal death of cells, potentially caused by disease or infection.

NEONICOTINOIDS, NEONICS. A class of insect neurotoxins—including clothianidin, thiamethoxam, and imidacloprid—that are in widespread use, especially on staple crops such as corn, and that have been associated with colony collapse disorder.

NEUROBRUCELLOSIS. Brucellosis that affects the central nervous system.

NEUROLOGIC. Pertaining to the nervous system.

NEUROTOXIN. A poisonous substance that acts on the central nervous system.

NEVUS. A mole.

NICOTINE. The addictive ingredient of tobacco, it acts on the nervous system and is both stimulating and calming.

NICOTINE REPLACEMENT THERAPY. A method of weaning a smoker away from both nicotine and the oral fixation that accompanies a smoking habit by giving the smoker smaller and smaller doses of nicotine in the form of a patch or gum.

NITROGEN DIOXIDE. With the chemical formula NO_2 (where N stands for nitrogen, and O for oxygen), a reddish-brown toxic gas that is one of several nitrogen oxides.

NITROGEN OXIDES. Any group of compounds consisting of a mixture of oxygen (O) and nitrogen (N).

NONGOVERNMENTAL ORGANIZATIONS (NGOS). Relief and development nonprofit organizations that work independently of governments.

NON-IONIZING RADIATION. Low-frequency electromagnetic radiation with insufficient energy to ionize atoms, including radio waves, microwaves, and radiofrequency from cell phones.

NON-NUCLEOSIDE REVERSE TRANSCRIPTASE INHIBITORS. The newest class of antiretroviral drugs that work by inhibiting the reverse transcriptase enzyme necessary for HIV replication.

NOROVIRUS. Norwalk virus; a large family of RNA viruses that are the most common cause of illness from contaminated food; often called "cruise ship disease" because outbreaks are common on cruise ships.

NOSEMA. A genus of fungal pathogens that live in the honeybee gut and may be associated with colony collapse disorder.

NOSOCOMIAL INFECTION. An infection acquired in a hospital during treatment for another condition.

NUCLEAR FISSION. A nuclear reaction that splits a heavy nucleus into lighter ones, or one atom into two. The reaction releases energy.

NUCLEAR POWER STATION. A thermal power station in which the heat source is a nuclear reactor. The heat produced is used to generate steam that drives a steam turbine connected to a generator that produces electricity.

NUCLEAR REACTION. A process, such as fission, fusion, or radioactive decay, in which the structure of an atomic nucleus is altered through release of energy or mass or by being broken apart.

NUCLEAR REACTOR. A device in which nuclear fission may be sustained and controlled in a self-supporting nuclear reaction. There are several varieties, but all incorporate certain features, such as fissionable material or fuel, a moderating material (to control the reaction), a reflector to conserve escaping neutrons, provisions for removal of heat, measuring and controlling instruments, and protective devices.

NUCLEIC ACIDS. The cellular molecules DNA and RNA that act as coded instructions for the production of proteins and are copied for transmission of inherited traits.

NUCLEOCAPSID. The combination of the capsid and viral genome.

NUCLEOSIDE ANALOGUES. The first group of effective anti-retroviral medications. They work by interfering with the AIDS virus' synthesis of DNA.

O

OBESITY. An abnormal accumulation of body fat, usually 20% or more above ideal body weight or a body mass index (BMI) of 30 or above.

OFF-LABEL USE. Drugs in the United States are approved by the Food and Drug Administration (FDA) for specific uses, periods of time, or dosages based on the results of clinical trials. However, it is legal for physicians to administer these drugs for other "off-label" or non-approved uses. It is not legal for pharmaceutical companies to advertise drugs for off-label uses.

OIL BARREL. A volume measure of 42 U.S. gallons or 19873 L.

OOCYST. A thick-walled spore that is the infective stage of certain waterborne illnesses, such as cryptosporidiosis.

OPEN READING FRAME (ORF). A stretch of DNA that translates into an amino acid sequence of a protein.

OPIATE BLOCKERS. A type of drug that blocks the effects of natural opiates in the system. This makes some people, including some people with autism, appear more responsive to their environment.

OPPORTUNISTIC INFECTION. An infection caused by an organism that does not cause disease in a person with a healthy immune system.

OPTICAL RADIATION. Light and infrared radiation.

ORAL REHYDRATION SOLUTION (ORS). A liquid preparation developed by the World Health Organization that can decrease fluid loss in persons with diarrhea. Originally developed to be prepared with materials available in the home, commercial preparations have recently come into use.

ORAL REHYDRATION THERAPY. oral administration of a solution of electrolytes and carbohydrates in the treatment of diarrhea-related dehydration.

ORCHITIS. Inflammation or swelling of the scrotal sac containing the testicles.

ORGANIC MERCURY. Poisonous compounds containing mercury and carbon, such as methylmercury, ethylmercury, and phenylmercury.

OSTEOPOROSIS. A disease in which the bones become extremely porous, are subject to fracture, and heal slowly.

OUTBREAK. A sudden increase in the incidence of a disease.

OVERWEIGHT. A body mass index (BMI) between 25 and 30.

OXIDATION. When a chemical element or compound loses an electron.

OXYGEN FREE RADICALS. Reactive molecules containing oxygen and can cause cell damage.

OZONE. A gaseous form of oxygen that has three oxygen (O) atoms per molecule with the chemical formula O_3.

P

PANDEMIC. The occurrence of a disease that in a short time infects a large percentage of the population over a wide geographical area.

PAP TEST. A screening test for cervical cancer devised by Giorgios Papanikolaou (1883–1962) in the 1940s.

PAPULES. Firm bumps on the skin.

PARALYSIS. The inability to voluntarily move.

PARAMYXOVIRUS. A genus of viruses that includes the causative agent of mumps.

PARASITE. An organism that survives by living with, on, or in another organism, usually to the detriment of the host.

PARESTHESIA. An altered sensation often described as burning, tingling, or pin pricks.

PARKINSON'S DISEASE. A neurological disorder caused by deficiency of dopamine, a neurotransmitter, that is a chemical that assists in transmitting messages between the nerves within the brain. It is characterized by muscle tremor or palsy and rigid movements.

PAROTITIS. Inflammation and swelling of the salivary glands.

PARTICULATE. From the word particle, particulate or particulate matter, is the term used to describe many of the tiny air pollutants that can gather in the air and cause problems when inhaled.

PARTICULATE MATTER. Fine liquid or solid particles that pollute the atmosphere by natural and human-made processes.

PATHOGEN. A causative agent of disease, such as a bacteria, virus, or parasite.

PCV. A vaccine against the pneumococcus that causes bacterial pneumonia.

PENICILLIUM. A group of fungi of major importance in the natural environment as well as in food and drug production. Members of the genus produce penicillin, which is used as an antibiotic to kill or stop the growth of certain kinds of bacteria in the body. *Penicillium* is a common indoor mold, and its spores can cause mold allergy.

PENTAGON. Headquarters of the U.S. Department of Defense, located in Arlington County, Virginia. The word *Pentagon* is often used to refer to the Department of Defense rather than the building itself.

PERFLUOROOCTANE SULFONATE (PFOS). A global persistent organic pollutant that was widely used in fabric protectors and stain repellents and that bioaccumulates in wildlife and humans and is associated with increased risk for chronic kidney disease.

PERMETHRIN. A common neurotoxic insecticide and insect repellent.

PERSONALIZED MEDICINE. Individualized medicine; the prediction, prevention, diagnosis, and/or treatment of a disease or condition based on a marker in the individual's DNA sequence.

PERTUSSIS. An infectious bacterial disease, especially of children, that is on the increase due to under-vaccination. Commonly called whooping cough.

PESTICIDE. An agent used to destroy pests such as insects that feed on crops.

PETECHIAE. Pinpoint size red spots caused by hemorrhaging under the skin.

PH. A measurement of the acidity or alkalinity of a fluid. A neutral fluid, neither acid nor alkali, has a pH of 7.

PHAGOCYTOSIS. The "ingestion" of a piece of matter by a cell.

PHARMACOGENOMICS. The effects of variations in DNA sequences on drug responses.

PHENYLKETONURIA (PKU). An enzyme deficiency present at birth that disrupts metabolism and causes brain damage. This rare inherited defect may be linked to the development of autism.

PHOBIA. An intense, abnormal, or illogical fear of something specific, such as heights or open spaces.

PHOTODYNAMIC THERAPY (PDT). A treatment for tumors in which a light-sensitive dye is injected into the blood (or skin) to be taken up selectively by the tumors. Light of a specific wavelength is then applied to the affected area to kill the tumors.

PHYSIOLOGICALLY BASED PHARMACOKINETICS (PBPK). A model developed by the U.S. Environmental Protection Agency to predict how chemicals travel through the body and concentrate in tissues and fluids.

PICA. An abnormal appetite or craving for non-food items, often such substances as chalk, clay, dirt, laundry starch, or charcoal.

PICARIDIN. A mosquito repellent that is applied directly to the skin.

PITUITARY GLAND. The master gland, located in the middle of the head, that controls most of the other glands by secreting stimulating hormones.

PLAGUE. A highly infectious and often fatal bacterial disease that is transmitted between humans and from rodents to humans by fleas.

PLASMID. A small loop of genetic material that is not part of a chromosome and can be easily transferred between bacteria.

PLATELETS. Circulating blood cells that are crucial to the mechanism of clotting.

PLEURAL EFFUSION. Pleural effusion is excess fluid that accumulates between the two pleural layers, the fluid-filled space that surrounds the lungs. Excessive amounts of such fluid can impair breathing by limiting the expansion of the lungs during ventilation.

PLEURAL PLAQUES. Pleural plaques are localized scars (fibrosis) consisting of collagen fiber deposits that form as a result of exposure to asbestos. They are the most common manifestation of exposure to asbestos. Normally, pleural plaque is found on the inside of the diaphragm, but in very rare cases it also can be found near the ribcage. Pleural plaques themselves are not associated with any symptoms. However, many people who develop pleural plaques also develop pleural effusion, asbestosis, malignant mesothelioma and other conditions associated with asbestos inhalation.

PNEUMOCOCCAL MENINGITIS. Meningitis caused by the bacterium *Streptococcus pneumoniae*.

PNEUMOCONIOSIS. Any chronic lung disease caused by inhaling particles of silica or similar substances that lead to loss of lung function.

PNEUMONITIS. Inflammation of lung tissue.

PNEUMOTHORAX. Air inside the chest cavity that may cause the lung to collapse. It is both a complication of pulmonary tuberculosis and a means of treatment designed to allow an infected lung to rest and heal.

POINT SOURCE DISCHARGE. A confined and discrete release of something directly into a specific source. For example, a point source discharge into water can be from a pipe into a river or stream.

POLIOMYELITIS. An infectious viral disease that was very widespread, especially among children, before the introduction of polio vaccines in the 1950s; it has been eradicated in most of the world through vaccines such as inactivated polio vaccine (IPV). Commonly known as polio.

POLLINATION. The process by which pollen is transferred during sexual reproduction in plants, often through the mediation of a pollinator such as honeybees.

POLYBROMINATED DIPHENYL ETHERS (PBDES). Compounds used as flame retardants that bioaccumulate in humans.

POLYCARBONATE (PC). Very strong, transparent, high-temperature-resistant plastics that may contain BPA; indicated by recycling number "7" (mixed or other).

POLYCHLORINATED BIPHENYLS. Any compound derived from biphenyl and containing chlorine (Cl), which is considered an hazardous environmental pollutant; with the abbreviation PCBs.

POLYETHYLENE (PE). Plastics with recycling numbers "1," "2," and "4," which generally do not contain BPA.

POLYPROPYLENE (PP). Plastics with recycling number "5," which generally do not contain BPA.

POLYVINYL CHLORIDE (PVC). Plastics with recycling number "3," which are manufactured using several harmful chemicals, sometimes including BPA.

POST-EXPOSURE PROPHYLAXIS (PEP). A four-week course of antiretroviral drugs given to people immediately following exposure to HIV infection from rape, unprotected sex, needlestick injuries, or sharing needles.

POST-TRAUMATIC STRESS SYNDROME (PTSS). A type of severe anxiety disorder that can develop after individuals experience traumatic events or situations.

POTABLE. Water or other liquid that is suitable for drinking.

POX. A pus-filled bump on the skin.

PREDIABETES. A condition characterized by blood glucose levels above normal, but lower than levels with diabetes; a precursor to type 2 diabetes.

PREFECTURE. A self-governing body or area. The administration of Japan consists of the nation, large area local governing units (prefectures), and basic local governing units (municipalities). Japan is divided into 47 prefectures.

PRENATAL. Before birth.

PRESSURE VESSEL. A strong-walled container housing the core of most types of power reactors.

PREVALENCE. The percentage of a population that is affected by a specific disease at a given time.

PREVALENCE RATE. The proportion of a population found to have a condition, such as a disease or a risk factor (e.g., smoking or seat-belt use). It is calculated by dividing the number of people found to have the condition by the total number of people studied, and is expressed as a ratio, as a percentage or as the number of cases per 10,000 or 100,000 people.

PRIMARY EXPLOSIVE. A very sensitive explosive used to ignite other types of more stable explosives.

PRIMARY SYSTEM. The cooling system used to remove energy from the reactor core and transfer that energy either directly or indirectly to the steam turbine.

PRION. An infectious protein that causes diseases such as Creutzfeldt-Jakob and mad cow.

PROBIOTICS. Food supplements containing live bacteria or other microbes intended to improve or restore the normal balance of microorganisms in the digestive tract.

PROCESS SLUDGES. Any one of many materials generated from industrial or municipal water treatment systems.

PROCTOSCOPE. An instrument consisting of a thin tube with a light source, used to examine the inside of the rectum.

PRODROME. Early symptoms or warning signs

PROTEASE INHIBITORS. The second major category of drug used to treat AIDS that works by suppressing the replication of the HIV virus.

PROTEOMICS. Analysis of the structures, functions, and interactions of the proteins in a particular cell, tissue, or organism, organization of the information in databases, and applications.

PROTOZOA. Single-celled microorganisms belonging to the subkingdom Protozoa that are more complex than bacteria. About 30 protozoa cause diseases in humans.

PRUSSIAN BLUE. The common name of potassium ferric hexacyanoferrate, a compound approved in the United States for treatment of thallium poisoning. Prussian blue gets its name from the fact that it was first used by artists in 1704 as a dark blue pigment for oil paints. It has also been used in laundry bluing and fabric printing.

PSORIASIS. A common recurring skin disease that is marked by dry, scaly, and silvery patches of skin that appear in a variety of sizes and locations on the body.

PULMONARY. Having to do with the lungs or respiratory system.

PULMONARY EDEMA. Fluid accumulation in the lungs; it is frequently a complication of heart disease and other medical disorders.

PULMONARY EMPHYSEMA. A progressive respiratory disorder that causes shortness of breath.

PURIFIED PROTEIN DERIVATIVE (PPD). An extract of tubercle bacilli that is injected into the skin to find out whether a person presently has or has ever had tuberculosis.

PYRETHROIDS. Synthetic insecticides that resemble pyrethrins from chrysanthemums.

Q

Q-FEVER. A disease marked by high fever, chills, and muscle pain. It is seen in North America, Europe, and parts of Africa. It may be spread by drinking raw milk or by tick bites.

QUADRIVALENT VACCINE. A vaccine that protects against four pathogens.

QUININE. One of the first treatments for malaria, a natural product made from the bark of the Cinchona tree. It was popular until being superseded by chloroquine in the 1940s. In the wake of widespread chloroquine resistance, however, it became popular again. Quinine, or its close relative quinidine, can be given intravenously to treat severe *Falciparum* malaria.

R

RABIES. A rare but serious viral disease transmitted to humans by the bite of an infected animal.

RADIATION. Particles (alpha, beta, neutrons) or photons (gamma) emitted from the nucleus of an unstable atom as a result of radioactive decay.

RADIATION THERAPY. Treatment using high-energy radiation from x-ray machines, cobalt, radium, or other sources.

RADIOACTIVE RADIATION. Radiation produced from radioactive substances.

RADIOACTIVITY. The act of emitting radiation spontaneously. This is done by an atomic nucleus that, for some reason, is unstable; it wants to give up some energy in order to shift to a more stable configuration.

RADIOFREQUENCY (RF). Low-frequency or low-energy radiation emitted by cell phones, radios, and televisions.

RADIOISOTOPE. An unstable isotope that emits radiation when it decays or returns to a stable state.

RADIOLOGICAL DISPERSION DEVICE (RDD). So-called dirty bomb, a weapon designed to spread radioactive material and terror.

RADIOTHERAPY. The use of ionizing radiation, either as x rays or radioactive isotopes, to treat disease.

RADON. A rare radioactive gas that occurs naturally as a decay product of the radioactive elements uranium and thorium.

RB51. A strain of *Brucella abortus* used to produce a cattle vaccine to prevent brucellosis.

RECREATIONAL WATER ILLNESS (RWI). An illness contracted by swallowing or contacting recreational waters during activities such as swimming and boating, and including pools, hot tubs, lakes, rivers, and oceans.

RED TIDE. A brownish-red coloration in seawater that is caused by increased plant-based plankton.

REDUCTION. When a chemical element or compound gains an electron.

REGISTRY. A collection of information such as names, locations, or other data.

REHYDRATION. The restoration of water or fluid to a body that has become dehydrated.

REITER'S SYNDROME. A group of symptoms that includes arthritis, inflammation of the urethra, and conjunctivitis, and develops as a late complication of infection with *Shigella flexneri*. The syndrome was first described by a German doctor named Hans Reiter in 1918.

REM. Short for roentgen equivalent in man, it is a dose equivalent radiation. One rem is equal to 0.01 Sievert (Sv).

REMISSION. A disappearance of a disease as a result of treatment. Complete remission means that all disease is gone; partial remission means that the disease is significantly improved by treatment, but residual traces are still present.

RENAL. Having to do with the kidneys.

RESECTION. The act of removing something surgically.

RESERVOIR. An animal species that harbors a virus, usually without symptoms of infection, and can transmit it to humans directly or via a vector.

RESPIRATORY DISTRESS SYNDROME. Also known as hyaline membrane disease, a condition of premature infants in which the lungs are imperfectly expanded due to a lack of a substance on the lungs that reduces tension.

RETICULOENDOTHELIAL SYSTEM. A group of cells located throughout the body that is part of the immune system with the ability to take up and sequester a variety of inert particles.

RETROVIRUS. A type of virus that uses RNA as its genetic material. After infecting a cell, a retrovirus uses an enzyme called reverse transcriptase to convert its RNA into DNA. The retrovirus then integrates its viral DNA into the DNA of the host cell, which allows the retrovirus to replicate. HIV, the virus that causes AIDS, is a retrovirus.

REVERSE TRANSCRIPTASE. A retroviral enzyme that produces DNA copies of genetic information encoded by RNA.

REVERSE TRANSCRIPTION-POLYMERASE CHAIN REACTION (RT-PCR). A method of polymerase-chain-reaction amplification of nucleic acid sequences that uses RNA as the template for transcribing the corresponding DNA using reverse transcriptase.

RHINORRHEA. A name for the common cold.

RIBAVIRIN. A drug used to combat viral infections.

RISK. The probability that exposure to a hazard will have a negative consequence. There are mathematical equations and computer programs that can be used to calculate risk in specific situations.

RODENTICIDE. A chemical used to kill rodents.

ROSE SPOTS. A pinkish rash across the trunk or abdomen that is a classic sign of typhoid fever.

ROTAVIRUS (RV). A genus of viruses, some of which are common causes of diarrhea and childhood death worldwide.

RUBELLA. German measles; a contagious viral disease that is milder than typical measles but is damaging to the fetus if it is contracted in early pregnancy.

S

SALMONELLA. A genus of bacteria that causes food poisoning, acute gastrointestinal inflammation, typhoid fever, and septicemia.

SALMONELLOSIS. Food poisoning caused by bacteria of the genus *Salmonella*, which usually leads to severe diarrhea and may be transmitted to a fetus.

SARCOIDOSIS. A chronic disease of unknown cause, characterized by the formation of nodules in the lungs, lymph nodes, and other organs.

SARS (SEVERE ACUTE RESPIRATORY SYNDROME). A potentially fatal viral respiratory illness that emerged from Asia in 2003.

SCHISTOSOMIASIS. A widespread disease caused by blood flukes (trematodes or flatworms) in the genus *Schistosoma* that are harbored by snails in contaminated water.

SEASONAL AFFECTIVE DISORDER (SAD). Depression that recurs in fall and winter as the hours of sunlight decrease.

SECONDARY EXPLOSIVE. A high explosive less sensitive than a primary explosive, but more sensitive than a tertiary explosive.

SECONDARY INFECTION. An infection in people whose resistance has been lowered by another disease or infection.

SECONDARY OR OPPORTUNISTIC INFECTION. An infection by a microbe that occurs because the body is weakened by a primary infection caused by a different kind of microbe.

SECONDARY SYSTEM. The steam generator tubes, steam turbine, condenser and associated pipes, pumps, and heaters used to convert the heat energy of the reactor coolant system into mechanical energy for electrical generation.

SECONDHAND SMOKE (SHS). Passive smoke; tobacco smoke given off by a cigarette or exhaled by a smoker and inhaled by others.

SECULAR. Not religious, having no religion basis.

SELECTIVE PRESSURE. Influence exerted by an antibiotic or other factor on natural selection to promote the survival of one group of organisms over another.

SELECTIVE SEROTONIN REUPTAKE INHIBITORS (SSRIS). A class of antidepressants that work by blocking the reabsorption of serotonin in the brain, raising the levels of serotonin. Examples include Prozac, Zoloft, and Paxil.

SENSITIVITY. The ease with which it can be detonated.

SEPSIS. An inflammatory response of the whole body to an infection. Listeriosis in newborns may take the form of sepsis.

SEPTICEMIA. The medical term for blood poisoning, in which bacteria have invaded the bloodstream and circulates throughout the body.

SEROCONVERSION. The development of detectable specific antibodies in a patient's blood serum as a result of infection or immunization.

SEVERE ACUTE RESPIRATORY SYNDROME (SARS). A serious infectious disease caused by a coronavirus that was the first emergent disease of the twenty-first century, arising from transmission events between animals and humans in Chinese markets.

SEXUALLY TRANSMITTED DISEASE (STD). An infectious disease that spreads from person to person during sexual contact. Sexually transmitted infections, such as syphilis, HIV infection, and gonorrhea, are caused by bacteria, parasites, and viruses.

SHELTER IN PLACE. A phrase used to describe remaining indoors in a safe location during an emergency rather than evacuating the area.

SHIGA TOXIN PRODUCING *E. COLI* (STEC). Strains of the common, normally harmless, intestinal bacterium *Escherichia coli* that can contaminate food with Shiga toxin; *E. coli* O157:H7 is the most commonly identified STEC in North America.

SHOCK. A state in which blood circulation is insufficient to deliver adequate oxygen to vital organs.

SICKLE CELL DISEASE. An inherited disorder characterized by a genetic flaw in hemoglobin production. (Hemoglobin is the substance within red blood cells that enables them to transport oxygen.) The hemoglobin that is produced has a kink in its structure that forces the red blood cells to take on a sickle shape, inhibiting their circulation and causing pain. This disorder primarily affects people of African descent.

SICKLE CELL TRAIT. A genetic factor that provides a person with the trait with a level of protective immunity against malaria.

SIDESTREAM SMOKE. The smoke that is emitted from the burning end of a cigarette or cigar, or that comes from the end of a pipe. Along with exhaled smoke, it is a constituent of second-hand smoke.

SIEVERT. Abbreviated Sv, it is a unit of dose equivalent radiation in the International System of Units (SI). One Sv is equal to 100 rem, or 100,000 millirem (mrem).

SILICA. A substance (silicon dioxide) occurring in quartz sand, sandstone, flint, and agate and other rocks. It is used in certain processes, such as making glass or pottery and scouring and grinding powders.

SILICOSIS. A lung disease caused by inhaling silica dust. Silicosis is considered a type of occupational lung disease because it is most often found in people who are working in hard-rock mining, tunneling, quarrying, and other jobs that expose them to silica dust. Natural disasters, such as volcanoes, which cause a large amount of silica dust, can also cause silicosis.

SINGLE NUCLEOTIDE POLYMORPHISM (SNP). A single-base variant in a DNA sequence.

SKIN APPENDAGES. Structures related to the integument such as hair follicles and sweat glands.

SKIN GRAFTING. A technique in which a piece of healthy skin from the patient's body (or a donor's body) is used to cover another part of the patient's body that has lost its skin.

SKIN SNIP BIOPSY. A procedure in which a small amount of suspicious skin is removed and examined for evidence of the parasite *Onchocerca volvulus*.

SMALLPOX. A highly contagious viral disease that has been eradicated through worldwide vaccination.

SMOG. A type of smoky fog that contains large amounts of air pollutants.

SOCIAL NORMS. laws (not considered to be formal) that govern a society's behaviors, that is, the rules that a group uses for appropriate and inappropriate values, beliefs, attitudes and behaviors. These rules may be explicit or implicit and result in social control. Failure to abide by the rules can result in severe punishments, the most feared of which is exclusion from the group. What is considered "normal" is relative to the location of the culture in which the social interaction is taking place. Norms in every culture create conformity that allows for people to become socialized to the culture in which they live.

SOMATOFORM DISORDERS. Any mental disorder characterized by symptoms that suggest physical illness or injury; however, with symptoms that cannot be completely explained by a medical condition, from exposure with a substance, or attributable to another mental disorder.

SORE. An open wound, bruise, or lesion on the skin.

SPECIFIC ABSORPTION RATE (SAR). The amount of radiofrequency absorbed by the body from cell phones in watts per kilogram of body weight.

SPECIFIC GRAVITY. The ratio of the density (mass of a unit volume) of a specific substance to the density of a reference substance.

SPIROCHETE. Any of a family of spiral- or coil-shaped bacteria known as Spirochetae. *L. interrogans* is a spirochete, as well as are the organisms that cause syphilis and relapsing fever.

SPIROMETRY. A test of the air capacity of a person's lungs and the amount of air that enters and leaves the lungs during breathing using a device called a spirometer.

SPORADIC. Rare and occasional in occurrence. Listeriosis in humans is a sporadic disease.

SPORE. A dormant form assumed by some bacteria, such as anthrax, that enable the bacterium to survive high temperatures, dryness, and lack of nourishment for long periods of time. Under proper conditions, the spore may revert to the actively multiplying form of the bacteria.

SPUTUM. Fluid-like matter that can be expectorated from the lungs and bronchi that are compromised by respiratory diseases. Sputum mostly is made up of mucus but also may contain pus, blood, or other materials.

STACHYBOTRYS. A group of molds with widespread distribution that inhabit materials high in cellulose. Certain species are known as "black mold" or "toxic black mold" in the U.S. and are frequently associated with poor indoor air quality arising from fungal growth on water-damaged building materials. Some species produce mycotoxins that are known to produce health symptoms, but it is not scientifically clear whether these mycotoxins affect human health during a mold infestation in a building.

STAPHYLOCOCCUS AUREUS. Also known as staph; a bacteria that can contaminate food.

STEAM GENERATOR. The heat exchanger used in some reactor designs to transfer heat from the primary (reactor coolant) system to the secondary (steam) system. This design permits heat exchange with little or no contamination of the secondary system equipment.

STIMULANTS. A class of drugs, including Ritalin, used to treat people with autism. They may make children calmer and better able to concentrate, but they also may limit growth or have other side effects.

STOCHASTIC HUMAN EXPOSURE AND DOSE SIMULATION (SHEDS). A model developed by the U.S. Environmental Protection Agency for estimating total chemical exposure in a population.

STOOL. Passage of fecal material; a bowel movement.

STORM SURGE. An abnormal rise in sea level caused by strong onshore winds.

STROKE. A sudden diminishing or loss of consciousness, sensation, or voluntary movement from a rupture or obstruction of a blood vessel in the brain.

SUBCUTANEOUS. Referring to the area beneath the skin.

SULFADOXONE/PYRIMETHAMINE (FANSIDAR). An antimalarial drug developed in the 1960s. It was the first drug tried in some parts of the world where chloroquine resistance is widespread. It has been associated with severe allergic reactions due to its sulfa component.

SULFUR DIOXIDE. With the chemical formula SO_2 (where S stands for sulfur, and O for oxygen), a toxic gas with a strong, irritating smell; in nature it is released from spewing volcanoes and it is also released by human-producing industrial processes.

SUPERBUG. An informal term for a bacterium that has become resistant to many different antibiotics. Bacteria that are resistant to several different drugs are also called multidrug-resistant or MDR bacteria.

SUPERFUND SITE. An abandoned hazardous waste site that have been identified for cleanup by the U.S. Environmental Protection Agency.

SYLVATIC. Pertaining to or living in the woods or forested areas. The form of yellow fever transmitted by mosquitoes to rainforest monkeys is called sylvatic yellow fever.

SYNDROME. Common features of a disease or features that appear together often enough to suggest they may represent a single, as yet unknown, disease entity. When a syndrome is first identified, an attempt is made to define it as strictly as possible, even to the exclusion of some cases, in order to identify samples to study. This process is most likely to identify a cause, a positive method of diagnosis, and a treatment. Later on, less typical cases can be considered.

SYSTEMIC DISEASE. Used to refer to a patient who has distant metastasis.

T

T CELL. A type of lymphocyte. There are two major types of T lymphocytes: CD8 cells (cytotoxic T lymphocytes) and CD4 cells (helper T lymphocytes); both T cell types are essential for a healthy immune system. HIV infects and destroys CD4 cells, gradually destroying the immune system.

TACHYPNEA. Increased respiration rate.

TASER. Also called a conducted electrical weapon or CEW, an electroshock device used by some police departments in various countries to subdue suspects who may be armed or otherwise dangerous without having to use lethal force. Tasers work by interfering with the capacity to control voluntary muscles. The name *taser* is an acronym for *Thomas A. Swift's Electric Rifle*, an adventure novel about a fictional weapon published in 1911.

TENESMUS. Ineffective spasms of the rectum or bladder accompanied by the desire to evacuate the rectum or pass urine but without being able to do so. Tenesmus is a characteristic feature of bacillary dysentery.

TEPHRA. The general term for rock particles and fragments produced by a volcanic eruption.

TERATOGEN. An agent that is known to disturb the development of an embryo or fetus.

TERATOGENIC. Having a tendency to produce birth defects in a child.

TERATOGENIC. Tending to cause birth defects.

TERMITICIDE. An insecticide used against termites.

TERTIARY EXPLOSIVE. A high explosive more stable than a secondary or primary explosive.

TESTOSTERONE. The primary male sex hormone.

TETANUS. An acute infectious disease caused by bacteria introduced into the body through a wound.

THIMEROSAL. A crystalline organic mercury compound used as an antifungal and antibacterial agent and present in very small amounts in some vaccines.

THRUSH. A yeast infection of the mouth characterized by white patches on the inside of the mouth and cheeks.

THYROXIN. The hormone secreted by the thyroid gland.

TINNITUS. Ringing in the ears.

TISSUE FACTOR. A glycoprotein involved in blood coagulation.

TOMOGRAPHY. Any of a number of medical imaging procedures that image sections of a body with the use of various types of penetrating waves, such as x rays.

TOPICAL. Referring to a medication or other preparation applied to the skin or the outside of the body.

TOXIC SUBSTANCES. Chemicals that are harmful or usually fatal to an individual.

TOXICANTS. Any type of poison made by humans or introduced into the environment by human activity, such as insecticides.

TOXICOLOGY. The study of the effects of chemicals on organisms.

TOXIN. A general term for something that harms or poisons the body **TOXOID.** A preparation made from inactivated exotoxin, used in immunization.

TOXOPLASMA GONDII. A very common parasite that can cause toxoplasmosis and is a leading cause of death from foodborne illness; although it infects large numbers of people, *T. gondii* is usually dangerous only in immunocompromised patients and in newly infected pregnant women.

TRACHEOTOMY. A surgical procedure in which a hole is cut through the neck to open a direct airway through an incision in the trachea (windpipe).

TRAUMA. A severe injury or shock to a person's body or mind.

TRAVELER'S DIARRHEA. An illness due to infection from a bacteria or parasite that occurs in persons traveling to areas where there is a high frequency of the illness. The disease is usually spread by contaminated food or water.

TREMOR. Shakiness or trembling.

TRIAGE. A method for determining the priority of patient treatment during a disaster or mass casualty event according to the severity of the injuries.

TRIGLYCERIDES. Neutral fats; lipids formed from glycerol and fatty acids that circulate in the blood as lipoprotein; elevated triglyceride levels are common in patients with chronic kidney disease.

TROPHOZOITE. The vegetative form of a protozoan, as opposed to the resting (cyst) or reproductive form.

TSUNAMI. A very large ocean wave that is caused by an underwater earthquake or volcanic eruption and often causes extreme destruction when it strikes land. Tsunamis can have heights of up to 30 meters (98 feet) or more and reach speeds of 950 kilometers (589 miles) per hour. They are characterized by long wavelengths of up to 200 km (124 mi) and long periods, usually between 10 and 60 minutes. Because of the long wave length, tsunami waves do not resemble normal breaking sea waves but may initially resemble a rapidly rising tide.

TUBERCULOMA. A tumor-like mass in the brain that sometimes develops as a complication of tuberculosis meningitis.

TUBERCULOSIS (TB). An chronic infectious disease of the respiratory system caused by bacteria, strains of which have become resistant to most of the effective drugs.

TUBEROUS SCLEROSIS. A genetic disease that causes skin problems, seizures, and mental retardation. Autism occurs more often in individuals with tuberous sclerosis.

TUMOR. An abnormal growth resulting from a cell that lost its normal growth control restraints and started multiplying uncontrollably.

TURBINE. A rotary engine made with a series of curved vanes on a rotating shaft. Usually turned by water or steam. Turbines are considered to be the most economical means to turn large electrical generators.

TYPHOID FEVER. A waterborne illness caused by the bacterium *Salmonella typhi*.

U

UNITED NATIONS. An international organization whose purpose is to facilitate cooperation in international law, international security, economic development, social progress, human rights, and achievement of world peace. The UN was founded in 1945 after World War II to replace the League of Nations, to stop wars between countries, and to provide a platform for dialogue. It contains multiple subsidiary organizations to carry out its missions.

U.S. ENVIRONMENTAL PROTECTION AGENCY (EPA). An agency of the U.S. federal government that was created to protect human health and the environment by writing and enforcing regulations based on laws passed by Congress. The EPA was proposed by President Richard Nixon and began operation on December 2, 1970.

UNPASTEURIZED. Products, especially dairy products, which have not been processed with heat to kill pathogenic bacteria.

UREA. Chemical formed during the body's metabolism of nitrogen and normally excreted by the kidney. Urea levels rise in the blood when kidney failure occurs.

UVA. Ultraviolet A, a long wave of ultraviolet radiation, with a wavelength of 400 to 315 nanometers and an energy level of 3.10 to 3.94 electron volts.

UVB. Ultraviolet B, a medium wave of ultraviolet radiation, with a wavelength of 315 to 280 nanometers and an energy level of 3.94 to 4.43 electron volts.

UVC. Ultraviolet C, a short wave of ultraviolet radiation, with a wavelength of 280 to 1000 nanometers and an energy level of 4.43 to 12.4 electron volts.

V

VACCINE. A preparation of killed or attenuated-live bacteria or virus that is administered to stimulate immunity against that disease-causing organism.

VARICELLA. A childhood disease caused by a herpes virus that may be reactivated later in life to cause herpes zoster or shingles. Commonly called chickenpox.

VARIEGATION. Patchy color variation.

VARIOLATION. The deliberate inoculation of an uninfected person with smallpox to protect against severe smallpox; widely used before the introduction of a vaccine.

VARROA. Mites—small insect-like organisms—that parasitize honeybees; the mite or a virus that it transmits to honeybees may be associated with colony collapse disorder.

VECTOR. An organism capable of transferring an infectious disease from one organism to a different organism.

VESSEL SANITATION PROGRAM (VSP). A program of the U.S. Centers for Disease Control and Prevention that is responsible for inspecting cruise ships and monitoring cruise ship health.

VIRAL LOAD. A measure of the severity of HIV infection, calculated by estimating the number of copies of the virus in a milliliter of blood.

VIRION. A single infectious virus particle.

VIROID. An unconventional virus that is made of uncoated RNA.

VIRUS. A parasitic microorganism that is smaller than a bacterium and has no independent metabolic activity. It is able to replicate only within a cell of a living plant or animal host.

VITAMIN D. A fat-soluble vitamin that is produced by the body through exposure to sunlight and can also be obtained from the diet and supplements.

VITAMIN G. A term used to describe green time—time spent outdoors in nature—that is essential for human health and well-being.

VITILIGO. A condition where the skin loses pigment and develops irregular white patches.

VOLATILE ORGANIC COMPOUNDS (VOCS). Any organic chemicals with a high vapor pressure at normal room temperature and pressure, such as formaldehyde, some of which are harmful to the health of humans and thus are regulated by governments.

VOLTAGE. The force necessary to drive an electric current between two specified points. A large voltage exerts a greater force, which moves more electrons through a wire at a given rate of time.

W

WART. A raised growth on the surface of the skin or other organ.

WASTING SYNDROME. A combination of weight loss and change in composition of body tissues that occurs in patients with HIV infection. Typically, the patient's body loses lean muscle tissue and replaces it with fat as well as losing weight overall.

WAVELENGTH. The distance between adjacent peaks or troughs of a wave.

WEST NILE VIRUS (WNV). A mosquito-transmitted flavivirus that can cause severe illness and whose geographical range is expanding rapidly.

WESTERN BLOT. A procedure that uses electrical current passed through a gel containing a sample of tissue extract in order to break down the proteins in the sample and detect the presence of antibodies for a specific disease. The Western blot method is used in HIV testing to confirm the results of an initial screening test.

WHEEZING. A whistling sound made by the flow of high-velocity air through narrowed airways; a symptom of several respiratory diseases including byssinosis and asthma.

WHITE BLOOD CELLS. A group of several cell types that occur in the bloodstream and are essential for a properly functioning immune system.

WINDOW PERIOD. The period of time between a person's getting infected with HIV and the point at which antibodies against the virus can be detected in a blood sample.

WIRELESS EMERGENCY ALERT (WEA). A nationwide system introduced in 2012 to send text-like emergency messages to WEA-capable mobile devices.

X

X RAYS. High-energy radiation used in high doses, either to diagnose or treat disease.

XENOBIOTICS. Chemicals that are foreign to living organisms, for example, pesticides.

Y

YELLOW FEVER. An infectious viral disease that is spread by mosquitoes and is most common in Central and South America and Central Africa.

Z

ZOONOSIS. A disease that can be transmitted from animals to humans under natural conditions.

GENERAL INDEX

The index is alphabetized using a word-by-word system. References to individual volumes are listed before colons; numbers following a colon refer to specific page numbers within that particular volume. **Boldface** references indicate main topical essays. Photographs and illustration references are highlighted with an *italicized* page number. Tables are also indicated with the page number followed by a lowercase, italicized *t*.

A

AAP (American Academy of Pediatrics), 1:423, 2:562, 563
AAPCC (American Association of Poison Control Centers), 2:531–532, 534
Abortive polio. *See* Polio
Abuse, drug. *See* Drug use
Abuse, stress response to. *See* Post-traumatic stress disorder
Accidents
 ammonia exposure, 1:35–36
 anthrax, 1:38
 background radiation, 1:73
 Bhopal, India, 1:86–89
 Chernobyl nuclear power station disaster, 1:154–160
 electric shock injuries, 1:252, 253, 254
 explosives, 1:289–290
 Exxon Valdez, 1:295–300
 Fukushima Daiichi nuclear power station disaster, 1:348–352
 Gulf oil spill, 1:368–376
 radiation injuries, 2:643
 Seveso, Italy, 2:682–684
 sulfur exposure from, 2:716
 Three Mile Island nuclear disaster, 2:724–729
Acclimatization, 1:27, 28, 29, 401
ACE inhibitors, 1:171
Acetaminophen, 1:152
Acetazolamide, 1:29
Acetone, 1:**1**
Acetylcholine, 1:444
Acetylcholinesterase, 1:445
Acetylcysteine, 1:152
Acid Deposition Act of 1980, 1:4
Acid rain, 1:**1–4**, *2,* 23, 177–178, 348
Acid reflux, 1:56
ACIP (Advisory Committee on Immunization Practices), 1:423

Acquired immune deficiency syndrome (AIDS). *See* AIDS
Acral lentiginous melanoma. *See* Melanoma
Acridine orange (AO), 2:503
Acrodermatitis chronica atrophicans, 1:496
ACS (American Cancer Society). *See* American Cancer Society (ACS)
Act Against AIDS Leadership Institute, 1:18–19
Activated charcoal, 1:151–152, 334, 409, 445, 2:531
Active Learning Network for Accountability and Performance in Humanitarian Action (ALNAP), 1:429
Activism
 AIDS, 1:18–19
 American Public Health Association, 1:34
 Chartered Institute of Environmental Health, 1:144–145
 Earth Day, 1:243–245
 Environmental Protection Agency, 1:278
 Love Canal, 1:490, 491, *491*
 nature deficit disorder, 2:562–563
 oil spills, 2:589
 Rivers and Harbors Act of 1899, 2:661
 Sierra Club, 2:692–693
 Toxic Substances Control Act, 2:735
Acupressure and acupuncture, 1:60, 2:545, 626, 712–713
Acupuncture. *See* Acupressure and acupuncture
Acute leukemia. *See* Leukemia
Acute lymphoblastic leukemia (ALL). *See* Leukemia
Acute mountain sickness, 1:27, 28, 29
Acute myeloid leukemia. *See* Leukemia

Acute myoblastic leukemia (AML). *See* Leukemia
Acute nonlymphoblastic leukemia. *See* Leukemia
Acute nonlymphocytic leukemia (ANLL) *See* Leukemia
Acute radiation syndrome, 1:158, 159, 2:639–640
Acute retroviral syndrome (ARS), 1:12, 13, 15
ADC (AIDS dementia complex), 1:12, 13, 18, 19
Adenocarcinoma. *See* Carcinoma
Adenoviruses, 2:809
ADHD (Attention deficit/hyperactivity disorder), 2:561, 562, 563
Adjuvant chemotherapy. *See* Chemotherapy
Advisory Committee on Immunization Practices (ACIP), 1:423
Aedes aegypti mosquitoes. *See* Mosquitoes
Aedes albopictus mosquitoes. *See* Mosquitoes
Aerosols, 1:2, 234, 438, 2:723, 724
Affordable Care Act, 1:34
Afghanistan, 2:570, 614
Africa
 AIDS in, 1:8–9, *9,* 10, 11
 amebiasis in, 1:30
 cholera in, 1:166
 drought in, 1:232–233
 ebola hemorrhagic virus in, 1:248–251
 endemic disease in, 1:271–272
 epidemiology in, 1:280
 hemorrhagic fevers in, 1:410
 Horn of Africa drought and famine in, 1:415–419
 plague in, 2:611
 river blindness in, 2:655, 656, 657
 sleeping sickness in, 2:699
 vector (mosquito) control in, 2:786

Africa *(continued)*
 water pollution in, 2:800
 yellow fever in, 2:825, 826
African Americans
 AIDS, 1:10, 11, 18, 19
 Hurricane Katrina, 1:456
 lead poisoning, 1:464
 leukemia, 1:476
 melanoma, 2:515
African mistletoe, 1:239
African Program for Onchocerciasis Control, 2:657
African trypanosomiasis. *See* Sleeping sickness
Age picture diagram. *See* Population pyramid
Aged people. *See* Older people
Agencies, government. *See specific agencies by name*
Agency for Toxic Substances and Disease Registry, 1:**4–5**
 on cadmium poisoning, 1:127
 Centers for Disease Control and Prevention and, 1:144
 on Love Canal, 1:490, 492
 Superfund Amendments and Reauthorization Act and, 2:718
Agent Orange, 1:148, *148*, 476
Agricola, Georgius, 1:108
Agricultural chemicals, 1:**5–8**, *147, 325*
 in Bhopal, India, 1:86
 in drinking water supply, 1:229, 231
 endocrine disruptors, 1:275
 Environmental Protection Agency on, 1:276
 in exposure science, 1:292
 Federal Insecticide, Fungicide and Rodenticide Act, 1:304–306
 food safety and, 1:336
 fungicides as, 1:354–355
 health effects of
  acid rain, 1:3
  ammonia exposure, 1:35
  chemical poisoning, 1:148, *148*, 149
  colony collapse disorder, 1:186–187, 188
  food contamination, 1:326, 327–328
  food poisoning, 1:332, 334, 335
  foodborne illness, 1:343, 345
  indoor air quality, 1:438
  leukemia, 1:476
  neurotoxins, 2:567
  sulfur exposure, 2:716
 Rachel Carson Council on, 2:631–632
 See also Insecticide poisoning; Insecticides
Agriculture
 agricultural chemicals, 1:5–8
 drought, 1:232–233, 234, *234*
 famine, 1:301–303

 food safety, 1:337
 heavy metal poisoning, 1:405
 Oxfam, 2:595, 596
 sanitation, 2:672
 Seveso, Italy, 2:683–683
 Soil Conservation Act, 2:714
 zoonoses, 2:834
AIDS, 1:**8–20**, *9*
 activism, 1:18–19
 American Public Health Association on, 1:34
 antimicrobial resistance, 1:41
 causes, 1:12
 comorbidities
  amebiasis, 1:30
  aspergillosis, 1:52, 53
  campylobacteriosis, 1:128
  dysentery, 1:240
  Legionnaires' disease, 1:468
  listeriosis, 1:485
  meningitis, 2:522
  tuberculosis, 2:753, 754, 757
 demographics, 1:10–12
 description, 1:8–10
 diagnosis, 1:12–13
 as emergent disease, 1:264
 epidemiology, 1:280
 history, 1:8–9
 from medical waste, 2:511, 512, 513
 in One Health Initiative, 2:593
 as pandemic, 2:601
 parasites and, 2:605
 prevention, 1:19
 prognosis, 1:19
 public health, 1:18–19
 sanitation and, 2:671
 symptoms, 1:12
 treatment, 1:13–18
 See also HIV (Human immunodeficiency virus)
AIDS dementia complex (ADC), 1:12, 13, 18, 19
Air, ambient. *See* Ambient air
Air embolism. *See* Decompression sickness
Air exchange, 1:438, 440
Air filtration, 1:438, 2:691
Air pollution, 1:**20–25**, *21, 21t*
 causes
  fracking, 1:347
  Iceland volcano eruption, 1:435, 436
  medical waste, 2:513
  mold, 2:536–537, 538
  9/11 terrorist attacks, 2:570–571
  oil spills, 2:587, 589–590
  Seveso, Italy accident, 2:682
  volcanic eruptions, 2:795, 796
 in exposure science, 1:291, 295
 health effects
  asthma, 1:54, 56
  benzene exposure, 1:80–81
  berylliosis, 1:82, 83

  bronchitis, 1:111, 113
  chemical poisoning, 1:147–148, 149–150
  emphysema, 1:269
  fibrosis, 1:309
  heavy metal poisoning, 1:404
  ozone exposure, 2:598–600
  sick building syndrome, 2:689–691
  Yokkaichi asthma, 2:829–830
 mercury in, 2:525, 526
 physical effects
  acid rain, 1:1–4
  ambient air, 1:30
  climate change, 1:*183, 184*
  drought, 1:233
  heat (stress) index, 1:401
  indoor air quality, 1:437–441
 regulation
  Clean Air Act, 1:176–178
  Environmental Protection Agency, 1:276, 279
  National Ambient Air Quality Standard, 2:549–551
 smog and, 2:705
 volatile organic compounds in, 2:793
Air pressure. *See* Barometric pressure
Air quality index, 2:598, 708
Air quality, indoor. *See* Indoor air quality
Air transportation, 1:435
Aircraft, 1:73–74, 2:572, *572*, 573, 574
Airplanes. *See* Aircraft
Airport malaria. *See* Malaria
Airports, 2:571
Akinetic mutism, 1:196
Alabama, 1:371, 455
Alaska
 earthquakes, 1:247
 Exxon Valdez, 1:295, 296, 297, 297–299, *298*
 national parks, 2:693
 tsunamis, 2:751
Alaska National Interest Conservation Act, 2:693
Albumin, 1:171
Alcohol use, 1:131, 2:621
Alcoholic beverages. *See* Liquor
Aldara. *See* Imiquimod
Aldehydes, 2:706
Aldesleukin, 2:518
Alemtuzumab, 1:479
Alexander, Hattie, 2:521
Algae, profusion of. *See* Algal bloom
Algal bloom, 1:**25–27**, *26*, 104, 326, 2:804
Alkalinity, 2:732
Alkylating agents, 1:424, 479
ALL (Acute lymphoblastic leukemia). *See* Leukemia
Allen, Thad, 1:370

Allergens
  in asthma, 1:55–56, 57, 61
  indoor air quality, 1:440
  mold as, 2:536–540
  patch testing for, 2:607–609
Allergic bronchopulmonary aspergillosis. *See* Aspergillosis
Allergies
  asthma, 1:55–56
  to mold, 2:536–540
  multiple chemical sensitivity, 2:540–543
  patch testing, 2:607–609
  to vaccinations, 2:779
Alliance Program, 2:586
ALNAP (Active Learning Network for Accountability and Performance in Humanitarian Action), 1:429
Aloe vera, 2:645
Alpha radiation. *See* Radiation
al-Qaeda, 2:570
ALS (Amyotrophic lateral sclerosis), 2:567–568
al-Shabaab, 1:415–416
Alternative energy, 1:351, 2:708
Alternative medicine. *See* Complementary and alternative medicine (CAM)
Altitude sickness, 1:**27–30**
Alumina, 2:731
Aluminum sulfate, 1:231
Alveoli, 1:268, 269, 308, 314, 2:723
Amantadine, 1:70, 384
Amazon River, 1:211–212
Ambient air, 1:**30**
  asbestos in, 1:47
  carbon monoxide poisoning, 1:138
  Clean Air Act, 1:176–177
  National Ambient Air Quality Standard, 2:549–551
Amebiasis, 1:**30–33**, 237, 238, 240, 2:809
Amebic dysentery. *See* Dysentery
Amelanonic melanoma. *See* Melanoma
American Academy of Pediatrics (AAP), 1:423, 2:562, 563
American Association of Poison Control Centers (AAPCC), 2:531–532, 534
American Biological Safety Association, 1:99
American Cancer Society (ACS)
  on cancer, 1:130, 131, 132, 134, 135
  on leukemia, 1:475
  on skin cancer, 2:696
American Conference of Governmental Industrial Hygienists, 1:164, 206
American Dietetic Association, 1:15
American Journal of Public Health, 1:34

American Lung Association, 1:111, 269, 2:550
American Medical Association, 1:321
American Psychiatric Association, 1:62, 64
American Public Health Association, 1:7, **33–35**, 420, 421
American Recovery and Reinvestment Act, 2:554
American Red Cross, 2:648, 649, 781
American Society of Clinical Oncology, 1:134
American Thoracic Society, 1:269, 2:758–759
American Trucking Association, 1:178
American trypanosomiasis. *See* Chagas disease
American Veterinary Medical Association (AVMA), 2:592
America's Great Outdoors, 2:562
Amikacin, 1:43
Amino acids, 1:90, 91
AML (Acute myoblastic leukemia). *See* Leukemia
Ammonia, 1:35–37, 163, 321
Ammonia exposure, 1:**35–37**
Ammonium hydroxide, 1:321
Ammonium nitrate-fuel oil mixture (ANFO), 1:288, 289
Amnesiac shellfish poisoning, 1:326
Amosite, 1:46
Amoxicillin, 1:497
Ampère, André-Marie, 1:252
Amperometric testing, 1:163
Amphotericin B, 1:53
Amyotrophic lateral sclerosis (ALS), 2:567–568
Analgesics, 2:565
Anaphylaxis, 1:76
Andrew, 1:*431,* 433
Anemia, 1:136, 137, 171, 2:501
  See also Aplastic anemia
Anesthesia and anesthetics, 1:280, 2:567
ANFO (Ammonium nitrate-fuel oil mixture), 1:288, 289
Angiotensin-converting enzyme (ACE) inhibitors, 1:171
Angiotensin-II receptor blockers, 1:171
Anhydrous ammonia. *See* Ammonia
Animal dander, 1:55, 56, 440
Animal feed, 1:6–7, 34, 42, 194, 195, 335
Animal testing, 1:38–39
Animals, domestic. *See* Domestic animals
Animals, farm. *See* Livestock
Animals, game. *See* Wildlife
Animals, wild. *See* Wildlife
Anion exchange, 1:208

ANLL (Acute nonlymphocytic leukemia). *See* Leukemia
Anopheles mosquitoes. *See* Mosquitoes
Anoxia. *See* Hypoxia
Antacids, 1:166–167
Antarctica, 1:449
Antelope. *See* Wildlife
Anthelminthics, 1:238
Anthracene, 1:79, 80
Anthracosis. *See* Black lung disease
Anthracycline, 1:478
Anthrax, 1:**37–41**, *38, 39, 101*
  in bioterrorism, 1:100, 101, 102, 103
  Centers for Disease Control and Prevention on, 1:144
  disease outbreaks of, 1:227
  as emergent disease, 1:265
  in exposure science, 1:294
  Gulf War syndrome and, 1:378
  in One Health Initiative, 2:592
Anthropogenic contamination, 1:404
Antibiotic resistance. *See* Antimicrobial resistance
Antibiotics
  in agricultural chemicals, 1:6, 7
  antimicrobial resistance, 1:41–45
  bioterrorism and, 1:102, 103
  microbial pathogens and, 2:536
  necrotizing fasciitis, 2:565
  as treatment for
    AIDS, 1:14
    anthrax, 1:39–40
    brucellosis, 1:118, 119
    campylobacteriosis, 1:128–129
    cholera, 1:168
    diphtheria, 1:219–220
    dysentery, 1:238, 239
    escherichia coli, 1:286
    giardiasis, 1:359
    Gulf War syndrome, 1:379
    Legionnaires' disease, 1:469
    leptospirosis, 1:472–473
    leukemia, 1:478
    listeriosis, 1:487
    Lyme disease, 1:497, 499
    malaria, 2:503
    meningitis, 2:522, 523, 524
    plague, 2:612
    rodent-borne diseases, 2:663
    shigellosis, 2:686, 687, 688
    smallpox, 2:702
    traveler's health, 2:742–743
    typhoid fever, 2:763
    typhus, 2:766–767
    whooping cough, 2:817
    zoonoses, 2:835
Antibodies
  AIDS, 1:13
  asthma, 1:55, 57
  dengue fever, 1:217
  measles, 2:509, 510
  viruses and, 2:791

Anticholinergics, 1:58
Anticonvulsants, 1:400
Antidepressants, 2:624, 711
Antidiarrheals, 1:238, 286, 327, 333, 2:688, 741–742
Antidotes, 1:152
Antifungals. *See* Fungicide
Antigens, 2:509, 519
Antihistamines, 1:122, 2:538
Anti-inflammatory drugs, 1:58, 2:746
Antimalarials, 2:503–505
Antimetabolites, 1:424
Antimicrobial resistance, 1:**41–46**
  in aspergillosis, 1:53
  in avian flu, 1:70
  in cholera, 1:168
  in emergent diseases, 1:265, 266
  of *escherichia coli,* 1:286–287
  to fungicide, 1:355
  in H1N1 influenza A, 1:384
  in Lyme disease, 1:497
  in malaria, 2:501, 503–504, 504
  in meningitis, 2:523
  of microbial pathogens, 2:536
  One Health Initiative and, 2:592
  in tropical disease, 2:746
  in tuberculosis, 2:753, 754, 757, 758, 759
  in typhoid fever, 2:763
Antioxidants, 1:153, 319, 2:645, 712
Antioxidants, synthetic. *See* Synthetic antioxidants
Antiparasitics, 2:605, 746
Antiretroviral drugs. *See* Antivirals
Antitoxins
  anthrax, 1:38–40
  diphtheria, 1:218, 219, 220
  food contamination, 1:327
  foodborne illness, 1:344
Antitrypanosomals, 2:700
Antivenins, 2:568
Antivirals
  for AIDS, 1:9, *9,* 14, 15, 17–18
  antimicrobial resistance, 1:41–45
  for avian flu, 1:69–70
  for flu pandemic, 1:314, 315, 316, 317
  for H1N1 influenza A, 1:384, 385
  for hantavirus infections, 1:394
  for hemorrhagic fevers, 1:412
  for meningitis, 2:523
  microbial pathogens and, 2:536
  for viruses, 2:791–792
Anxiety. *See* Mental health
AO (Acridine orange), 2:503
APHA (American Public Health Association). *See* American Public Health Association
Aplastic anemia, 1:80, 81, 476
Apoptosis, 2:519
Appia, Louis, 2:648

Aquatic ecosystems
  detriments to
    algal blooms, 1:25–26
    biotoxins, 1:104
    climate change, 1:184
    dams, 1:210
    drought, 1:233
    Fukushima Daiichi nuclear power station disaster, 1:350
    Gulf oil spill, 1:368–376
    heavy metal poisoning, 1:404–406
    mercury, 2:525, 526
    poor sanitation, 2:671
    toxic sludge spill in Hungary, 2:732
    water pollution, 2:799, 801, 802
  in exposure science, 1:293–294
  Federal Water Act on, 1:306, 307
  in low-temperature environments, 1:493
  water quality in, 2:804
Aquifers, 1:232, 234, 404, 2:667, 668
Aralen. *See* Chloroquine
Arbor Vita Corporation, 1:69
Arboviruses, 1:215, 216–217
Archaea, 1:45
Archaeocins, 1:45
Arenaviridae. *See* Arenaviruses
Arenaviruses, 1:411, 2:746
Argentinean hemorrhagic fever. *See* Hemorrhagic fevers
Arilvax, 2:828–829
Armed forces, 1:377–379, 2:620, 621
Aromatherapy, 1:60, 2:712
Aromatic hydrocarbons. *See* Hydrocarbons
ARS (Acute retroviral syndrome), 1:12, 13, 15
Arsenic
  in chronic kidney disease, 1:173
  in heavy metal poisoning, 1:404, 406, 407, 408, 409
  in leukemia, 1:480
  Safe Drinking Water Act on, 2:668
  in sanitation, 2:671
  for sleeping sickness, 2:700
  toxicology of, 2:737
Arsenicosis, 2:671
Artemisinin, 2:504
Arterial gas embolism. *See* Decompression sickness
Arthritis, 1:496
Arthropods, 1:410, 2:604
Artificial colors, 1:149, 319, 320
Artificial flavors, 1:319
Artificial sweeteners, 1:149
Arzerra. *See* Ofatumumab
Asbestos, 1:**46–48,** *47, 48*
  air pollution from, 1:24
  in asbestosis, 1:48–51
  in exposure science, 1:294

  in indoor air quality, 1:438, 439
  Toxic Substances Control Act on, 2:734
Asbestosis, 1:46, **48–51,** 308
Ascorbic acid. *See* Vitamin C
Aseptic meningitis. *See* Meningitis
Ash, fly. *See* Fly ash
Ash, volcanic. *See* Volcanic ash
Asia
  AIDS in, 1:10, 11
  avian flu in, 1:68–69
  drought in, 1:234
  endemic disease in, 1:272
  flu pandemic in, 1:314
  hantavirus infections in, 1:392
  hemorrhagic fevers in, 1:410, 411, 412, 413
  plague in, 2:610, 611
  severe acute respiratory syndrome in, 2:679–681
  water pollution in, 2:800
Asian Americans, 1:10
Asian flu, 1:382
Asian tiger mosquitoes. *See* Mosquitoes
Aspartame. *See* Artificial sweeteners
Asperger, Hans, 1:62
Asperger syndrome. *See* Autism
Aspergilloma, 1:52, 53
Aspergillosis, 1:**51–54,** 2:537
Aspergillus, 1:51–54, 2:522
Aspirin, 2:509
Asthma, 1:**54–61,** *55, 56*
  adult-onset, 1:54, 55–56
  air pollution, 1:23
  in byssinosis, 1:121
  causes, 1:56
  child-onset, 1:54, 55, 58, 59, 60–61
  demographics, 1:54
  development, 1:54–55
  diagnosis, 1:57
  exercise-induced, 1:54, 56
  food additives, 1:321
  housing and, 1:421
  Iceland volcano eruption, 1:436
  mold, 2:537
  9/11 terrorist attacks, 2:571
  prevention, 1:61
  prognosis, 1:60–61
  risk factors, 1:55
  symptoms, 1:56–57
  treatment, 1:57–60
  See also Yokkaichi asthma
Asthma, Yokkaichi. *See* Yokkaichi asthma
Astringent drugs, 1:239
AT (Ataxia telangiectasia), 1:446
Ataxia, 1:196
Ataxia telangiectasia (AT), 1:446
Athlete's foot. *See* Tinea pedis
Atlantic Ocean, 1:433, 2:750, 751

Atmospheric pressure. *See* Barometric pressure
Atomic bombs
   background radiation from, 1:73
   explosives in, 1:289
   in exposure science, 1:294
   ionizing radiation from, 1:446
   radiation exposure from, 2:638, *638*
   radiation injuries from, 2:641–642
Atopy, 1:55
Atropine, 1:152, 445
Atta, Mohamed, 2:570
Attention deficit/hyperactivity disorder (ADHD), 2:561, 562, 563
Atypical nevus syndrome, 2:516
Audiologists, 2:574
Audubon Society, 2:561
Australia, 1:166, 234, 274, 347–348, 2:819
Australian Red Cross, 2:649
Autism, 1:**61–67**, *62, 63t*
   causes, 1:63
   classification, 1:62
   definition, 1:61
   demographics, 1:63
   diagnosis, 1:64
   measles and, 2:510
   mumps and, 2:546
   prognosis, 1:66
   public health, 1:66
   risk factors, 1:62–63
   symptoms, 1:63–64
   treatment, 1:64–66
Autism spectrum disorders. *See* Autism
Autoclaves, 2:514
Automobiles
   air pollution from, 1:22, 23, 24
   benzene exposure from, 1:80–81
   Clean Air Act on, 1:177, 178
   noise pollution from, 2:572–573, 574
   smog from, 2:707
   See also Vehicle safety
Avian flu, 1:**67–71**, *68, 264,* 314, 315, 2:592
Avicides. *See* Agricultural chemicals
AVMA (American Veterinary Medical Association), 2:592
Axelrod, David, 1:490
Ayurvedic medicine. *See* Complementary and alternative medicine (CAM)

B

B cells. *See* Blood cells
B methylamino-1-alanine, 2:568
Babesiosis, 1:499, 2:663
Babies. *See* Children
Bacillary dysentery. *See* Shigellosis

Bacilli. *See* Microbial pathogens
Bacillus anthracis. See Anthrax
Bacillus Calmette-Guérin (BCG), 2:759
Bacillus subtilis, 1:355
Background radiation, 1:**73–74**, 446, 447, 2:634
Bacon, Roger, 1:290
Bacteremia, 1:237
Bacteria. *See* Microbial pathogens
Bacterial meningitis. *See* Meningitis
Bacteriophages. *See* Microbial pathogens
Badham, Charles, 1:110
Bake-out, 1:441
BAL. *See* Dimercaprol
Balantidiasis, 1:237
Bald eagles. *See* Birds
Bang, Bernhard L. F., 2:699
Bangladesh, 1:161, 303
Bang's disease. *See* Brucellosis
Bans. *See* Government regulation
Barley, 1:*147*
Barometric pressure
   decompression sickness, 1:212–213, 214
   drought, 1:234
   hurricanes, 1:431, 432
   tornadoes and cyclones, 2:730–731
Barr, Robert, 2:706
Barton, Clara, 2:648, *648*
Basal cell skin cancer. *See* Skin cancer
Bats, fruit. *See* Fruit bats
Batteries, 1:125, 126, 127
Battle fatigue. *See* Post-traumatic stress disorder
Bauxite, 2:731
Bayer CropScience, 1:188
Bayou virus, 1:392
BCG (Bacillus Calmette-Guérin), 2:759
BCNU (carmustine), 2:519
Beaches. *See* Coastal areas
Beaver fever. *See* Giardiasis
Bed Bug Registry, 1:78
Bedbug infestation, 1:**74–78**
Bedbugs, 1:*75*
Beef. *See* Meat
Bees. *See* Honeybees
Beijing, China, 1:23, 2:707
Belarus, 1:154–155, 156, 158
Belladonna, 2:545
Belo Monte Dam, 1:211–212
Bendamustine, 1:479
Bends. *See* Decompression sickness
Benzene, 1:**78–79**
   exposure, 1:79–81
   from fracking, 1:347, 348
   leukemia from, 1:481
   in sick building syndrome, 2:690
   toxicology of, 2:737

Benzene and benzene derivatives exposure, 1:**79–82**
Benzocaine, 2:534, 535
Benzodiazeprines, 2:625
Benzo(a)pyrene, 1:**82**
Berberine, 2:606
Bernard, Claude, 1:136
Berylliosis, 1:**82–85**, 308
Beryllium, 1:82–85
Beryllium lymphocyte proliferation test, 1:84, 85
Beta agonists, long-acting. *See* Long-acting beta agonists
Beta radiation. *See* Radiation
Beta-carotene, 2:645
Beta-receptor agonists
   for asthma, 1:57, 58, 59, 60
   for bronchitis, 1:112
   for byssinosis, 1:122
   for emphysema, 1:270
Beverages, alcoholic. *See* Liquor
BHA (Butylated hydroxyanisole), 1:149
Bhopal, India, 1:**86–89**, *87,* 257, 396
BHT (Butylated hydroxytoluene), 1:149
Bicarbonate ions, 1:3
Bilharz, Theodor, 2:676
Bilharzial dysentery. *See* Schistosomiasis
Bilharziasis. *See* Schistosomiasis
Bill and Melinda Gates Foundation, 2:747, 772
Biltricide. *See* Praziquantel
bin Laden, Osama, 2:570
Bioaccumulation
   in exposure science, 1:292
   in heavy metal poisoning, 1:293, 404, 405, 406, 407
   of mercury, 2:526
   in mercury poisoning, 2:528
   in toxicology, 2:736
Bioaerosols. *See* Aerosols
Bioavailability, 1:404
Biodiversity. *See* Global public health
Biofeedback, 1:60
Biohazardous waste. *See* Medical waste
Bioinformatics, 1:**89–94**
Biological response modifiers, 1:133
Biological safety. *See* Biosafety
Biological warfare. *See* Bioterrorism
Biological weapons. *See* Bioterrorism
Biomagnification, 1:405
Biomethylation, 1:405
Biomolecules, 1:90
Biomonitoring, 1:**94–96**
   for byssinosis, 1:122
   in chlorination, 1:163
   escherichia coli in, 1:284
   in exposure science, 1:291–292, 295

Biopsy. *See* Diagnostic testing
Bioremediation. *See*
  Phytoremediation
Biorepositories, 1:92
Biosafety, 1:*97*, **97–100**
Biostatistics, 1:362
Biosurveillance
  for bioterrorism, 1:102
  of byssinosis, 1:122
  of campylobacteriosis, 1:175
  of chronic wasting disease, 1:128
  of noroviruses, 2:584
  for pandemic, 2:602
  of smallpox, 2:704
Biotechnology, 1:414, 2:748
Bioterrorism, 1:**100–103**
  anthrax in, 1:37, 38, 39, 40–41
  biosafety and, 1:99
  biotoxins in, 1:103
  brucellosis in, 1:118
  Centers for Disease Control and
    Prevention on, 1:144
  disease outbreaks from, 1:226
  emergent diseases for, 1:265
  in exposure science, 1:294
  food contamination as, 1:324
  food poisoning in, 1:330
  food safety and, 1:336
  in global public health, 1:363
  hemorrhagic fevers in, 1:413
  in One Health Initiative, 2:592
  plague in, 2:612
  smallpox for, 2:701, 703
  typhus in, 2:767
  vaccination and, 2:782
Biotoxins, 1:**103–104**, 324, 336
Bioturbation, 1:405
Bird flu. *See* Avian flu
Birds
  antimicrobial resistance, 1:45
  avian flu in, 1:67, 68–69, 70
  campylobacteriosis from, 1:128, 129
  endocrine disruptors on, 1:274–275
  Exxon Valdez, 1:297, 298, 299
  in flu pandemic, 1:315, 317
  food contamination from, 1:324, 325
  food poisoning from, 1:330
  food safety, 1:337, 338–339
  foodborne illness from, 1:341, 343
  fungicide on, 1:354
  in Gulf oil spill, 1:372, *373*
  hemorrhagic fevers from, 1:411
  leptospirosis from, 1:470
  listeriosis from, 1:484, 485
  in One Health Initiative, 2:592
  in West Nile virus, 2:812, 813
  zoonoses from, 2:834
Birnbaum, Linda S., 2:556
Birth control. *See* Contraception
Birth defects, 1:273, 274, 490

Birth rates, 1:161, 2:619–620, 832
Bisexuality. *See* Sexual behavior
Bismuth subsalicylate, 2:742, 743
Bison (wild). *See* Wildlife
Bisphenol A, 1:**104–108**, 293
Bitter melon, 2:606
Black Creek Canal virus, 1:392
Black Death. *See* Plague
Black lung disease, 1:23, *108*, **108–110**, 308
Black powder. *See* Gunpowder
Blackflies, 2:655–656, 657, 658
Blast cells. *See* Blood cells
Bleach and bleaching agents, 1:320, 2:583
Bleeding, 1:410, 411, 412
Blindness, 1:*87*, 88, 196
Blindness, river. *See* River blindness
Bliss, Russell M., 2:729
Blisters. *See* Skin
BLM (Bureau of Land Management), 2:693
Bloch, Bruno, 2:607
Blood
  AIDS, 1:8, 10, 11, 14
  air pollution, 1:23
  decompression sickness, 1:212–213, 214
  dengue fever, 1:216–217
  Food and Drug Administration on, 1:322, 323
  malaria, 2:501, 502
  methemoglobinemia, 2:534–535
Blood cells
  in AIDS, 1:12, 14, 19
  in asthma, 1:55, 58
  in benzene exposure, 1:79–80
  benzene on, 1:79
  in cancer, 1:134
  Chernobyl nuclear power station disaster on, 1:157
  in cyanosis, 1:206
  in hemorrhagic fevers, 1:413
  in Legionnaires' disease, 1:468
  in leukemia, 1:474–481
  in listeriosis, 1:485
  in malaria, 2:502–503
  in melanoma, 2:518
  parasites on, 2:605
  radiation exposure on, 2:640
  in silicosis, 2:694
  in talcosis, 2:721
Blood cholesterol, 1:16
Blood pressure, high. *See* Hypertension
Blood transfusions, 1:157
  Creutzfeldt-Jakob disease from, 1:194
  for hemorrhagic fevers, 1:412
  for leukemia, 1:478
  for methemoglobinemia, 2:535
  for radiation injuries, 2:645

Blood vessels, 1:216, 2:757
Blood-brain barrier, 2:521, 813, 814
Blowout preventers, 1:369, 370
Blue baby syndrome. *See* Cyanosis
Blue River virus, 1:392
Body fat, 1:16
Boiling, 2:811
Bolivian hemorrhagic fever. *See* Hemorrhagic fevers
Bombs, atomic. *See* Atomic bombs
Bombs, hydrogen. *See* Hydrogen bombs
Bone marrow
  benzene exposure, 1:79–80
  cancer, 1:134
  Chernobyl nuclear power station disaster on, 1:157, 158
  leukemia, 1:474, 475, 479
Bone scan. *See* Gallium scan
Bones, 1:127, 2:756, 797
Bordatella pertussis, 2:816, 817, 818
Bordeaux mixture, 1:354
Boron, 1:6
Boron-10, 2:636
Borrelia burgdorferi, 1:494, 495, 496, 497
Botanical medicine. *See* Complementary and alternative medicine (CAM)
Botox, 2:567
Bottled water. *See* Drinking water supply
Bottom kill, 1:370
Botulinum, 1:327, 378, 2:567
Botulism, 1:102, 326, 327, 331–332, 344, 345
Bovine spongiform encephalopathy (BSE). *See* Creutzfeldt-Jakob disease
Boxing Day Tsunami, 1:247, 2:751
BP, 1:368–372, 374
BPA. *See* Bisphenol A
Brain
  altitude sickness, 1:28–29
  autism, 1:*62,* 63
  benzene exposure, 1:80
  bisphenol A on, 1:105, 106
  cellular phones on, 1:140, 141
  chronic wasting disease, 1:174–175
  Creutzfeldt-Jakob disease, 1:194, 195, 196
  post-traumatic stress disorder, 2:622
Brazil, 1:31, 211–212
Brazilian hemorrhagic fever. *See* Hemorrhagic fevers
Breastfeeding
  AIDS from, 1:8, 10, 11
  in child survival revolution, 1:161
  escherichia coli on, 1:286
  food contamination on, 1:329

Breastfeeding *(continued)*
  food safety on, 1:340
  foodborne illness on, 1:345
  for protein-energy malnutrition, 2:629–630
  UNICEF on, 2:771
Breasts, 1:134
Breathing methods, 1:60
Breslow system, 2:517
Brevetoxins, 1:326
Brill-Zinsser disease. *See* Typhus
British Columbia Cancer Agency, 2:681
Bronchi, 1:54–55, 110, 268–269
Bronchioles, 1:268, 269
Bronchitis, 1:**110–113**
  in black lung disease, 1:108
  in byssinosis, 1:122
  emphysema with, 1:268, 269
  in Yokkaichi asthma, 2:831
Bronchoconstriction, 1:54, 55
Bronchodilators. *See* Beta-receptor agonists
Bronchoscopy. *See* Diagnostic testing
Brookhaven National Laboratory, 2:725
Brown lung disease. *See* Byssinosis
Brown, Michael, 1:489
Brown tides, 1:326
Brownfield sites, 1:**113–115,** *114*
Bruce, David, 1:115–116, 2:699
Bruce, Mary Elizabeth Steele, 2:699
Brucella, 1:115, 117, 118
Brucellosis, 1:39, **115–120,** *116,* 333, 2:592, 699
Brune, Michael, 2:692
Brushfires. *See* Wildfires
Bryonia, 2:545
BSE (Bovine spongiform encephalopathy). *See* Creutzfeldt-Jakob disease
Bubonic plague. *See* Plague
Buffalo (wild). *See* Wildlife
Building codes. *See* Government regulation
Buildings and building materials
  acid rain on, 1:3, 4
  air pollution on, 1:23
  asbestos in, 1:47–48
  asbestosis from, 1:48, 49–50, 51
  biosafety of, 1:99
  mold in, 2:536–537, 538–539
  See also Sick building syndrome
Bulbar polio. *See* Polio
Bullets, 1:464, 465
Bunyaviridae. *See* Bunyaviruses
Bunyaviruses, 1:411–412
Bupropion hydrochloride, 2:711
Bureau of Labor Statistics, 1:282
Bureau of Land Management (BLM), 2:693

Bureau of Land Management Organic Act, 2:693
Burgdorfer, Willy, 1:494
Burkina Faso, 1:161
Burkitt's lymphoma, 1:12
Burns, 1:254, 2:516, 697
Buruli ulcer, 2:746
Burundi, 2:766
Bush fires. *See* Wildfires
Bush, George H. W., 1:177
Bush, George W., 1:102, 178, 279, 458, 2:570
Butylated hydroxyanisole (BHA), 1:149
Butylated hydroxytoluene (BHT), 1:149
Buxton, Dorothy, 2:674, 675
Byrd, Robert, 1:177
Byssinosis, 1:**120–123,** 308

C

Cadmium, 1:**125**
  in air pollution, 1:22
  in chronic kidney disease, 1:173
  in fungicide, 1:354–355
  in heavy metal poisoning, 1:404, 406, 407, 408
  poisoning, 1:125–127
  toxicology of, 2:738
Cadmium poisoning, 1:**125–127,** 406, 408
Caesium. *See* Cesium
Caffeine, 1:60
CAIR (Clean Air Interstate Rule), 2:526, 708
Cairo, Egypt, 1:23
Caisson disease. *See* Decompression sickness
Calcium, 1:6, 466, 2:769
Calcium hypochlorite, 1:162
Caldera, 1:435
Caldicott, Helen, 2:727, *727*
Calendula, 2:545–546
CaliciNet, 2:581
Caliciviruses, 1:237, 241
  See also Noroviruses
California, 1:225, 246, 247, 439, 2:713
CAM (Complementary and alternative medicine). *See* Complementary and alternative medicine (CAM)
Camels, 1:*414*
Cameron, James, 1:245
Camp Lejeune, 1:229
Campath. *See* Alemtuzumab
Campylobacter
  antimicrobial resistance of, 1:45
  in campylobacteriosis, 1:128, 129

  food contamination from, 1:325, 327
  food poisoning from, 1:331
  food safety, 1:337
  foodborne illness from, 1:343, 344
  in traveler's health, 2:740
  as waterborne illness, 2:809
Campylobacteriosis, 1:**128–129**
Canada
  acid rain, 1:2
  AIDS, 1:10
  bisphenol A, 1:105
  cholera, 1:166
  listeriosis, 1:484
  manganese exposure, 2:506
  severe acute respiratory syndrome, 2:679, 680, 681
  water quality standards, 2:806, 807
Cancer, 1:**130–135**
  bioinformatics, 1:91, 92, 93
  causes, 1:131
    acetone, 1:1
    AIDS, 1:12, 14
    air pollution, 1:24
    asbestos, 1:46, 47
    background radiation, 1:74
    benzene, 1:79
    benzene exposure, 1:80
    benzo(a)pyrene, 1:82
    berylliosis, 1:82–83, 85
    campylobacteriosis, 1:128
    cellular phones, 1:140, 141
    chemical poisoning, 1:149
    Chernobyl nuclear power station disaster, 1:156, 158
    chlorination, 1:163
    cutting oil exposure, 1:205
    drinking water supply, 1:229, 231
    endocrine disruptors, 1:273
    food additives, 1:320, 321
    fracking, 1:347–348
    Fukushima Daiichi nuclear power station disaster, 1:350
    human papilloma virus, 1:425, 426, 427
    indoor air quality, 1:437
    ionizing radiation, 1:446–447
    Love Canal, 1:490
    mercury poisoning, 2:532
    9/11 terrorist attacks, 2:571
    non-ionizing radiation, 2:576–577
    radiation exposure, 2:638, 639, 640
    radiation injuries, 2:641–642
    smog, 2:706
    Three Mile Island nuclear disaster, 2:726
    viruses, 2:788, 790
  demographics, 1:130
  diagnosis, 1:132–133
  epidemiology, 1:280, 281
  HPV vaccination, 1:422–423

Cancer *(continued)*
  National Institute of Environmental Health Sciences, 2:556, 557
  prevention, 1:134
  prognosis, 1:134
  public health, 1:135
  Rachel Carson Council, 2:631
  radiation, 2:633, 634–635, 635–636
  See also specific types of cancer
Cancer Genome Atlas, 1:92
Candida albicans, 1:353
Candidiasis, oral. *See* Thrush
Candidiasis, vaginal. *See* Vaginal candidiasis
Cannibalism, 1:194
Cantaloupe, 1:484
Cap-and-trade systems, 1:4, 178
Capreomycin, 1:43
Capsids, 2:788
Carbamate poisoning. *See* Insecticide poisoning
Carbaryl, 1:86
Carbon, 1:74, 288
Carbon dioxide
  in acid rain, 1:1
  Clean Air Act on, 1:178
  in climate change, 1:184
  in explosives, 1:288
  from Iceland volcanic eruption, 1:435, 436
  in indoor air quality, 1:438
  in sick building syndrome, 2:690
Carbon monoxide
  in air pollution, 1:22, 23
  chemical poisoning from, 1:148
  Clean Air Act on, 1:176, 177, 178
  in indoor air quality, 1:438
  in National Ambient Air Quality Standard, 2:549, 550, 551
  poisoning, 1:135–139
  in sick building syndrome, 2:690
Carbon monoxide poisoning, 1:**135–139**, 311
Carbonous oxide. *See* Carbon monoxide
Carboxyhemoglobin, 1:137, 138
Carcinogens. *See* Cancer
Carcinoma, 1:46, 130
Cardiovascular disease
  Centers for Disease Control and Prevention on, 1:144
  in chronic kidney disease, 1:170
  cyanosis in, 1:207
  epidemiology of, 1:280, 281
  from noise pollution, 2:573
  from smoking, 2:711
Carmustine (BCNU), 2:519
Carpal tunnel syndrome, 1:282
Carpets, 1:148
Carriers of disease. *See* Disease transmission

Carrying capacity, 1:301, 310
Cars. *See* Automobiles
Carson, Rachel, 2:618, 631, 632, *632*, 784
Cartagena Protocol on Biosafety, 1:99
Carter, Jimmy, 1:366, 421, 490
Carter, Rosalynn, 1:421
Casein, 1:65–66
Castor oil, 2:582
CAT (Computerized axial tomography scans). *See* Diagnostic testing; Radiation
Cat scratch fever, 2:592
Catalytic converters, 2:706
Cataracts, 2:576
Catastrophes, 1:259
Cats, domestic. *See* Domestic animals
Cattle. *See* Livestock
Caucasians, 1:10, 11, 18, 476, 2:515
Cavities (dental). *See* Tooth decay
CD4 cells. *See* Blood cells
CD38, 1:477
CDC (Centers for Disease Control and Prevention). *See* Centers for Disease Control and Prevention
Ceftriaxone, 1:472, 2:763
Cell phones. *See* Cellular phones
Cells, blood. *See* Blood cells
Cellular phones, 1:**139–143**, 451, 2:576–577
Censuses, 2:619
Center for Biologic Evaluation and Research, 1:322
Center for Chronic Disease Prevention and Health Promotion, 1:143
Center for Devices and Radiological Health, 1:323
Center for Drug Evaluation and Research, 1:262, 323
Center for Environmental Health and Injury Control, 1:143
Center for Food Safety and Applied Nutrition, 1:323
Center for Health, Environment and Justice, 1:491
Center for Infectious Diseases, 1:143
Center for Science in the Public Interest, 1:321
Center for the Evaluation of Risks to Human Reproduction, 1:105
Center for Tobacco Products, 1:323
Center for Veterinary Medicine, 1:323
Centers for Disease Control and Prevention, 1:**143–145**
  on disasters
    drought, 1:235
    emergency preparedness, 1:261, 262
    Haiti earthquake, 1:389, 390
    Hurricane Katrina, 1:457

    9/11 terrorist attacks, 2:571
    oil spills, 2:588
    Times Beach, 2:730
  on diseases and disorders
    AIDS, 1:9, 10, 11, 12, 18–19
    altitude sickness, 1:29
    anthrax, 1:40–41
    antimicrobial resistance, 1:42
    aspergillosis, 1:52, 54
    avian flu, 1:68, 70
    bedbug infestation, 1:77
    bronchitis, 1:111, 112
    campylobacteriosis, 1:129
    carbon monoxide poisoning, 1:136, 138
    chemical poisoning, 1:150
    cholera, 1:168, 169
    chronic wasting disease, 1:175
    cryptosporidiosis, 1:202
    dengue fever, 1:216
    disease outbreaks, 1:228
    dysentery, 1:236, 239
    emphysema, 1:269
    escherichia coli infection, 1:284, 287
    flu pandemic, 1:314, 316
    food contamination, 1:324, 328
    food poisoning, 1:330, 334
    foodborne illness, 1:341, 344
    giardiasis, 1:357
    heat disorders, 1:398
    heavy metal poisoning, 1:408
    human papilloma virus, 1:425, 428
    lead poisoning, 1:463, 464, 465
    leptospirosis, 1:471
    leukemia, 1:480–481
    listeriosis, 1:487
    Lyme disease, 1:494–495, 498–499
    malaria, 2:501, 504
    measles, 2:510
    meningitis, 2:523
    mercury poisoning, 2:529
    mumps, 2:544
    necrotizing fasciitis, 2:564, 566
    noroviruses, 2:578, 579, 580
    pandemic, 2:601–602
    parasites, 2:603, 604
    plague, 2:610–611
    polio, 2:614
    radiation injuries, 2:642
    rodent-borne diseases, 2:664
    severe acute respiratory syndrome, 2:680–681
    shigellosis, 2:687
    smallpox, 2:702
    tropical disease, 2:747
    tuberculosis, 2:753, 758
    typhoid fever, 2:761–762, 763–764
    West Nile virus, 2:812, 815
    whooping cough, 2:816
    zoonoses, 2:833

Centers for Disease Control and Prevention *(continued)*
  on health issues and threats
    biomonitoring, 1:95
    biosafety, 1:98, 99
    bioterrorism, 1:100, 102–103
    bisphenol A, 1:105
    cellular phones, 1:141
    drinking water supply, 1:230
    epidemiology, 1:280–281
    ergonomics, 1:283
    food safety, 1:336
    housing, 1:422
    HPV vaccination, 1:422
    One Health Initiative, 2:592
    smoking, 2:710
    traveler's health, 2:739, 741–742, 743
    vaccination, 2:781
    vector (mosquito) control, 2:786
    water fluoridation, 2:799
    water quality, 2:504–805
  National Institute for Occupational Safety and Health and, 2:554
  Public Health Service and, 2:630
Central America, 1:272, 2:657, 670
Central Intelligence Agency (CIA), 2:675
Central nervous system. *See* Nervous system
Cephalosporins, 1:43, 45, 286
CEQ (Council on Environmental Quality), 2:552, 553, 554
Cercariae, 2:676
CERCLA (Comprehensive Environmental Response, Compensation, and Liability Act). *See* Comprehensive Environmental Response, Compensation, and Liability Act (CERCLA)
Ceroperazone, 2:763
Cervarix, 1:423, 428
Cervical intraepithelial neoplasia (CIN), 1:427
Cervids. *See* Wildlife
Cervix, 1:134, 422, 423, 425, 426, 427
Cesium, 1:156, 159, 350
CFCs (Chlorofluorocarbons), 1:178, 2:598, 734
CFR (Code of Federal Regualtions), 1:395–396
CGL (Chronic granulocytic leukemia). *See* Leukemia
Chad, 1:303, 367
Chadwick, Edwin, 1:145, 2:672, 803
Chagas disease, 1:272, 2:603, 604, 745, 746
Chang Jiang. *See* Yangtze River
Change.org, 2:786
Chantix. *See* Verenicline

Charcoal, 1:288
  See also Activated charcoal
Chartered Institute of Environmental Health, 1:**145–146**
Cheese. *See* Dairy products
Chelation therapy
  for cadmium poisoning, 1:126
  for chemical poisoning, 1:152
  for heavy metal poisoning, 1:407, 408, 409
  for lead poisoning, 1:465–466
  for manganese exposure, 2:506, 507
  for mercury poisoning, 2:531
  for neurotoxins, 2:568
Chemet. *See* Succimer
Chemical coagulation, 1:231
Chemical dispersants. *See* Dispersants
Chemical elements. *See specific elements by name*
Chemical explosives. *See* Explosives
Chemical Manufacturers Association, 1:259
Chemical poisoning, 1:**146–154**, *147*
  alternative therapy, 1:152–153
  causes, 1:150
    food contamination, 1:327
    food poisoning, 1:331, 332, 333–335
    foodborne illness, 1:344, 345
    fungicide, 1:354–355
  demographics, 1:150
  diagnosis, 1:151
  prevention, 1:153
  public health, 1:153–154
  results, 1:153
  symptoms, 1:150–151
  treatment, 1:151–152
  types, 1:146–150
  See also specific types of poisoning by causative chemical
Chemical Safety and Hazard Investigation Board, 1:260
Chemicals. *See specific chemicals by name*
Chemicals, agricultural. *See* Agricultural chemicals
Chemicals, biological monitoring of. *See* Biomonitoring
Chemotherapy
  for AIDS, 1:14
  in aspergillosis, 1:52
  for cancer, 1:133
  for leukemia, 1:478–480, 481
  leukemia from, 1:476
  for melanoma, 2:517, 518–519
  for skin cancer, 2:698
Chen, Johnny, 2:679
Chernobyl nuclear power station disaster, 1:**154–160**, *156*
  causes, 1:156–157
  demographics, 1:155–156
  diseases and disorders from, 1:157–159

  prevention, 1:160
  prognosis, 1:159–160
  public health, 1:159
  radiation injuries, 2:643
  timeline, 1:154–155
  treatment, 1:157
Chickenpox, 1:*190*
Chickens. *See* Birds
Chiggers. *See* Parasites
Child survival revolution, 1:**160–162**
Childhood disintegrative disorder, 1:64
Children
  advocacy organizations
    Centers for Disease Control and Prevention, 1:144
    Oxfam, 2:596
    Save the Children, 2:674–675
    UNICEF, 2:771–775
  disasters
    Chernobyl nuclear power station disaster and, 1:155, *156*, 153, 159
    disaster preparedness, 1:221, 222
    famine, 1:*302*
    Horn of Africa drought and famine, 1:416, 418
    Japanese earthquake, 1:452, 453
    Love Canal, 1:490
    oil spills, 2:587
    Seveso, Italy accident, 2:683
    Three Mile Island nuclear disaster, 2:726, 727
  diseases and disorders
    AIDS, 1:*9*, 10, 11, 13
    altitude sickness, 1:27
    amebiasis, 1:30, 31
    asthma, 1:54, 55, 58, 59, 60–61
    autism, 1:62–66
    cadmium poisoning, 1:126
    carbon monoxide poisoning, 1:136
    chemical poisoning, 1:146, 148, 150, 151
    cholera, 1:166, 167
    cyanosis, 1:207
    diphtheria, 1:220
    dysentery, 1:236, 237, 239, 240, 241
    electric shock injuries, 1:256
    escherichia coli infection in, 1:284, 285, 286, 287
    food poisoning, 1:330, 331, 332, 333, 334
    foodborne illness, 1:342, 343
    giardiasis, 1:360
    H1N1 influenza A, 1:382
    heat disorders, 1:398, 399
    heavy metal poisoning, 1:406, 407, 408, 409
    hemorrhagic fevers, 1:411
    human papilloma virus, 1:426
    lead poisoning, 1:463, 464–465, 466

Children *(continued)*
  Legionnaires' disease, 1:468
  leukemia, 1:474, 475, 476, 479–481
  listeriosis, 1:485, 486, 487
  Lyme disease, 1:496–497
  malaria, 2:501
  manganese exposure, 2:506
  measles, 2:508, *508,* 509, 510
  meningitis, 2:521, 522
  mercury poisoning, 2:528, 529, 530, 532–533
  methemoglobinemia, 2:534, 535
  mumps, 2:543, 544, 545, 546
  nature deficit disorder, 2:560–563
  noroviruses, 2:581, 582
  ozone exposure, 2:599
  post-traumatic stress disorder, 2:621, 622
  protein-energy malnutrition, 2:627–630
  radiation exposure, 2:639
  radiation injuries, 2:642–643
  schistosomiasis, 2:677
  shigellosis, 2:684–685
  talcosis, 2:721
  whooping cough, 2:816, 818
 health issues and threats
  air pollution, 1:23
  biomonitoring, 1:95
  bisphenol A, 1:104, 105–107
  cellular phones, 1:141
  child survival revolution, 1:160–161
  endocrine disruptors, 1:274
  exposure science, 1:292, 293, 294
  food contamination, 1:327, 329
  food safety, 1:339–340
  housing, 1:420, 421
  HPV vaccination, 1:423
  indoor air quality and, 1:438
  lead, 1:462
  mercury, 2:526
  parasites, 2:605
  population pyramids, 2:619–620
  smog, 2:707
  vaccination, 2:778, 779, 780, 781, 782
  water fluoridation, 2:797, 798–799

Children & Nature Network, 2:562

Chile, 1:247, 2:752

Chimpanzees. *See* Primates

China
 acid rain, 1:4
 agricultural chemicals, 1:6–7
 dams, 1:210, *210,* 212
 earthquakes, 1:247
 famine, 1:301
 heavy metal poisoning, 1:407
 lead poisoning, 1:466
 mercury, 2:526
 sanitation, 2:671
 severe acute respiratory syndrome, 2:679, 680, 681
 water pollution, 2:801

Chinese medicine. *See* Complementary and alternative medicine

Chisso, 2:531

Chloracne, 2:683

Chloramination, 1:163

Chloramines, 1:162, 163

Chlorinated hydrocarbons. *See* Hydrocarbons

Chlorinated tris, 1:293

Chlorination, 1:**162–164**, 162*t*
 for amebiasis, 1:33
 for cholera, 1:168
 of drinking water supply, 1:230, 231
 for giardiasis, 1:357
 in sanitation, 2:671
 for waterborne illness, 2:808, 811

Chlorine
 in agricultural chemicals, 1:6
 in air pollution, 1:22
 in chlorination, 1:162–164
 in drinking water supply, 1:230
 exposure, 1:164–165
 noroviruses and, 2:583
 ozone and, 2:598

Chlorine exposure, 1:**164–165**

Chlorobenzene, 1:79

Chlorofluorocarbons (CFCs), 1:178, 2:598, 734

Chloroform, 1:163, 2:690

Chloroquine, 2:503, 505

Cholera, 1:**166–169**, *167*
 in bioterrorism, 1:101
 Centers for Disease Control and Prevention on, 1:144
 as communicable disease, 1:190
 disease outbreaks of, 1:226–227
 from drinking water supply, 1:229
 as endemic, 1:272
 epidemiology of, 1:280–281
 from food contamination, 1:326
 Haiti earthquake, 1:*388,* 388–389, 390, 391
 Horn of Africa drought and famine, 1:418
 as pandemic, 2:601
 in population and disease, 2:618
 sanitation on, 2:670, 671
 in traveler's health, 2:739
 as tropical disease, 2:745, 746
 water quality on, 2:803
 as waterborne illness, 2:808

Chongqing, China, 1:23

Christie, Chris, 1:260, 432

Chromium, 1:404, 406, 407

Chromosomes, 1:476, 477, 478, 479, 480, 490
 See also Philadelphia chromosome

Chronic beryllium disease. *See* Berylliosis

Chronic fatigue syndrome, 1:378

Chronic granulocytic leukemia (CGL). *See* Leukemia

Chronic kidney disease, 1:**170–174,** 287

Chronic leukemia. *See* Leukemia

Chronic lymphocytic leukemia. *See* Leukemia

Chronic lymphocytic leukemia (CLL). *See* Leukemia

Chronic myelogenous leukemia (CML). *See* Leukemia

Chronic myeloid leukemia (CML). *See* Leukemia

Chronic myelomonocytic leukemia (CMML). *See* Leukemia

Chronic obstructive pulmonary disease (COPD). *See* Emphysema

Chronic wasting disease, 1:**174–176,** 194, 265

Churchill County, Nevada, 1:480–481

CIA (Central Intelligence Agency), 2:675

Cidofovir, 1:426

Cigarette smoking. *See* Smoking

Ciguatera fish poisoning, 1:326

Ciguatoxin, 1:326

Cilia, 1:111, 2:816

Cimicidae. See Bedbug infestation

CIN (Cervical intraepithelial neoplasia), 1:427

Cinnabar. *See* Mercury

Ciprofloxacin, 1:472

Cisplatin, 2:519

Cities. *See* Urban areas

Citizens' Clearinghouse for Hazardous Wastes. *See* Center for Health, Environment and Justice

Citrus seed extract, 2:606

Civil war. *See* War

CJD (Creutzfeldt-Jakob disease). *See* Creutzfeldt-Jakob disease

Clades, 2:701

Clarke system, 2:517

Clean Air Act (1963, 1970, 1977, 1990), 1:**176–179**
 on acid rain, 1:4
 on benzene, 1:79
 Earth Day, 1:245
 on endocrine disruptors, 1:275
 Environmental Protection Agency, 1:278
 on mercury, 2:526
 National Ambient Air Quality Standard, 2:549–551
 National Environmental Policy Act, 2:553–554
 on noise pollution, 2:574
 on ozone exposure, 2:600

Clean Air Act *(continued)*
   Sierra Club, 2:693
   on smog, 2:708
Clean Air Act (UK), 2:706
Clean Air Interstate Rule (CAIR), 2:526, 708
Clean Air Mercury Rule, 2:526
Clean Air Scientific Advisory Committee, 2:549
Clean Water Act (1972, 1977, 1987), 1:**179–182**, *180*
   Earth Day, 1:245
   on endocrine disruptors, 1:275
   Environmental Protection Agency, 1:278, 279
   Exxon Valdez, 1:299
   Federal Water Act, 1:306–307
   Rivers and Harbors Act of 1899, 2:661
   on water pollution, 2:802
   on water quality standards, 2:806
Cleaning and cleaning products
   in chemical poisoning, 1:148–149
   in chlorine exposure, 1:164, 165
   on indoor air quality, 1:440
   in lead poisoning, 1:466
   for mold, 2:538, 540
   for noroviruses, 2:583
Cleanup, environmental. *See* Environmental cleanup
Clear Skies Act of 2003, 1:178
Cleavers, 2:545–546
Cleopatra, 1:365
Climate change, 1:**182–185**, *183, 184*
   from air pollution, 1:22, 23–24
   algal bloom from, 1:26
   American Public Health Association on, 1:34
   Clean Air Act on, 1:178
   from dams, 1:211
   disease outbreaks from, 1:226
   drought from, 1:232, 234
   emergent diseases from, 1:266
   Environmental Protection Agency on, 1:279
   food contamination from, 1:324
   on food safety, 1:336
   global public health on, 1:362
   heat (stress) index from, 1:402
   Horn of Africa drought and famine from, 1:417
   hurricanes from, 1:432, 433
   Iceland volcano eruption from, 1:435
   malaria from, 2:501
   One Health Initiative on, 2:592
   Oxfam on, 2:595–596, *596*
   tornadoes and cyclones from, 2:731
   tropical disease from, 2:745
   volatile organic compounds on, 2:793
   water pollution from, 2:802
   waterborne illness from, 2:808
   zoonoses from, 2:834

Climbing, mountain. *See* Mountain climbing
Clindamycin, 1:43
Clinical staging, 2:517
Clinical trials, 1:323, 2:519–520, 556, 759
Clinton, Bill, 1:181, 2:553
CLL (Chronic lymphocytic leukemia). *See* Leukemia
Clostridium botulinum, 1:326, 331–332, 340, 343, 345
Clostridium difficile, 1:43
Clostridium perfingens, 1:337, 343
Clothianidin, 1:188
CML (Chronic myelogenous leukemia). *See* Leukemia
CML (Chronic myeloid leukemia). *See* Leukemia
CMML (Chronic myelomonocytic leukemia). *See* Leukemia
Coal, 1:4, 21, 22, 108–110, 2:705
Coal gas. *See* Carbon monoxide
Coal miners and mining, 1:108–109, 149, 181, 290, 442–443, 2:801
Coal Workers' Health Surveillance Program, 1:109
Coal worker's pneumoconiosis. *See* Black lung disease
Coastal areas
   algal bloom, 1:25, *26*
   Exxon Valdez, 1:297–298, *299*
   Federal Water Act, 1:306, 307
   Gulf oil spill, 1:368–376
   Japanese earthquake, 1:449, *450*, *450*, 453
   Sierra Club, 2:693
   water pollution, 2:801
Cobalt, 1:404, 406
Cobalt-60, 2:636
Cockroaches, 1:56, 61
Code of Federal Regualtions (CFR), 1:395–396
Codes, building. *See* Government regulation
Coffee, 1:60
Cognitive-behavioral therapy. *See* Psychotherapy
Cohort Study of Mobile Phone Use and Health (COSMOS), 2:577
Coliforms, 2:718
Colitis, 1:30, 31, 237, 238, 240
Collier, R. John, 1:39
Colon, 1:30, 31, 32, 134, 237
Colony collapse disorder, **1:185–189**
Color Additives Amendment, 1:320
Colorado, 1:174, 175, 484
Colorado River, 1:*209*, 211
Colors, artificial. *See* Artificial colors
Columbia University, 1:412
Combustion, 1:21, 22, 81, 82, 404, 438

Communicable Disease Center, 1:143–144
Communicable diseases, 1:**189–191**, *190*
   as endemic, 1:271–272
   global public health on, 1:361–362
   from Haiti earthquake, 1:387
   in population and disease, 2:618
   Public Health Service on, 2:630
   See also specific diseases by name
Communication, 1:63–64, 65, 140, 260, 451
Community action
   on brownfield sites, 1:113, 114–115
   Chernobyl nuclear power station disaster, 1:159
   Comprehensive Environmental Response, Compensation, and Liability Act, 1:192
   in disaster preparedness, 1:224
   on drought, 1:235
   Emergency Planning and Community Right-to-Know Act, 1:257–259
   for guinea worm disease, 1:367–368
   Healthy Cities, 1:396–397
   housing, 1:421–422
   Oxfam on, 2:595
Compassion fatigue. *See* Post-traumatic stress disorder
Compensation, legal. *See* Settlements and damages
Complementary and alternative medicine (CAM)
   for AIDS, 1:18
   for asthma, 1:59–60
   for autism, 1:65–66
   for avian flu, 1:70
   for bronchitis, 1:112
   for chemical poisoning, 1:152–153
   for dysentery, 1:239
   for guinea worm disease, 1:367
   for Gulf War syndrome, 1:379
   for H1N1 influenza A, 1:384–385
   for heavy metal poisoning, 1:407
   heavy metal poisoning from, 1:406, 409
   lead poisoning from, 1:464
   for Lyme disease, 1:497–498
   for malaria, 2:504
   for measles, 2:509
   for melanoma, 2:519
   for mercury poisoning, 2:531
   for methemoglobinemia, 2:535
   for mumps, 2:545
   for noroviruses, 2:582
   for parasites, 2:605–606
   for post-traumatic stress disorder, 2:625
   for radiation injuries, 2:645
   for smoking cessation, 2:711–713
Compliance, government. *See* Government regulation

Compounding pharmacies. *See* Pharmacies
Comprehensive Environmental Response, Compensation, and Liability Act (CERCLA), 1:**191–193**
 Agency for Toxic Substances and Disease Registry, 1:4–5
 Environmental Protection Agency, 1:278–279
 Love Canal, 1:491–492
 Resource Conservation and Recovery Act, 2:652
 Sierra Club, 2:693
 Superfund Amendments and Reauthorization Act, 2:717–718
Computational molecular biology. *See* Bioinformatics
Computed tomography (CT) scans. *See* Diagnostic testing; Radiation
Computerized axial tomography (CAT) scans. *See* Diagnostic testing; Radiation
Computerized axial tomography (CT) scans. *See* Diagnostic testing; Radiation
Concern (organization), 1:390
Condoms, 1:11, 19, 428
Condylox. *See* Podofilox
Conjugation, 1:42
Conservation
 brucellosis, 1:118
 drought, 1:235
 land use, 1:461
 national parks, 2:559
 Rachel Carson Council, 2:631
 Resource Conservation and Recovery Act, 2:650–652
 Sierra Club, 2:692–693
 Soil Conservation Act, 2:714
Conservationism. *See* Activism
Consumer Product Safety Commission (CPSC), 1:138, 466
Consumer Product Safety Control Act, 1:462
Consumer protection, 1:324
Consumption. *See* Tuberculosis
Contact dermatitis, 2:607–609
Contagious diseases. *See* Communicable diseases
Containment, 1:368, 369, 370, 371, 376
Contamination of drinking water. *See* Drinking water supply
Contamination of drugs. *See* Food contamination
Contamination of food. *See* Food contamination
Contamination of waterways. *See* Water pollution
Continental shelves, 2:751
Contraception, 1:144, 161, 425
 See also Family planning
Control, disease. *See* Disease control

Convention on the Rights of the Child, 2:771–772
Cooke, W. E., 1:46
Cooking, 1:338–339, 485, 487, 2:835
Cooling, 1:338
COPD (Chronic obstructive pulmonary disease). *See* Emphysema
Copper, 1:6, 404, 406, 407, 2:668, 804
Cor pulmonale, 1:109
Cordyceps, 1:384
Corexit, 1:298
Coriolis effect, 1:431
Corn, 1:7, 355
Coronary artery disease. *See* Cardiovascular disease
Coronaviruses, 2:679, 681
Corporate responsibility
 Bhopal, India, 1:86, 88, 89
 Comprehensive Environmental Response, Compensation, and Liability Act, 1:192
 Earth Day, 1:244
 Emergency Planning and Community Right-to-Know Act, 1:258–259
 Exxon Valdez, 1:295–300
 Gulf oil spill, 1:368–376
 hazardous waste, 1:396
 Hurricane Katrina, 1:458
 Japanese earthquake, 1:452
 Love Canal, 1:488, 489, 491
 mercury poisoning, 2:531
 Oxfam, 2:596
 Seveso, Italy accident, 2:684
Corpses, 1:169, 451
Corrosivity, 1:395
Corticosteroids
 for aspergillosis, 1:52, 53
 for asthma, 1:58, 59
 for berylliosis, 1:84, 85
 for byssinosis, 1:122
 for fibrosis, 1:309
 HPV vaccination and, 1:424
 for leukemia, 1:479
 for meningitis, 2:523–524
 for mold allergy, 2:538
Cortisol, 2:560
Corynebacterium diphtheriae, 1:218
Cosmetics, 1:464, 2:529
Cosmic rays, 1:73–74
COSMOS (Cohort Study of Mobile Phone Use and Health), 2:577
Costa Concordia (ship), 1:198–199
Costs, health care. *See* Health care costs
Costs, social. *See* Social costs
Cotton, 1:120–121, 122
Coughing, paroxysmal. *See* Whooping cough
Council on Environmental Quality (CEQ), 2:552, 553, 554, 733

Counting Technique, 2:626
Cowpox, 2:702, 704, 777
Cows. *See* Livestock
CPSC (Consumer Product Safety Commission), 1:138, 466
Creutzfeldt-Jakob disease, 1:**193–198,** *194, 195*
 causes, 1:195–196
 chronic wasting disease and, 1:174
 demographics, 1:195
 diagnosis, 1:196–197
 in One Health Initiative, 2:593
 prevention, 1:197
 public health, 1:197
 symptoms, 1:196
 treatment, 1:197
 as virus, 2:790
 as zoonosis, 2:835
Crimean-Congo hemorrhagic fever. *See* Hemorrhagic fevers
Critical Mass Energy Project, 1:278
Cromolyn, 1:58
Crop rotation, 2:714
Cross-State Air Pollution Rule, 1:279
Cross-State Air Pollution Rule (CSAPR), 2:708
Crude oil
 in exposure science, 1:293–294
 from fracking, 1:346, 347, 348
 in Yokkaichi asthma, 2:829, 830
 See also Oil spills, health effects of
Cruise ship health, 1:**198–202**
 dysentery, 1:237
 food poisoning, 1:332
 food safety, 1:337
 foodborne illness, 1:341
 noroviruses, 2:579–580
Cryogenics, 1:493
Cryonics, 1:493
Cryosurgery, 2:698
Cryotherapy, 1:427
Cryptococcal meningitis. *See* Meningitis
Cryptococcus gattii, 1:265, 266
Cryptosporidiosis, 1:**202–204**
 as dysentery, 1:237, 238, 240
 in One Health Initiative, 2:592
 sanitation in, 2:670
 water quality in, 2:804
 as waterborne illness, 2:809, 810
Cryptosporidium
 in cryptosporidiosis, 1:202, 203
 food contamination from, 1:326
 food poisoning from, 1:332
 as parasite, 2:604
 in traveler's health, 2:740
 waterborne illness from, 2:809
CSAPR (Cross-State Air Pollution Rule), 2:708
CT (Computed tomography) scans. *See* Diagnostic testing; Radiation
Cullen, Mark R., 2:541

Cultures (medical tests). *See* Diagnostic testing
Cuprimine. *See* Penicillamine
Curettage, 2:698
Curie, Marie, 2:641
Curie, Pierre, 2:641
Cutaneous anthrax. *See* Anthrax
Cutaneous diphtheria. *See* Diphtheria
Cutting oil exposure, 1:**204–206**
Cyanobacteria, 1:25
Cyanosis, 1:**206–208,** 308, 2:534
Cyclones. *See* Tornado and cyclone
Cyclosarin, 1:377
Cyclospora, 1:200, 326, 2:740
Cyprus fever. *See* Brucellosis
Cysticercosis, 2:603, 604, 745
Cysts, 1:*358,* 359
Cytarabine, 1:478
Cytogenetic analysis, 1:477
Cytotoxics, 1:424

D

Dacarbazine (DTIC), 2:519
Daichi Petrochemical Complex, 2:830
Dairy products
 brucellosis from, 1:116–117, 119
 Chernobyl nuclear power station disaster on, 1:158, 159
 escherichia coli in, 1:287
 food poisoning from, 1:330, 333
 foodborne illness from, 1:343
 listeriosis from, 1:484, 487
Dallas, Texas, 2:786
Damages, legal. *See* Settlements and damages
Dampness. *See* Humidity
Dams, 1:*209,* **209–212,** *210, 211*
 drought from, 1:232
 flooding and, 1:311, 312
 Omnibus Flood Control Act, 2:591
 Rivers and Harbors Act of 1899, 2:659
 See also Hydroelectricity
Dander, animal. *See* Animal dander
Danish Cohort Study, 1:141
Danube River, 2:731–732
Dark Winter, 2:705
Databases
 on anthrax, 1:41
 for bioinformatics, 1:92
 on disease outbreaks, 1:228
 on insecticide poisoning, 1:445
 on Lyme disease, 1:498
 on mercury poisoning, 2:532
 on necrotizing fasciitis, 2:566
 on noroviruses, 2:581
DCS (Decompression sickness). *See* Decompression sickness

DDE (Dichlorodiphenyl-dichloroethylene), 1:274
DDT (Dichlorodiphenyltrichloroethane)
 for bedbug infestation, 1:75
 as endocrine disruptor, 1:274, 275
 for malaria, 2:504
 Rachel Carson Council on, 2:632
 for river blindness, 2:658
 for typhus, 2:765
 for vector (mosquito) control, 2:784
Dechlorination, 1:163
Decibels, 2:572
Decompression sickness, 1:**212–214**
Decongestants, 2:538
Decontamination, environmental. *See* Environmental cleanup
Deepwater Horizon Joint Investigation, 1:372
Deepwater Horizon oil spill. *See* Gulf oil spill
Deer. *See* Wildlife
Deer mice. *See* Rodents
DEET (N,N-diethyl-m-toluamide), 2:785
Deflagration, 1:288
Deforestation. *See* Forests
Dehydration and rehydration
 altitude sickness, 1:29
 cadmium poisoning, 1:128
 child survival revolution, 1:161
 cholera, 1:166, 167–168, 169
 cruise ship health, 1:200
 dysentery, 1:238, 239
 food contamination, 1:327, 329
 food poisoning, 1:333, 334
 foodborne illness, 1:343, 344
 heat disorders, 1:398, 399–400
 noroviruses, 2:582
 traveler's health, 2:741, 742
 UNICEF on, 2:771
 waterborne illness, 2:809
Delaney Clause, 1:320
Delhi, India, 2:670
Delongueville, Diane, 2:*753*
Dementia, 1:174, 193, 194, 196
 See also AIDS dementia complex (ADC)
Democratic Republic of Congo, 2:761
Dengue fever, 1:**214–218,** *215*
 disease outbreaks of, 1:227
 as emergent disease, 1:266
 as hemorrhagic fever, 1:410, 411
 as tropical disease, 2:745, 746, 748
 vector (mosquito) control for, 2:783–784, 785
Dengue hemorrhagic fever-dengue shock syndrome (DHF-DSS), 1:411, 412–412
Denisovans, 1:93
Dental caries. *See* Tooth decay

Dental professionals. *See* Medical personnel
Department of Agriculture (U.S.). *See* U.S. Department of Agriculture
Depen. *See* Penicillamine
Dependency syndrome, 1:159
Deposition, acid. *See* Acid rain
Depression (mental illness). *See* Mental health
Dermatitis, contact. *See* Contact dermatitis
DES (Diethylstilbestrol), 1:7, 274
Des Voeux, Henry Antoine, 2:705
Desalinization, 1:234
Desert fires. *See* Wildfires
Desertification, 1:234
Deserts, 1:*414,* 2:801
Detonation, 1:288
Detoxification diet, 1:152
Developing countries
 disasters
  Bhopal, India, 1:88, 89
  drought, 1:232
  famine, 1:301, 303–304
 diseases and disorders
  AIDS, 1:11
  amebiasis, 1:30, 31, 32
  anthrax, 1:38
  berylliosis, 1:85
  black lung disease, 1:109
  brucellosis, 1:117
  byssinosis, 1:120, 122
  cholera, 1:166, 168, 169
  chronic kidney disease, 1:170, 172–173
  communicable diseases, 1:190
  dengue fever, 1:215, 216, 217
  dysentery, 1:236
  emergent diseases, 1:267
  endemic disease, 1:272
  food poisoning, 1:330, 331
  foodborne illness, 1:341
  giardiasis, 1:357
  goiter, 1:365
  guinea worm disease, 1:366, 367–368
  H1N1 influenza A, 1:381, 385
  lead poisoning, 1:465
  leptospirosis, 1:473
  malaria, 2:501
  measles, 2:508, 509, 510
  meningitis, 2:521
  noroviruses, 2:578
  pandemic, 2:601
  protein-energy malnutrition, 2:627, 628, 629–630
  schistosomiasis, 2:676
  shigellosis, 2:685
  tropical disease, 2:744–745
  tuberculosis, 2:754, 759
  typhoid fever, 2:762
  typhus, 2:767
 health issues and threats

Developing countries *(continued)*
    air pollution, 1:22
    antimicrobial resistance, 1:44
    bedbug infestation, 1:75
    child survival revolution, 1:160–161
    cruise ship health, 1:198
    drinking water supply, 1:228, 230
    food contamination, 1:326
    food safety, 1:337
    global public health, 1:361–363
    Healthy Cities, 1:397
    parasites, 2:602
    population pyramid, 2:619
    sanitation, 2:670–671
    traveler's health, 2:739
    water pollution, 2:800
    zero population growth, 2:832
  Oxfam, 2:594–597
Developmental disorders. *See specific disorders by name*
Devices, medical. *See* Medical devices
DHF-DSS (Dengue hemorrhagic fever-dengue shock syndrome), 1:412–412
Diabetes, 1:15, 170
Diagnostic and Statistical Manual of Mental Disorders, 1:62
Diagnostic testing
    AIDS, 1:12, 13, 19
    amebiasis, 1:31–32
    asbestosis, 1:49
    aspergillosis, 1:52–53
    asthma, 1:57
    autism, 1:64
    avian flu, 1:69
    berylliosis, 1:84, 85
    bioinformatics for, 1:91
    black lung disease, 1:109
    bronchitis, 1:111–112
    brucellosis, 1:117
    byssinosis, 1:121–122
    campylobacteriosis, 1:128
    cancer, 1:132–133, 134
    carbon monoxide poisoning, 1:137
    chemical poisoning, 1:151
    cholera, 1:167
    chronic kidney disease, 1:171
    chronic wasting disease, 1:175
    Creutzfeldt-Jakob disease, 1:196–197
    cryptosporidiosis, 1:203
    dengue fever, 1:216–217
    dysentery, 1:237
    ebola hemorrhagic fever, 1:251
    electric shock injuries, 1:254
    emphysema, 1:270
    escherichia coli infections, 1:285–286
    fibrosis, 1:309
    food poisoning, 1:333
    foodborne illness, 1:344
    giardiasis, 1:359
    goiter, 1:365
    H1N1 influenza A, 1:383–384
    hantavirus infections, 1:393
    heat disorders, 1:399
    heavy metal poisoning, 1:407–408
    hemorrhagic fevers, 1:412
    human papilloma virus, 1:426–427
    indoor air quality, 1:439
    insecticide poisoning, 1:445
    ionizing radiation in, 1:447
    lead poisoning, 1:465
    Legionnaires' disease, 1:468–469
    leptospirosis, 1:472
    leukemia, 1:476–478, 477
    listeriosis, 1:486–487
    Lyme disease, 1:496–497
    malaria, 2:503
    measles, 2:509
    melanoma, 2:516–517
    meningitis, 2:522–523
    mercury poisoning, 2:530–531
    multiple chemical sensitivity, 2:542
    mumps, 2:544–545
    noroviruses, 2:581–582
    parasite infections, 2:605
    patch testing, 2:607–609
    plague, 2:611–612
    polio, 2:615
    post-traumatic stress disorder, 2:623–624
    protein-energy malnutrition, 2:629
    radiation exposure, 2:638, 640
    radiation in, 2:633, 634–635
    radiation injuries, 2:642–643, 645
    river blindness, 2:656–657
    rodent-borne diseases, 2:662
    schistosomiasis, 2:677
    severe acute respiratory syndrome, 2:681
    shigellosis, 2:686
    silicosis, 2:695
    skin cancer, 2:697
    sleeping sickness, 2:700
    smallpox, 2:702
    sulfur exposure, 2:716
    traveler's health, 2:741
    tuberculosis, 2:754, 757–758
    typhoid fever, 2:763
    typhus, 2:766
    viruses, 2:791
    waterborne illness, 2:809
    West Nile virus, 2:814
    whooping cough, 2:817
    yellow fever, 2:827
    zoonoses, 2:834–835
Dialysis, kidney. *See* Kidney dialysis
Dianin, Alexander P., 1:104
Diarrhea
    AIDS, 1:15
    amebiasis, 1:31
    antimicrobial resistance and, 1:43
    campylobacteriosis, 1:128
    cholera, 1:166, 167
    cryptosporidiosis, 1:202
    dysentery, 1:237
    from *escherichia coli,* 1:284–285
    food poisoning, 1:331, 332, 333, 334
    giardiasis, 1:357, 360
    listeriosis, 1:485
    sanitation on, 2:671
    shigellosis, 2:684, 685, 686
    water quality on, 2:804
Diarrhea, traveler's. *See* Dysentery; Shigellosis; Traveler's health
Dichlorodiphenyldichloroethylene (DDE), 1:274
Dichlorodiphenyltrichloroethane (DDT). *See* DDT (Dichlorodiphenyltrichloroethane)
Diesel fuel, 1:348
Diet and nutrition
    for AIDS, 1:15, 16, 17
    in altitude sickness, 1:29
    for asthma, 1:59–60
    for autism, 1:65–66
    in cancer, 1:131
    for chemical poisoning, 1:152
    in chronic kidney disease, 1:171
    in colony collapse disorder, 1:188, 189
    for dysentery, 1:239
    in global public health, 1:362–363
    in goiter, 1:364, 365
    housing and, 1:421
    in lead poisoning, 1:466
    in manganese exposure, 2:505, 506, 507
    for measles, 2:509
    in mercury poisoning, 2:532–533
    for mumps, 2:545
    for parasites, 2:606
    for protein-energy malnutrition, 2:627–630
    for radiation injuries, 2:645
    smoking and, 2:710
Diethylstilbestrol (DES), 1:7, 274
Diethyltoluamide, 1:77
Dietitians, 1:15
Digoxin, 1:152
Digoxin immune fab, 1:152
Dike. *See* Levee
Dimercaprol, 1:465
Dimercaptosuccinic acid (DMSA), 1:126, 152
Dimethylbenzene. *See* Xylene
Dimethylglycine (DMG), 1:65
Dingell, John, 1:177
Dioscorides, 2:735
Dioxin
    in air pollution, 1:22
    in chemical poisoning, 1:148
    as endocrine disruptor, 1:274, 275
    from Seveso, Italy accident, 2:682, 683
    in Times Beach, 2:729–730
Diphtheria, 1:**218–221**
Disabled persons, 2:773–774

Disaster preparedness, 1:**221–226**
  aftercare, 1:224
  anthrax, 1:40–41
  bioterrorism, 1:101–102, 103
  Chernobyl nuclear power station disaster, 1:156–157, 159
  climate change, 1:184–185
  community preparedness, 1:224
  description, 1:221–224
  flooding, 1:312
  Fukushima Daiichi nuclear power station disaster, 1:350
  Haiti earthquake, 1:387, 388–389
  Hurricane Katrina, 1:455, 457, 458
  Japanese earthquake, 1:451–453
  National Institute for Occupational Safety and Health, 2:555
  public health, 1:225
  Red Cross, 2:646–649
  results, 1:224–225
  Seveso, Italy accident, 2:683–684
  tsunamis, 2:750–751
  volcanic eruptions, 2:795, 796
  See also Emergency preparedness

Disaster relief. *See* Humanitarian aid

Disasters. *See* Disaster preparedness; *specific disasters by name*

Discharged effluents. *See* Water pollution

Disease and population. *See* Population and disease

Disease control
  in child survival revolution, 1:160–161
  in disasters
    bioterrorism, 1:101–102, 103
    Haiti earthquake, 1:388, 390–391
    Japanese earthquake, 1:452
    oil spills, 2:589–590
  by disease or disorder
    anthrax, 1:38, 40–41
    avian flu, 1:68, 70
    bronchitis, 1:112
    brucellosis, 1:116, 117, 118, 119
    campylobacteriosis, 1:129
    cholera, 1:168
    chronic wasting disease, 1:175
    communicable diseases, 1:190
    Creutzfeldt-Jakob disease, 1:197
    cruise ship health, 1:198, 200–201, 201
    cryptosporidiosis, 1:203
    diphtheria, 1:220–221
    dysentery, 1:239, 241
    escherichia coli infections, 1:286, 287
    fibrosis, 1:309
    flu pandemic, 1:316–317
    food poisoning, 1:334
    foodborne illness, 1:345
    fungal infections, 1:354
    giardiasis, 1:359, 360
    guinea worm disease, 1:366, 367–368
    H1N1 influenza A, 1:384, 385
    hantavirus infections, 1:394
    hemorrhagic fevers, 1:413
    human papilloma virus, 1:427–428
    lead poisoning, 1:466–467
    Legionnaires' disease, 1:469, 470
    leptospirosis, 1:473
    leukemia, 1:481
    listeriosis, 1:487
    Lyme disease, 1:498–499
    malaria, 2:504–505
    manganese exposure, 2:507
    measles, 2:510
    melanoma, 2:520
    meningitis, 2:524
    mercury poisoning, 2:532–533
    methemoglobinemia, 2:535
    mold exposure, 2:540
    multiple chemical sensitivity, 2:543
    necrotizing fasciitis, 2:565–566
    noroviruses, 2:583
    for parasitic infections, 2:606–607
    plague, 2:612–613
    polio, 2:616–617
    post-traumatic stress disorder, 2:626
    radiation exposure, 2:640
    river blindness, 2:657, 658
    schistosomiasis, 2:678
    severe acute respiratory syndrome, 2:680–682
    shigellosis, 2:687–688
    skin cancer, 2:698
    sleeping sickness, 2:700
    smallpox, 2:703–704
    talcosis, 2:722–723
    traveler's health, 2:743
    tropical disease, 2:747–748
    tuberculosis, 2:752–753, 758, 759–760
    typhoid fever, 2:763–764
    typhus, 2:767
    viruses, 2:792
    waterborne illness, 2:811
    West Nile virus, 2:815
    whooping cough, 2:818
    zoonoses, 2:835
  in disease outbreaks, 1:227–228
  for drinking water supply, 1:228–231, 230
  for food contamination, 1:327–329, 327t
  in food safety, 1:338–340
  in housing, 1:422
  for medical waste, 2:511, 513–514
  methods
    chlorination, 1:162–164
    sanitation, 2:672–673
    ultraviolet radiation, 2:769
    vaccination, 2:777–782
    vector (mosquito) control, 2:783–787
  organizational support for Centers for Disease Control and Prevention, 1:144–146
  Oxfam, 2:595
  UNICEF, 2:771

Disease ecology, 2:617

Disease gaol. *See* Typhus

Disease outbreaks, 1:**226–228**, 2:546
  causes, 1:100–103
    climate change, 1:184
    drinking water supply, 1:229
    drought, 1:232, 233
    escherichia coli, 1:284
    flooding, 1:311–312
    food contamination, 1:325–326
    food safety, 1:336, 337, 339
    Haiti earthquake, 1:387–388, 390
    Horn of Africa drought and famine, 1:418
    housing, 1:420–421
    Japanese earthquake, 1:452
    medical waste, 2:512
    parasites, 2:602–603
    population and disease, 2:617–619
    sanitation, 2:669–670
  by disease
    anthrax, 1:38, 40–41
    bronchitis, 1:111
    cholera, 1:166, 168
    communicable diseases, 1:190
    cruise ship health, 1:198, 199–201
    cryptosporidiosis, 1:202
    dengue fever, 1:216, 217
    diphtheria, 1:218
    ebola hemorrhagic virus, 1:248, 251
    emergent diseases, 1:264
    food poisoning, 1:330–331, 334
    foodborne illness, 1:341, 342, 343
    giardiasis, 1:357, 359–360
    H1N1 influenza A, 1:381, 382, 383
    hemorrhagic fevers, 1:410, 413
    Legionnaires' disease, 1:467, 468
    leptospirosis, 1:473
    leukemia, 1:480–481
    listeriosis, 1:484
    malaria, 2:501
    measles, 2:508
    meningitis, 2:523
    mumps, 2:544
    necrotizing fasciitis, 2:566
    noroviruses, 2:577, *578*, 579–580, 581–582
    plague, 2:611
    polio, 2:613
    shigellosis, 2:685
    smallpox, 2:701
    tropical disease, 2:745

Disease outbreaks *(continued)*
    tuberculosis, 2:754
    typhoid fever, 2:761, 762
    typhus, 2:765, 766, 767
    West Nile virus, 2:812–813, 815
    whooping cough, 2:816
    zoonoses, 2:833–834
  organizational support for
    Centers for Disease Control and Prevention on, 1:144–146
    UNICEF, 2:775
    World Health Organization, 2:823
  pandemic *vs.*, 2:601–602
  See also Flu pandemic

Disease prevention. *See* Disease control

Disease reservoirs, 1:410, 411

Disease transmission
  causes
    antimicrobial resistance, 1:42, 44
    bioterrorism, 1:101–102
    cruise ship health, 1:198, 200
    flooding, 1:311
    flu pandemic, 1:314, 315
    food contamination, 1:324–326
    food safety, 1:336, 337
    Japanese earthquake, 1:451
    medical waste, 2:511, 512–513
    parasites, 2:603, 604–605
    population and disease, 2:617–619
    rodents, 2:662–663
    sanitation, 2:669–673
    water quality, 2:803
  by disease
    AIDS, 1:8, 9–10, 11, 19
    amebiasis, 1:31, 32
    anthrax, 1:37, 38, 39
    avian flu, 1:67, 68–69
    brucellosis, 1:115, 116–117, 118
    cholera, 1:166, 169
    chronic wasting disease, 1:174–175
    communicable diseases, 1:189–191
    Creutzfeldt-Jakob disease, 1:193–196
    cryptosporidiosis, 1:202, 203
    dengue fever, 1:215, 216, 217
    diphtheria, 1:218
    dysentery, 1:236
    ebola hemorrhagic virus, 1:248, 251
    emergent diseases, 1:264–267
    endemic diseases, 1:272
    escherichia coli infections, 1:284, 285
    food poisoning, 1:330, 331, 332, 334
    foodborne illness, 1:341
    fungal infections, 1:352, 354
    giardiasis, 1:357, *358*, 359
    guinea worm disease, 1:366–367
    H1N1 influenza A, 1:382
    hantavirus infections, 1:391, *392*
    hemorrhagic fevers, 1:410, 411
    human papilloma virus, 1:425, 426
    Legionnaires' disease, 1:467–468, 468
    leptospirosis, 1:470–471
    listeriosis, 1:484, 485, 487
    Lyme disease, 1:494, 495
    malaria, 2:501–502
    measles, 2:508
    meningitis, 2:521–522, 523
    mumps, 2:543–544
    noroviruses, 2:577, 578–579, 583
    plague, 2:611
    polio, 2:614–615
    river blindness, 2:655–656
    schistosomiasis, 2:676, 678
    severe acute respiratory syndrome, 2:679–682
    shigellosis, 2:685, 686
    sleeping sickness, 2:699
    smallpox, 2:702
    tropical disease, 2:744, 745–746
    tuberculosis, 2:752, 755–756
    typhoid fever, 2:761, 762, 763
    viruses, 2:789–790
    waterborne illness, 2:807–809
    yellow fever, 2:825, 826
    zoonoses, 2:832–833, 834
  in epidemiology, 1:279–281
  Public Health Service on, 2:630

Diseases. *See specific diseases by name*

Disinfection. *See* Disease control

Dispersants, 1:371–372, 2:589

Displaced people. *See* Population displacement

Disseminated histoplasmosis, 1:353

Disseminated intravascular coagulation, 1:216

Dissociation, 2:621

Diuretics, 1:399

Divers Alert Network, 1:213, 214

Diving, 1:212–214

Djibouti, 1:415

DMG (Dimethylglycine), 1:65

DMSA (Dimercaptosuccinic acid), 1:126, 152

DNA
  anthrax, 1:39
  bioinformatics, 1:89–93
  cancer, 1:131
  cellular phones, 1:140, 141
  Creutzfeldt-Jakob disease, 1:195–196
  radiation injuries on, 2:641
  uses, 2:788, 789
  See also Mutation

DND (N,N- Diethyl-p-phenylenediamine), 1:163

Dobrava virus, 1:412

Doctors. *See* Medical personnel

Doctors Without Borders, 1:407, 430

Dogs, domestic. *See* Domestic animals

Doll, Richard, 1:280

Dolphins, 1:372

Domestic animals
  asthma from, 1:55, 56, 61
  brucellosis from, 1:116, 119
  food poisoning in, 1:335
  fungal infections from, 1:353
  hemorrhagic fevers from, 1:411
  indoor air quality and, 1:440
  leptospirosis from, 1:470–471, 473
  mercury poisoning in, 2:531
  in One Health Initiative, 2:592
  parasites in, 2:607
  plague from, 2:611, 612
  Rachel Carson Council on, 2:632
  West Nile virus in, 2:813
  zoonoses from, 2:834, 835

Domoic acid, 1:326

Donovan v. A.A. Beiro (1984), 2:586

Down syndrome, 1:475, 481

Doxycycline, 1:43, 118, 119, 168, 497, 2:657

Dracunculiasis. *See* Guinea worm disease

Drills, emergency. *See* Emergency preparedness

Drinking water illness. *See* Waterborne illness

Drinking Water State Revolving Fund, 2:668

Drinking water supply, 1:**228–232**
  conditions
    algal bloom, 1:26
    antimicrobial resistance, 1:44
    chlorination, 1:162–164
    climate change, 1:184
    disease outbreaks, 1:226, 227
    drought, 1:233, 234, 235
    flooding, 1:311, 312
    fluoridation, 2:797–799
    food contamination, 1:324, 325
    fracking, 1:346–347, 346–348, *347,* 348
    housing, 1:421
    sanitation, 2:672
    volcanic eruptions, 2:796
    water pollution, 2:800, 802
    water quality, 2:802–805
    water quality standards, 2:805–807
  contaminants
    agricultural chemicals, 1:7
    asbestos, 1:47
    biotoxins, 1:103, 104
    escherichia coli, 1:284
    lead, 1:462
    mercury, 2:526
    parasites, 2:604

Drinking water supply *(continued)*
disasters
Bhopal, India, 1:88
bioterrorism, 1:103
Camp Lejeune, 1:229
Haiti earthquake, 1:387, 389
Horn of Africa drought and famine, 1:417, 418
Japanese earthquake, 1:451, 452
diseases and disorders
amebiasis, 1:32, 33
asbestosis, 1:50
chlorine exposure, 1:164, 165
cholera, 1:166, 168, 169
communicable diseases, 1:189
cryptosporidiosis, 1:202
cyanosis, 1:207, 208
dysentery, 1:236, 240, 241
food poisoning, 1:330, 331, 332
giardiasis, 1:357, 359, 360
guinea worm disease, 1:366–367, 368
lead poisoning, 1:464, 466, 467
leptospirosis in, 1:473
manganese exposure, 2:505, 506, 507
methemoglobinemia, 2:535
traveler's health, 2:739, 743
typhoid fever, 2:761
waterborne illness, 2:807–808
zoonoses, 2:833
in exposure science, 1:295
organizational support
Centers for Disease Control and Prevention, 1:144
Environmental Protection Agency, 1:276
Oxfam, 2:594, 595, 596
Safe Drinking Water Act, 2:667–668
Drought, 1:**232–235**, *233, 234*
from climate change, 1:183, 184, 185
famine and, 1:302
Drug abuse. *See* Drug use
Drug contamination. *See* Food contamination
Drug interactions, 1:17–18, 424, 469, 479, 2:737
Drug overdoses. *See* Drug use
Drug resistance. *See* Antimicrobial resistance
Drug side effects, 1:58, 59, 398, 399
Drug use
AIDS from, 1:8, 10, 11, 13, 19
chemical poisoning from, 1:151, 152
post-traumatic stress disorder and, 2:621, 623, 624
talcosis from, 2:721, 722, 723
toxicology and, 2:736
tuberculosis and, 2:754
Drugs (medications)
antimicrobial resistance, 1:42
Food and Drug Administration, 1:322–324

Japanese earthquake, 1:452
medical waste, 2:513
National Institute of Environmental Health Sciences, 2:557
Oxfam on, 2:595, 596
toxicology of, 2:737
See also specific drugs by name or class
Drugs, off-label use of. *See* Off-label drug use
DTIC (Dacarbazine), 2:519
Ducks. *See* Birds
Dufour, Guillaume Henri, 2:648
Duluth, MN, 1:47
Dumping, 1:47, 488–489, 2:801, 804
Dunant, Henry, 2:648, 649
Duncan, Kirsty, 1:314
Dust
byssinosis from, 1:120–121, 122
emphysema, 1:269
exposure science, 1:293
lead poisoning, 1:464
mold exposure, 2:538
parasites in, 2:603
Dust mites, 1:54, 55, 56, 61, 440
Dust storms, 2:714
Dynamite, 1:288
Dysentery, 1:**235–241**
amebiasis as, 1:30, 31
causes, 1:236–237
demographics, 1:236
description, 1:235–236
diagnosis, 1:238
escherichia coli in, 1:284
prevention, 1:240–241
prognosis, 1:240
public health, 1:239–240
risk factors, 1:236
sanitation in, 2:670
as shigellosis, 2:685, 686
symptoms, 1:237
in traveler's health, 2:739
treatment, 1:238–239
Dysplastic nevus syndrome, 2:516
Dyspnea, 1:121

E

E. coli. *See* Escherichia coli
Eagles. *See* Birds
Earth Day, 1:**243–245**, *244*
Earthquakes, 1:**245–248**, *246*
disaster preparedness for, 1:225
Fukushima Daiichi nuclear power station disaster, 1:349, 350
tsunamis from, 2:750–751
See also Haiti earthquake; Japanese earthquake (2011); Tsunamis
Earth's temperature. *See* Climate change

East Indian medicine. *See* Complementary and alternative medicine (CAM)
Ebola hemorrhagic fever, 1:103, **248–252**, *249t–250t*, 264–265, 267, 410, 412
EBV (Epstein-Barr virus), 1:425
Echinacea, 1:384, 497, 2:545
Economic impact
after 9/11 terrorist attacks, 2:570
brownfield sites, 1:115
Chernobyl nuclear power station disaster, 1:232, 233
drought, 1:159
famine, 1:301, 302–303, 304
global public health, 1:362
Gulf oil spill, 1:369, 370
Hurricane Katrina, 1:458
Iceland volcano eruption, 1:436
One Health Initiative, 2:592
population and disease, 2:618
severe acute respiratory syndrome, 2:680
Ecosystems, aquatic. *See* Aquatic ecosystems
Ecotherapy, 2:562
Ectoparasites. *See* Parasites
Edema, 2:518
Edetate calcium disodium (EDTA calcium), 1:465
Edison, Thomas Alva, 1:252
EDTA (Ethylenediamine tetraacetic acid), 1:126, 152
EDTA calcium (Edetate calcium disodium), 1:465
Education
in autism, 1:65
from Chartered Institute of Environmental Health, 1:144–145
on endemic disease, 1:272
in global public health, 1:362
on guinea worm disease, 1:367
Oxfam on, 2:595, 596
Save the Children on, 2:675
on smoking, 2:710
UNICEF on, 2:774
Edwards Dam, 1:*211*
Efficiency, 2:573–574
Effluents. *See* Water pollution
Eflornithine, 2:700
eGFR (Estimated glomerular filtration rate), 1:171
Eggs, 2:546
Egypt, 1:31
Ehrlich, Paul R., 2:832
EIS (Environmental impact statements), 2:553–554
El Salvador, 1:172
Elderly people. *See* Older people
Electric power plants
acid rain from, 1:2, 4

Electric power plants *(continued)*
  air pollution from, 1:24
  background radiation from, 1:73
  cadmium poisoning from, 1:126–127
  chlorination and, 1:162
  Clean Air Act on, 1:178
  Safe Drinking Water Act on, 2:667
  smog, 2:708
Electric shock injuries, 1:**252–257**
  causes, 1:253
  demographics, 1:253
  description, 1:252–253
  diagnosis, 1:254
  from flooding, 1:311
  prevention, 1:255–256
  prognosis, 1:255
  public health, 1:255
  symptoms, 1:253–254
  treatment, 1:254
Electric utilities. *See* Electric power plants
Electricity, water-generated. *See* Hydroelectricity
Electroconvulsive therapy, 1:252
Electrocution. *See* Electric shock injuries
Electrodessication, 2:698
Electrodialysis, 1:208
Electrolytes. *See* Dehydration and rehydration
Electromagnetic fields. *See* Cellular phones; Ionizing radiation; Non-ionizing radiation; Radiation; Radiation exposure; Radiation injuries; Radiofrequency energy
Electromagnetic radiation, ionizing. *See* Ionizing radiation
Electromagnetic radiation, medical. *See* Radiation
Electromagnetic radiation, non-ionizing. *See* Non-ionizing radiation
Electromagnetic waves, 1:446
Electronic media, 2:560, 561, 562, 563
Electronics industry, 1:24, 437
Elemental mercury. *See* Mercury
Elements, chemical. *See specific elements by name*
Elephantiasis, 2:746
ELISA (Enzyme-linked immunosorbent assays). *See* Diagnostic testing
Elk. *See* Wildlife
Ellenbog, Ulrich, 1:442
EM (Erythema migrans), 1:496
Emergencies, 1:259
Emergency Planning and Community Right-to-Know Act (1986), 1:**257–259**
Emergency preparedness, 1:**259–263**
  Chernobyl nuclear power station disaster, 1:156–157, 159
  disease outbreaks, 1:228
  drought, 1:234–235
  Emergency Planning and Community Right-to-Know Act, 1:257–259
  flu pandemic, 1:316
  Gulf oil spill, 1:376
  H1N1 influenza A, 1:384, 385
  Haiti earthquake, 1:387, 388–389, 391
  Horn of Africa drought and famine, 1:415, 418–419
  humanitarian aid, 1:429–430
  Japanese earthquake, 1:451–453
  National Institute for Occupational Safety and Health, 2:555
  National Institute of Environmental Health Sciences, 2:558
  9/11 terrorist attacks, 2:571
  pandemic, 2:602
  Seveso, Italy accident, 2:683–684
  Three Mile Island nuclear disaster, 2:727, 728–729
  volcanic eruptions, 2:795
  See also Disaster preparedness
Emergency relief. *See* Humanitarian aid
Emergent diseases (human), 1:**263–268**
  causes, 1:266
  demographics, 1:266
  hermorrhagic fevers, 1:410
  necrotizing fasciitis, 2:566
  population and disease, 2:619
  prevention, 1:267
  prognosis, 1:266–267
  public health, 1:266
  severe acute respiratory syndrome, 2:679
  symptoms, 1:266
  whooping cough, 2:816
  zoonoses, 2:833
Emissions. *See* Air pollution
Emotional Freedom Techniques, 2:626
Emphysema, 1:**268–271**
  black lung disease, 1:108, 109
  bronchitis, 1:110, 111, 112, 113
  Yokkaichi asthma, 2:830, 831
Encephalitis, 1:98, 2:509, 510, 544
  See also Western equine encephalitis
Encephalitis, West Nile. *See* West Nile virus
ENCODE (Encyclopedia of DNA Elements), 1:93
Encyclopedia of DNA Elements (ENCODE), 1:93
End stage renal disease. *See* Chronic kidney disease
Endangered Species Act, 1:245, 278
Endemic, 1:**271–273**
  amebiasis, 1:31, 32
  antimicrobial resistance, 1:43
  dengue fever, 1:215, 216
  emergent diseases, 1:264
  guinea worm disease, 1:366
  hemorrhagic fevers, 1:410
  malaria, 2:501, 502, 503
  plague, 2:610
  polio, 2:614
  river blindness, 2:657
  tropical disease, 2:744, 745, 746
  yellow fever, 2:825, 826
Endemic typhus. *See* Typhus
Enders, John F, 2:508
Endocarditis, 1:486, 487
Endocrine Disruptor Screening Program, 1:275
Endocrine disruptors, 1:**273–276**
Endoparasites. *See* Parasites
Endosomes, 2:789
Endotoxins, 1:120
Energy, alternative. *See* Alternative energy
Engines, 1:2
England, 1:420, 2:777
English Factory Acts, 1:443
Entamoeba dispar, 1:31, 32
Entamoeba histolytica
  ameobiasis, 1:30–33
  cruise ship health and, 1:200
  dysentery, 1:236, 237, 239, 240
  food contamination, 1:326
  as parasite, 2:604, 607
  traveler's health, 2:740
  waterborne illness, 2:809
Enterobacter, 1:200
Enterococcus faecalis, 1:43
Enterotoxins, 1:237, 285
Enteroviruses, 2:522
Entry inhibitors. *See* Fusion inhibitors
Environmental cleanup
  Agency for Toxic Substances and Disease Registry, 1:4–5
  brownfield sites, 1:113–115
  Chernobyl nuclear power station disaster, 1:155, 158–159
  Comprehensive Environmental Response, Compensation, and Liability Act, 1:191–193
  Environmental Protection Agency, 1:*277,* 278–279
  Exxon Valdez, 1:*297,* 297–299, *298*
  Fukushima Daiichi nuclear power station disaster, 1:351–352
  Gulf oil spill, 1:371–372, 374
  heavy metal poisoning, 1:407
  Japanese earthquake, 1:453–454
  lead poisoning, 1:466
  Love Canal, 1:490–491, 492
  oil spills, 2:587–590
  Seveso, Italy, 2:683
  Sierra Club, 2:693

Environmental cleanup *(continued)*
  Superfund Amendments and Reauthorization Act, 2:717–718
  Three Mile Island nuclear disaster, 2:727
  toxic sludge spill in Hungary, 2:732
  water pollution, 2:801

Environmental impact statements (EIS), 2:553–554

Environmental Protection Agency (EPA), 1:**276–279**, *277*
  on disasters and events
    Earth Day, 1:245
    Gulf oil spill, 1:371, 372, 373
    Love Canal, 1:490, 491
    9/11 terrorist attacks, 2:571
    oil spills, 2:590
    Three Mile Island nuclear disaster, 2:725
    Times Beach, 2:730
  on diseases and disorders
    ammonia exposure, 1:37
    asbestosis, 1:49–50
    berylliosis, 1:82
    carbon monoxide poisoning, 1:138
    colony collapse disorder, 1:188
    cyanosis, 1:208
    fibrosis, 1:309
    food poisoning, 1:334, 335
    heavy metal poisoning, 1:407
    insecticide poisoning, 1:444, 445
    lead poisoning, 1:466
    mercury poisoning, 2:532–533
    methemoglobinemia, 2:535
    ozone exposure, 2:600
    radiation exposure, 2:639
    sulfur exposure, 2:716
  on environmental conditions
    acid rain, 1:4
    bedbug infestation, 1:77
    brownfield sites, 1:113
    chlorination, 1:163
    drinking water supply, 1:229, 231
    food safety, 1:337
    fracking, 1:348
    indoor air quality, 1:437–438, 440
    noise pollution, 2:573, 574
    sick building syndrome, 2:689–690, 691
    smog, 2:708
    vector (mosquito) control, 2:785
    water pollution, 2:801
    water quality, 2:804
  on exposure science, 1:292
  on hazards
    biotoxins, 1:104
    cellular phones, 1:140
    endocrine disruptors, 1:275
    hazardous waste, 1:395–396
    lead, 1:462
    medical waste, 2:511, 512
    mercury, 2:526
    mold, 2:537
    neurotoxins, 2:568
    rodenticides, 2:664
  on legislation and regulation
    Clean Air Act, 1:176–177, 178
    Clean Water Act, 1:180, 181, 182
    Comprehensive Environmental Response, Compensation, and Liability Act, 1:192–193
    Emergency Planning and Community Right-to-Know Act, 1:257, 258
    Federal Insecticide, Fungicide and Rodenticide Act, 1:304–306
    Federal Water Act, 1:306, 307
    National Ambient Air Quality Standard, 2:549–551
    Resource Conservation and Recovery Act, 2:650–652
    Rivers and Harbors Act of 1899, 2:661
    Safe Drinking Water Act, 2:667–668
    Superfund Amendments and Reauthorization Act, 2:717–718
    Toxic Substances Control Act, 2:733–735
    water quality standards, 2:807
  on organizations
    Agency for Toxic Substances and Disease Registry, 1:4
    Rachel Carson Council, 2:631
    Sierra Club, 2:693

Environmental Working Group, 1:49

Environmentalism. *See* Activism

Enzyme-linked immunosorbent assays (ELISA). *See* Diagnostic testing

Enzymes, 1:481

Eosinophils. *See* Blood cells

EPA (Environmental Protection Agency). *See* Environmental Protection Agency (EPA)

EPA, Massachusetts v. (2007), 1:178

Ephedra, 1:60

Ephedrine, 1:60

Epidemic Intelligence Service, 1:280

Epidemic typhus. *See* Typhus

Epidemic yellow fever. *See* Yellow fever

Epidemics. *See* Disease outbreaks; Epidemiology

Epidemics, global. *See* Pandemic

Epidemiology, 1:**279–281**
  Centers for Disease Control and Prevention on, 1:143, 144
  of communicable diseases, 1:190
  of Creutzfeldt-Jakob disease, 1:195
  in exposure science, 1:291
  of flu pandemic, 1:313–317
  in global public health, 1:362
  of Lyme disease, 1:494
  of noroviruses, 2:581–582
  population and disease in, 2:617–619
  of severe acute respiratory syndrome, 2:679, 680
  in toxicology, 2:736

Epidemiology Program Office, 1:143

Epigenetic regulation, 1:91

Epinephrine, 2:70

Epithelium, 1:130

Epstein-Barr virus (EBV), 1:425

Equipment, protective. *See* Protective equipment

Ergonomics, 1:**281–283**

Eritrea, 1:415, 417

Erosion, 2:714

Erythema migrans (EM), 1:496

Erythrocytes. *See* Blood cells

Erythromycin, 1:128, 220, 469, 2:817

Erythropoietin, 1:27

Erythrosine, 1:321

Escherich, Theodor, 1:284

Escherichia coli, 1:**283–288**
  antimicrobial resistance, 1:43
  biosafety, 1:98
  causes, 1:284
  cruise ship health, 1:200
  demographics, 1:284
  description, 1:283–284
  diagnosis, 1:285–286
  disease outbreaks, 1:226
  in emergent diseases, 1:265
  food contamination from, 1:325, 327
  food poisoning from, 1:331
  in food safety, 1:337
  foodborne illness from, 1:342, 344
  meningitis from, 2:522
  prevention, 1:286
  public health, 1:284
  shigellosis and, 2:685
  swimming advisories for, 2:718
  symptoms, 1:284–285
  in traveler's health, 2:740
  treatment, 1:286–287
  in waterborne illness, 2:808–809, 810, 811

Estimated glomerular filtration rate (eGFR), 1:171

Estrogen, 1:105, 107

Estuaries, 2:804

Ethambutol, 2:758

Ethane, 1:348

Ethics, 1:262

Ethics in the Science Classroom, 1:489

Ethiopia
  famine in, 1:301
  guinea worm disease in, 1:367
  Horn of Africa drought and famine in, 1:415, 416, 417, 418

Ethiopia *(continued)*
    Oxfam in, 2:596
    typhus in, 2:766
Ethylbenzene, 1:80, 348
Ethylenediamine tetraacetic acid (EDTA), 1:126, 152
EU (European Union). *See* European Union (EU)
Eucalyptus, 1:385
Europe
    acid rain, 1:3, 4
    AIDS, 1:10
    air pollution, 1:21
    bioterrorism, 1:100
    bisphenol A, 1:105, 106
    bronchitis, 1:110, 111
    Chernobyl nuclear power station disaster, 1:155, 156
    cholera, 1:166
    colony collapse disorder, 1:188
    Creutzfeldt-Jakob disease, 1:194
    drinking water supply, 1:228
    emergent diseases, 1:264
    endocrine disruptors, 1:274
    food additives, 1:320
    hantavirus infections, 1:392
    Healthy Cities, 1:397
    housing, 1:421
    Iceland volcano eruption, 1:435–436
    listeriosis, 1:484
    Lyme disease, 1:494
    meningitis, 2:524
    noise pollution, 2:573
    noroviruses, 2:580
    patch testing, 2:607
    plague, 2:610
    Seveso, Italy accident, 2:683–684
    tuberculosis, 2:753
    typhus, 2:765
    water quality standards, 2:806–807
European Commission, 1:320, 321, 2:684
European Food Safety Authority, 1:106, 321
European Union (EU)
    biosafety, 1:98
    bisphenol A, 1:105
    Creutzfeldt-Jakob disease, 1:194
    Horn of Africa drought and famine, 1:418–419
    Hurricane Katrina, 1:458
    Seveso, Italy accident, 2:683–684
    water quality standards, 2:806–807
Euthyroid goiter. *See* Goiter
Eutrophication, 1:25, 2:671, 801, 804
Evacuation
    disaster preparedness, 1:222–223
    emergency preparedness, 1:261
    Fukushima Daiichi nuclear power station disaster, 1:350, 351
    Hurricane Katrina, 1:455, 456, 457
    Japanese earthquake, 1:451–452
    mold, 2:538

Three Mile Island nuclear disaster, 2:726, 737
Times Beach, 2:730
tsunamis, 2:750–751
volcanic eruptions, 2:796
Evans, Alice Catherine, 1:333
Evaporation, 1:210–211
Every Beat Matters, 2:675
EVERY ONE, 2:675
Evolution, 1:42, 90
Exanthem. *See* Measles
Excisional biopsy. *See* Diagnostic testing
Exercise
    asthma, 1:56, 60, 61
    autism, 1:66
    cancer, 1:131
    chemical poisoning, 1:152
    heat disorders, 1:400
Exercises, emergency. *See* Emergency preparedness
Exhaustion, heat. *See* Heat disorders
Exobiology, 1:97
Exotoxin, 1:218, 219
Explosives, 1:**288–291**, *289*
Exposome, 1:291–292
Exposure, ammonia. *See* Ammonia exposure
Exposure, benzene. *See* Benzene and benzene derivatives exposure
Exposure, chlorine. *See* Chlorine exposure
Exposure, cutting oil. *See* Cutting oil exposure
Exposure, manganese. *See* Manganese exposure
Exposure, occupational. *See* Workplace safety
Exposure, ozone. *See* Ozone exposure
Exposure, radiation. *See* Radiation exposure
Exposure science, 1:**291–295**
    Exxon Valdez, 1:298–299
    Gulf oil spill, 1:373
    in risk assessment, 2:653–655
    in toxicology, 2:735, 736, 737
Exposure, sulfur. *See* Sulfur exposure
Exserohilum rostatum, 2:522
Extermination, pest. *See* Pest control
Extrapulmonary tuberculosis. *See* Tuberculosis
Extremophiles, 1:493
Exxon Mobil Corporation, 1:295, 297, 298, 299
Exxon Valdez, 1:**295–300**, *296, 297, 298*
    in exposure science, 1:294
    Gulf oil spill *vs.*, 1:370
    as oil spill, 2:587–588
Eye Movement Desensitization and Reprocessing, 2:625
Eyes
    chemical poisoning, 1:151
    chlorine exposure, 1:164, 165
    meningitis, 2:520
    river blindness, 2:655–658, *656*
    West Nile virus, 2:813
Eyjafjallajökull, 1:435–436, *436*

F

Factories. *See* Manufacturing
Fair trade, 2:585, 586
Falciparum malaria. *See* Malaria
False sago plant, 2:567–568
Family disaster plans, 1:222
Family planning, 2:619, 620
    See also Contraception
Family Smoking Prevention and Tobacco Control Act, 1:323
Family therapy. *See* Psychotherapy
Famine, 1:**301–304**, *303*
    from drought, 1:232–233
    in Horn of Africa, 1:415–419
    Oxfam on, 2:594, 595, 596, 597
    protein-energy malnutrition during, 2:628, 629
FAO (Food and Agricultural Organization), 1:320, 321, 2:526, 835
Farm animals. *See* Livestock
Farmer's lung. *See* Aspergillosis
Farming. *See* Agriculture
Fasting, 1:153
Fat, body. *See* Body fat
Fatal familial insomnia, 1:194, 196
Faults (geology), 1:246, 386, 450
FCC (Federal Communications Commission), 1:139–140
FDA (Food and Drug Administration). *See* Food and Drug Administration
FDA v. Brown & Williamson Tobacco Corp. (2000), 1:323
FD&C Red No. 3. *See* Erythrosine
FD&C Yellow No. 5. *See* Tartrazine
Feces
    amebiasis in, 1:30, 31–32, 33
    cholera in, 1:166, 169
    cryptosporidiosis in, 1:202, 203
    in dysentery, 1:237, 238
    escherichia coli in, 1:284
    food contamination from, 1:324, 325, 326
    food poisoning from, 1:331
    foodborne illness from, 1:341, 344
    giardiasis in, 1:357, 359
    noroviruses in, 2:577, 581
    sanitation and, 2:669, 670, 671, 672, 673
    swimming advisories due to, 2:718–719
    waterborne illness from, 2:808

Federal Coal Mine Health and Safety Act of 1969, 1:108, 109
Federal Communications Commission (FCC), 1:139–140
Federal Disaster Assistance Administration, 1:491
Federal Emergency Management Agency (FEMA)
  Agency for Toxic Substances and Disease Registry and, 1:5
  on disaster preparedness, 1:225
  on emergency preparedness, 1:259–261
  humanitarian aid from, 1:430
  on Hurricane Katrina, 1:455, 457, 458
  on hurricanes, 1:432
  on levees, 1:483
Federal Emergency Response Agency, 2:571
Federal Food, Drug and Cosmetic Act, 1:275, 320, 322, 323
Federal Insecticide, Fungicide and Rodenticide Act (1972), 1:275, **304–306**
Federal Trade Commission (FTC), 1:323
Federal Water Act (1972), 1:**306–307**, 2:806
Federal Water Pollution Control Act of 1972. *See* Clean Water Act (1972, 1977, 1987)
Federal-state relations
  Clean Air Act, 1:176–177
  Clean Water Act, 1:180, 181, 182
  Comprehensive Environmental Response, Compensation, and Liability Act, 1:192
  Environmental Protection Agency, 1:276, 279
  Gulf oil spill, 1:373–374
  National Ambient Air Quality Standard, 2:551
  Resource Conservation and Recovery Act, 2:650, 651
  Safe Drinking Water Act, 2:667, 668
  Superfund Amendments and Reauthorization Act, 2:718
  water quality standards, 2:806
Feed, animal. *See* Animal feed
FEMA (Federal Emergency Management Agency). *See* Federal Emergency Management Agency (FEMA)
Fertilizers. *See* Agricultural chemicals
Fibromyalgia, 1:378
Fibrosis, 1:**308–309**
  berylliosis, 1:84
  black lung disease, 1:109
  silicosis, 2:694
  talcosis, 2:721
Filoviridae. *See* Filoviruses

Filoviruses, 1:248, 410–411, 412–413, 2:746
Filtration, air. *See* Air filtration
Filtration, water. *See* Water treatment
Fingernails, 1:353
Firefighters, 1:*432*, 2:*819, 820*, 821
Fires, 1:21
Fires, wild. *See* Wildfires
Fireworks, 1:287, 290
First responders. *See* Disaster preparedness; Emergency preparedness
Fish
  acid rain on, 1:3
  algal bloom on, 1:25
  chemical poisoning from, 1:149, 153
  endocrine disruptors on, 1:274–275
  Exxon Valdez disaster on, 1:297, 298, 299
  food contamination in, 1:326, 327
  food poisoning from, 1:330, 332, 334–335
  food safety and, 1:337, 339
  foodborne illness from, 1:343, 345
  fungicide in, 1:355
  Gulf oil spill on, 1:372
  heavy metal poisoning in, 1:406–407
  listeriosis from, 1:485, 487
  mercury in, 2:526
  mercury poisoning from, 2:528, 529, 531, 532–533
  neurotoxins in, 2:567
  oil spills on, 2:589
  in toxic sludge spill in Hungary, 2:732
  water pollution on, 2:*800,* 802
  water quality on, 2:804
  water quality standards on, 2:806
  See also Shellfish
Fish (animals). *See* Fish
Fish (food). *See* Fish
Fisher-Price, 1:466
Fission, 1:289
Five-day measles. *See* Measles
Flame retardants, 1:293
Flash floods. *See* Flooding
Flashbacks, 2:620, 621, 623
Flatworm infestation. *See* Schistosomiasis
Flatworms. *See* Parasites
Flaviviridae. *See* Flaviviruses
Flaviviruses, 1:411, 2:746
Flavonoids, 1:59, 2:712
Flavors, artificial. *See* Artificial flavors
Fleas, 1:*366,* 367, 2:603, 610–613, 662, 835
Flesh-eating disease. *See* Necrotizing fasciitis

Flies, 1:31, 191, 2:663
  See also Blackflies; Sand flies; Tsetse flies
Flight (aviation), 1:212, 213
Flood Control Acts. *See* Omnibus Flood Control Act (1936)
Flood embankment. *See* Levee
Flooding, 1:*310*, **310–312**
  dams in, 1:210, 212
  disaster preparedness for, 1:225
  emergency preparedness for, 1:260
  famine and, 1:302, 303
  from Hurricane Katrina, 1:455, 456–457
  from hurricanes, 1:431–433
  from Japanese earthquake, 1:449, 451
  levees in, 1:483–484
  of Love Canal, 1:489–490
  Omnibus Flood Control Act on, 2:591
  of Times Beach, 2:730
  from tsunamis, 2:748
  waterborne illness from, 2:808
  yellow fever from, 2:825
Florida, 2:512
Flu, avian. *See* Avian flu
Flu, H1N1. *See* H1N1 influenza A
Flu, Hong Kong. *See* Hong Kong flu
Flu pandemic, 1:*313,* **313–317**, *315*
  avian flu, 1:68–69, 70
  Centers for Disease Control and Prevention on, 1:144
  communicable diseases, 1:190
  disease outbreaks, 1:226, 227
  emergent diseases, 1:264, 267
  epidemiology, 1:280
  H1N1 influenza A, 1:381, 382, 383
  medical waste, 2:512
Flu shots. *See* Vaccination
Flu, Spanish. *See* Flu pandemic
Flu, stomach. *See* Foodborne illness
Flu, swine. *See* H1N1 influenza A
Fluke infestation. *See* Schistosomiasis
Flukes. *See* Parasites
Flumandine. *See* Rimantadine
Fluorescent lighting, 1:82
Fluoridation. *See* Water fluoridation
Fluoride
  drinking water supply, 1:230–231
  sanitation, 2:671
  water fluoridation, 2:797–799
Fluorine, 2:598
Fluoroquinolones, 1:129, 265, 286, 2:523
Fluoroscopy. *See* Diagnostic testing
Fluorosis, 2:671, 797, 798
Fly ash, 1:22
Fog, volcanic. *See* Volcanic fog
Folk medicine. *See* Complementary and alternative medicine (CAM)

Food additives, 1:**318–322,** 318*t*–319*t*, 338
  See also specific additives by name
Food Additives Amendment, 1:320
Food and Agricultural Organization (FAO), 1:320, 321, 2:526, 835
Food and Drug Administration, 1:**322–324**
  on conditions
    antimicrobial resistance, 1:45
    drinking water supply, 1:230
    emergency preparedness, 1:262
    food contamination, 1:324
    food safety, 1:337, 338, 339
    HPV vaccination, 1:423, 424
    low-temperature environments, 1:493
    smoking, 2:709
    vector (mosquito) control, 2:787
  on diseases and disorders
    AIDS, 1:13
    asbestosis, 1:50
    asthma, 1:58, 60
    avian flu, 1:69, 70
    disease outbreaks, 1:228
    food poisoning, 1:334
    lead poisoning, 1:466
    Lyme disease, 1:496
    manganese exposure, 2:507
    meningitis, 2:523, 524
    mercury poisoning, 2:529, 532–533
    methemoglobinemia, 2:535
    radiation injuries, 2:642
  on hazards
    agricultural chemicals, 1:7
    biotoxins, 1:104
    bisphenol A, 1:105, 106
    cellular phones, 1:141
    endocrine disruptors, 1:274
    food additives, 1:318, 320, 321
    mercury, 2:526
    neurotoxins, 2:567
Food chains, 1:405, 406, 407, 2:526, 785
Food contamination, 1:**324–330,** *325*, 327*t*
  biosafety, 1:97
  causes, 1:326–327
    algal bloom, 1:25, 26
    bioterrorism, 1:103
    biotoxins, 1:103, 104
    chemical poisoning, 1:148, 149
    Chernobyl nuclear power station disaster, 1:158–159
    cholera, 1:166
    escherichia coli, 1:283, 284, 285
    flooding, 1:311
    Fukushima Daiichi nuclear power station disaster, 1:351
    fungicide, 1:355
    Japanese earthquake, 1:451
    lead poisoning, 1:464
    listeriosis, 1:484, 485
    mercury poisoning, 2:528, 529, 531, 532–533
    noroviruses, 2:577, 579, 580, 581, 582
    oil spills, 2:589
    typhoid fever, 2:761, 762
  in communicable diseases, 1:190
  in cruise ship health, 1:198, 200
  demographics, 1:324
  description, 1:324–326
  diseases from
    brucellosis, 1:116–117, 119
    campylobacteriosis, 1:128, 129
    Creutzfeldt-Jakob disease, 1:194, 197
    cryptosporidiosis, 1:202
    food poisoning, 1:330, 331–332, 334
    foodborne illness, 1:341, 343
    giardiasis, 1:357
    meningitis, 2:523
    parasitic infections, 2:603, 604
    shigellosis, 2:686
  food safety and, 1:336–340, 338
  parental concerns, 1:329
  prevention, 1:327–329
  prognosis, 1:327
  symptoms, 1:327
  in traveler's health, 2:740
  treatment, 1:327
Food Drug, and Cosmetic Act. *See* Federal Food, Drug and Cosmetic Act
Food irradiation, 1:286, 328, 336, 338, 345
Food poisoning, 1:**330–335**
  causes, 1:331–332
    bioterrorism, 1:103
    biotoxins, 1:104
    escherichia coli, 1:283
    food contamination, 1:324, 326, 327
  demographics, 1:330–331
  diagnosis, 1:333
  in dysentery, 1:236
  food safety and, 1:336, 337, 339
  as foodborne illness, 1:341–345
  listeriosis as, 1:485, 487
  prevention, 1:335
  prognosis, 1:334–335
  public health, 1:334
  risk factors, 1:330
  symptoms, 1:331–332
  treatment, 1:333–334
Food preservatives. *See* Food additives
Food processing
  food contamination during, 1:324, 326, 328
  food poisoning from, 1:334, 335
  food safety in, 1:336, 337, 338
  foodborne illness from, 1:341, 343, 345
Food Quality Protection Act, 1:275

Food safety, 1:327*t*, **336–341,** 336*t*
  Centers for Disease Control and Prevention, 1:144
  complications, 1:339
  Food and Drug Administration, 1:322–324
  in global public health, 1:363
  government regulation of, 1:337–338
  methods, 1:338–339
  parental concerns, 1:339–340
  precautions, 1:339
  purpose, 1:336
  threats to, 1:336
    agricultural chemicals, 1:6–7
    amebiasis, 1:32
    anthrax, 1:37, 39, 40
    asbestos, 1:47
    bisphenol A, 1:105, 106–107
    chemical poisoning, 1:149
    cholera, 1:169
    dysentery, 1:239, 241
    endocrine disruptors, 1:275
    escherichia coli, 1:286, 287
    food additives, 1:320–321
    food contamination, 1:325–329, 327*t*
    food poisoning, 1:330, 331–332, 334
    foodborne illness, 1:341, 345
    Japanese earthquake, 1:452
    lead poisoning, 1:464, 466, 467
    listeriosis, 1:487
    low-temperature environments, 1:493, 494
    manganese exposure, 2:505, 506
    mercury poisoning, 2:532–533
    noroviruses, 2:583
    parasites, 2:607
    typhoid fever, 2:764
  in traveler's health, 2:739, 740
Food Safety and Inspection Service, 1:320, 337, 339
Food Safety Modernization Act, 1:337, 345
Food shortages. *See* Famine
Food webs, 1:275
Foodborne illness, 1:**341–346,** 342*t*
  causes, 1:341–343
    escherichia coli, 1:284
    food contamination, 1:324–325, 324–326, 326, 327
    listeriosis, 1:484, 485, 487
    mold, 2:536
    noroviruses, 2:577, 579
    zoonoses, 2:833
  demographics, 1:341
  description, 1:341
  diagnosis, 1:344
  disease outbreaks of, 1:226, 227, 228
  as emergent diseases, 1:266
  food poisoning as, 1:330–335
  food safety and, 1:336, 337, 339

Foodborne illness *(continued)*
  in global public health, 1:363
  prevention, 1:344–345
  prognosis, 1:344–345
  symptoms, 1:343–344
  in traveler's health, 2:740
  treatment, 1:344
  See also specific illnesses by name
Foodbourne illness. *See* specific illnesses by name
FoodNet, 1:129, 334
Forced migration. *See* Population displacement
Foreign aid. *See* Humanitarian aid
Forensic toxicology. *See* Toxicology
Forest fires. *See* Wildfires
Forests
  acid rain, 1:3
  drought, 1:232, 234
  in epidemiology, 1:281
  Haiti earthquake, 1:387
  Sierra Club, 2:693
  tropical disease, 2:745
Formaldehyde, 1:5, 24, 437, 438, 2:690
Fossil fuels, 1:1, 21, 24, 80–81, 126
4-methylimidazole, 1:321
Fournier's gangrene. *See* Necrotizing fasciitis
Fracking, 1:**346–348**, *347*
Fracturing, hydraulic. *See* Fracking
Franz, Andrew, 2:659–660
Frasch process, 2:715
Free radical scavengers. *See* Antioxidants
Free radicals, 2:710
Freezing. *See* Refrigeration and freezing
Frequency (waves), 2:575
Freshwater ecosystems. *See* Aquatic ecosystems
Frostbite, 1:493
Frosting, 1:493
Fruit bats, 1:248, 251, 265
Fruits. *See* Food
Fruits and vegetables, 1:484, 485, 487, 2:583, 607
FTC (Federal Trade Commission), 1:323
Fuel, automotive. *See* Diesel fuel; Gasoline
Fuel Relief Fund, 1:430
Fukushima Daiichi nuclear power station disaster, 1:**348–352**, *349*
  cancer from, 1:131
  earthquakes and, 1:247
  on food safety, 1:336
  Japanese earthquake and, 1:449, 452, 453–454
  radiation injuries from, 2:643

Fukushima Nuclear Accident Commission, 1:350
Fulminant colitis. *See* Colitis
Fumigation, 1:77
Fungal balls. *See* Aspergilloma
Fungal infections, 1:*352*, **352–354**, 355
  See also specific infections by name
Fungal meningitis. *See* Meningitis
Fungi
  in emergent diseases, 1:265
  in fungal infections, 1:352–354
  fungicide for, 1:354–355
  mold as, 2:536–540
  zoonoses from, 2:833
Fungicide, 1:**354–355**
  for AIDS, 1:14
  antimicrobial resistance, 1:41–45
  for aspergillosis, 1:52, 53
  in colony collapse disorder, 1:187
  Federal Insecticide, Fungicide and Rodenticide Act, 1:304–306
  for fungal infections, 1:353, 354
  for meningitis, 2:523
  mercury poisoning from, 2:527, 528
Furnaces, 1:22
Fusion, 1:289
Fusion inhibitors, 1:14

G

Gadjusek, Carleton, 1:193
Gallbladder, 2:763
Gallium scan, 1:478
Galveston-Houston Association for Smog Prevention (GHASP), 2:708
Gaman, 1:453
Game animals. *See* Wildlife
Gamma radiation. *See* Radiation
Gangrene. *See* Necrotizing fasciitis
Ganz, Michael, 1:66
GAO (General Accounting Office), 1:5
Gardasil, 1:423, 428
Garlic, 1:466, 497
Gas embolism. *See* Decompression sickness
Gas, natural. *See* Natural gas
Gasoline, 1:81, 294, 462, 464, 465, 466
Gastrectomy, 1:166
Gastric lavage, 1:151, 152, 409, 445
Gastritis, 1:166
Gastroenteritis. *See* Food poisoning
Gastrointestinal disorders. *See* specific disorders by name
GAVI Alliance, 2:772, 773
GenBank, 1:92
Gene therapy. *See* Genetic engineering
Gene transfer, 1:42, 43
General Accounting Office (GAO), 1:5

Genes. *See* Genetics
Genesee River, 2:669
Genetic engineering
  on agricultural chemicals, 1:6
  Food and Drug Administration, 1:322, 323, 324
  on food safety, 1:337
  in tropical disease, 2:748
  in vector (mosquito) control, 2:785, 787
  viruses in, 2:789
Genetic testing, 1:134
Genetically modified food. *See* Genetic engineering
Genetics
  autism, 1:62
  avian flu, 1:68
  bioinformatics, 1:89–93
  cancer, 1:131, 134
  Creutzfeldt-Jakob disease, 1:194, 196
  emphysema, 1:269, 271
  H1N1 influenza A, 1:382
  leukemia, 1:481
  melanoma, 2:515, 516, 519
  methemoglobinemia, 2:534
  noroviruses, 2:577
  population and disease, 2:619
  post-traumatic stress disorder, 2:621
  smoking, 2:710
  See also Chromosomes; DNA; Mutation; RNA
Genital warts, 1:422–423, 425, 426–427
Genomes. *See* Genomics
Genomics, 1:93*t*
  in bioinformatics, 1:89–91, 92–93
  in exposure science, 1:291–292
  of severe acute respiratory syndrome, 2:681
  of viruses, 2:788, 789, 791, 792
Gentamicin, 1:287
Geological Survey (U.S.). *See* U.S. Geological Survey
Geology, 1:346, 348
Geotrichosis, 1:*352*
Geranium mexicanum, 1:239
German measles, 2:507–508, *508*, 779, 781
Germany, 1:35–36, 100
Gerstmann-Straussler-Scheinker disease, 1:194, 196
Ghana, 2:529, 670
Giard, Alfred, 1:357
Giardia
  cruise ship health, 1:200
  dysentery, 1:236
  food contamination, 1:326
  food poisoning, 1:239, 332
  giardiasis, 1:357, 359
  as parasite, 2:604, 606
  traveler's health, 2:740
  waterborne illness, 2:808, 809

Giardiasis, 1:**357–361**, *358*
   as dysentery, 1:237, 238
   in One Health Initiative, 2:592
   water quality in, 2:804
   as waterborne illness, 2:808, 809, 810
Gibbs, Lois, 1:490, 491, *491*
Gibraltar fever. *See* Brucellosis
Ginger, 1:384
Gingko biloba, 1:29
Ginkgo, 1:60
Glacier National Park, 2:693
Glaciers, 1:21
Gleevec. *See* Imatinib
Glioma, 1:131
Global Autism Public Health Initiative, 1:66
Global Campaign for Education, 2:596
Global Early Warning System for Major Animal Diseases, 2:835
Global Plan to Stop Tuberculosis, 2:758
Global Polio Eradication Initiative, 2:613
Global Positioning System (GPS), 1:248
Global public health, 1:**361–364**
   child survival revolution, 1:160–161
   cholera, 1:168
   cruise ship health, 1:198
   dams, 1:210
   emergent diseases, 1:263–267
   endemic disease, 1:272
   famine, 1:303–304
   flu pandemic, 1:317
   food contamination, 1:325
   guinea worm disease, 1:366
   H1N1 influenza A, 1:381, 385
   World Health Organization, 2:822–823
Global warming. *See* Climate change
Glucose, 1:141, 171
Glutathione, 1:152
Gluten, 1:65–66
Glycopyrrolate, 1:445
Goiter, 1:**364–366**
Gold, 2:529
Goldenseal, 1:497
Goldfarb, Theodore, 1:489
Gonococcus. *See* Neisseria gonorrhoeae
Gonorrhea, 1:41, 43, 45, 265
Google, 1:452
Gorillas. *See* Primates
Gorsuch, Ann, 2:693
Government agencies. *See specific agencies by name*
Government regulation
   biosafety, 1:98–99
   Clean Air Act, 1:176–178
   Clean Water Act, 1:179–182
   Comprehensive Environmental Response, Compensation, and Liability Act, 1:191–193
   disasters
      Bhopal, India, 1:88, 89
      Chernobyl nuclear power station disaster, 1:157, 160
      earthquakes, 1:247
      flooding, 1:312
      Gulf oil spill, 1:375–376
      Japanese earthquake, 1:453
      Love Canal, 1:491–492
      oil spills, 2:589
      Seveso, Italy accident, 2:683–684
      Three Mile Island nuclear disaster and, 2:728–729
   diseases and disorders
      asbestosis, 1:51
      benzene exposure, 1:81
      black lung disease and, 1:108, 109
      byssinosis and, 1:122
      cadmium poisoning, 1:127
      chemical poisoning, 1:149
      chlorine exposure, 1:164
      colony collapse disorder, 1:188
      Creutzfeldt-Jakob disease, 1:194–195, 197
      cruise ship health, 1:198–199
      cutting oil exposure, 1:205, 206
      cyanosis, 1:207, 208
      escherichia coli infections, 1:284, 286
      food poisoning, 1:334
      foodborne illness, 1:345
      heavy metal poisoning, 1:407, 409
      insecticide poisoning, 1:445
      lead poisoning, 1:465
      malaria, 2:504
      manganese exposure, 2:507
      meningitis, 2:523–524
      mercury poisoning, 2:527, 529
      methemoglobinemia, 2:535
      mumps, 2:544
      ozone exposure, 2:600
      plague, 2:612
      radiation injuries, 2:642
      severe acute respiratory syndrome, 2:680–681
      silicosis, 2:695
      sulfur exposure, 2:716
      thesaurosis, 2:723, 724
      waterborne illness, 2:811
      Yokkaichi asthma, 2:831
   Emergency Planning and Community Right-to-Know Act, 1:257–259
   environmental conditions and hazards
      acid rain, 1:4
      bisphenol A, 1:104, 105, 106
      drinking water supply, 1:229–230, 231
      endocrine disruptors, 1:274, 275
      explosives, 1:290
      food additives, 1:318, 320–321
      food safety, 1:337–338
      fracking, 1:346–348
      hazardous waste, 1:395–396
      housing, 1:421, 422
      indoor air quality, 1:437–438, 439
      ionizing radiation, 1:447
      lead, 1:462
      levees, 1:483
      medical waste, 2:511, 512, 513
      mercury, 2:526
      mold, 2:537
      neurotoxins, 2:567, 568
      smog, 2:707–708
      ultraviolet radiation, 2:770
      water pollution, 2:800, 801, 802
      water quality, 2:803, 804–807
   Environmental Protection Agency, 1:276–279
   exposure science in, 1:292, 293, 294
   Federal Insecticide, Fungicide and Rodenticide Act, 1:304–306
   Food and Drug Administration, 1:322–324
   on National Ambient Air Quality Standard, 2:549–551
   National Environmental Policy Ac, 2:552–554
   Occupational Safety and Health Act, 2:585
   Occupational Safety and Health Administration, 2:585–586
   Rachel Carson Council, 2:631
   Resource Conservation and Recovery Act, 2:650–652
   risk assessment and, 2:653
   Rivers and Harbors Act of 1899, 2:658–661
   Safe Drinking Water Act, 2:667–668
   Superfund Amendments and Reauthorization Act, 2:717–718
   Toxic Substances Control Act, 2:733–735
   toxicology in, 2:736, 737
   of vaccination, 2:780, 782
GPS (Global Positioning System), 1:248
Gram's stain, 1:219
Grand Challenges in Global Health, 2:785
Grand Teton National Park, 2:693
Grant, Ulysses S., 2:559
Granulocytes. *See* Blood cells
Granulomas, 2:721
Granulomatosis infantisepticum, 1:486
Granulomatous reaction, 2:676
Grass fires. *See* Wildfires
Graves' disease, 1:364
Great East Japan Earthquake. *See* Japanese Earthquake (2011)
Great Smog of 1952. *See* Smog

Greece, 1:120–121
Green Revolution, 1:7
Greenhouse effect. *See* Climate change
Greenhouse gases. *See specific gases by name*
Greenland, 1:21
Groundwater
   dams on, 1:210
   drinking water supply and, 1:228, 229
   drought on, 1:233
   fracking on, 1:348
   heavy metal poisoning on, 1:404
   Safe Drinking Water Act on, 2:667, 668
   sanitation on, 2:670
   water pollution in, 2:801
   water quality of, 2:803–804
   waterborne illness from, 2:808
Group A strep, 2:566
Group B strep, 1:265, 2:522
Growth monitoring, 2:771
Guangzhou, China, 1:23
Guided imagery, 1:498
Guillain-Barré syndrome, 1:128, 344
Guinea worm disease, 1:*366*, **366–368**
   sanitation and, 2:671
   as tropical disease, 2:746, 747
   as waterborne illness, 2:809
Guinea-Bissau, 1:190
Gulf Coast Claims Facility, 1:370
Gulf Long-Term Follow-Up Study, 2:588–589
Gulf of Mexico, 1:368–376, *369*
Gulf oil spill, 1:**368–377**, *369, 373*
   causes, 1:372
   demographics, 1:370–371
   description, 1:368–370
   environmental impact, 1:371–372
   in exposure science, 1:293
   as oil spill, 2:587, 588–589, 590
   Oxfam on, 2:597
   prevention, 1:375–376
   prognosis, 1:374–375
   public health, 1:373–374
   treatment, 1:372–373
   on water quality, 2:805
Gulf War syndrome, 1:**377–380**
Gunpowder, 1:288, 290
Guo, Peng, 2:831
Gustav, Angelina, 1:159

H

H1N1 influenza A, 1:**381–385**
   Centers for Disease Control and Prevention and, 1:144
   as communicable disease, 1:190
   disease outbreak of, 1:227
   as emergent disease, 1:264

   epidemiology of, 1:280
   as flu pandemic, 1:313, 314–315
H5N1 influenza. *See* Avian flu
HAART (Highly active antiretroviral therapy)
   for AIDS, 1:9, 14, 15, 16, 17–18, 19
   for dysentery, 1:240
Habitat for Humanity, 1:421–422
Haemagglutinin, 1:68
Hague Conventions, 1:100
Hair, 1:408
Hair spray, 2:723–724
Haiti, 1:166, 168, 2:670
   See also Haiti earthquake
Haiti earthquake, 1:247, *386*, **386–391**, *388*
   Centers for Disease Control and Prevention and, 1:144
   cholera and, 1:168
   sanitation and, 2:670
   tsunami from, 2:752
   typhoid fever and, 2:761
Haiti Ministry of Public Heath and Population, 1:388, 389, 390
Haiti National Public Health Laboratory, 1:388
Halliburton, 1:372, 374
Halofantrine, 2:504
Halogenated methanes, 1:163
Hamilton, Alice, 1:191, *191*, 443
Hand, foot, and mouth virus, 1:265
Hand washing. *See* Personal hygiene
Hantaan virus, 1:392, 412
Hantavirus infections, 1:**391–395**, *392*
   as emergent disease, 1:265
   as hemorrhagic fevers, 1:412
   in One Health Initiative, 2:592
Hantavirus pulmonary syndrome (HPS), 1:391, 392, 393, 394, 2:662
Harbors, 2:658–661
Hard measles. *See* Measles
Harmful algal bloom. *See* Algal bloom
Harvard School of Public Health, 1:62
Hatmakers, 1:407, 2:527
Hawaii, 1:471, 2:751
Hawaiian eruptions. *See* Volcanic eruptions
Hayes, Denis, 1:243, 244
Hazardous and Solid Waste Amendments, 2:651, 652
Hazardous waste, 1:*395*, **395–396**
   at brownfield sites, 1:113, *114*
   cellular phones as, 1:140
   Comprehensive Environmental Response, Compensation, and Liability Act, 1:191–193
   in drinking water supply, 1:229, 231
   Environmental Protection Agency, 1:*277*, 278–279
   heavy metal poisoning from, 1:404, 407

   from Japanese earthquake, 1:451, 453
   at Love Canal, 1:488–492
   medical waste as, 2:511
   National Institute of Environmental Health Sciences, 2:558
   noroviruses and, 2:584
   Resource Conservation and Recovery Act, 2:650, 651
   risk assessment, 2:653
   Superfund Amendments and Reauthorization Act, 2:717–718
   from toxic sludge spill in Hungary, 2:731–732
   in water pollution, 2:801
   See also Medical waste
Hazardous work environment. *See* Workplace safety
Hazards, biological. *See* Medical waste
Hazelwood, Joseph, 1:297, 299
HCFCs (Hydrochlorofluorocarbons), 1:178
Health Alert Network, 1:262
Health care costs, 1:44
Health care reform, 1:34
Health care workers. *See* Medical personnel
Health inspections. *See* Sanitation
Health Physics Society, 1:351
Health, public. *See* Public health
Healthy Cities, 1:**396–398**
Healthy Homes, 1:422
Healthy People 2020, 1:112, 269–270
Hearing, 2:572, 573, 574
Heart, 1:23, 107, 218, 252, 254
Heart disease. *See* Cardiovascular disease
Heat cramps. *See* Heat disorders
Heat disorders, 1:**398–401**, 402, 403
Heat exhaustion. *See* Heat disorders
Heat index. *See* Heat (stress) index
Heat (stress) index, 1:**401–403**, 402*t*
Heat stroke. *See* Heat disorders
Heat wave. *See* Heat disorders
Heavy metal poisoning, 1:**403–410**
   See also specific types of poisoning by name
Heavy metals, 1:148, 152, 403–409, 2:567, 732
Helicobacter pylori, 1:166
Helsinki, Finland, 1:397
Hemagglutin, 1:383
Hemodialysis. *See* Kidney dialysis
Hemoglobin
   carbon monoxide poisoning, 1:136–137, 138
   chronic kidney disease, 1:171
   cyanosis, 1:206
   methemoglobinemia, 2:534–535

Hemolytic uremic syndrome (HUS)
  dysentery, 1:237
  escherichia coli infections, 1:285, 286, 287
  from food contamination, 1:327
  foodborne illness, 1:344
  shigellosis, 2:686
Hemophilus influenzae, 2:521, 522
Hemoptysis, 1:52, 53
Hemorrhagic fever with renal syndrome (HFRS), 1:391–393, 394, 412, 2:662
Hemorrhagic fevers, 1:**410–413**
  from hantavirus infections, 1:391–392
  as tropical disease, 2:746
Heparin, 1:412
Hepatitis
  disease outbreaks, 1:227
  from food contamination, 1:326
  from medical waste, 2:511, 512, 513
  sanitation and, 2:670
  water quality and, 2:804
  as waterborne illness, 2:809
Herbal medicine. *See* Complementary and alternative medicine (CAM)
Herbicides. *See* Agricultural chemicals
Herd immunity, 2:510, 777, 782
Heredity. *See* Genetics
Heroin, 1:152, 2:567
Herpes, 2:521, 523
HF (Hemorrhagic fevers). *See* Hemorrhagic fevers
HFRS (Hemorrhagic fever with renal syndrome), 1:391–393, 394
HI (Heat index). *See* Heat (stress) index
High blood pressure. *See* Hypertension
High explosives. *See* Explosives
High temperature environments, 1:*414*, **414–415**, 2:578, 744
High test hypochlorite. *See* Calcium hypochlorite
High-altitude cerebral edema, 1:27, 28–29
High-altitude pulmonary edema, 1:27, 28, 29
Highly active antiretroviral therapy (HAART). *See* HAART (Highly active antiretroviral therapy)
Hippocrates, 1:442, 2:564, 591
Hiroshima, Japan, 2:638, *638*
Hispanic Americans, 1:10, 19, 464
Histadine-rich protein II (HRP2), 2:503
Histamine, 1:55, 59
Histamine blockers, 1:166–167
HIV (Human immunodeficiency virus)
  antimicrobial resistance, 1:34
  biosafety and, 1:98
  as communicable disease, 1:190

epidemiology of, 1:280
from medical waste, 2:511, 512–513
mumps and, 2:546
in One Health Initiative, 2:593
as pandemic, 2:601
parasites and, 2:605
sanitation and, 2:671
tuberculosis and, 2:754, 755, 757, 760
See also AIDS
Hodgkin's disease, 1:12
Hoffman-LaRoche, 2:683
Home, Francis, 2:508
Homelessness, 1:421
Homeopathic medicine. *See* Complementary and alternative medicine (CAM)
Homosexuality. *See* Sexual behavior
Honeybees, 1:185–188
Hong Kong, 1:23, 68, 2:679, 680, 681
Hong Kong flu, 1:313, 314, 382
The Honoring America's Veterans and Caring for Camp Lejeune Families Act of 2012, 1:229
Hooker Chemical Corporation, 1:488–489, 491
Hookworms. *See* Parasites
Hoover Dam, 1:*209*
Hormone therapy, 1:134
Hormones, 1:105, 107, 273–275
  See also specific hormones by name
Horn of Africa drought and famine, 1:**415–419**, *416*
Horses, 2:813, 834
Hospitals
  antimicrobial resistance in, 1:41, 42, 43, 45
  bioterrorism and, 1:101, 103
  bronchitis in, 1:112
  in Chernobyl nuclear power station disaster, 1:159
  emergent diseases in, 1:265, 266
  escherichia coli in, 1:284
  in Haiti earthquake, 1:388, 389, 390
  in Japanese earthquake, 1:451, 452
  medical waste from, 2:511, 513–514
  sanitation in, 2:669
  for tuberculosis, 2:752–753
Hosts (disease)
  dengue fever, 1:215, 216
  ebola hemorrhagic fever, 1:248, 251
  guinea worm disease, 1:366
  Lyme disease, 1:494
  parasites and, 2:602, 603, 605
  viruses and, 2:788–790
  yellow fever, 2:825
Household products, 1:147–149, 439
Household safety, 1:421
Household waste disposal. *See* Sanitation
Housing, 1:**420–422**
  Haiti earthquake, 1:390
  Healthy Cities, 1:397

Hurricane Katrina, 1:457, 458
lead poisoning in, 1:464
HPS (Hantavirus pulmonary syndrome), 1:391, 392, 393, 394, 2:662
HPV. *See* Human papilloma virus
HPV vaccination, 1:**422–424**, 427, 428
HRP2 (Histadine-rich protein II), 2:503
HSI (Heat stress index). *See* Heat (stress) index
HTLV-I (Human T-cell leukemia virus), 1:476
Human Factors Society, 1:282
Human Genome Project, 1: 90–91, 291
Human immunodeficiency virus (HIV). *See* AIDS; HIV (Human immunodeficiency virus)
Human Microbiome Project, 1:92–93
Human papilloma virus (HPV), 1:131, 134, 422–424, **425–429**
Human remains. *See* Corpses
Human rights
  Oxfam on, 2:595, 596
  Save the Children, 2:674–675
  UNICEF on, 2:771–772, 773–775
Humanitarian aid, 1:**429–431**, *430*
  famine, 1:303
  Fukushima Daiichi nuclear power station disaster, 1:351
  Haiti earthquake, 1:388, 389, 390
  Horn of Africa drought and famine, 1:415–416, 417, 418–419
  housing, 1:421
  Hurricane Katrina, 1:457–458
  Japanese earthquake, 1:451–452, 453
  Oxfam, 2:594–597
  Red Cross, 2:646–649
  UNICEF, 2:771, 774
Humidity
  heat (stress) index, 1:401, 402–403, 402*t*
  indoor air quality, 1:438, 439
  mold, 2:536–537, 540
Hungary, 2:731–732
Hunger. *See* Famine
Hunting, 1:175
Hurricane Andrew. *See* Andrew
Hurricane Ike. *See* Ike
Hurricane Ivan. *See* Ivan
Hurricane Katrina. *See* Katrina
Hurricane Rita. *See* Rita
Hurricane Sandy. *See* Sandy
Hurricane Tomas. *See* Tomas
Hurricane Wilma. *See* Wilma
Hurricanes, 1:**431–433**
  Centers for Disease Control and Prevention and, 1:145
  cholera from, 1:166
  climate change on, 1:185
  disaster preparedness, 1:224–225
  flooding from, 1:310
  Oxfam on, 2:597

Hurricanes *(continued)*
  sanitation after, 2:670
  See also Katrina; Sandy
HUS (Hemolytic uremic syndrome). *See* Hemolytic uremic syndrome (HUS)
HVAC systems. *See* Ventilation
Hydraulic fracturing. *See* Fracking
Hydrocarbons
  in air pollution, 1:22
  benzene and, 1:79, 80–81, 82
  Clean Air Act on, 1:177
  in National Ambient Air Quality Standard, 2:549
  as neurotoxins, 2:567
  in smog, 2:707
  as volatile organic compounds, 2:793
Hydrochloric acid, 1:22
Hydrochlorofluorocarbons (HCFCs), 1:178
Hydroelectricity, 1:210, *210*, 211, 212
Hydrogen, 1:349
Hydrogen bombs, 1:73
Hydrogen sulfide, 2:715
Hydro-Québec, 1:255–256
Hydrostatic kill. *See* Static kill
Hydrotherapy, 1:60
Hydroxybenzene. *See* Phenol
Hygiene, industrial. *See* Industrial hygiene
Hygiene, personal. *See* Personal hygiene
Hyperarousal, 2:623
Hyperbaric oxygen therapy. *See* Oxygen therapy
Hypersensitivity pneumonitis, 2:537
Hypertension, 1:170, 171
Hyperthermia. *See* Heat disorders
Hyperthyroid goiter. *See* Goiter
Hyperventilation, 1:27
Hypnotherapy, 2:711
Hypochlorite ion, 1:162
Hypochlorous acid, 1:162
Hypothermia, 1:493
Hypothyroid goiter. *See* Goiter
Hypoxemia, 1:27
Hypoxia
  from algal bloom, 1:26
  in altitude sickness, 1:27, 28
  from carbon monoxide poisoning, 1:136
  from Gulf oil spill, 1:374
  in heavy metal poisoning, 1:405

I

IARC (International Agency for Research on Cancer), 2:642, 769
Ice, 1:310
Iceland, 1:435, 436
Icelandic volcano eruption (2010), 1:**435–437**, *436*
IFRC (International Federation of Red Cross and Red Crescent Societies). *See* Red Cross
Ignitability, 1:395
Ike, 1:433
Illinois, 2:669
Imaginative play, 1:64
Imaging, medical. *See* Diagnostic testing
Imatinib, 1:479
Imiquimod, 1:427, 2:698
Immigrants, 1:236, 2:602–603, 630
Immune system
  AIDS, 1:8, 12, 19
  aspergillosis, 1:51–52, 53, 54
  benzene exposure on, 1:80
  campylobacteriosis and, 1:128
  cancer, 1:133
  cryptosporidiosis, 1:203
  escherichia coli on, 1:287
  fungal infections, 1:352, 354
  hemorrhagic fevers, 1:412
  human papilloma virus on, 1:425
  listeriosis, 1:485
  malaria, 2:503
  mumps, 2:546
  necrotizing fasciitis, 2:564, 565
  parasites on, 2:603, 604
  skin cancer and, 2:697, 698
  sleeping sickness, 2:700
Immunization. *See* Vaccination
Immunodeficiency. *See* Immune system
Immunoglobulins, 1:469, 477
Immunomodulating agents, 1:133
Immunosuppressants, 1:476
Immunotherapy, 2:517, 518–520, 538
Inactivated polio vaccine (IPV), 2:614, 616–617
Incineration, 1:22, 2:513
India
  byssinosis in, 1:120
  cholera, 1:169
  endemic disease in, 1:272
  famine in, 1:303
  sanitation in, 2:671
  severe acute respiratory syndrome, 2:680
  smallpox in, 2:701
  See also Bhopal, India
Indian Ocean, 1:247, 2:750
Indian Ocean Tsunami. *See* Boxing Day Tsunami
Indian tobacco. *See* Lobelia
Indiana, 1:392
Indonesia, 2:751, 820, *820*
Indoor air pollution. *See* Air pollution
Indoor air quality, 1:**437–442**
  air pollution, 1:23, 24
  asthma, 1:61
  chemical poisoning, 1:147–148
  of housing, 1:420
  mold on, 2:536–527
  sick building syndrome, 2:689–691
  volatile organic compounds on, 2:793
Industrial accidents. *See* Accidents
Industrial diseases. *See specific diseases by name*
Industrial Hygiene, 1:*442*, **442–444**
  biomonitoring, 1:96
  disasters
    Bhopal, India, 1:88, 89
    Chernobyl nuclear power station disaster, 1:156–157
    Seveso, Italy accident, 2:684
    Three Mile Island nuclear disaster, 2:728–729
  diseases and disorders
    berylliosis, 1:82
    byssinosis, 1:120, 122
    cadmium poisoning, 1:126, 127
    chlorine exposure, 1:164, 165
    cutting oil exposure, 1:205–206
    fibrosis, 1:309
    food contamination, 1:324, 326, 327, 328
    food poisoning, 1:334, 335
    foodborne illness, 1:345
  food safety in, 1:338
  ionizing radiation in, 1:447
  National Institute of Environmental Health Sciences, 2:558–559
  Occupational Safety and Health Act, 2:585
  Occupational Safety and Health Administration, 2:585–586
  See also Workplace safety
Industrial medicine, 1:443
Industrial pollution. *See* Air pollution; Water pollution
Industrial production. *See* Manufacturing
Industries. *See specific industries by name*
Infants. *See* Children
Infection control. *See* Disease control
Infections. *See specific infections by name*
Infectious diarrhea. *See* Foodborne illness
Infectious diseases. *See* Communicable diseases
Infestation, bedbug. *See* Bedbug infestation
Infestation, mold. *See* Mold
Infiltration, 1:440
Influenza. *See specific types of influenza by name*
Influenza A, 1:67, 68, 2:791–792
  See also H1N1 influenza A

Influenza, avian. *See* Avian flu
Influenza pandemic. *See* Flu pandemic
Influenza vaccination. *See* Vaccination
Influenzal meningitis. *See* Meningitis
Information technology, 1:89–93
Infrared radiation. *See* Non-ionizing radiation
INH. *See* Isoniazid
Inhalation anthrax. *See* Anthrax
Inhalation disease. *See* Asbestosis
Inhalers, 1:58–59
Inheritance (genetics). *See* Genetics
Injuries, electric shock. *See* Electric shock injuries
Injuries, household. *See* Household safety
Innocenti Research Centre (IRC), 2:773
Inorganic mercury. *See* Mercury
Insect bites
    bedbug infestation, 1:75, 76, 78
    Lyme disease, 1:494, 495, 496
    malaria, 2:501–502
    parasites from, 2:603, 604
    sleeping sickness, 2:609
    tropical disease, 2:744
    zoonoses, 2:833, 834
Insect repellents. *See* Insecticides
Insecticide poisoning, 1:**444–446**
    bedbug infestation and, 1:78
    as chemical poisoning, 1:149, 152
    from vector (mosquito) control, 2:784
Insecticides
    for bedbug infestation, 1:75, 76–78
    emergent disease and, 1:266
    as endocrine disruptors, 1:274, 275
    Federal Insecticide, Fungicide and Rodenticide Act, 1:304–306
    heavy metal poisoning from, 1:409
    indoor air quality, 1:438
    for parasites, 2:605
    Rachel Carson Council on, 2:632
    river blindness and, 2:657, 658
    for tropical disease, 2:747, 748
    for vector (mosquito) control, 2:784–786
    for West Nile virus, 2:815
Insects. *See specific insects by name*
Inspections, health. *See* Sanitation
Institute for Altitude Medicine, 1:28
Institute of Medicine (IOM), 1:476
Insulin resistance, 1:16
Insurance, 1:260
Integrase inhibitors, 1:14
Integrated pest management, 1:7–8, 2:784–785
Intelligence, 1:23
Intelligence Reform and Terrorism Prevention Act, 2:571

Interactions, drug. *See* Drug interactions
Interferon, 1:479, 2:518–519, 698, 792, 828
Interleukin-2. *See* Aldesleukin
International Agency for Research on Cancer (IARC), 2:642, 769
International Air Transport Association, 1:436
International Association for Medical Assistance to Travellers, 2:766
International Atomic Energy Agency, 1:352
International Classification of Diseases, 2:823
International Council of Cruise Lines, 2:580
International Federation of Red Cross and Red Crescent Societies (IFRC). *See* Red Cross
International Labor Organization, 1:443
International Mother Earth Day. *See* Earth Day
International Society of Infectious Diseases, 2:580
Intestinal anthrax. *See* Anthrax
Intestinal parasites. *See* Parasites
Iodine, 1:157, 364, 365
    See also Radioactive iodine
Iodine-131. *See* Radioactive iodine
IOM (Institute of Medicine), 1:476
Ionizing radiation, 1:**446–448**
    exposure, 2:638
    in exposure science, 1:294
    injuries, 2:641–646
    leukemia from, 1:476, 481
    non-ionizing radiation *vs.*, 2:576
    See also Background radiation
Ipecac syrup. *See* Syrup of ipecac
IPV (Inactivated polio vaccine), 2:614, 616–617
Iran, 2:649
Iraq, 2:527, 529, 570, 703
IRC (Innocenti Research Centre), 2:773
Ireland, 1:301
Iron, 1:466
Iron (element), 1:6, 404, 406
Irradiation, food. *See* Food irradiation
Irrigation, 1:235, 2:672
Isolation and quarantine (disease control)
    for antimicrobial resistance, 1:44
    for diphtheria, 1:221
    for plague, 2:612
    for radiation exposure, 2:640
    for severe acute respiratory syndrome, 2:679, 680–681
    for smallpox, 2:704

    for tuberculosis, 2:752–753, 758
    for viruses, 2:792
Isoniazid, 1:43, 2:758, 759–760
Israel, 2:649
Itai-itai disease, 1:126, 406
Italy, 1:247
Itraconazole, 1:53
Ivan, 1:432
Ivermectin, 2:657
Ixtoc 1 oil spill, 1:370

J

Jadassohn, Joseph, 2:607
Jail fever. *See* Typhus
James L. Zadroga 9/11 Health and Compensation Act, 2:570, 571
Japan
    bioterrorism in, 1:100
    cadmium poisoning in, 1:126
    cholera in, 1:166
    earthquakes in, 1:247
    Fukushima Daiichi nuclear power station disaster, 1:348–352
    heavy metal poisoning in, 1:406–407
    Japanese earthquake, 1:449–454
    mercury in, 2:526
    mercury poisoning in, 1:355, 2:528, *528*, 529, 531
    tsunamis in, 2:*749*, 750, 752
    Yokkaichi asthma in, 2:829–832
Japanese earthquake (2011), 1:**449–454**, *450*, *452*
    See also Fukushima Daiichi nuclear power station disaster
Japanese Ministry of Health, Labour, and Welfare, 1:452
Japanese puffer fish, 1:332, 2:567
Jarisch-Herxheimer reaction, 1:472–473
Jastrzebowski, Wojciech, 1:282
Jebb, Eglantyne, 2:674, 675
Jenner, Edward, 2:702, 704, 777
Jets. *See* Aircraft
Jock's itch. *See* Tinea cruris
Joint Commission, 1:112
Joint Monitoring Programme for Water Supply and Sanitation, 2:673
Joplin, Missouri, 2:731, *731*
JO-RRP (Juvenile-onset recurrent respiratory paillomatosis). *See* Laryngeal papillomatosis
The Journal of Environmental Health, 2:552
Junk shot, 1:370
Juvenile-onset recurrent respiratory papillomatosis (JO-RRP). *See* Laryngeal papillomatosis

K

Kabul, Afghanistan, 1:23
Kalur v. Resor (1971), 2:661
Kanamycin, 1:43
Kaneko, Youji, 2:*528*
Kanner, Leo, 1:62
Kaposi's sarcoma, 1:12
Karenia brevis, 1:326
Kartulis, S., 1:30
Katayama fever, 2:677
Katrina, 1:5, 432, **455–459,** *456*
  cholera from, 1:166
  disaster preparedness for, 1:225
  flooding from, 1:311, 312
  levees in, 1:*483,* 484
Kefauver-Harris Amendments, 1:323
Kemeny Commission, 2:726, 727
Kennebec River, 1:*211*
Kenya, 1:415, 416, 417, 418, 2:*753*
Ketamine, 2:622
Ketones, 2:706
Key West, FL, 2:787
Kida, Hirotaka, 2:831
Kidney dialysis, 1:126, 173, 394
Kidney disease, chronic. *See* Chronic kidney disease
Kidney failure
  dysentery, 1:170–173, 238
  escherichia coli, 1:285
  food poisoning, 1:335
  Legionnaires' disease, 1:468, 469, 470
  tuberculosis, 2:756
Kimchi, 1:70
Kings Canyon National Park, 2:693
Kiva, 1:430
Kmart, 1:466
Koch, Heinrich Hermann Robert, 2:752
Koch, Robert, 1:166, 189, 272, 2:669
Koplik's spots, 2:508, 509
Korean War, 2:621
Kostina, Yulia, 1:*156*
Krakatoa, 2:751
Kurds, 2:527
Kuru, 1:194
Kwan, Sui-Chu, 2:679
Kwashiorkor. *See* Protein-energy malnutrition
Kyoto Protocol, 1:22
Kyrgyzstan, 2:526

L

Labeling, 1:275, 2:653
Laboratories, 1:98, 99
Lacour, Michael, 2:541
Lactobacillus acidophilus, 1:497, 498, 2:582
Lake Louise Score, 1:29
Lake Mead, 1:211
Lake Ontario, 1:488
Lake Powell, 1:211
Lake Superior, 1:47
Lakes, 1:3, 2:804
Lambl, Vilem Dusan, 1:357
Lancisi, Giovanni Maria, 2:591–592
Land and Water Conservation Fund, 2:693
Land use, 1:**461–462,** *462,* 2:592, 596, 692–693
Language. *See* Communication
Large intestine. *See* Colon
Larvicides. *See* Insecticides
Laryngeal diphtheria. *See* Diphtheria
Laryngeal papillomatosis, 1:426
Larynx, 1:219
Lasers, 1:427
Lassa fever, 1:411, 412, 2:*661,* 662
Last Child in the Woods: Saving Our Children from Nature-Deficit Disorder, 2:560
Latency, 1:46, 49
Latino Americans. *See* Hispanic Americans
Latrines. *See* Sanitation
Latvia, 1:397
Lava, 1:435, 2:793, 794
Law Concerning Compensation for Pollution-Related Health Damages and Other Measures (Japan), 2:831–832
Law Concerning Special Measures for the Relief of Pollution-Related Patients (Japan), 2:831
Lawn chemicals. *See* Yard chemicals
Laws. *See specific laws by name*
Lawsuit settlements and damages. *See* Settlements and damages
Laying Waste: The Poisoning of America by Toxic Chemicals, 1:489
Lead, 1:*462*
  air pollution, 1:23
  Clean Air Act on, 1:176, 177, 178
  drinking water supply, 1:230, 231
  in exposure science, 1:294
  heavy metal poisoning, 1:404, 406, 407, 408, 409
  indoor air quality, 1:439
  industrial hygiene for, 1:442
  lead poisoning, 1:463–467
  National Ambient Air Quality Standard, 2:549, 550
  poisoning, 1:148
  toxicology of, 2:736, 737
Lead poisoning, 1:*463,* **463–467**
  Centers for Disease Control and Prevention and, 1:144
  as chemical poisoning, 1:148
  from drinking water supply, 1:231
  as heavy metal poisoning, 1:406, 407, 408
  from housing, 1:420
  lead in, 1:462
League of Nations, 1:100
Lederberg, Esther, 1:42
Lederberg, Joshua, 1:42
Leeuwenhoek, Anton van, 1:357
Legal settlements. *See* Settlements and damages
Legal settlements and damages. *See* Settlements and damages
Legionella
  cruise ship health, 1:200
  Legionnaires' disease, 1:467–468, 469
  water quality and, 2:804
  as waterborne illness, 2:809
Legionellosis, 1:468
Legionnaires' disease, 1:438, **467–470,** 2:804
Legislation. *See specific laws by name*
Leishmaniasis, 2:663, 745
Lentigo maligna melanoma. *See* Melanoma
Leprosy, 2:746
Leptospira, 1:470, 472, 473
Leptospirosis, 1:**470–474,** 2:662, 746
Leukemia, 1:131, **474–482**
  from benzene, 1:79
  causes, 1:476
  Chernobyl nuclear power station disaster, 1:158
  demographics, 1:475–476
  description, 1:474–475
  diagnosis, 1:476–478
  public health, 1:480–481
  from radiation exposure, 2:639
  symptoms, 1:476
  from Three Mile Island nuclear disaster, 2:726
  treatment, 1:478–480
Leukocytes. *See* Blood cells
Leukotriene receptor agonists, 1:58
Leukotrienes, 1:55, 2:538
Levee, 1:*483,* **483–484**
  Hurricane Katrina, 1:455, 457, 458
  hurricanes and, 1:432–433
  Omnibus Flood Control Act and, 2:591
  Rivers and Harbors Act of 1899, 2:659
Levine, Peter, 2:625
Libby, MT, 1:47
Lice. *See* Parasites
Licorice, 1:60
Licorice root, 2:712
Light radiation. *See* Non-ionizing radiation
Lightning. *See* Electric shock injuries

Lima, Henrique da Rocha, 2:765
Lindane, 1:149
Linezolid, 1:43
Lipodystrophy, 1:16, 18
Liquor, 1:464
Lister, Joseph, 1:484
Listeria
    food contamination, 1:325–326
    food safety and, 1:337, 341
    foodborne illness, 1:343
    listeriosis, 1:484–487
    meningitis, 2:521, 522
Listeria infections. *See* Listeriosis
Listeriosis, 1:**484–488**
    from food contamination, 1:325–326, 327
    food safety and, 1:337
    as foodborne illness, 1:343
Liu, Jianlun, 2:679
Liver
    amebiasis, 1:30, 31, 32
    dysentery, 1:238, 239, 240
    food poisoning, 1:335
    manganese exposure, 2:506, 507
    schistosomiasis, 2:676, 677
Livestock
    disasters
        drought, 1:233
        Horn of Africa drought and famine, 1:417
        Iceland volcano eruption, 1:436
        Seveso, Italy, 2:683
    diseases
        anthrax, 1:37, 38, 39, 40
        brucellosis, 1:115, 116, 117, 118, 119
        Creutzfeldt-Jakob disease, 1:194–195
        flu pandemic, 1:314, 317
        leptospirosis, 1:470–471, 473
        listeriosis, 1:484, 485
        zoonoses, 2:834, 835
    environmental hazards
        agricultural chemicals, 1:6, 7
        antimicrobial resistance, 1:42, 45
        escherichia coli, 1:285
    in exposure science, 1:293
    in One Health Initiative, 2:592, 593
Lloyd, Wray, 2:827
Loa loa, 2:657
Lobelia, 2:712
Loeffler's medium, 1:219
London, England
    air pollution in, 1:21, 22
    disease outbreaks in, 1:226–227
    drinking water supply in, 1:229
    epidemiology in, 1:280
    sanitation in, 2:669
    smog in, 2:*705*, 705–706
    water pollution in, 2:802
    water quality in, 2:803
Long-acting beta agonists, 1:58
Los Angeles, CA, 1:22, 2:705, 706–707

Losch, Fedor Aleksandrovich, 1:30
Lou Gehrig's disease. *See* Amyotrophic lateral sclerosis (ALS)
Louisiana
    Gulf oil spill on, 1:371, 372, 373
    hantavirus infections in, 1:392
    Hurricane Katrina in, 1:455–458
    hurricanes in, 1:432, 433
Louse-borne typhus. *See* Typhus
Louv, Richard, 2:560, 561
Love Canal, 1:**488–493**, *489, 491*
    causes, 1:490
    Centers for Disease Control and Prevention on, 1:144
    Comprehensive Environmental Response, Compensation, and Liability Act, 1:192
    demographics, 1:490
    description, 1:488–490
    hazardous waste in, 1:396
    prevention, 1:491–492
    prognosis, 1:490–491
    public health and, 1:490
    results, 1:490
    treatment of, 1:490
Love, William T., 1:488
Low explosives. *See* Explosives
Low-temperature environments, 1:**493–494**, 2:578
Lumbar puncture. *See* Diagnostic testing
Lungs
    acid rain, 1:4
    altitude sickness, 1:27
    anthrax, 1:39
    asbestos, 1:46, 47
    asbestosis, 1:48–51
    aspergillus, 1:51–54
    asthma, 1:54–61
    avian flu, 1:69
    berylliosis, 1:82–85
    black lung disease, 1:108–110
    bronchitis, 1:110–113
    byssinosis, 1:120–122
    chlorine exposure, 1:164–165
    cutting oil exposure, 1:205
    emphysema, 1:268–271
    fibrosis, 1:308–309
    fungal infections, 1:353
    Legionnaires' disease, 1:468
    mold, 2:537
    9/11 terrorist attacks, 2:571
    ozone exposure, 2:599
    silicosis, 2:694–695
    tuberculosis, 2:756
Lyme disease, 1:**494–500**, *495*
    causes, 1:495
    demographics, 1:494
    description, 1:494–495
    diagnosis, 1:496–497
    as emergent disease, 1:265, 266
    epidemiology of, 1:281
    in One Health Initiative, 2:592

    prevention, 1:499
    prognosis, 1:499
    public health, 1:498–499
    from rodents, 2:663
    symptoms, 1:495–496
    treatment, 1:497–498
    as zoonosis, 2:835
Lymph, 1:475, 2:514–515
Lymph nodes, 1:474, 475, 2:515, 516, 517–518, 520
Lymphatic filariasis, 2:746
Lymphatic system, 1:474–475, 2:639–640
Lymphatic vessels, 1:475
Lymphoblasts. *See* Blood cells
Lymphoma, 1:131
Lynch, Kenneth M, 1:46

M

Ma huang, 1:60
MAC (*Mcobacterium avium* complex), 2:757
Macronutrients, 1:6
Macroparasites. *See* Parasites
Macrophages. *See* Blood cells
Mad cow disease. *See* Creutzfeldt-Jakob disease
Magen David Adom, 2:649
Magma, 2:793, 794
Magnesium, 1:6
Magnetic resonance imaging (MRI). *See* Diagnostic testing; Radiation
Mail, 1:40
Maitotoxin, 1:326
Make-believe. *See* Imaginative play
Malaria, 2:**501–505**, *502*, 503*t*
    amebiasis and, 1:31
    antimicrobial resistance, 1:41
    as communicable disease, 1:189
    disease outbreaks of, 1:227
    as emergent disease, 1:266
    as endemic, 1:271–272
    in flooding, 1:311
    sanitation and, 2:672
    in traveler's health, 2:739–740
    as tropical disease, 2:745, 746, 747, 748
    vector (mosquito) control for, 2:783, 784, 786
    water quality and, 2:804
Malaria ague, 2:502
Malaysia, 2:800
Mali, 1:303, 367
Malignancy. *See* Cancer
Malignant melanoma. *See* Melanoma
Mallon, Mary, 2:762
Malnutrition, protein-energy. *See* Protein-energy malnutrition
Malta fever. *See* Brucellosis

Manganese, 1:6, 404, 406, 2:505–507
Manganese exposure, 2:**505–507**
Mantoux test, 2:757
Manufacturing
 acid rain from, 1:2
 berylliosis from, 1:83
 climate change, 1:*184*
 Federal Insecticide, Fungicide and Rodenticide Act, 1:304–306
 food safety and, 1:338
 water pollution from, 2:801
Manville Corporation, 1:47
Marasmus. *See* Protein-energy malnutrition
Marburg virus, 1:248, 251, 410, 412
Marine ecosystems. *See* Aquatic ecosystems
Marlow syndrome. *See* Shigellosis
Marshall Islands, 2:671
Massachusetts v. EPA (2007), 1:178, 279
Massage, 1:60
Mast cells. *See* Blood cells
Mattel, 1:466
Maunoir, Theodore, 2:648
Mauritania, 1:*233*
Mayo Clinic, 2:761
McKay, Frederick S., 2:797
MCS (Multiple chemical sensitivity). *See* Multiple chemical sensitivity
MDGs (Millennium Development Goals), 2:672, 754, 781
MDR TB (Multi drug-resistant tuberculosis), 2:757, 758, 759
Meadowsweet, 2:582
Measles, 1:265, 2:**507–511**
 Horn of Africa drought and famine, 1:418
 as pandemic, 2:601
 vaccination, 2:778, 779, 781–782
Measles and Rubella (MR) Initiative, 2:781–782
Meat
 brucellosis from, 1:117
 Creutzfeldt-Jakob disease from, 1:193, 194–195, 197
 escherichia coli in, 1:285, 286, 287
 food contamination in, 1:325, 326
 in food poisoning, 1:330
 food safety and, 1:337, 338–339
 foodborne illness from, 1:341, 342, 343
 listeriosis from, 1:484, 485, 487
 mercury poisoning, 2:528
 parasites from, 2:604, 607
 zoonoses from, 2:833, 835
Médecins Sans Frontières. *See* Doctors Without Borders
Medical devices, 1:323
Medical imaging. *See* Diagnostic testing; Radiation
Medical personnel

 antimicrobial resistance and, 1:42
 Japanese earthquake and, 1:451, 452
 medical waste and, 2:512, 513
 severe acute respiratory syndrome, 2:679
 toxicology and, 2:737
 water fluoridation and, 2:799
Medical records, 1:452
Medical testing. *See* Diagnostic testing
Medical toxicology. *See* Toxicology
Medical waste, 2:**511–514**, *512*
 biosafety, 1:97–99
 Resource Conservation and Recovery Act on, 2:650, 651
Medical Waste Tracking Act, 2:511, 513
Medically unexplained illnesses. *See* Gulf War syndrome
Medications. *See* Drugs (medications)
Medicines. *See* Drugs (medications)
Mediterranean fever. *See* Brucellosis
Mediterranean Sea, 2:750
Meeting the MDG Drinking Water and Sanitation Target, 2:673
Mefloquine, 2:504, 505
Megavitamins. *See* Vitamin therapy
Melamine, 1:6–7
Melanin, 2:514, 515
Melanocytes, 2:514, 515
Melanoma, 2:**514–520**, *515*
 as cancer, 1:130, 131
 causes, 2:515
 clinical staging, 2:517
 clinical trials, 2:519–520
 demographics, 2:515
 description, 2:514–515
 diagnosis, 2:516
 from non-ionizing radiation, 2:576
 prevention, 2:520
 prognosis, 2:519
 as skin cancer, 2:696
 symptoms, 2:516
 treatment, 2:517–519
 from ultraviolet radiation, 2:769
Melanoma Intergroup Committee, 2:517
A Memory of Solferino, 2:648
Men
 AIDS, 1:10, 11, 19
 altitude sickness, 1:28
 amebiasis, 1:31, 32
 antimicrobial resistance, 1:41
 bisphenol A and, 1:105, 106
 lead poisoning, 1:465
 leukemia, 1:476
 melanoma, 2:514, 515
 population pyramids, 2:619, 620
 post-traumatic stress disorder, 2:621, 622
 skin cancer, 2:696

Meninges, 2:520, 521, 522, 523, 757
Meningitis, 1:227, 2:**520–525**
 from antimicrobial resistance, 1:43
 causes, 2:521–522
 demographics, 2:521
 description, 2:521–522
 diagnosis, 2:522–523
 as emergent disease, 1:265
 from *escherichia coli*, 1:284, 286, 287
 in leptospirosis, 1:471, 472, 473
 in listeriosis, 1:487
 from mumps, 2:544
 in polio, 2:615
 prevention, 2:524
 prognosis, 2:524
 public health, 2:523–524
 symptoms, 2:522
 treatment, 2:523
Meningitis, West Nile. *See* West Nile virus
Meningoencephalitis, West Nile. *See* West Nile virus
Mental health
 asthma, 1:54, 56, 57
 Chernobyl nuclear power station disaster, 1:158
 electric shock injuries, 1:252
 Gulf oil spill, 1:373–374
 Gulf War syndrome, 1:378, 379
 housing and, 1:421
 Hurricane Katrina, 1:457, 458
 Japanese earthquake, 1:453
 multiple chemical sensitivity, 2:542–543
 nature deficit disorder and, 2:561–563
 9/11 terrorist attacks, 2:570–571
 noise pollution, 2:573, 574
 oil spills, 2:587, 588, 589, 590
 post-traumatic stress disorder, 2:620–626
 Three Mile Island nuclear disaster, 2:727
Mercalli scale, 1:246, 247
Merck, 2:657
Mercuric chloride, 2:527, 532
Mercuric oxide, 2:527, 532
Mercury, 2:**525–527**
 chemical poisoning from, 1:149, 153
 in fungicides, 1:354–355
 in heavy metal poisoning, 1:404, 405, 406, 407, 408, 409
 in medical waste, 2:513
 poisoning, 2:527–533
 toxicology of, 2:737
Mercury poisoning, 2:**527–534**, *528*
 causes, 2:529
 demographics, 2:529
 description, 2:527–529
 diagnosis, 2:530–531
 as heavy metal poisoning, 1:406–407, 408

Mercury poisoning *(continued)*
  mercury in, 2:525–526
  prevention, 2:532–533
  prognosis, 2:532
  public health, 2:531–532
  symptoms, 2:529–530
  treatment, 2:531
Mercury Poisoning Linked to Skin Products, 2:529
Mesothelioma, 1:46, 49
Metabolomics, 1:90
Metallic mercury. *See* Mercury
Metalloids. *See* Heavy metals
Metalworkers, 1:204, 205
Metamorphic rocks. *See* Rocks
Metamorphism, 1:415
Metastasis, 2:514, 515, 516, 517, 518, 519
Methacholine, 1:122
Methadone, 1:152
Methamphetamine, 1:10
Methane, 1:347, 348
Methemoglobin, 2:534–535
Methemoglobinemia, 1:207, 2:**534–536**
Methicillin-resistant *staphylococcus aureus* (MRSA), 1:43, 265, 266, 2:565
Methyl chloroform, 1:178
Methyl isocyanate, 1:86–88
Methylbenzene. *See* Toluene
Methylene blue, 2:534, 535
Methylmercury. *See* Mercury
Methyl-t-butyl ether (MTBE), 2:668
Metrifonate, 2:677, 678
Metronidazole, 1:32, 2:606
Mexico, 1:31, 190, 272, 381–382, 458
Mexico City, Mexico, 1:23, 2:707
MHSA (Mine Safety and Health Administration), 1:109, 2:695
Mice. *See* Rodents
Microbes, drug-resistant. *See* Antimicrobial resistance
Microbial pathogens, 2:**536**
  antimicrobial resistance of, 1:45
  biosafety and, 1:97–99
  brucellosis, 1:116
  cholera, 1:166–167, 168
  communicable diseases, 1:189, 190
  diphtheria, 1:218, 219
  disease outbreaks, 1:226
  drinking water supply, 1:229, 230
  drought, 1:233
  dysentery, 1:236, 237–238
  emergent diseases, 1:265
  epidemiology, 1:279–281
  exposure science, 1:292
  food additives and, 1:318–319
  food contamination from, 1:324–327, 328
  food poisoning, 1:330, 331–332, 334
  food safety and, 1:336, 337
  foodborne illness, 1:341–343, 342*t*, 344, 345
  Gulf oil spill, 1:374
  Gulf War syndrome, 1:378
  heavy metal poisoning, 1:405
  high temperature environments, 1:414
  indoor air quality, 1:438
  Legionnaires' disease, 1:467, 468
  leptospirosis, 1:470, 471
  listeriosis, 1:484–485
  low-temperature environments, 1:493
  meningitis, 2:520–521, 521–522
  necrotizing fasciitis, 2:564, 565
  ozone on, 2:598
  from rodents, 2:662–663
  sanitation on, 2:671–672
  sick building syndrome, 2:690
  toxic sludge spill in Hungary, 2:732
  traveler's health, 2:739, 740
  tropical disease, 2:744, 745–746, 747, 748
  tuberculosis, 2:752
  typhoid fever, 2:761, 762
  water pollution from, 2:799–800
  water quality standards on, 2:806, 807
  waterborne illness from, 2:807, 808–809
  zoonoses from, 2:833
  See also specific pathogens by name
Microbiome, 1:292
Microbiomics, 1:90
Microlending, 1:430
Micronesia, 2:671
Micronutrients, 1:6, 406
Microparasites. *See* Parasites
Microscopy, diagnostic. *See* Diagnostic testing
Microvilli, 2:572, 573
Microwave radiation. *See* Non-ionizing radiation
Middle East, 1:69, 272
Migration, forced. *See* Population displacement
Mildew. *See* Mold
Military conflict. *See* War
Military forces. *See* Armed forces
Military tuberculosis. *See* Tuberculosis
Milk. *See* Dairy products
Milk thistle, 1:152, 153
Millennium Development Goals (MDGs), 2:672, 754, 781
Milwaukee River, 1:*180*
Milwaukee, Wisconsin, 2:670
Minamata disease, 1:406–407, 2:526, 528, *528*, 531
Mind/body medicine. *See* Complementary and alternative medicine (CAM)
Mine fields, 1:*289*
Mine Safety and Health Administration (MHSA), 1:109, 2:695
Minerals, 1:74
Miners, coal. *See* Coal miners and mining
Mining, coal. *See* Coal miners and mining
Miracidium, 2:676
Miscarriage. *See* Pregnancy
Mississippi, 1:455
Missouri, 2:729–730
Mitchell, George, 1:177
Mites. *See* Parasites
Mitigation (environmental), 1:259–260, 371–372
Miyako City, Japan, 2:*749*
MMR (Mumps, measles, rubella) vaccination, 2:510, 546, 779
Mobile phones. *See* Cellular phones
Model Food Code, 1:129
Modified vaccinia Ankara 85A (MVA85A), 2:759
Mohammed, Khalid Sheikh, 2:570
Mohs' surgery, 2:698
Moisture in the air. *See* Humidity
Mold, 2:**536–540**
  asthma, 1:56
  from flooding, 1:311
  food contamination from, 1:326
  indoor air quality, 1:437, 438, 439
Molecular modeling. *See* Protein modeling
Moles, 2:514, 515–516
Molina, Mario J., 2:556
Molybdenum, 1:404, 406, 407
Monarch of the Seas (ship), 1:199
Monkeypox, 2:593
Monkeys. *See* Primates
Monoclonal antibodies, 1:479
Monocytes. *See* Blood cells
Monongahela virus, 1:392
Monosodium glutamate (MSG), 1:149, 321
Montagu, Mary Wortley, 2:777
Montelukast, 2:538
Moose. *See* Wildlife
Morphine, 1:152
Mortality rates, 1:161, 2:619–620, 675, 832
MOSOP (Movement for the Survival of the Ogoni People), 2:589
Mosquitoes
  communicable diseases, 1:189
  dengue fever from, 1:214–217
  emergent diseases, 1:265, 266, 267

Mosquitoes *(continued)*
  epidemiology, 1:281
  hemorrhagic fevers from, 1:410, 413
  Hurricane Katrina, 1:457
  malaria from, 2:501–505
  One Health Initiative, 2:592
  as parasites, 2:604
  tropical disease, 2:745, 748
  vector (mosquito) control, 2:783–787
  West Nile virus, 2:812
  yellow fever, 2:825
Motion, 2:575
Motor vehicles. *See* Automobiles
Mould, Richard, 1:156–157
Mount Rainier, 2:693
Mount St. Helens, 2:*795*
Mountain climbing, 1:27, 28, 29
Movement for the Survival of the Ogoni People (MOSOP), 2:589
Moynier, Gustave, 2:648
MR (Measles and Rubella Initiative), 2:781–782
MRI (Magnetic resonance imaging). *See* Diagnostic testing; Radiation
MRSA (Methicillin-resistant *staphylococcus aureus*), 1:43, 265, 266, 2:565
MSG (Monosodium glutamate), 1:149, 321
MTBE (Methyl-t-butyl ether), 2:668
Mucormycosis, 2:731
Muir, John, 2:693
Multi drug-resistant tuberculosis (MDR TB), 2:757, 758, 759
Multidrug-resistant bacteria. *See* Antimicrobial resistance
Multiple chemical sensitivity, 1:438, 2:**540–543**
Mumps, 2:**543–547**
Mumps, measles, rubella (MMR) vaccination, 2:510, 546, 779
Murine typhus. *See* Typhus
Murrell, Hugh, 1:282
Museums, 1:24, 437
Mushrooms, 1:330, 332, 334–335, 343, 345
Muskie, Edmund, 1:176
Mutation
  antimicrobial resistance and, 1:42, 43
  in avian flu, 1:68
  background radiation and, 1:74
  from benzene exposure, 1:80, 81
  bioinformatics and, 1:91
  in cancer, 1:131
  chlorination and, 1:163
  in Creutzfeldt-Jakob disease, 1:196
  of emergent diseases, 1:264, 266–267
  in flu pandemic, 1:313–314, 315
  from ionizing radiation, 1:446
  in melanoma, 2:516
  in noroviruses, 2:580
  from radiation injuries, 2:643
  of viruses, 2:791
MVA85A (Modified vaccinia Ankara 85A), 2:759
Mycobacteria. *See* Microbial pathogens
Mycobacterium avium complex (MAC), 2:757
Mycobacterium tuberculosis, 2:752, 757
Mycoplasma fermentans, 1:378, 379
Mycoses. *See* Fungal infections
Mycotoxins, 2:536
Myocarditis, 1:218, 220
Myoclonus, 1:196
Myopia, 2:561

N

NAAQS (National Ambient Air Quality Standard). *See* National Ambient Air Quality Standard (NAAQS)
NACDG (North American Contact Dermatitis Group), 2:607
Nader, Ralph, 1:278, *278*
Nagal, Isamu, 2:*528*
Nagana disease, 2:699
Nagasaki, Japan, 2:638, *638*
Nail infections, 1:353
Nails, 2:520
Nairoviruses, 1:411–412
Naloxone, 1:152
Nanotubes, 1:48
NAPAP (National Acidic Precipitation Assessment Program). *See* National Acidic Precipitation Assessment Program (NAPAP)
Naphthalene, 1:79, 80
NASA (National Aeronautics and Space Administration), 1:401
Nasal diphtheria. *See* Diphtheria
National Academy of Engineers, 1:230
National Academy of Sciences, 1:321
National Acidic Precipitation Assessment Program (NAPAP), 1:4
National Aeronautics and Space Administration (NASA), 1:401
National Ambient Air Quality Standard (NAAQS), 2:**549–551**
  Clean Air Act and, 1:176–177, 178
  on lead, 1:462
  on smog, 2:708
National Biomonitoring Program, 1:95–96
National Brownfield Association, 1:115
National Brucellosis Eradication Program, 1:118
National Capital Poison Center, 1:150
National Center for Health Statistics, 1:111
National Center for PTSD, 2:626
National Center for Toxicological Research, 1:322, 2:558
National Children's Study, 1:95
National Clearinghouse for Worker Safety and Health Training, 2:558, 559
National Commission on the BP *Deepwater Horizon* Oil Spill and Offshore Drilling, 1:372, 375–376
National Commission on Water Quality, 1:181
National Counterterrorism Center, 2:571
National Disaster Medical System, 1:373
National Environmental Education Foundation, 2:562–563
National Environmental Health Association, 2:**551–552**
National Environmental Policy Act (1969), 1:278, 2:**552–554**, 693
National Guard, 1:261
National Institute for Occupational Safety and Health, 1:**554–555**
  on acetone, 1:1
  on asbestos, 1:46
  on asbestosis, 1:50
  on black lung disease, 1:109
  on bronchitis, 1:112
  on carbon monoxide poisoning, 1:138
  on cellular phones, 1:141
  Centers for Disease Control and Protection and, 1:143
  on chlorine exposure, 1:164
  on cutting oil exposure, 1:206
  on emphysema, 1:271
  on ergonomics, 1:283
  on Gulf oil spill, 1:374
  on indoor air quality, 1:437–438
  on insecticide poisoning, 1:445
  on Love Canal, 1:492
  National Institute of Environmental Health Sciences and, 1:558–559
  on sick building syndrome, 2:691
  on silicosis, 2:695
  on talcosis, 2:722
National Institute of Environmental Health Sciences (Research Triangle Park, NC), 1:105, 2:**556–559**
National Institute of Mental Health (NIMH), 2:622
National Institutes of Health (NIH)
  on AIDS, 1:19
  on biosafety, 1:98
  on cancer, 1:135

National Institutes of Health (NIH) (continued)
  National Institute of Environmental Health Sciences and, 2:556
  on oil spills, 2:588–589
  population pyramid from, 2:619
  on typhoid fever, 2:762
National Notifiable Diseases Surveillance System, 1:394
National Occupational Research Agenda (NORA), 2:555
National Oceanic and Atmospheric Administration (NOAA), 1:222, 403
National Park Service, 2:559, 693
National parks, 2:**559–560**
  brucellosis in, 1:118
  Clean Air Act, 1:177
  emergent disease in, 1:265
  hemorrhagic fevers in, 1:412
  Sierra Club and, 2:692, 693
  See also specific parks by name
National Pharmaceutical Stockpile, 1:38
National Poison Data System, 2:532
National Pollutant Discharge Elimination System (NPDES), 2:802
National Priorities List, 1:278–279, 2:717, 718
National Red Cross Societies. *See* Red Cross
National Safety Council, 1:255
National Toxicology Program (NTP), 1:105, 106, 141, 2:556, 557–558
National Vietnam Veteran Readjustment Survey, 2:621
National Weather Service (NWS), 1:311, 401, 2:731
National Wilderness Preservation System, 2:693
National Wildlife Federation (NWF), 2:561, 562, 563
National Wildlife Health Center, 1:175
Native Americans
  AIDS and, 1:10
  bioterrorism against, 1:100
  communicable diseases and, 1:189
  post-traumatic stress disorder in, 2:621, 625
  Safe Drinking Water Act and, 2:668
  smoking among, 2:710
Natural disasters. *See* Disaster preparedness; *specific disasters by name*
Natural gas, 1:346, 347, 348
Natural killer (NK) cells. *See* Blood cells
Natural selection, 1:42
Natural toxins. *See* Toxins
The Nature Conservancy, 2:561
Nature deficit disorder, 2:**560–564**

The Nature Principle: Human Restoration and the End of Nature-Deficit Disorder, 2:561
Naturopathic medicine. *See* Complementary and alternative medicine (CAM)
Navigation, 2:658–661
NDD (Nature deficit disorder). *See* Nature deficit disorder
Neanderthals, 1:93
Near ultraviolet radiation. *See* Ultraviolet radiation
Nearsightedness. *See* Myopia
Nebulizers, 1:53, 122
Necrosis. *See* Necrotizing fasciitis
Necrotizing colitis. *See* Colitis
Necrotizing fasciitis, 1:43, 2:**564–566**
Nedocromil, 1:58
Neglected tropical diseases (NGDs). *See* Tropical disease
NEHA (National Environmental Health Association). *See* National Environmental Health Association
Neisseria gonorrhoeae, 1:43
Neisseria meningitidis, 1:265, 2:522, 523
Nelson, Gaylord, 1:243
Nematicides. *See* Agricultural chemicals
Nematodes. *See* Parasites
Neoadjuvant chemotherapy. *See* Chemotherapy
Neonicotinoids. *See* Neonics
Neonics, 1:186–187, 188
NEPA (National Environmental Policy Act). *See* National Environmental Policy Act (1969)
Nepal, 1:357
Nephropathia epidemica, 1:392
Nerve agents, 1:377, 378
Nerve toxin. *See* Neurotoxin
Nervous system
  benzene exposure, 1:80
  electric shock injuries, 1:254
  Gulf War syndrome, 1:378
  heavy metal poisoning, 1:407, 408
  insecticide poisoning, 1:444
  listeriosis, 1:485, 486
  manganese exposure, 2:506–507
  neurotoxins, 2:567–568
  parasites, 2:604–605
Neuraminidase, 1:68, 383
Neurobrucellosis. *See* Brucellosis
Neurotoxic shellfish poisoning, 1:26, 326
Neurotoxin, 2:**567–568**
  algal bloom, 1:25, 26
  chemical poisoning, 1:148
  drinking water supply, 1:231
  food contamination, 1:326
  food poisoning, 1:331, 332
  Gulf War syndrome, 1:377, 378
New Delhi, India, 1:23

New England Compounding Center, 2:523, 524
New Jersey, 1:439
New Orleans, LA
  flooding, 1:311, 312
  Hurricane Katrina, 1:455–458
  hurricanes, 1:432
  levees, 1:*483*, 484
New Source Performance Standards, 1:177
New York, 1:443, 488–492
New York City Department of Health and Mental Hygiene, 2:570
New York, NY, 2:568–571, *569*
New York State Department of Health, 1:490
New York virus, 1:392
New Zealand, 1:357, 387
NF (Necrotizing fasciitis). *See* Necrotizing fasciitis
NGDs (Neglected tropical diseases). *See* Tropical disease
NGOs (Nongovernmental organizations). *See specific organizations by name*
Niagara Falls, NY, 1:488–492
Niagara River, 1:488
Nicaragua, 1:172
Nickel, 1:404, 406, 407
Nicotine, 2:709, 710, 712
Nicotine replacement therapy, 2:711
Niemann-Pick C1, 1:251
Niger, 1:303
Nigeria, 1:407, *463*, 2:589, 614
Nightmares, 2:620, 623
NIH (National Institutes of Health). *See* National Institutes of Health (NIH)
NIMH (National Institute of Mental Health), 2:622
La Niña, 1:234
9/11 Commission, 2:570
9/11 terrorist attacks, 2:**568–571**, *569*
El Niño, 1:234, 433
NIOSH (National Institute for Occupational Safety and Health). *See* National Institute for Occupational Safety and Health
Nipah virus, 1:265
Nitazoxanide, 1:238
Nitrates
  chemical poisoning, 1:149
  cyanosis, 1:207, 208
  drinking water supply, 1:231
  methemoglobinemia, 2:534, 535
Nitric acid, 1:1, 2, 4, 2:706
Nitrites
  cyanosis, 1:207, 208
  drinking water supply, 1:231
  food additives, 1:321
  methemoglobinemia, 2:534

Nitrogen, 1:6, 212–214, 2:804
Nitrogen dioxide, 1:23, 176, 2:706
Nitrogen oxides
    acid rain, 1:1, 4
    air pollution, 1:21, 22, 23, 24
    Clean Air Act on, 1:177, 178
    explosives, 1:288
    indoor air quality, 1:437, 438
    National Ambient Air Quality Standard, 2:549, 550
    smog, 2:707, 708
    volatile organic compounds and, 2:793
Nitroglycerin, 1:288, 290
Nitrosamines, 1:320
Nixon, Richard M., 1:176, 179, 276, 2:661
NK (Natural killer) cells. *See* Blood cells
N,N- Diethyl-p-phenylenediamine (DND), 1:163
N,N-diethyl-m-toluamide (DEET), 2:785
No Child Left Inside Coalition, 2:562
NOAA (National Oceanic and Atmospheric Administration), 1:222, 403
Nobel, Alfred, 1:288
Noda, Yoshihiko, 1:453
Noise pollution, 2:**571–575,** *572*
Nongovernmental organizations (NGOs). *See specific organizations by name*
Non-Hodgkins' lymphoma, 1:476
Non-ionizing radiation, 1:140, 2:**575–577,** 597
    See also Radiofrequency energy
Nonlymphocytic leukemia. *See* Leukemia
Non-nucleoside reverse transcriptase inhibitors, 1:14
Non-point source pollution
    Clean Water Act, 1:181, 182
    drinking water supply, 1:229, 230, 231
    drought, 1:233
    Federal Water Act, 1:306
    from fracking, 1:348
    Rivers and Harbors Act of 1899, 2:661
    as water pollution, 2:801, 802
    on water quality, 2:803–804
    water quality standards for, 2:806
Nonprofit organizations. *See specific organizations by name*
NORA (National Occupational Research Agenda), 2:555
Normix. *See* Rifamixin
Noroviruses, 2:**577–584**
    causes, 2:580
    in children, 2:578
    cruise ship health, 1:198, 199, 200, 201
    demographics, 2:577
    description, 2:578–580
    diagnosis, 2:581–582
    in dysentery, 1:237
    food contamination from, 1:325
    food poisoning from, 1:332
    food safety and, 1:338
    foodborne illness from, 1:341, 344
    prevention, 2:583–584
    prognosis, 2:582–583
    public health, 2:582
    symptoms, 2:580–581
    treatment, 2:582
    water quality and, 2:804
    as waterborne illnesses, 2:809
North America, 1:2, 3, 197
North American Contact Dermatitis Group (NACDG), 2:607
Norwalk agent, 2:740
Norwalk viruses. *See* Noroviruses
Nosocomial infections, 1:41, 44
NPDES (National Pollutant Discharge Elimination System), 2:802
NRC (U.S. Nuclear Regulatory Commission). *See* U.S. Nuclear Regulatory Commission
NRDC (U.S. Natural Resources Defense Council), 2:526
NTP (National Toxicology Program). *See* National Toxicology Program
Nuclear and Industrial Safety Agency, 1:350
Nuclear bombs. *See* Atomic bombs
Nuclear explosives. *See* Atomic bombs
Nuclear power stations, 1:144, 149, 2:642, 643
    See also Chernobyl nuclear power station disaster; Fukushima Daiichi nuclear power station disaster; Three Mile Island nuclear disaster
Nuclear radiation, medical. *See* Radiation
Nuclear reactors. *See* Nuclear power stations
Nuclear Safety Commission (Japan), 1:452
Nucleic acids. *See* DNA; RNA
Nucleocapsids, 2:788
Nucleoside reverse transcriptase inhibitors, 1:14
Nurses. *See* Medical personnel
Nutrient additives, 1:320
Nutrition. *See* Diet and nutrition
NWF (National Wildlife Federation), 2:561, 562, 563
NWS (National Weather Service), 1:311, 401, 2:731

O

Obama, Barack
    on Clean Air Act, 1:178
    on Clean Water Act, 1:181
    on emergency preparedness, 1:260
    on food safety, 1:337
    on Gulf oil spill, 1:372
    on hurricanes, 1:432, 2:570
    on 9/11 terrorist attacks, 2:570
Obama, Michelle, 2:561, 562
Obesity, 1:170, 272, 2:560, 561, 562
Occidental Petroleum, 1:491
Occupational diseases. *See specific diseases by name*
Occupational health and safety. *See* Workplace safety
Occupational hygiene. *See* Industrial hygiene
Occupational medicine. *See* Industrial medicine
Occupational Safety and Health Act (1970), 2:**585**
    Environmental Protection Agency and, 1:278
    National Institute for Occupational Safety and Health and, 2:555
    Occupational Safety and Health Administration and, 2:585, 586
Occupational Safety and Health Administration, 1:**585–587**
    on ammonia exposure, 1:35
    on asbestos, 1:47
    on asbestosis, 1:50
    on berylliosis, 1:84
    on byssinosis, 1:122
    on carbon monoxide poisoning, 1:137, 138
    on chlorine exposure, 1:164
    on electric shock injuries, 1:255
    on ergonomics, 1:282
    on exposure science, 1:291
    on fibrosis, 1:309
    on Gulf oil spill, 1:373
    on heavy metal poisoning, 1:409
    on indoor air quality, 1:437, 439
    on ionizing radiation, 1:447
    on lead poisoning, 1:466
    on Love Canal, 1:492
    on manganese exposure, 2:507
    on medical waste, 2:513
    National Institute for Occupational Safety and Health and, 2:555
    on neurotoxins, 2:568
    on noise pollution, 2:573
    Occupational Safety and Health Act and, 1:585
    on silica, 2:695
    on talcosis, 2:722
Oceans, 2:801, 805

Ofatumumab, 1:479
Office of Noise Abatement and Control (ONAC), 2:574
Office of Regulatory Affairs, 1:322
Off-label drug use, 1:42
Offshore drilling, 1:375–376
See also Oil spills, health effects of
Ogoni people, 2:589
OHI (One Health Initiative). See One Health Initiative
Ohio, 1:443
Oil, crude. See Crude oil
Oil Pollution Act, 1:299
Oil spills, health effects of, 2:**587–590**
    in exposure science, 1:293–294
    Federal Water Act, 1:307
    Rivers and Harbors Act of 1899, 2:661
    See also Crude oil; *Exxon Valdez*; Gulf oil spill
Oklahoma, 1:392
Older people
    AIDS in, 1:10, 11–12, 18, 19
    amebiasis in, 1:30, 31, 32
    asthma in, 1:59
    carbon monoxide poisoning, 1:136
    cholera in, 1:166, 167
    dysentery in, 1:240
    escherichia coli in, 1:285, 287
    food contamination and, 1:327
    food poisoning in, 1:330, 331
    global public health on, 1:362
    heat disorders in, 1:398, 399
    leukemia in, 1:474, 475
    listeriosis in, 1:485
    meningitis in, 2:522
    in population pyramids, 2:619–620
    post-traumatic stress disorder in, 2:621
    protein-energy malnutrition in, 2:627
    skin cancer in, 2:696, 697
    smog and, 2:707
    tuberculosis in, 2:754
    typhus in, 2:767
    West Nile virus in, 2:813
Olin Corporation, 1:488
Olympic National Park, 2:693
Omnibus Flood Control Act (1936), 1:483, 2:**591**
ONAC (Office of Noise Abatement and Control), 2:574
Onchocerca volvulus, 2:655, 656, 657
Onchocerciacis Control Programme, 2:657
Onchocerciasis. See River blindness
Onchocerciasis Elimination Program for the Americas, 2:657
One Health Initiative, 2:**591–594**
Oophoritis, 2:544
Opium, 1:239

Optical radiation. See Non-ionizing radiation
OPV (Oral polio vaccine), 2:616, 617
Oral candidiasis. See Thrush
Oral polio vaccine (OPV), 2:616, 617
Oral rehydration therapy. See Dehydration and rehydration
Oral thrush. See Thrush
Orchitis, 2:544, 545
Orders of prohibition, 1:45
Organ and tissue transplants
    for aspergillosis, 1:52
    for chronic kidney disease, 1:170
    Creutzfeldt-Jakob disease from, 1:194
    for emphysema, 1:270
    for fibrosis, 1:309
    for leukemia, 1:478, 479, 480
    parasites from, 2:604
Organic food. See Food
Organic mercury. See Mercury
Organizing for emergencies. See Emergency preparedness
Organophosphates. See Insecticides
Osaka Prefectural Institute of Public Health, 2:581
Oseltamivir, 1:70, 384
OSHA (Occupational Safety and Health Administration). See Occupational Safety and Health Administration
Osler, William, 1:30, 2:592
Osteoarthritis, 1:283
OTC (Over-the-counter) drugs. See Drugs (medications)
Outbreak Surveillance and Response in Humanitarian Emergencies, 2:767
Outdoor education, 2:560–563
Ovaries, 2:544, 756
Overdoses, drug. See Drug use
Overpopulation, 1:301–302
Over-the-counter drugs. See Drugs (medications)
Oxamniquine, 2:677–678
Oxfam, 1:390, 415, 2:**594–597**
Oxfam America, 2:596–597
Oxford University, 2:759
Oxidation, 1:162, 405, 2:598, 705, 706
Oxitec, 2:785, 787
Oxygen
    algal bloom, 1:26
    altitude sickness, 1:27–29
    carbon monoxide poisoning, 1:136–137, 138
    cyanosis, 1:206, 207
    food poisoning, 1:331
    ozone, 2:598, 599
    water pollution, 2:802
    water quality, 2:803
Oxygen therapy
    for bronchitis, 1:112

    for byssinosis, 1:122
    for carbon monoxide poisoning, 1:138
    for decompression sickness, 1:213
    for emphysema, 1:270
    for methemoglobinemia, 2:535
Oysters. See Shellfish
Ozone, 2:**597–598**
    acid rain and, 1:3
    Clean Air Act on, 1:176, 178
    exposure, 2:598–600
    heat (stress) index and, 1:401
    indoor air quality, 1:438
    National Ambient Air Quality Standard, 2:549, 550
    from oil spills, 2:590
    smog, 2:706, 707
    ultraviolet radiation and, 2:769, 770
    volatile organic compounds and, 2:793
Ozone exposure, 2:**598–600**

P

Pacemakers, 1:142, 220
Pacific Islands, 2:670–671
Pacific Ocean, 1:234, 350, 2:750, 751, 752
Pacific Tsunami Warning Center, 2:751, 752
Pain, 1:252
Paints, 1:294, 463–464, 465
Pakistan, 1:247, 311, 362, 367, 2:529, 614
Palua, 2:672
PAN (Peroxyacetyl nitrate), 1:23, 2:706
Pan American Health Organization, 1:34
Pandemic, 2:**601–602**
    AIDS, 1:8–9, 10
    cholera, 1:166
    plague, 2:610
    See also Flu pandemic
Pap smear, 1:427
Papanikolaou test. See Pap smear
Paracelsus, 1:443, 2:527, 735
Paralysis, 1:332, 2:613–614, 615, 616, 813–814
Paralytic polio. See Polio
Paralytic shellfish poisoning, 1:326
Paramyxovirus, 2:508, 544
Paraquat, 1:444
Parasites, 2:*602*, **602–607**, 603*t*
    AIDS, 1:11
    amebiasis, 1:30–33
    causes, 2:604
    cryptosporidiosis, 1:202
    demographics, 2:602–603

Parasites *(continued)*
   description, 2:603–604
   diagnosis, 2:605
   dysentery, 1:235, 236, 237–238, 240–241
   emergent diseases, 1:265
   food contamination, 1:324, 325, 326
   food poisoning, 1:332
   giardiasis, 1:357, 359
   guinea worm disease, 1:366–367
   malaria, 2:501–502, 503, 504
   as microbial pathogens, 2:536
   prevention, 2:606–607
   river blindness, 2:655, 656
   sanitation on, 2:671, 673
   symptoms, 2:604–605
   treatment, 2:605–606
   tropical disease, 2:745–746
   typhus, 2:765–766
   waterborne illness, 2:809
   zoonoses, 2:833, 835
   See also specific parasites by name
Parasitoids, 2:605
Paregoric, 1:239
Park, national. *See* National park
Parkinson's disease, 2:567
Parotid glands. *See* Salivary glands
Paroxysmal coughing. *See* Whooping cough
Partial pressure, 1:27
Particulates. *See* Air pollution
Partnership for Maternal, Newborn, and Child Health, 1:161
Parvoviruses, 2:740
Pasig River, 2:800–801
Passive smoking. *See* Smoking
Pasteur, Louis, 1:38
Pasteurella pestis. See Yersinia pestis
Pasteurellosis, 2:592
Pasteurization
   brucellosis, 1:116, 117, 119
   escherichia coli, 1:286
   food poisoning, 1:330, 333
   foodborne illness, 1:345
   listeriosis, 1:485, 487
Patch testing, 2:**607–610**
Pathogens, microbial. *See* Microbial pathogens
Patrick, William, 1:102
Pavillion, WY, 1:348
PCBs (Polychlorinated biphenyls), 1:22, 275, 2:734, 738
PCR (Polymerase chain reaction testing). *See* Diagnostic testing
PDT (Photodynamic therapy), 1:426
Peak flow meters, 1:57, 59
Peebles, Thomas C, 2:508
PEM (Protein-energy malnutrition). *See* Protein-energy malnutrition
Pemethrin, 1:77
Penicillamine, 1:465–466

Penicillin, 1:42, 43, 220, 286, 2:523
Pennsylvania, 1:392, 2:724, 725, 726, 727
Pentagon (building), 2:568–571
Pentamidine, 2:700
Peppermint, 1:385
Pepto-Bismol. *See* Bismuth subsalicylate
Perception, sensory. *See* Sensory perception
Perfluorooctane, 1:170
Perfluorooctane sulfonate, 1:293
Peritonitis, 2:762
Permethrin, 2:785
Permits. *See* Government regulation
Peroxyacetyl nitrate (PAN), 1:23, 2:706
Persistent organic pollutants, 1:275
Personal hygiene
   amebiasis, 1:33
   anthrax, 1:40
   antimicrobial resistance, 1:42, 43, 45
   bronchitis, 1:113
   campylobacteriosis, 1:129
   Creutzfeldt-Jakob disease, 1:197
   cruise ship health, 1:198, 199, 200, 201
   cryptosporidiosis, 1:203
   drought, 1:233
   dysentery, 1:239–240, 241
   escherichia coli, 1:286, 287
   flu pandemic, 1:316
   food contamination, 1:326
   food poisoning, 1:332, 334, 335
   food safety, 1:338
   foodborne illness, 1:343, 345
   fungal infections, 1:354
   giardiasis, 1:360
   H1N1 influenza A, 1:385
   lead poisoning, 1:466
   listeriosis, 1:487
   meningitis, 2:524
   necrotizing fasciitis, 2:566
   noroviruses, 2:579, 583–584
   parasites, 2:604, 606–607
   sanitation, 2:672, 673
   shigellosis, 2:685, 686, 687–688
   typhoid fever, 2:761, 762
   viruses, 2:782
   waterborne illness, 2:811
   See also Industrial hygiene
Pertussis. *See* Whooping cough
Pest control, 1:75–76, 77–78, 355
Pest management, integrated. *See* Integrated pest management
Pesticide poisoning. *See* Insecticide poisoning
Pesticide Registration Improvement Act, 1:306
Pesticides. *See* Agricultural chemicals
PET (Positron emission tomography scans). *See* Diagnostic testing; Radiation

Petechiae, 1:216, 393, 410, 411
Petrochemicals, 2:829, 830
Petroleum. *See* Crude oil
Pets. *See* Domestic animals
pH scale, 1:1, 2, 2:732
Phage therapy, 1:45
Phages, bacterial. *See* Microbial pathogens
Phagocytes, 2:762
Phagocytosis, 1:468
Pharmacies, 2:523–524
Pharyngeal diphtheria. *See* Diphtheria
Pharynx, 1:219
Phenol, 1:80, 348
Philadelphia chromosome, 1:476, 477, 478, 480
Philippines, 2:800–801
Phleboviruses, 1:411, 2:746
Phones, cellular. *See* Cellular phones
Phosphorus, 1:6, 171
Phosphorus-32, 2:636
Photochemical smog. *See* Smog
Photochemicals, 1:22
Photodynamic therapy, 2:698
Photodynamic therapy (PDT), 1:426
Physicians. *See* Medical personnel
Physicians for Social Responsibility, 2:727
Physiologically based pharmacokinetic model, 1:292
Phytolacca, 2:545
Phytoremediation, 1:407
Pica, 1:464
Pickling, 1:318–319
Pilots, 1:212
Pinworms. *See* Parasites
Plague, 2:**610–613**
   as bioterrorism, 1:100, 102
   as emergent disease, 1:264
   as pandemic, 2:601
   from rodents, 2:662
   as zoonosis, 2:833, 835
Planning, disaster. *See* Disaster preparedness
Planning, emergency. *See* Emergency preparedness
Plants (organisms)
   acid rain on, 1:2–3
   agricultural chemicals on, 1:5–8
   for dysentery, 1:239
   fungicide on, 1:355
   heavy metal poisoning of, 1:406, 407
   in low-temperature environments, 1:493
   parasites in, 2:605
Plasmids, 1:42
Plasmodium, 1:265, 2:501, 502–504, 783
Plastics, 1:22, 104–105, 2:723–724

Platelets. *See* Blood cells
Play, 2:560–563
Play, imaginative. *See* Imaginative play
Plinian eruptions. *See* Volcanic eruptions
Pliny the Elder, 1:442
Pliny the Younger, 2:793
Plumbing, 1:231, 294, 464
Pneumoconioses. *See* Silicosis
Pneumocystis jirovecii, 1:12, 14
Pneumonia
    AIDS, 1:12, 14, 18
    aspergillosis, 1:52
    avian flu, 1:69
    flu pandemic, 1:315, 316
    H1N1 influenza A, 1:381, 385
    Legionnaires' disease as, 1:467–470
    severe acute respiratory syndrome, 2:679, 680, 681
Pneumonic plague. *See* Plague
Podofilox, 1:427
Point source pollution, 2:801, 802
Poison centers
    for chemical poisoning, 1:146, 150, 151, 153–154
    for mercury poisoning, 2:531–532, 534
    for toxicology, 2:737
Poisoning. *See specific types of poisoning by causative substance*
Poisons. *See* Toxins and toxic substances
Poke root. *See* Phytolacca
Poland, 1:157, *442,* 2:800
Polio, 2:**613–617,** 779, 782, 809
Politics, 1:362, 415–416, 417, 418
Pollen, 1:55, 56, 440
Pollination, 1:185–186
Pollutants. *See specific pollutants by name*
Pollution, air. *See* Air pollution
Pollution control
    Clean Air Act, 1:176–178
    Clean Water Act, 1:179–182
    Environmental Protection Agency, 1:276, 277, 279
    Federal Water Act, 1:306–307
    water pollution, 2:800, 801
    water quality standards, 2:805–807
Pollution, noise. *See* Noise pollution
Pollution, non-point source. *See* Non-point source pollution
Pollution Prevention Act, 1:104, 278
Pollution, water. *See* Water pollution
Poly(vinylpolypyrrolidone) (PVP), 2:723
Polybrominated diphenyl ethers, 1:293
Polycarbonate plastics. *See* Plastics
Polychlorinated biphenyls (PCBs), 1:22, 275, 2:734, 738

Polycyclic aromatic hydrocarbons. *See* Hydrocarbons
Polymerase chain reaction (PCR) testing. *See* Diagnostic testing
Pontiac fever, 1:438, 468
Poor. *See* Poverty
Poor Law Amendment Act (UK), 2:672
Population and disease, 2:**617–619**
    child survival revolution, 1:160–161
    endemic diseases, 1:272
    epidemiology, 1:279–281
    global public health, 1:361–363
Population displacement
    by dams, 1:210, 212
    by drought, 1:233
    by ebola hemorrhagic fever, 1:251
    by Fukushima Daiichi nuclear power station disaster, 1:351
    in global public health, 1:362, 363
    by Horn of Africa drought and famine, 1:416, *416,* 417
    by Hurricane Katrina, 1:458
    by Japanese earthquake, 1:452, 453
    by levees, 1:484
    in Love Canal, 1:490, 491
    shigellosis and, 2:685
    by tropical disease, 2:745
    by tuberculosis, 2:753
    by typhus, 2:767
    vaccination and, 2:781
Population growth, zero. *See* Zero population growth
Population pyramid, 2:**619–620**
Porcine reproductive and respiratory syndrome (PRRS), 2:593
Pork. *See* Meat
Positron emission tomography (PET) scans. *See* Diagnostic testing; Radiation
Post-exposure prophylaxis, 1:14, 119
Post-polio syndrome, 2:616
Post-traumatic stress disorder, 2:**620–627**
    causes, 2:622–623
        Chernobyl nuclear power station disaster, 1:158
        Hurricane Katrina, 1:458
        9/11 terrorist attacks, 2:570, 571
    demographics, 2:621–622
    description, 2:620–621
    diagnosis, 2:623–624
    Gulf War syndrome, 1:378
    prevention, 2:626
    prognosis, 2:626
    public health, 2:626
    symptoms, 2:623
    treatment, 2:624–626
Potable water. *See* Drinking water supply

Potassium, 1:6
Potassium iodide, 1:157, 159, 452
Potassium nitrate, 1:288
Poultry. *See* Birds
Poverty
    Haiti earthquake, 1:387
    Horn of Africa drought and famine, 1:418
    housing and, 1:420, 421
    Hurricane Katrina, 1:456
    One Health Initiative on, 2:593
    Oxfam on, 2:594, 595
    post-traumatic stress disorder, 2:621
    sanitation and, 2:672
    smoking and, 2:710
    UNICEF on, 2:771, 772
Power plants, electric. *See* Electric power plants
Power plants, nuclear. *See* Nuclear power stations
Poxviruses, 2:520, 701
PPD (Purified protein derivative), 2:757, 760
Pralidoxime, 1:445
Pranayama, 1:60
Praziquantel, 2:677
Precipitation, 1:183, 310–311
    See also Acid rain; Drought
Prednisone, 1:84
Pregnancy
    disaster impacts
        Love Canal, 1:490
        oil spills, 2:587, 589–590
        Seveso, Italy accident, 2:683
        Three Mile Island nuclear disaster, 2:727
    disease impacts
        AIDS, 1:10, 11, 13
        brucellosis, 1:117
        chemical poisoning, 1:148, 149, 150
        foodborne illness, 1:342, 343
        H1N1 influenza A, 1:382
        listeriosis, 1:484, 485, 486, 487
        Lyme disease, 1:497
        malaria, 2:503
        measles, 2:509, 510
        meningitis, 2:522
        mercury poisoning, 2:527, 528, 532–533
        mumps, 2:546
    health issues and threats
        bisphenol A, 1:105, 106
        endocrine disruptors, 1:273, 274, 275
        food safety, 1:339–340
        parasites, 2:607
        smoking, 2:710
        vaccination, 2:779
Prehistoric era, 1:21
Preparedness, disaster. *See* Disaster preparedness

Preparedness, emergency. *See* Emergency preparedness
Prescription drugs. *See* Drugs (medications)
Preservatives, food. *See* Food additives
Presidential Special Oversight Board for Department of Defense Investigations of Gulf War Chemical and Biological Incidents, 1:377
President's Cancer Panel, 2:639
Pressure, barometric. *See* Barometric pressure
Pressure gradient, 1:431
Pressure, partial. *See* Partial pressure
Prevention, disease. *See* Disease control
Priestley, Joseph, 1:136
Prilocaine, 2:534
Primaquine, 2:504
Primates
 AIDS in, 1:8
 ebola hemorrhagic fever in, 1:248, 251
 emergent diseases in, 1:264–265
 epidemiology, 1:280
 hemorrhagic fevers in, 1:411
 severe acute respiratory syndrome in, 2:681
 shigellosis in, 2:685
Prince William Sound, 1:295, *297*, *297*–299, *299*
Prion diseases. *See* Creutzfeldt-Jakob disease
Prions, 1:195–196, 2:790–791
Pritchard, Michael S., 1:489
Probiotics, 1:238, 498, 2:606
Product recalls, 1:336, 337, 338, 466, 2:523
Product testing, 1:305, 321, 322–324
Progress on Sanitation and Drinking-water, 2010 Update, 2:673
Progressive massive fibrosis. *See* Black lung disease
Prohibition, orders of. *See* Orders of prohibition
Prophylaxis, post-exposure. *See* Post-exposure prophylaxis
Prospect Hill virus, 1:392
Protease inhibitors, 1:14
Protective equipment
 for avian flue, 1:70
 for biosafety, 1:98, 99
 for brucellosis, 1:119
 for byssinosis, 1:122
 for cadmium poisoning, 1:127
 for chlorine exposure, 1:165
 for cutting oil exposure, 1:205–206
 for ebola hemorrhagic fever, 1:251
 for electric shock injuries, 1:254, 255–256
 in flu pandemic, 1:316
 for heavy metal poisoning, 1:409
 in industrial hygiene, 1:442
 for insecticide poisoning, 1:445
 for leptospirosis, 1:473
 for malaria, 2:504
 in oil spills, 2:589
 for radiation exposure, 2:640
 for radiation injuries, 2:646
 for skin cancer, 2:698
 for sulfur exposure, 2:717
 for vector (mosquito) control, 2:784
Protein modeling, 1:90
Protein-calorie malnutrition. *See* Protein-energy malnutrition
Protein-energy malnutrition, 2:**627–630**
Proteins, 1:89, 90, 91, 251, 466, 477
 See also specific proteins by name
Proteomics, 1:89, 90, 91
Proton pump inhibitors, 1:166–167
Protozoa, parasitic. *See* Parasites
Proviruses. *See* Viruses
PrP, 1:196
PRRS (porcine reproductive and respiratory syndrome), 2:593
Prusiner, Stanley, 1:196
Pseudomonas, 1:43, 2:809
Pseudonitzschia, 1:326
Psychodynamic psychotherapy. *See* Psychotherapy
Psychological health. *See* Mental health
Psychotherapy, 2:624
Psychrophilic organisms. *See* Extremophiles
PTSD (Post-traumatic stress disorder). *See* Post-traumatic stress disorder
Public health
 disasters
  Bhopal, India, 1:88
  drought, 1:232–233, 234—235
  Exxon Valdez, 1:298–299
  famine, 1:301, 302–303
  flooding, 1:311–312
  Fukushima Daiichi nuclear power station disaster, 1:350, 351
  Gulf oil spill, 1:373–374
  Haiti earthquake, 1:387
  Horn of Africa drought and famine, 1:418
  Iceland volcano eruption, 1:436
  Japanese earthquake, 1:451–453
  Love Canal, 1:490
  9/11 terrorist attacks, 2:570–571
  oil spills, 2:587, 588
  Three Mile Island nuclear disaster, 2:726–727
  Times Beach, 2:730
  toxic sludge spill in Hungary, 2:732
  volcanic eruptions, 2:795, 796
 diseases and disorders
  AIDS, 1:18–19
  altitude sickness, 1:29
  amebiasis, 1:31, 32
  anthrax, 1:40–41
  asbestosis, 1:49–50
  aspergillosis, 1:54
  autism, 1:66
  avian flu, 1:70–71
  berylliosis, 1:84
  bioterrorism, 1:103
  bronchitis, 1:112
  brucellosis, 1:118
  byssinosis, 1:122
  cadmium poisoning, 1:126, 127
  cancer, 1:135
  carbon monoxide poisoning, 1:138
  chemical poisoning, 1:153–154
  cholera, 1:168
  chronic kidney disease, 1:172–173
  chronic wasting disease, 1:175
  communicable diseases, 1:189–190
  Creutzfeldt-Jakob disease, 1:197
  cruise ship health, 1:201
  dengue fever, 1:217
  diphtheria, 1:219, 220, 221
  disease outbreaks, 1:227–228
  dysentery, 1:239–240
  ebola hemorrhagic fever, 1:251
  emergent diseases, 1:266
  emphysema, 1:270
  endemic disease, 1:272
  flu pandemic, 1:316
  food poisoning, 1:330–331, 334
  foodborne illness, 1:341, 345
  fungal infections, 1:352
  giardiasis, 1:359–360
  guinea worm disease, 1:367–368
  Gulf War syndrome, 1:379
  H1N1 influenza A, 1:384, 385
  hantavirus infections, 1:393–394
  heavy metal poisoning, 1:409
  insecticide poisoning, 1:445
  lead poisoning, 1:466
  Legionnaires' disease, 1:469
  leptospirosis, 1:473
  leukemia, 1:480
  Lyme disease, 1:498–499
  measles, 2:510–511
  meningitis, 2:523–524
  mercury poisoning, 2:531–532
  methemoglobinemia, 2:535
  mumps, 2:546
  nature deficit disorder, 2:562–563
  necrotizing fasciitis, 2:566
  noroviruses, 2:582
  pandemic, 2:601–602
  plague, 2:612
  population and disease, 2:617–619
  post-traumatic stress disorder, 2:626

Public health *(continued)*
- river blindness, 2:657
- severe acute respiratory syndrome, 2:679–682
- shigellosis, 2:687
- smallpox, 2:702–703
- sulfur exposure, 2:716
- tuberculosis, 2:758–759
- typhus, 2:767
- West Nile virus, 2:815
- yellow fever, 2:828
- Yokkaichi asthma, 2:831

hazards
- agricultural chemicals, 1:7–8
- air pollution, 1:24
- algal bloom, 1:26
- antimicrobial resistance, 1:41, 44–45
- asbestos, 1:47–48
- background radiation, 1:74
- bedbug infestation, 1:77–78
- bioterrorism, 1:101–102
- cellular phones, 1:140
- climate change, 1:184–185
- drinking water supply, 1:230
- endocrine disruptors, 1:275
- *escherichia coli*, 1:284
- housing, 1:420–422, 421–422
- indoor air quality, 1:439
- low-temperature environments, 1:493–494
- medical waste, 2:511–512, 513
- mold, 2:538–539
- noise pollution, 2:574
- smog, 2:707–708
- smoking, 2:713
- volatile organic compounds, 2:793
- water pollution, 2:801
- wildfires, 2:820–821

legislation
- National Environmental Policy Act, 2:553–554
- Rivers and Harbors Act of 1899, 2:659–660
- Safe Drinking Water Act, 2:667

methods
- biomonitoring, 1:95, 96
- biosafety, 1:99
- disaster preparedness, 1:225
- emergency preparedness, 1:261–262
- epidemiology, 1:279–281
- ergonomics, 1:283
- exposure science, 1:292–293
- Healthy Cities, 1:396–397
- risk assessment, 2:653–655
- vaccination, 2:781–782
- vector (mosquito) control, 2:786–787
- water fluoridation, 2:797–799
- water quality, 2:804, 805

organizations
- American Public Health Association, 1:33–34
- Centers for Disease Control and Prevention, 1:144–146
- Food and Drug Administration, 1:322–324
- Public Health Service, 2:630
- UNICEF, 2:775

See also Global public health

Public Health Act of 1848, 1:145
Public Health Security and Bioterrorism Preparedness and Response Act of 2002, 1:99, 102
Public Health Service, 1:229, 2:556, **630**
Public housing. *See* Housing
Pulmonary dust disorders. *See* Talcosis
Pulmonary fibrosis, 1:308–309
Pulmonary hypertension, 2:721, 722
Pulmonary thesaurosis. *See* Thesaurosis
Pulmonary tuberculosis. *See* Tuberculosis
Pulse field gel electrophoresis, 1:281
PulseNet, 2:687
Pure Food and Drug Act, 1:144, 323
Purified protein derivative (PPD), 2:757, 760
Purine analogs, 1:478–479
Puumala virus, 1:392, 412
Pu'u'O'o Cone of Kilauea Volcano, 2:*794*
PVP (Poly(vinylpolypyrrolidone)), 2:723
Pyrazinamide, 2:758
Pyrethroids, 2:784
Pyriostigmine bromide, 1:378

Q

Qiinghaosu. *See* Artemisinin
Qingdao, China, 1:*26*
Quarantine. *See* Isolation and quarantine (disease control)
Quercetin, 1:59
Quicksilver. *See* Mercury
Quinine, 2:503

R

Rabbits, 2:521
Rabies, 2:592, 835
Rachel Carson Council, 2:**631–633**
Radiation, 2:**633–637**
- for AIDS, 1:14
- for anthrax, 1:40
- cancer from, 1:131, 133
- Centers for Disease Control and Prevention on, 1:144
- chemical poisoning from, 1:149
- in drinking water supply, 1:230
- Environmental Protection Agency on, 1:276
- exposure, 2:637–640
- Food and Drug Administration, 1:323
- injuries, 2:641–646
- from Japanese earthquake, 1:449, 451, 452, 453–454
- leukemia and, 1:476, 478, 479, 480
- in medical waste, 2:511, 512, 513
- melanoma and, 2:517, 519
- skin cancer and, 2:697, 698
- in toxic sludge spill in Hungary, 2:731–732

See also Background radiation; Ionizing radiation; Ultraviolet radiation

Radiation Effects Research Foundation (RERF), 2:638
Radiation exposure, 2:634, *637*, **637–641**
- background radiation, 1:73
- from Chernobyl nuclear power station disaster, 1:154–160
- in exposure science, 1:294
- from Fukushima Daiichi nuclear power station disaster, 1:350–351
- from Japanese earthquake, 1:449, 451, 452–453
- leukemia from, 1:481
- from Three Mile Island nuclear disaster, 2:726

See also Acute radiation syndrome

Radiation injuries, 2:**641–646**
Radiation of food. *See* Food irradiation
Radiation sickness. *See* Acute radiation syndrome
Radio radiation. *See* Non-ionizing radiation
Radio stations, 1:222
Radioactive iodine, 1:157, 158, 350, 351, 2:636
Radiofrequency energy, 1:139–142
Radioisotopes. *See* Radiation
Radionuclides, 1:74, 350, 2:668
Radiotherapy. *See* Radiation
Radon
- air pollution, 1:24
- background radiation, 1:74
- chemical poisoning from, 1:148
- drinking water supply, 1:230
- earthquakes, 1:247
- indoor air quality, 1:437, 438, 439, 440–441
- radiation exposure from, 2:639
- Safe Drinking Water Act on, 2:668

Ragpicker's disease. *See* Anthrax
Rain, acid. *See* Acid rain
Rainfall. *See* Precipitation
Ramazzini, Bernardino, 1:443, 2:527

Rapid Alert System for Food and Feed (RASFF), 2:580
RASFF (Rapid Alert System for Food and Feed), 2:580
Rashes
  bedbug infestation, 1:75, 76
  Lyme disease, 1:496
  measles, 2:507, *508,* 508–509
  schistosomiasis, 2:677
  smallpox, 2:702
  typhoid fever, 2:762, 763
Rats. *See* Rodents
Rays, cosmic. *See* Cosmic rays
RCRA (Resource Conservation and Recovery Act). *See* Resource Conservation and Recovery Act
Reactivity, 1:396
Reactors, nuclear. *See* Nuclear power stations
Reagan, Ronald, 1:177, 2:693
Rebuilding. *See* Redevelopment
Recalls, product. *See* Product recalls
Recovery Act. *See* American Recovery and Reinvestment Act
Recreational water illness. *See* Waterborne illness
Recycling, 1:235, 2:513–514, 652
Red blood cells. *See* Blood cells
Red Cross, 2:**646–650**
  on emergency preparedness, 1:261
  Haiti earthquake, 1:389
  humanitarian aid from, 1:429, 430
  Hurricane Katrina, 1:457
  Japanese earthquake, 1:451–452
Red measles. *See* Measles
Red tides, 1:25, 26, 326
Redevelopment
  brownfield sites, 1:113–115
  Environmental Protection Agency on, 1:278–279
  Hurricane Katrina, 1:457, 458
  Japanese earthquake, 1:453
Redwood National Work, 2:693
Reflexology, 1:60
Refrigeration and freezing
  ammonia exposure, 1:35, 36
  food safety, 1:338
  foodborne illness, 1:343, 345
  listeriosis, 1:485
  low-temperature environment, 1:493–494
Refugees. *See* Population displacement
Refuse Act. *See* Rivers and Harbors Act of 1899
Registries, 1:4–5
Regulation, government. *See* Government regulation
Rehydration. *See* Dehydration and rehydration
Reiter's syndrome, 1:237, 240
Relaxation training, 2:625

Relenza. *See* Zanamivir
Relief programs. *See* Humanitarian aid
Relief wells, 1:368–369, 370
Relocation. *See* Population displacement
Remediation, environmental. *See* Environmental cleanup
Remission, 1:478, 481
Renal disease, chronic. *See* Chronic kidney disease
Renewable energy. *See* Alternative energy
Reoviruses, 2:809
Repellents, insect. *See* Insecticides
Replacement level of fertility. *See* Zero population growth
Report on an Inquiry into the Sanitary Condition of the Labouring Population of Great Britain, 2:803
Reproductive system, 1:106
RERF (Radiation Effects Research Foundation), 2:638
Research
  by Agency for Toxic Substances and Disease Registry, 1:5
  on air pollution, 1:23
  by American Public Health Association, 1:34
  on anthrax, 1:39–40
  on antimicrobial resistance, 1:45
  on autism, 1:66
  on bioinformatics, 1:89–93
  biomonitoring in, 1:94–96
  on biosafety, 1:98–99
  on bioterrorism, 1:100
  on bisphenol A, 1:104, 105–106
  on cancer, 1:133
  on cellular phones, 1:140–141, *141*
  by Centers for Disease Control and Prevention, 1:144–145
  by Environmental Protection Agency, 1:277, 279
  on hemorrhagic fevers, 1:412
  on ionizing radiation, 1:447
  by National Institute for Occupational Safety and Health, 2:554–555
  by National Institute of Environmental Health Sciences, 2:556–559
  on nature deficit disorder, 2:560
  on tropical disease, 2:747
  on tuberculosis, 2:759
Reserve Mining Company, 1:47
Reservoirs (water), 1:210, 211, 2:591
Reservoirs, disease. *See* Disease reservoirs
Resistance, antibiotic. *See* Antimicrobial resistance
Resource Conservation and Recovery Act, 1:277, 395, 396, 2:**650–653**

Respiratory diseases. *See specific diseases by name*
Respiratory syncytial virus (RSV), 1:111
Restitution. *See* Settlements and damages
Retroviruses. *See* Viruses
Reverse osmosis, 1:208
Reverse transcriptase, 2:789, 792
Rewrite the Future, 2:675
Reye's syndrome, 2:509
RHA (Rivers and Harbors Act of 1899). *See* Rivers and Harbors Act of 1899
Rhinitis, 1:56
Ribavirin, 1:394, 412, 2:828
Rice, 1:127, 303, 406
Richter scale, 1:246, 247
Rickettsia, 2:765
Rifamixin, 2:742
Rifampin, 1:43, 118, 119, 469, 2:758
Rift Valley fever, 1:411, 413
Rimantadine, 1:70, 384
Ring of Fire, 2:794
Ringworm, 1:353
Riparian habitats, 1:210
Risk assessment, 2:**653–655**
  emergency preparedness and, 1:260
  by Environmental Protection Agency, 1:277
  Federal Insecticide, Fungicide, and Rodenticide Act, 1:304–305
  in toxicology, 2:736
Risk reduction, 1:260, 277
Rita, 1:5, 432
Rituxan. *See* Rituximab
Rituximab, 1:479
River blindness, 1:272, 2:**655–658,** *656,* 746
Rivers
  dams and, 1:209–212
  Rivers and Harbors Act of 1899, 2:658–661
  water pollution in, 2:800–801, 802
  water quality of, 2:804
Rivers and Harbors Act of 1899, 2:591, **658–661**
RNA
  bioinformatics, 1:89–93
  Creutzfeldt-Jakob disease, 1:195–196
  emergent diseases, 1:266–267
  noroviruses, 2:577, 580, 581
  viruses, 2:788, 789
Robertson, F. L., 2:797
Robock, Alan, 1:435
Rochester, NY, 2:669
Rock, 1:346, 347, 348
Rock fever. *See* Brucellosis
Rocks, 1:415

Rocky Mountain spotted fever, 2:663, 664
Rodbell, Martin, 2:556
Rodenticides, 1:149, 394, 409, 2:664
Rodents, 2:*661*, **661–665**
    agricultural chemicals and, 1:6
    in emergent diseases, 1:265
    hantavirus infections from, 1:391–392
    hemorrhagic fevers from, 1:410, 411, 413
    leptospirosis from, 1:470–471, 473
    in One Health Initiative, 2:592
    in plague, 2:610–613
    zoonoses from, 2:835
Roentgen, 2:641
Rolfing, 1:60
Roll Back Malaria, 2:784
Rome (ancient), 1:21
Rose spots, 2:762, 763
Rotaviruses, 1:237, 241, 326, 2:581, 740
Roundworms. *See* Parasites
Royal Commission of Enquiry on the English Poor Laws, 2:672
Royal Dutch Shell Group, 2:589
RSV (Respiratory syncytial virus), 1:111
Rubber, 1:23
Rubella. *See* German measles
Rubeola. *See* Measles
Runoff. *See* Non-point source pollution
Runway malaria. *See* Malaria
Rural areas
    sanitation in, 2:671, 672
    water pollution in, 2:800
Rush, Benjamin, 1:215
Russia
    anthrax in, 1:38
    bioterrorism by, 1:100, 101, 102
    diphtheria in, 1:218
    endemic disease in, 1:272
    famine in, 1:301
    hantavirus infections in, 1:392
    smallpox in, 2:702, 703
    water pollution in, 2:800
    wildfires in, 2:819
    See also Chernobyl nuclear power station disaster
Russian State Centre of Virology and Biotechnology (VECTOR), 2:702

S

Sabin, Albert Bruce, 2:778
Sabin vaccine. *See* Oral polio vaccine (OPV)
Saccharin. *See* Artificial sweeteners
SAD (Seasonal affective disorder), 2:560

Safe Drinking Water Act (1974), 2:**667–669**
    drinking water supply and, 1:229–230
    on endocrine disruptors, 1:275
    Environmental Protection Agency and, 1:278
    on *escherichia coli*, 1:284
    on water quality, 2:805
Safety, biohazard. *See* Biosafety
Safety, food. *See* Food safety
Safety, household. *See* Household safety
Safety, industrial. *See* Workplace safety
Safety, occupational. *See* Workplace safety
Safety, vehicle. *See* Vehicle safety
Safety, workplace. *See* Workplace safety
Saffir-Simpson hurricane scale, 1:431–432
Salinity, 2:801
Salivary glands, 2:543, 544, 545
Salk, Jonas E., 2:614
Salk vaccine. *See* Inactivated polio vaccine (IPV)
Salmon. *See* Fish
Salmonella
    biosafety, 1:98
    bioterrorism, 1:101, 200, 226, 228
    emergent diseases, 1:265
    epidemiology of, 1:280, 281
    food contamination from, 1:325
    food poisoning from, 1:330, 331
    food safety and, 1:337, 340
    foodborne illness from, 1:342
    typhoid fever, 2:761, 762, 763, 764
    waterborne illness from, 2:809
Salmonellosis, 1:325, 337, 342, 343
Salts, 1:318, 2:801
Samoan islands, 2:751
Sanatoriums, 2:752–753
Sand flies, 2:745
Sandy, 1:145, 185, 260, 432, *432*
The Sanitary Conditions of the Laboring Population, 2:672
Sanitation, 1:47, 2:**669–674**
    amebiasis, 1:30, 32–33
    anthrax, 1:40
    antimicrobial resistance and, 1:44
    avian flu, 1:70
    Chartered Institute of Environmental Health and, 1:145–146
    chlorine exposure, 1:164
    chlorine for, 1:162
    cholera, 1:166, 169
    communicable diseases, 1:189, 191
    cruise ship health, 1:198, 199, 200, 201
    demographics, 2:671

    description, 2:669–674
    disease outbreaks, 1:226
    drinking water supply, 1:228, 230
    drought, 1:233
    dysentery, 1:236
    endemic disease, 1:272
    epidemiology, 1:281
    flooding, 1:311
    flu pandemic, 1:316
    food contamination, 1:326
    food poisoning, 1:332, 334
    foodborne illness, 1:343
    giardiasis, 1:357
    global public health, 1:363
    guinea worm disease, 1:367–368
    Haiti earthquake, 1:*386*, 387, 389, 390
    Horn of Africa drought and famine, 1:418
    housing, 1:420–421
    listeriosis, 1:487
    for medical waste, 2:511, *512*
    noroviruses, 2:579, 580, 583
    Oxfam on, 2:594, 595, 596
    parasites in, 2:602, 604
    public health, 2:671–673
    Resource Conservation and Recovery Act on, 2:650–652
    rodent-borne diseases, 2:664
    schistosomiasis, 2:676
    traveler's health, 2:739, 743
    tropical disease, 2:748
    tuberculosis, 2:753
    typhoid fever, 2:762, 764
    UNICEF on, 2:774
    vector (mosquito) control, 2:785
    water pollution, 2:800
    waterborne illness, 2:808
    West Nile virus, 2:815
    See also Industrial hygiene; Personal hygiene
Santiago, Chile, 1:23
Sapovirus, 2:581
SARA (Superfund Amendments and Reauthorization Act). *See* Superfund Amendments and Reauthorization Act (1986)
Sarcoidosis, 1:84, 2:571
Sarcoma, 1:131
Sarin, 1:377
Saro-Wiwa, Ken, 2:589, *589*
SARS. *See* Severe acute respiratory syndrome (SARS)
Satellites, 1:248
Save the Children, 1:390, 415, 2:**674–676**
Sawyer, Wilbur Augustus, 2:827
Saxitoxins, 1:326
SBA (U.S. Small Business Administration), 1:260, 432
SBRP (Superfund Basic Research Program), 2:558–559

SBS (Sick building syndrome). *See* Sick building syndrome
Scandinavian Committee for Standardization of Routine Patch Testing, 2:607
SCC (Society of Cosmetic Chemists of Great Britain), 2:724
Schaudin, Fritz, 1:30
Schistosoma haematobium, 2:677
Schistosoma intercalatum, 2:676
Schistosoma japonicum, 2:676
Schistosoma mansoni, 2:676
Schistosoma mekongi, 2:676
Schistosomes, 2:676
Schistosomiasis, 2:**676–678**
  in AIDS, 1:11
  as dysentery, 1:236–237, 238, 240–241
  as endemic, 1:272
  sanitation for, 2:672
  as waterborne illness, 2:809
Scombroid, 1:326
Scrapie, 1:194, 195
Screening, medical. *See* Diagnostic testing
Scrotum, 2:544, 545
Scrub typhus. *See* Typhus
Scuba diving. *See* Diving
SDWA (Safe Drinking Water Act). *See* Safe Drinking Water Act (1974)
Sea levels, 1:183, 184
Seafood. *See* Fish
Seafood industry, 1:26
Seal Up! Trap Up! Clean Up!, 2:664
Seashores. *See* Coastal areas
Seasonal affective disorder (SAD), 2:560
Secondhand smoke. *See* Smoking
Sedgwick, William Thompson, 1:34
Sediment, 1:210–211, 404, 405, 2:525, 526
Seibert, Florence B., 2:754
Seismology. *See* Earthquakes
Selective pressure, 1:42
Selenium, 1:404, 406, 407, 2:645
Senegal, 1:303
SENSOR-Pesticides (Sentinel Event Notification System for Occupational Risks-Pesticides Program), 1:445
Sensory perception, 1:63, 64
Sentinel Event Notification System for Occupational Risks-Pesticides Program (SENSOR-Pesticides), 1:445
Sentinel lymph node mapping, 2:518
Seoul National University, 1:70
Seoul virus, 1:392, 412
September 11 Victim Compensation Fund, 2:571

September 11th Commission. *See* 9/11 Commission
September 11th terrorist attacks. *See* 9/11 terrorist attacks
Septic systems. *See* Sanitation
Septicemic plague. *See* Plague
Sequences, DNA. *See* DNA
Sequoia National Park, 2:693
Seroconversion, 1:12
Serum (blood), 1:217, 219, 2:521
Settlements and damages
  in Bhopal, India, 1:86
  Exxon Valdez, 1:299
  from Gulf oil spill, 1:370, 372, 374
  from Love Canal, 1:491
  from 9/11 terrorist attacks, 2:570, 571
  for Yokkaichi asthma, 2:831, 832
Severe acute respiratory syndrome (SARS), 2:**679–682**
  Centers for Disease Control and Prevention on, 1:144
  disease outbreaks of, 1:227
  as emergent disease, 1:265, 266
  in One Health Initiative, 2:593
  pandemic, 2:601
Seveso, Italy, 1:396, 2:**682–684**
Sevin. *See* Carbaryl
Sewage. *See* Wastewater
Sewers. *See* Sanitation
Sexual behavior
  AIDS, 1:8, 9–10, 11–12, 18, 19
  amebiasis, 1:31
  antimicrobial resistance, 1:45
  cancer, 1:131
  cryptosporidiosis, 1:202
  dysentery, 1:241
  human papilloma virus, 1:425, 427, 428
  shigellosis, 2:686
Sexually transmitted diseases (STDs). *See specific diseases by name*
Shale. *See* Rock
Shanghai, China, 2:550
SHARE (Supporting Horn of Africa Resilience), 1:419
Shave biopsy. *See* Diagnostic testing
Sheep. *See* Livestock
Shell shock. *See* Post-traumatic stress disorder
Shellfish
  algal bloom on, 1:25, 26
  biotoxins in, 1:104
  in communicable diseases, 1:190
  food contamination in, 1:324, 326, 327
  food poisoning from, 1:330, 332
  food safety and, 1:337
  foodborne illness from, 1:341, 343–344
  heavy metal poisoning from, 1:406–407

  mercury poisoning from, 2:528, 529, 532–533
  noroviruses from, 2:579, 580, 583, 584
  oil spills on, 2:589
  water quality standards on, 2:806
Sheltering in place, 1:223, 261, 351, 452, 2:727
Shelters. *See* Evacuation
Shiga, Kiyoshi, 2:684
Shiga toxin-producing *E. coli* (STEC). *See Escherichia coli*
Shigella
  cruise ship health, 1:200
  dysentery, 1:236–237
  emergent diseases, 1:265
  food contamination, 1:326
  food poisoning, 1:332
  foodborne illness, 1:343
  shigellosis, 2:684–686, 688
  traveler's health, 2:740
Shigellosis, 2:**684–688**, 685
  as dysentery, 1:236–237, 238, 239, 240
  in traveler's health, 2:739
  water quality and, 2:804
Shock, 1:216, 393, 2:565
Shock, anaphylactic. *See* Anaphylaxis
Shock injuries, electric. *See* Electric shock injuries
Shorelines. *See* Coastal areas
Shortages, food. *See* Famine
Shortages, water. *See* Drought
Siberia, 1:93
Sick building syndrome, 1:420, 438, 2:689, **689–692**
Sierra Club, 2:692, **692–694**
Sierra Leone, 2:670
Sierra Nevada mountains, 2:692
Silent Spring, 2:618, 631, 632, 784
Silica, 1:109, 2:694, 695
Silicosis, 1:308, 2:**694–696**, 721
Siltation, 2:804
Silver, 1:404
Sin Nombre virus (SNV), 1:392, 412
Singapore, 2:681
Single nucleotide polymorphisms, 1:91
Single proton emission computed tomography (SPECT). *See* Diagnostic testing; Radiation
Sinusitis, 1:56
Skimming, 1:371
Skin
  AIDS, 1:12
  anthrax, 1:37, 38, 39, 40
  chemical poisoning, 1:151
  Chernobyl nuclear power station disaster, 1:158
  chlorine exposure, 1:164, 165
  cutting oil exposure, 1:204, 205, 206
  diphtheria, 1:219

Skin *(continued)*
  electric shock injuries, 1:253–254
  listeriosis, 1:485
  low-temperature environments, 1:493
  melanoma, 2:514–520, *515*
  mercury poisoning, 2:529
  necrotizing fasciitis, 2:564–566
  patch testing of, 2:607–609
  radiation injuries, 2:645
  Seveso, Italy accident, 2:683
Skin cancer, 1:130, 131, 2:**696–698**
  melanoma as, 2:514–520
  from non-ionizing radiation, 2:576
  from ultraviolet radiation, 2:769
Slaughterhouses, 1:116, 117
Sleeping sickness, 1:272, 2:**699–701**, 745
Slippery elm, 2:582
Sludge, toxic. *See* Hazardous waste
Small intestine, 1:167
Smallpox, 2:*701*, **701–704**
  bioterrorism, 1:100, 102
  Centers for Disease Control and Prevention on, 1:144
  as communicable disease, 1:190
  measles *vs.*, 2:508
  as pandemic, 2:601
  vaccination, 2:777
Smith, Stephen, 1:34
Smog, 2:*550, 705*, **705–709**
  as air pollution, 1:22, 23, 24
  bronchitis from, 1:110
  ozone exposure and, 2:598, 599
Smoke, 1:21, 22, 23, 56, 61, 2:820–821
Smoking, 2:**709–714**
  asbestosis, 1:50–51
  asthma, 1:56
  benzene exposure, 1:81
  benzo(a)pyrene from, 1:82
  black lung disease, 1:108
  bronchitis, 1:111, 112–113
  byssinosis, 1:120, 121, 122
  cancer, 1:131
  carbon monoxide poisoning, 1:137, 138
  causes, 2:710
  Centers for Disease Control and Prevention on, 1:144
  children and, 2:710
  chronic kidney disease, 1:171
  demographics, 2:710
  description, 2:709–710
  diagnosis, 2:711
  emphysema, 1:269, 270–271
  epidemiology of, 1:280
  in exposure science, 1:294
  Food and Drug Administration, 1:322, 323
  human papilloma virus, 1:425
  indoor air quality, 1:438, 439
  leukemia, 1:476, 481
  population and disease, 2:618
  public health, 2:713
  sick building syndrome, 2:691
  symptoms, 2:710–711
  treatment, 2:711–713
Smoking cessation aides, 2:711
Snail fever. *See* Schistosomiasis
Snails, 2:676, 678
Snow, 1:310
Snow, John, 1:227, 229, 280, 2:618, 669, 803
SNV (Sin Nombre virus), 1:392, 412
Soapstone. *See* Talc
Sobrero, Ascanio, 1:290
Social costs
  antimicrobial resistance, 1:44
  disease outbreaks, 1:227
  drought, 1:233
  guinea worm disease, 1:367
  housing, 1:421
  medical waste, 2:512
  pandemic, 2:601
  water pollution, 2:801
  water quality, 2:804–805
Social interaction, 1:63, 64, 65
Social justice
  in One Health Initiative, 2:593
  Oxfam on, 2:594, 595, 596, 597
Society of Cosmetic Chemists of Great Britain (SCC), 2:724
Socioeconomics, 2:618
Sodium hypochlorite, 1:162
Soil
  acid rain on, 1:3
  agricultural chemicals on, 1:6, 7
  background radiation on, 1:74
  cadmium poisoning on, 1:126
  Chernobyl nuclear power station disaster on, 1:158–159
  communicable diseases in, 1:189
  drought, 1:232–233, 234
  flooding and, 1:310
  heavy metal poisoning in, 1:404, 406, 407
  in high temperature environments, 1:415
  Japanese earthquake on, 1:454
  lead poisoning from, 1:464, 466
  in Seveso, Italy, 2:682–683
  Soil Conservation Act on, 2:714
  water pollution from, 2:801
Soil Conservation Act (1935), 2:**714–715**
Soil Conservation Service, 2:714
Solar energy. *See* Sun and sunlight
Soldiers. *See* Armed forces
Solid waste disposal. *See* Sanitation
Solid Waste Disposal Act, 2:650, 652
Solvents, 1:23, 24, 437
Somalia, 1:301, *302*, 415–416, 418, 2:701
Soman, 1:378
Somatic Experiencing, 2:625
Soper, George A., 2:762
Sores. *See* Skin
Sorghum, 1:7
Sound, 2:571–574
South Africa, 1:*9*, 10, 2:759
South America
  cholera in, 1:166
  endemic disease in, 1:272
  Japanese earthquake and, 1:449
  plague in, 2:611
  river blindness in, 2:655, 656, 657
  water pollution in, 2:800
  yellow fever in, 2:825, 826
South American hemorrhagic fevers. *See* Hemorrhagic fevers
South Korea, 1:70
South Pacific Environment Programme (SPREP), 2:670
South Sudan, 1:367
Soviet Union. *See* Russia
Soybeans, 1:7
Spacers, 1:58
Spanish influenza. *See* Flu pandemic
Speciation, 1:404–405
Specific absorption rate, 1:139, 140, 141, 142
SPECT (Single proton emission computed tomography). *See* Diagnostic testing; Radiation
Speech. *See* Communication
Spilanthes, 1:497
Spinal tap. *See* Diagnostic testing
Spirituality, 2:625
Spirometry. *See* Diagnostic testing
Spleen, 1:474
Spores, 1:37, *38*, 352, 2:536
SPREP (South Pacific Environment Programme), 2:670
Sputum, 1:112, 2:757
Squamous cell skin cancer. *See* Skin cancer
Sri Lanka, 1:172–173
St. Jude's Children's Hospital, 1:480–481
Stabilizing agents. *See* Thickening agents
Stable ecosystems model, 2:672
Staging, clinical. *See* Clinical staging
Standards, government. *See* Government regulation
Staphylococcus aureus
  antimicrobial resistance of, 1:43, 44
  in emergent diseases, 1:265
  in food contamination, 1:325
  food safety for, 1:337
  in foodborne illness, 1:343, 345
Starbucks Coffee, 2:596
Startle response, 2:623
Starvation. *See* Famine
State-federal relations. *See* Federal-state relations

Static kill, 1:370
Status asthmaticus, 1:57
STDs (Sexually transmitted diseases). *See specific diseases by name*
Steam pasteurization. *See* Pasteurization
STEC (Shiga toxin-producing *E. coli*). *See Escherichia coli*
Steel, 2:505–506
Steele, James H., 2:592
Stem cells. *See* Blood cells
Sterilization, 2:513–514
Steroids (medications). *See* Corticosteroids
Stillbirth. *See* Pregnancy
Stochastic Human Exposure and Dose Simulation model, 1:292
Stomach acid, 1:166–167
Stomach flu. *See* Food poisoning
Stool. *See* Feces
Stop TB Partnership, 2:758
Storage disease. *See* Thesaurosis
Storm surge. *See* Flooding
Storms
   algal bloom from, 1:25
   electric shock injuries from, 1:256
   flooding from, 1:310–311
   housing and, 1:420
   hurricanes from, 1:431
Streamside habitats. *See* Riparian habitats
Street noise. *See* Noise pollution
Streptococcal sepsis, 2:592
Streptococcus, 1:265, 2:522, 565
Streptomycin, 1:118, 2:612, 753, 758
Stress
   in asthma, 1:54, 56, 60
   in colony collapse disorder, 1:187
   Gulf War syndrome and, 1:377, 378
   nature deficit disorder and, 2:560
   from noise pollution, 2:573, 574
Stress, post-traumatic. *See* Post-traumatic stress disorder
Stroke. *See* Cardiovascular disease
Stroke, heat. *See* Heat disorders
Strombolian eruptions. *See* Volcanic eruptions
Subacute sclerosing panencephalitis, 2:509
Subsidies, 2:714
Substance abuse. *See* Drug use
Subungal melanoma. *See* Melanoma
Succimer, 1:465
Sudan, 2:572
Suenaga, Masami, 2:831
Sugar industry, 1:172
Suicide, 1:151, 406, 409, 2:626
Sulfate aerosols, 1:436
Sulfides, 1:24, 125

Sulfur
   acid rain, 1:3
   air pollution, 1:21, 22
   explosives, 1:288
   exposure, 2:715–716
   as fungicide, 1:354
   from Iceland volcano eruption, 1:436
   smog, 2:706
Sulfur dioxide
   acid rain, 1:1, 2, 4
   air pollution, 1:21, 22, 23, 24
   Clean Air Act on, 1:177–178
   explosives, 1:288
   National Ambient Air Quality Standard, 2:549, 550
   smog, 2:705, 708
   sulfur exposure, 2:715
   Yokkaichi asthma, 2:830
Sulfur exposure, 2:**715–717**
Sulfur oxide, 1:23, 2:829, 830
Sulfur trioxide, 2:715
Sulfuric acid, 1:1, 2, 4, 2:706
Sulfuryl fluoride, 1:77
Sumatra, 2:751
Summer smog. *See* Smog
Sun and sunlight
   climate change, 1:183–184
   melanoma, 2:515, 516, 520
   nature deficit disorder, 2:560
   non-ionizing radiation from, 2:576
   radiation injuries from, 2:642
   skin cancer, 2:696, 697, 698
   smog, 2:706, 707
   ultraviolet radiation, 2:769, 770
Sunblock. *See* Sunscreen and sunblock
Sunburn, 2:576
Sunscreen and sunblock, 2:520, 698, 770
Sunstroke. *See* Heat disorders
Superbugs, 1:43
Superfund. *See* Comprehensive Environmental Response, Compensation, and Liability Act (CERCLA)
Superfund Amendments and Reauthorization Act (1986), 1:5, 2:**717–718**
   Comprehensive Environmental Response, Compensation, and Liability Act, 1:192–193
   Emergency Planning and Community Right-to-Know Act, 1:257
   Environmental Protection Agency, 1:278
   National Institute of Environmental Health Sciences, 2:558
Superfund Basic Research Program (SBRP), 2:558–559

Supplements, dietary. *See* Diet and nutrition
Supplements, livestock. *See* Agricultural chemicals
Supplements, nutritional. *See* Diet and nutrition
Supplements, vitamin. *See* Vitamin therapy
Supply kits, disaster. *See* Disaster preparedness
Supply kits, emergency. *See* Emergency preparedness
Supporting Horn of Africa Resilience (SHARE), 1:419
Supreme Court of India, 1:88–89
Suramin, 2:700
Surgery
   for cancer, 1:133
   for dysentery, 1:238
   for emphysema, 1:270
   Haiti earthquake and, 1:389
   for human papilloma virus, 1:426, 427
   for melanoma, 2:517–518
   for tuberculosis, 2:758
Surgical debridement, 2:565
Surtseyan eruptions. *See* Volcanic eruptions
Sushi. *See* Fish
Sustainable development, 2:594
Swamping, 1:211
Swansea, Wales, 1:397
Swimming
   advisories, 2:718–719
   cryptosporidiosis from, 1:202, 203
   dysentery from, 1:241
   escherichia coli from, 1:284
   Exxon Valdez, 1:295
   giardiasis from, 1:357, 360
   leptospirosis from, 1:473
Swimming advisories, 2:**718–719**
Swine. *See* Livestock
Swine flu. *See* H1N1 influenza A
Switzerland, 2:648–649
Sylvatic fever. *See* Yellow fever
Symadine. *See* Amantadine
Symmetrel. *See* Amantadine
Synthetic antioxidants, 1:149
Synthetic substances. *See specific substances by name*
Syrup of ipecac, 1:151

T

T cells. *See* Blood cells
Tachypnea, 1:121
Taenia, 1:326
Tailings, 1:47
Taiwan, 2:681

Talc, 2:721, 722–723
Talcosis, 2:**721–723**
Talcum powder. *See* Talc
Taliban, 2:570
Tamiflu. *See* Oseltamivir
Tamoxifen, 2:519
Tanning beds, 2:642
Tanzania, 1:*234*
Tapas Acupressure Technique, 2:626
Tapeworms. *See* Parasites
Tar, 2:709
Tarballs. *See* Crude oil
Tartars, 1:100
Tartrazine, 1:321
Tasers, 1:252
TB (Tuberculosis). *See* Tuberculosis
TCDD (2,3,7,8-tetrachlorodibenzo-p-dioxin), 2:682, 683
Tea, 1:60
Tea tree oil, 2:606
Technology, 1:180
Tectonic plates
   earthquakes, 1:245–246, 248
   Haiti earthquake, 1:386
   high temperature environments, 1:414, 415
   Japanese earthquake, 1:450–451
   tsunamis, 2:750, 751
   volcanic eruptions, 2:794, 795
Telephones, cellular. *See* Cellular phones
Temperature
   food safety, 1:338–339
   foodborne illness, 1:343, 345
   heat disorders, 1:398–400
   heat (stress) index and, 1:401–403, 402*t*
   high temperature environments, 1:414–415
   housing and, 1:420
   indoor air quality, 1:438, 441
   listeriosis and, 1:485, 487
   low-temperature environments, 1:493–494
   mold and, 2:536–537
Temperature change. *See* Climate change
Tephra, 1:435, 2:793, 794
Teratogen, 2:**723**
   benzene exposure, 1:80
   mercury, 2:526
   oil spills, 2:590
Terrorism, 2:568–571
Terrorism, biological. *See* Bioterrorism
Terrorist attacks on World Trade Center. *See* 9/11 terrorist attacks
Testicles, 2:544
Testing, diagnostic. *See* Diagnostic testing
Testing, product. *See* Product testing

Testosterone, 1:107
Tetracycline, 1:168, 469, 2:503
Texas, 1:233, 392, 433
Textile workers, 1:120–122
TF (tissue factor), 1:412
Thallium, 1:406, 408, 409
Thames River, 2:802
Theiler, Max, 2:825
Theophylline, 1:60
Thermophiles, 1:414
Thesaurosis, 2:**723–724**
Thiamine, 1:466
Thickening agents, 1:320
Thimerosal, 2:528
Third World countries. *See* Developing countries
Thornburgh, Richard, 2:726, 727
Thought Field Therapy, 2:626
Threat of Mercury Poisoning Rises with Gold Mining Boom, 2:529
Three Gorges Dam, 1:210, *210*, 212
Three Mile Island nuclear disaster, 2:**724–729**, *725*
Three-day measles. *See* German measles
Thrombocytes. *See* Blood cells
Thrombocytopenic purpura, 1:285, 286
Thrush, 1:12, 14, 18, 353
Thunderstorms. *See* Storms
Thymus, 1:474
Thyroid gland, 1:157, 158, 364–365
Thyroid-stimulating hormone, 1:364, 365
Thyroxin, 1:364, 365
Ticks
   emergent diseases, 1:265
   epidemiology, 1:281
   hemorrhagic fevers, 1:410
   Lyme disease, 1:494–499
   in One Health Initiative, 2:592
   as parasites, 2:*602*, 603, 604, 607
   rodents and, 1:662–663
   zoonoses, 2:835
Tidal waves. *See* Tsunamis
Times Beach, 1:491–492, 2:**729–730**
Tin, 1:404
Tinea capitis, 1:353
Tinea corporis, 1:353
Tinea cruris, 1:353
Tinea pedis, 1:352
Tinea unguium, 1:353
Tinidazole, 1:238
Tinnitus, 2:573
Tissue factor (TF), 1:412
Title III. *See* Emergency Planning and Community Right-to-Know Act (1986)
TKI (Tyrosine kinase inhibitors), 1:478, 479, 480

TNT (Trinitrotoluene), 1:288, 289
Tobacco smoke. *See* Smoking
Tobacco use. *See* Smoking
Toenails, 1:353
Toes, 1:*352*
Tohoku-Pacific Ocean earthquake. *See* Japanese Earthquake (2011)
Toilets. *See* Sanitation
Tokyo Electric Power Company, 1:348–349, 350, 351
Toluene, 1:79, 80, 347
Tomas, 2:670
Tomography. *See* Radiation
Tonsils, 1:474
Tooth decay, 1:230–231, 2:797–799
Top kill, 1:370
Topsoil. *See* Soil
Tornado and cyclone, 2:*730*, **730–731**, *731*
Torture, 1:252
Toxic megacolon, 2:686, 741
Toxic sludge. *See* Hazardous waste
Toxic sludge spill in Hungary, 2:**731–733**
Toxic Substances Control Act (1976), 1:275, 278, 462, 2:**733–735**
Toxic waste. *See* Hazardous waste
Toxicity, 1:407–408
Toxicity, waste. *See* Hazardous waste
Toxicology, 2:**735–739**
   chemical poisoning and, 1:153–154
   food additives and, 1:320, 321
   National Institute of Environmental Health Sciences, 2:556, 557–558
Toxicovigilance, 1:154
Toxins and toxic substances
   Agency for Toxic Substances and Disease Registry on, 1:4–5
   algal bloom, 1:25
   anthrax, 1:39–40
   in Bhopal, India, 1:86–89
   biomonitoring of, 1:94–96
   chemical poisoning, 1:147–150
   Clean Water Act on, 1:179, 180
   drinking water supply, 1:230
   Emergency Planning and Community Right-to-Know Act on, 1:257–259
   exposure science, 1:291–295
   food contamination, 1:324–328
   food poisoning, 1:331, 332, 333–334, 334–335
   food safety, 1:336
   foodborne illness, 1:343–344, 345
   from Gulf oil spill, 1:371–373
   heavy metal poisoning, 1:404, 405, 406
   housing, 1:420
   at Love Canal, 1:488–492
   medical waste, 2:511, 512, 513
   mold, 2:536

Toxins and toxic substances (continued)
  National Institute of Environmental Health Sciences on, 2:556, 557–558
  necrotizing fasciitis, 2:565
  from 9/11 terrorist attacks, 2:570, 571
  Occupational Safety and Health Administration on, 2:586
  from smoking, 2:709
  Toxic Substances Control Act on, 2:733–735
  toxicology, 2:735–738
  water pollution, 2:801
  waterborne illness, 2:809, 811
  See also specific toxins by name
Toxocariasis, 2:592, 603
Toxoid, 1:221, 378
Toxoplasma gondii, 1:325, 337, 342, 2:604–605
Toxoplasmosis, 1:325, 342, 2:603, 605
Toys, 1:466
Trace elements, 1:404
Trachoma, 2:672, 746
Tracking Network, 1:228
Traditional Chinese medicine. See Complementary and alternative medicine (CAM)
Traditional East Indian medicine. See Complementary and alternative medicine (CAM)
Traffic noise. See Noise pollution
Training, emergency. See Emergency preparedness
Transfusions, blood. See Blood transfusions
Translocation, 1:406
Transmissible diseases. See Communicable diseases
Transmissible spongiform encephalopathies (TSEs). See Creutzfeldt-Jakob disease
Transmission of disease. See Disease transmission
Transocean Ltd., 1:372, 374, 375
Transplantation, bone marrow. See Bone marrow
Transplants, organ. See Organ and tissue transplants
Transplants, stem cell. See Organ and tissue transplants
Transplants, tissue. See Organ and tissue transplants
Transportation Security Administration (TSA), 2:571
Traumatic Incident Reduction, 2:626
Travel. See Traveler's health
Traveler's diarrhea. See Dysentery; Shigellosis; Traveler's health
Traveler's health, 2:**739–744**
  antimicrobial resistance, 1:44
  bedbug infestation, 1:78
  causes, 2:740
  communicable diseases, 1:190–191
  complications, 2:741
  demographics, 2:740
  dengue fever, 1:215
  description, 2:739–740
  diagnosis, 2:741
  dysentery, 1:236, 239, 241
  escherichia coli, 1:284
  hemorrhagic fevers, 1:413
  malaria, 2:501, 504–505
  measles, 2:508, 509, 510–511
  mercury poisoning, 2:529
  mumps, 2:544
  noroviruses, 2:579–580
  One Health Initiative, 2:592
  parasites, 2:602–603
  plague, 2:610
  prevention, 2:743–744
  prognosis, 2:743
  public health, 2:743
  schistosomiasis, 2:678
  severe acute respiratory syndrome, 2:679, 680, 682
  shigellosis, 2:684, 688
  symptoms, 2:740–741
  treatment, 2:741–743
  tropical disease, 2:745, 746
  tuberculosis, 2:753
  typhoid fever, 2:761–762, 763–764
  typhus, 2:766
  vaccination, 2:777, 779
  waterborne illness, 2:809
  yellow fever, 2:825, 826
  See also Cruise ship health
Treanda. See Bendamustine
Trees, 1:2
  See also Forests
Trematodes. See Parasites
Treponematoses, 2:746
Trichinella spiralis, 1:326
Trichinellosis, 2:592
Trichloreothylene, 1:231
Trichomonas, 2:605
Trichomoniasis, 2:603
Trichuriasis, 2:746
Trick or Treat for UNICEF, 2:772
Triglycerides, 1:18, 171
Trihalomethanes, 1:163
Trihalomines, 1:231
Trinitrotoluene (TNT), 1:288, 289
Tris-BP, 1:293
Trophozoites, 1:30, 31, 237, *358, 359*
Tropical disease, 2:**744–748**
  See also specific diseases by name
Trypanosoma, 2:699, 700
Trypanosomiasis, African. See Sleeping sickness
Trypanosomiasis, American. See Chagas disease
TSA (Transportation Security Administration), 2:571
TSCA (Toxic Substances Control Act). See Toxic Substances Control Act (1976)
TSEs (Transmissible spongiform encephalopathies). See Creutzfeldt-Jakob disease
Tsetse flies, 2:699, 745
Tsunamis, 2:**748–752**, *749*
  flooding from, 1:310
  Fukushima Daiichi nuclear power station disaster, 1:349, 350
  Japanese earthquake, 1:449, 450, *450,* 451
  See also Earthquakes
Tuberculin skin test, 2:754, 757, 758, 760
Tuberculosis, 2:**752–761**, *753, 755*
  AIDS, 1:12
  antimicrobial resistance of, 1:41, 43
  causes, 2:755–756
  as communicable disease, 1:190
  demographics, 2:754–755
  description, 2:752–753
  diagnosis, 2:757–758
  as emergent disease, 1:265, 267
  as endemic disease, 1:272
  history, 2:753–754
  in One Health Initiative, 2:592
  prevention, 2:759–760
  prognosis, 2:759
  public health, 2:758–759
  risk factors, 2:754–755
  silicosis, 2:694, 695
  symptoms, 2:756–757
  as tropical disease, 2:746
Tularemia, 1:39, 103, 2:662
Tumors, malignant. See Cancer
Tumpey, Terrence, 1:*313*
Tungsten, 1:480, 481
Turkeys. See Birds
24/7 Wall St., 1:23
Twins, 1:476
2011 Japanese Earthquake. See Japanese Earthquake (2011)
2,3,5-TCP (2,4,5-trichlorophenol), 2:682, 683
2,3,7,8-tetrachlorodibenzo-p-dioxin (TCDD), 2:682, 683
2,4,5-trichlorophenol (TCP), 2:682, 683
Typhoid fever, 1:191, 2:**761–765**
  drinking water supply, 1:230
  as emergent disease, 1:265
  epidemiology of, 1:280
  sanitation and, 2:669, 672
  traveler's health, 2:740
Typhus, 2:**765–768**
  disease outbreaks of, 1:226
  from rodents, 2:663
  as tropical disease, 2:746
Tyrosine kinase inhibitors (TKI), 1:478, 479, 480
Tyzzer, Edward, 1:202

U

Ukraine, 1:155, 156, 158
Ulaanbaatar, Mongolia, 1:23
Ultrasonography, medical. *See* Diagnostic testing
Ultraviolet radiation, 2:**769–770**
  cancer from, 1:131
  injuries, 2:642
  melanoma, 2:516
  as non-ionizing radiation, 2:576
  ozone and, 2:597–598
  skin cancer from, 2:696
UN (United Nations). *See* United Nations (UN)
Underdeveloped countries. *See* Developing countries
Underground storage tanks, 2:650, 651
Undulant fever. *See* Brucellosis
Unemployment, 2:620
UNICEF, 2:**771–776**
  on AIDS, 1:11
  child survival revolution, 1:160–161
  description, 2:771–772
  on guinea worm disease, 1:366
  public health, 2:775
  purpose, 2:773–775
  on sanitation, 2:673
  on vaccination, 2:781
Union Carbide, 1:89
United Kingdom
  Chartered Institute of Environmental Health in, 1:145–146
  Creutzfeldt-Jakob disease in, 1:194, 195
  cryptosporidiosis in, 1:202
  escherichia coli in, 1:285
  H1N1 influenza A in, 1:384
  measles in, 2:510
  sanitation in, 2:672
United Nations (UN)
  on air pollution, 1:22
  on Earth Day, 1:243, 244
  on Horn of Africa drought and famine, 2:415–416
  humanitarian aid from, 1:429, 430–431
  on measles, 2:510
  on sanitation, 2:672–673
  on tsunamis, 2:751
  on water pollution, 2:800
  World Health Organization and, 2:822
United Nations Children's Fund (UNICEF). *See* UNICEF
United Nations Development Program, 1:366
United Nations Emergency Relief, 1:430
United Nations Environment Programme, 2:600

United Nations Foundation, 2:781
United Nations International Children's Emergency Fund (UNICEF). *See* UNICEF
United Nations Scientific Committee on the Effects of Atomic Radiation, 1:446
United States
  disasters
    Bhopal, India, 1:86, 88
    drought, 1:232, 233
    flooding, 1:311
    Haiti earthquake and, 1:389
    Horn of Africa drought and famine, 1:415, 416
    Hurricane Katrina, 1:458
    hurricanes, 1:432–433
    Japanese earthquake, 1:449
    Love Canal, 1:491–492
    9/11 terrorist attacks, 2:568–571
    oil spills, 2:587–590
    tornadoes, 2:730
    tsunamis, 2:750
    wildfires, 2:819, 820
  diseases and disorders
    AIDS, 1:9, 10, 11, 18–19
    amebiasis, 1:30, 31
    ammonia exposure, 1:35
    anthrax, 1:37–38, 40
    asbestosis, 1:48
    asthma, 1:54
    avian flu, 1:70
    berylliosis, 1:83, 84–85
    black lung disease, 1:108, 109
    bronchitis, 1:111
    brucellosis, 1:116, 117, 118
    byssinosis, 1:120, 122
    cancer, 1:130, 131
    carbon monoxide poisoning, 1:136
    chemical poisoning, 1:150
    chlorine exposure, 1:164
    cholera, 1:166
    chronic kidney disease, 1:170
    chronic wasting disease, 1:174
    colony collapse disorder, 1:185–186, 188
    communicable disease, 1:190
    Creutzfeldt-Jakob disease, 1:194–195
    cruise ship health, 1:198, 199, 200, 201
    cryptosporidiosis, 1:202
    cutting oil exposure, 1:206
    diphtheria, 1:218
    dysentery, 1:236
    emergent disease, 1:264, 265, 266
    emphysema, 1:269, 270–271
    endemic disease, 1:272
    flu pandemic, 1:313, 314
    food poisoning, 1:334
    foodborne illness, 1:341, 342, 345
    fungal infections, 1:353

    giardiasis, 1:357, 359
    H1N1 influenza A, 1:381, 382, 384
    hantavirus infections, 1:392
    heat disorders, 1:398
    heavy metal poisoning, 1:407, 409
    hemorrhagic fevers, 1:411, 412
    human papilloma virus, 1:425, 428
    insecticide poisoning, 1:445
    lead poisoning, 1:463–465, 466
    Legionnaires' disease, 1:467–468, 469
    leptospirosis, 1:473
    leptospirosis in, 1:471
    leukemia, 1:475
    listeriosis, 1:484, 487
    Lyme disease, 1:494–495, 498–499
    malaria, 2:501
    manganese exposure, 2:507
    measles, 2:508, 510
    melanoma, 2:515
    meningitis, 2:521, 523–524
    mercury poisoning, 2:529, 531–532, 532–533
    methemoglobinemia, 2:534, 535
    mumps, 2:543–544, 546
    nature deficit disorder, 2:561
    necrotizing fasciitis, 2:564, 566
    noroviruses, 2:578
    plague, 2:610–611
    post-traumatic stress disorder, 2:621, 622, 626
    protein-energy malnutrition, 2:627–628
    radiation exposure, 2:*637*, 638–639
    rodent-borne diseases, 2:662, 663
    severe acute respiratory syndrome, 2:680–681
    shigellosis, 2:685, 687
    silicosis, 2:694, 695
    skin cancer, 2:696
    smallpox, 2:702, 703
    sulfur exposure, 2:716
    traveler's health, 2:739–740, 741–742
    tropical disease, 2:745, 747
    tuberculosis, 2:753–754, 755, 756, 757, 758–759
    typhoid fever, 2:763
    typhus, 2:765, 766, 767
    waterborne illness, 2:808
    West Nile virus, 2:812, 815
    whooping cough, 2:816, 818
    yellow fever, 2:825
  hazards
    acid rain, 1:2, 4
    agricultural chemicals, 1:7
    air pollution, 1:21, 24
    antimicrobial resistance, 1:41, 43, 45

United States (continued)
asbestos, 1:47
background radiation, 1:73–74
bedbug infestation, 1:75–76
bioterrorism, 1:100, 101–102, 103
biotoxins, 1:104
bisphenol A, 1:105–106
brownfield sites, 1:113–115
cellular phones, 1:139–140, 142
climate change, 1:184–185
endocrine disruptors, 1:274, 275
escherichia coli, 1:284
explosives, 1:289–290
food additives, 1:318, 320
food contamination, 1:324, 325–326
fracking, 1:346–347
hazardous waste, 1:395–396
ionizing radiation, 1:447
medical waste, 2:511, 512, 513
mercury, 2:526
parasites, 2:603, 604–605
sick building syndrome in, 2:689
smog, 2:707–708
smoking, 2:710, 713
water pollution, 2:799–800, 801
health issues
biomonitoring, 1:95–96
biosafety, 1:98–99
chlorination, 1:162–164
disaster preparedness, 1:224–225
drinking water supply, 1:229–231
Earth Day, 1:243–245
emergency preparedness, 1:259–262
ergonomics, 1:282
exposure science, 1:291, 292, 293–294
food safety, 1:336, 337–338
Healthy Cities, 1:397
heat (stress) index, 1:403
housing, 1:420, 421
indoor air quality, 1:437–438, 439
industrial hygiene, 1:443
land use, 1:461
levees, 1:483–484
National Ambient Air Quality Standard, 2:549–551
national parks, 2:559
noise pollution, 2:572, 573
patch testing, 2:607
population pyramid, 2:619
risk assessment, 2:653–655
toxicology, 2:737–738
vaccination, 2:777–279, 780, 782
vector (mosquito) control, 2:784, 786–787
water fluoridation, 2:797–799
water quality, 2:803–804, 804–805
water quality standards, 2:806, 807

legislation
Clean Air Act, 1:176–178
Clean Water Act, 1:179–182
Emergency Planning and Community Right-to-Know Act, 1:257–259
Federal Water Act, 1:306–307
National Environmental Policy Act, 2:551–552
Occupational Safety and Health Act, 1:585
Omnibus Flood Control Act, 2:591
Resource Conservation and Recovery Act, 2:650–652
Rivers and Harbors Act of 1899, 2:658–661
Safe Drinking Water Act, 2:667–668
Superfund Amendments and Reauthorization Act, 2:717–718
organizations
Centers for Disease Control and Prevention, 1:144–146
Environmental Protection Agency, 1:276–279
National Environmental Health Association, 2:551–552
National Institute for Occupational Safety and Health, 2:554–555
Occupational Safety and Health Administration, 1:585–586, 2:585–586
Red Cross in, 2:648, 649
Sierra Club, 2:692–693
University of California-Irvine, 2:785
University of Kentucky, 1:75
University of Pittsburgh Center for Biomedical Informatics, 1:102
Unsafe at Any Speed, 1:278
Unyango, Elisha, 2:753
Uptake, 1:406
Uranium, 1:74
Urban areas
air pollution in, 1:20, 21, 22–23
Clean Air Act in, 1:178
drought in, 1:235
flooding in, 1:311
Healthy Cities, 1:396–397
nature deficit disorder in, 2:561
noise pollution in, 2:573
ozone exposure in, 2:599
post-traumatic stress disorder in, 2:621
smog in, 2:705–707
tuberculosis in, 2:753
water fluoridation in, 2:797
water pollution in, 2:800
water quality in, 2:803
See also specific urban areas or cities by name
Urban yellow fever. *See* Yellow fever

Urbani, Carlo, 2:679, 680, *680*
Urinary tract, 2:676, 677
Urine, 1:171, 470
U.S. Agency for International Development, 1:161
U.S. Agricultural Research Service, 1:188
U.S. Air Force, 1:457
U.S. Army, 1:98
U.S. Army Corps of Engineers, 1:179, 181, 483, 2:591, 659, 661
U.S. Census Bureau, 2:573
U.S. Coast Guard, 1:457
U.S. Department of Agriculture (USDA)
on agricultural chemicals, 1:7
on avian flu, 1:70
on campylobacteriosis, 1:129
on food poisoning, 1:334, 335
on food safety, 1:337
Soil Conservation Act, 2:714
U.S. Department of Defense, 1:38, 377, 378
U.S. Department of Education, 1:457
U.S. Department of Energy, 1:144, 2:725, 726
U.S. Department of Health and Human Services, 2:**776**
on flu pandemic, 1:316
on Gulf oil spill, 1:373–374
National Institute of Environmental Health Sciences and, 2:556
on oil spills, 2:588
on Three Mile Island nuclear disaster, 2:726
U.S. Department of Health, Education and Welfare. *See* U.S. Department of Health and Human Services
U.S. Department of Homeland Security, 1:103, 261, 2:570, 571
U.S. Department of Housing and Urban Development, 2:573
U.S. Department of Labor, 1:457
U.S. Department of the Interior, 1:337, 375
U.S. Department of Transportation, 1:98
U.S. Department of Veterans Affairs (VA), 1:377, 378, 379, 476
U.S. Geological Survey (USGS), 1:7, 246, 247, 346, 435
U.S. Marine Corps, 1:229
U.S. National Academy of Sciences, 1:156
U.S. National Center for Emerging and Zoonotic Infectious Diseases, 1:266
U.S. National Pest Management Association, 1:75

U.S. Natural Resources Defense Council (NRDC), 2:526
U.S. Navy, 1:*430*, 457
U.S. Nuclear Regulatory Commission (NRC), 2:642, 643, 725, 726, 728–729
U.S. Postal Service, 1:98, 144
U.S. Small Business Administration (SBA), 1:260, 432
U.S. Supreme Court, 1:178
U.S. v. Standard Oil Company (1966), 2:660
U.S. vs. Republic Steel Corp. (1980), 2:660
USDA (U.S. Department of Agriculture). *See* U.S. Department of Agriculture (USDA)
USGS (U.S. Geological Survey). *See* U.S. Geological Survey (USGS)
Utilities, electric. *See* Electric power plants
UV radiation. *See* Ultraviolet radiation
UV-A radiation. *See* Ultraviolet radiation
UV-B radiation. *See* Ultraviolet radiation
UV-C radiation. *See* Ultraviolet radiation
Uveitis, 1:472, 473

V

VA (U.S. Department of Veterans Affairs), 1:377, 378, 379, 476
Vaccination, 2:**777–783**, *778*
  AIDS, 1:6, 19
  anthrax, 1:38, 40
  antimicrobial resistance, 1:44
  avian flu, 1:70
  bioterrorism and, 1:102, 103
  brucellosis, 1:116, 117, 119
  Centers for Disease Control and Prevention on, 1:143, 144, 145
  in child survival revolution, 1:161
  cholera, 1:169
  communicable diseases, 1:190
  cruise ship health and, 1:201
  description, 2:777–778
  diphtheria, 1:218, 220–221
  disease outbreaks, 1:227–228
  dysentery, 1:241
  emergent diseases, 1:265, 267
  flooding and, 1:312
  flu pandemic, 1:313, 314, 315, 316, 317
  Food and Drug Administration on, 1:322
  global public health, 1:362
  Gulf War syndrome, 1:378
  H1N1 influenza A, 1:382, 385
  hantavirus infections, 1:394
  hemorrhagic fevers, 1:413
  Horn of Africa drought and famine, 1:418
  interactions, 2:780–781
  leptospirosis, 1:473
  Lyme disease, 1:499
  malaria, 2:504
  measles, 2:508, 509, 510–511
  melanoma, 2:519–520
  meningitis, 2:521, 524
  mumps, 2:543–544, 545, 546
  noroviruses, 2:584
  pandemic and, 2:601
  plague, 2:612–613
  polio, 2:613, 616–617
  precautions, 2:779
  public health, 2:781–782
  purpose, 2:777
  schistosomiasis, 2:678
  side effects, 2:780
  smallpox, 2:701, 702–704
  for traveler's health, 2:739, 741–742, 743
  tropical disease, 2:744
  tuberculosis, 2:759
  typhoid fever, 2:763–764
  UNICEF on, 2:771, 772, 773
  for viruses, 2:788, 792
  West Nile virus, 2:815
  whooping cough, 2:816, 818
  World Health Organization on, 2:823
  yellow fever, 2:825, 826, *826*, 827, 828–829
  zoonoses, 2:835
  See also HPV vaccination
Vaccine Adverse Event Reporting System (VAERS), 2:780
Vaccines. *See* Vaccination
VAERS (Vaccine Adverse Event Reporting System), 2:780
Vaginal candidiasis, 1:353
Vanadium, 1:404, 406
Vancomycin, 1:43, 265
Vancomycin-resistant staph (VRSA), 1:43
Vanguard Study, 1:95
Vaporization, 1:414, 415, 2:525, 527, 530
Variant Creutzfeldt-Jakob disease. *See* Creutzfeldt-Jakob disease
Variola, 2:701, 702, 704
Variolation. *See* Vaccination
Varroa destructor mites, 1:186
VECTOR (Russian State Centre of Virology and Biotechnology), 2:702
Vector (mosquito) control, 2:**783–787**
  for dengue fever, 1:217
  in dengue fever, 1:215
  for emergent diseases, 1:267
  for hemorrhagic fevers, 1:413
  Hurricane Katrina and, 1:457
  for malaria, 2:504
  for tropical disease, 2:748
  for West Nile virus, 2:815
  for yellow fever, 2:829
Vectors
  dengue fever, 1:215
  endemic disease, 1:272
  hemorrhagic fevers, 1:410
  Lyme disease, 1:494
  parasites as, 2:603
  tropical disease, 2:744
  yellow fever, 2:825
Veendam (ship), 1:199
Vegetables. *See* Fruits and vegetables
Vegetation fires. *See* Wildfires
Vehicle safety, 1:144, 278
Vehicles, motorized. *See* Automobiles
Venezuelan hemorrhagic fever, 1:411
Ventilation
  for cadmium poisoning, 1:126–127
  for cutting oil exposure, 1:205
  heat disorders and, 1:400
  housing, 1:420
  indoor air quality, 1:438, 439, 440–441
  sick building syndrome, 2:689, 690, 691
Verenicline, 2:711
Vermiculite, 1:47
Vermont, 1:225
Verotoxin, 1:285
Vessel Sanitation Program, 1:199, 200, 201
Veterans, 1:377–379, 476, 2:620, 621, 622
Veterans Administration (VA), 1:476, 2:622
Veterinary medicine, 2:592–593
VHF (Viral hemorrhagic fevers). *See* Hemorrhagic fevers
Vibrio, 1:166–169, 326, 343, 2:808
Vicarious tramatization, 2:622
Victims' rights, 1:86, 88–89
Vietnam, 1:148, *148,* 265
Vietnam War, 1:476, 2:620, 621
Vinyl chloride, 2:737
Violence, stress response to. *See* Post-traumatic stress disorder
Viral hemorrhagic fever. *See* Yellow fever
Viral hemorrhagic fevers. *See* Hemorrhagic fevers
Viral hemorrhagic fevers (VHF). *See* Hemorrhagic fevers
Viral meningitis. *See* Meningitis
Virchow, Rudolf, 2:592
Virions, 2:788, 789
Viroids, 2:788
Viruses, 2:**788–793**
  antimicrobial resistance of, 1:42, 45
  biosafety, 1:98

Viruses *(continued)*
  as biotoxins, 1:103
  in bronchitis, 1:111
  in cancer, 1:131
  causes, 2:791
  Centers for Disease Control and Prevention on, 1:144
  in colony collapse disorder, 1:186
  as communicable diseases, 1:190
  description, 2:788
  diagnosis, 2:791
  in emergent diseases, 1:265
  function, 2:788–789
  health role, 2:789–790
  in meningitis, 2:520, 521–522
  as microbial pathogens, 2:536
  as parasites, 2:603
  prevention, 2:792
  symptoms, 2:791
  treatment, 2:791–792
  in tropical disease, 2:746
  in zoonoses, 2:833
  See also specific viruses by name
Vistula River, 2:800
Vitamin A, 2:509
Vitamin B_6, 1:65
Vitamin C, 2:535, 645
Vitamin D, 2:561, 769
Vitamin deficiency. *See* Diet and nutrition
Vitamin E, 2:645
Vitamin K, 1:412
Vitamin therapy
  asthma, 1:59–60
  autism, 1:65
  chemical poisoning, 1:153
  dysentery, 1:239
  Lyme disease, 1:497
  smoking cessation, 2:713
  See also specific vitamins by name
VOC (Volatile organic compound). *See* Volatile organic compound
Vog. *See* Volcanic fog
Volatile chemicals, 1:147–148
Volatile organic compound, 2:**793**
  acetone from, 1:1
  in air pollution, 1:22
  Clean Air Act on, 1:178
  from fracking, 1:347
  in housing, 1:420
  in indoor air quality, 1:438, 439, 441
  from oil spills, 2:587, 588, 590
  in sick building syndrome, 2:690
  in smog, 2:707
Volcanic ash, 1:435–436, *436,* 2:794, 795
Volcanic eruptions, 2:**793–796**, *794, 795*
  Icelandic volcano eruption, 1:435–436, *436*
  tsunamis and, 2:751
Volcanic fog, 2:795
Volcanoes, 1:414, 2:793–796
Voles. *See* Rodents

Volga River, 2:800
Voriconzole, 2:524
VRSA (Vancomycin-resistant staph), 1:43
Vulcanian eruptions. *See* Volcanic eruptions

W

Wagner, Christopher, 1:46
WAND (Women's Action for Nuclear Disarmament), 2:727
War
  Horn of Africa drought and famine, 1:415–416, 417, 418
  Red Cross, 2:648–649
  UNICEF, 2:774
Warfare, biological. *See* Bioterrorism
Warfarin, 2:664
Warning systems, 2:750–751, 795, 796, 835
Washington, DC, 2:568–571
Washington University, 2:584
Waste disposal. *See* Sanitation
Waste, hazardous. *See* Hazardous waste
Waste management. *See* Sanitation
Waste, medical. *See* Medical waste
Waste, toxic. *See* Hazardous waste
Wastewater
  chlorination of, 1:162–163, 164, 166, 168
  cholera from, 1:169
  Clean Water Act and, 1:179–180, 181
  escherichia coli in, 1:285
  Federal Water Act and, 1:306–306
  food poisoning from, 1:332
  as hazardous waste, 1:396
  Rivers and Harbors Act of 1899 and, 2:658–661
  sanitation and, 2:669–673
  water pollution in, 2:801
Wastewater treatment. *See* Water treatment
Wasting (weight loss). *See* Weight loss
Wasting disease, chronic. *See* Chronic wasting disease
Water, bottled. *See* Drinking water supply
Water chlorination. *See* Chlorination
Water conservation. *See* Conservation
Water contamination (drinking water). *See* Drinking water supply
Water contamination (waterways). *See* Water pollution
Water, diseases from. *See* Waterborne illness

Water, drinking. *See* Drinking water supply
Water fluoridation, 1:230–231, 2:**797–799**
Water pollution, 2:**799–802,** *800*
  acid rain in, 1:1, 3
  agricultural chemicals in, 1:7
  algal bloom from, 1:25
  asbestos in, 1:47
  cadmium poisoning, 1:126
  chemical poisoning, 1:150
  from Chernobyl nuclear power station disaster, 1:159
  from chlorination, 1:162–164
  cholera, 1 166, 168, 169
  Clean Water Act on, 1:179–182
  Environmental Protection Agency on, 1:276, 279
  from *Exxon Valdez,* 1:295–300
  Federal Water Act on, 1:306–307
  from flooding, 1:311
  from fracking, 1:346, 347, 348
  from Fukushima Daiichi nuclear power station disaster, 1:350, 351
  giardiasis from, 1:357, 359
  global public health, 1:363
  from Gulf oil spill, 1:368–376
  heavy metal poisoning, 1:404, 407
  Legionnaires' disease, 1:468
  from medical waste, 2:512, 513
  mercury in, 2:525, 526
  noroviruses, 2:583–584
  from oil spills, 2:587
  Rivers and Harbors Act of 1899 and, 2:658–661
  Safe Drinking Water Act and, 2:667–668
  sanitation and, 2:669–673
  from toxic sludge spill in Hungary, 2:731–732
  water quality and, 2:803–804, *804*
  water quality standards on, 2:806
Water Pollution Control Act of 1948. *See* Clean Water Act (1972, 1977, 1987)
Water Pollution Control Amendments of 1972. *See* Clean Water Act (1972, 1977, 1987)
Water quality, 2:**802–805**
  algal bloom on, 1:25, 26
  Centers for Disease Control and Prevention on, 1:144
  chlorination on, 1:162–164
  Clean Water Act, 1:179–182
  climate change and, 1:184
  dams and, 1:210–211
  in disease outbreaks, 1:226
  of drinking water supply, 1:228
  in drought, 1:233
  Safe Drinking Water Act, 2:667–668
  sanitation on, 2:669–673
  standards, 1:179–182, 2:805–807
  water pollution and, 2:799–802

Water Quality Act of 1965. *See* Clean Water Act (1972, 1977, 1987)
Water quality standards, 2:**805–807**
  Clean Water Act on, 1:179–182
  Environmental Protection Agency on, 1:279
  Federal Water Act on, 1:306–307
  Safe Drinking Water Act on, 2:667–668
  for water pollution, 2:801
  on water quality, 2:802, 803, 804–805
  waterborne illness and, 2:811
Water Resources Development Act, 2:591
Water shortages. *See* Drought
Water supply, for drinking. *See* Drinking water supply
Water treatment
  for amebiasis, 1:33
  Clean Water Act on, 1:179–180
  drinking water supply, 1:228–231
  Federal Water Act on, 1:307
  Fukushima Daiichi nuclear power station disaster and, 1:351
  ozone in, 2:598
  Rivers and Harbors Act of 1899 on, 2:659
  Safe Drinking Water Act on, 2:667, 668
  for sanitation, 2:671, 672
  for schistosomiasis, 2:678
  for water pollution, 2:799, 801, 802
  water quality and, 2:804
  for waterborne illness, 2:811
Waterborne illness, 2:**807–812**
  causes, 2:808
  demographics, 2:808
  description, 2:807–808
  diagnosis, 2:809
  in drinking water supply, 1:228–230
  from *escherichia coli*, 1:284
  in global public health, 1:363
  from Horn of Africa drought and famine, 1:418
  from Japanese earthquake, 1:451
  noroviruses, 2:577, 579, 581, 582
  prevention, 2:811
  prognosis, 2:811
  sanitation and, 2:669–673
  swimming advisories and, 2:718–719
  in traveler's health, 2:739
  treatment, 2:810
  tropical disease and, 2:745, 746, 748
  from water pollution, 2:799–800
  water quality and, 2:804–805
  zoonoses as, 2:833
  See also specific diseases by name
Water-generated electricity. *See* Hydroelectricity
Watt, James, 2:693

Wavelengths, 1:183–184, 446, 2:575
Waves, tidal. *See* Tsunamis
Waxman, Henry, 1:177
Weapons, biological. *See* Bioterrorism
Weather
  climate change, 1:182–185
  drought, 1:232, 233–234
  flooding, 1:310–311
  Horn of Africa drought and famine, 1:417
  hurricanes and, 1:431, 432, 433
  smog, 2:705–707, 707
  tornadoes and cyclones, 2:730–731
Weight loss
  AIDS, 1:16–17, 18
  chronic wasting disease, 1:174–175
Weil, Adolf, 1:470
Weil's syndrome, 1:472
Wells, from fracking. *See* Fracking
Wells, H. G., 1:101
West Nile encephalitis. *See* West Nile virus
West Nile fever. *See* West Nile virus
West Nile meningitis. *See* West Nile virus
West Nile meningoencephalitis. *See* West Nile virus
West Nile virus, 2:**812–816**
  as emergent disease, 1:265, 266
  Hurricane Katrina and, 1:457
  in One Health Initiative, 2:592, 593
  vector (mosquito) control for, 2:784, 785, 786
Western blot test. *See* Diagnostic testing
Western equine encephalitis, 2:663, 664
Westinghouse, George, 1:252
Wetlands, 1:179, 306, 307, 372, 433, 473
WFP (World Food Progam), 1:415–416, 418
Whalen, Robert P, 1:492
What the Yuck: Mercury Poisoning from Sushi, 2:528
Wheat, 1:7
Wheezing, 1:54, 56, 111, 120, 121
Whipworm disease. *See* Trichuriasis
Whipworms. *See* Parasites
White blood cells. *See* Blood cells
White House Office on Environmental Policy, 2:553
WHO (World Health Organization). *See* World Health Organization
Whooping cough, 1:265, 2:**816–819**
Wild, Christopher, 1:291
Wild hops. *See* Bryonia
Wilderness Act, 2:693
Wildfires, 1:233, 310, 2:*819*, **819–822**, 820

Wildlife
  brucellosis in, 1:115, 117, 118
  chronic wasting disease in, 1:174–175
  Creutzfeldt-Jakob disease in, 1:194
  in emergent diseases, 1:265
  endocrine disruptors on, 1:273, 274–275
  in epidemiology, 1:281
  Exxon Valdez, 1:297, 298, 299
  Gulf oil spill, 1:372
  hemorrhagic fevers from, 1:411
  leptospirosis from, 1:470–471
  listeriosis from, 1:484
  in low-temperature environments, 1:493
  Lyme disease from, 1:494–495
  in national parks, 2:559
  in One Health Initiative, 2:
  plague from, 2:611
  in Seveso, Italy, 2:683
  tropical disease from, 2:744
  water quality standards on, 2:806
  zoonoses from, 2:833, 834, 835
Wildlife conservation. *See* Conservation
Wilma, 1:432
Wilson, B., 2:564
Wind, 1:431–432, 2:730–731
Window period, 1:13
Winter smog. *See* Smog
Winter vomiting disease. *See* Noroviruses
Wireless phones. *See* Cellular phones
WNV (West Nile virus). *See* West Nile virus
Wolman, Abel, 1:163
Women
  AIDS, 1:10, 11, 19
  altitude sickness, 1:28
  amebiasis, 1:30, 31
  bisphenol A on, 1:105, 106
  Centers for Disease Control and Prevention on, 1:144
  global public health on, 1:361
  lead poisoning, 1:465
  leukemia, 1:476
  melanoma, 2:514, 515
  Oxfam on, 2:595, 596
  populaton pyramids, 2:619, 620
  post-traumatic stress disorder, 2:621, 622
  skin cancer, 2:696
  water fluoridation and, 2:797
  See also Pregnancy
Women's Action for Nuclear Disarmament (WAND), 2:727
Wool-sorter's disease. *See* Anthrax
The Work of the International Steering Committee for the Study of the Health Effects of the Seveso Accident: Its Methodology, Its Issues and Its Conclusions, 2:683

Workplace safety, 1:191
  Centers for Disease Control and Prevention, 1:143, 144
  disasters
    Bhopal, India, 1:88, 89
    Chernobyl nuclear power station disaster, 1:155–158
    Gulf oil spill, 1:372–373, 374, 375–376
    heat disorders, 1:399
    Japanese earthquake, 1:449, 451
    Love Canal, 1:492
    9/11 terrorist attacks, 2:570, 571
    oil spills, 2:587–590
    Three Mile Island nuclear disaster, 2:727
    wildfires, 2:821
  diseases and disorders
    ammonia exposure, 1:35–36, 35–37
    anthrax, 1:38, 40
    asbestosis, 1:48–49, 50, 51
    asthma, 1:61
    benzene exposure, 1:81
    berylliosis, 1:82, 83, 84–85
    black lung disease, 1:108–109
    bronchitis, 1:111
    brucellosis, 1:116
    byssinosis, 1:120–122
    cadmium poisoning, 1:126, 127
    chemical poisoning, 1:149
    chlorine exposure, 1:164, 165
    cutting oil exposure, 1:204206
    electric shock injuries, 1:252, 255–256
    emphysema, 1:269, 270
    fibrosis, 1:309
    heavy metal poisoning, 1:406, 407, 408, 409
    lead poisoning, 1:464, 466, 467
    manganese exposure, 2:505–506, 507
    mercury poisoning, 2:527
    post-traumatic stress disorder, 2:622–623
    radiation injuries, 2:642
    silicosis, 2:694, 695
    talcosis, 2:721
    thesaurosis, 2:723, 724
  hazards
    acetone, 1:1
    asbestos, 1:46–47
    bisphenol A, 1:106
    endocrine disruptors, 1:274
    explosives, 1:289
    ionizing radiation, 1:447
    medical waste, 2:512, 513
    mercury, 2:525–526
    neurotoxins, 2:568
    noise pollution, 2:573–574
    ultraviolet radiation, 2:769
  health issues
    biomonitoring, 1:96
    ergonomics, 1:281–283
    exposure science, 1:291, 294
    fibrosis, 1:308
    indoor air quality, 1:437–438
    industrial hygiene, 1:442–443
    toxicology, 2:736, 737
  National Institute for Occupational Safety and Health, 2:554–555
  National Institute of Environmental Health Sciences, 2:558–559
  Occupational Safety and Health Act, 2:585
  Occupational Safety and Health Administration, 2:585–586
World Bank, 1:366, 390, 2:596, 772
World Conference on National Parks, 2:560
World Food Progam (WFP), 1:415–416, 418
World Health Organization, 2:**822–823**
  disasters
    Chernobyl nuclear power station disaster, 1:158
    Fukushima Daiichi nuclear power station disaster, 1:351
    toxic sludge spill in Hungary, 2:732
  diseases and disorders
    AIDS, 1:8
    asbestosis, 1:48–49
    avian flu, 1:68, 69, 70
    black lung disease, 1:109
    bronchitis, 1:112
    cancer, 1:131
    chemical poisoning, 1:153
    cholera, 1:166, 168, 169
    chronic kidney disease, 1:173
    Creutzfeldt-Jakob disease, 1:197
    cyanosis, 1:207–208
    dengue fever, 1:217
    disease outbreaks, 1:227
    ebola hemorrhagic fever, 1:248, 251
    emergent diseases, 1:266
    emphysema, 1:269, 270
    flu pandemic, 1:314, 316
    guinea worm disease, 1:366
    H1N1 influenza A, 1:381, 385
    heavy metal poisoning, 1:407
    leptospirosis, 1:473
    malaria, 2:501, 503t, 504
    measles, 2:510
    melanoma, 2:517
    ozone exposure, 2:599–600
    pandemic, 2:601–602
    plague, 2:612
    polio, 2:613, 614, 616
    river blindness, 2:655
    schistosomiasis, 2:676, 678
    severe acute respiratory syndrome, 2:679–680
    shigellosis, 2:685
    smallpox, 2:701, 703, 704
    traveler's health, 2:742
    tropical disease, 2:744, 747
    tuberculosis, 2:753, 754, 755, 758
    typhoid fever, 2:761
    typhus, 2:766, 767
    West Nile virus, 2:812
    yellow fever, 2:826, 828
    zoonoses, 2:833, 835
  hazards
    cellular phones, 1:141
    food additives, 1:320, 321
    medical waste, 2:513, 514
    noise pollution, 2:573
    non-ionizing radiation, 2:576
    sick building syndrome, 2:689
    ultraviolet radiation, 2:769
  health issues
    antimicrobial resistance, 1:41, 43, 44
    child survival revolution, 1:161
    drinking water supply, 1:228, 230
    global public health, 1:361, 363
    Healthy Cities, 1:396–397
    industrial hygiene, 1:443
    population and disease, 2:617
    sanitation, 2:673
    vaccination, 2:781, 782
    vector (mosquito) control, 2:784–785, 786
    water quality, 2:804
    water quality standards, 2:806
  UNICEF, 2:771, 772, 773, 774
World Summit for Children, 2:772
World Trade Center, 2:568–571, 569
World Trade Center Health Program, 2:570
World Trade Organization, 2:596
World War I, 1:100, 314, 315
World War II, 1:100, 2:621, 638, 638
Worms, parasitic. See Parasites
Wormwood, 2:504, 606
Wounds. See Skin
Wyoming, 1:174

X

X rays. See Diagnostic testing; Radiation
Xylene, 1:80, 348

Y

Yangtze River, 1:210, 210, 212
Yard chemicals, 1:149
Yaws, 2:746
Yeast, 1:265

Yeast infections, 1:353
Yellow fever, 2:**825–829**, *826*
  as emergent disease, 1:266, 267
  as hemorrhagic fever, 1:411, 413
  in traveler's health, 2:743
  vector (mosquito) control for, 2:783–784
Yellow Fever Initiative, 2:828
Yellowstone National Park, 1:118, 2:559
Yemen, 2:655, 656
Yersinia enterocolitica, 1:326, 343
Yersinia pestis, 2:611
Yoga, 1:60
Yokkaichi asthma, 2:**829–832**
Yokkaichi, Japan, 2:829–832
Yokoyama, Kazuhito, 2:831

York, England, 1:*310*
Yosemite National Park, 1:412, 2:559, 692
Young people. *See* Children
Youth. *See* Children
Youth bulge, 2:620
Youth in the Great Outdoors, 2:562
Yugoslavia, 2:701

Z

Zadroga Act. *See* James L. Zadroga 9/11 Health and Compensation Act
Zaire, 2:685
Zanamivir, 1:70, 384

ZAP-70, 1:477
Zero discharge, 1:180, 181
Zero population growth, 1:161, 2:**832**
Zinc, 1:168, 239, 404, 406, 407, 466
Zoonoses, 2:**832–836**
  American Public Health Association on, 1:34
  as emergent diseases, 1:264–265, 266
  One Health Initiative and, 2:591–593
  parasites from, 2:603
  as viruses, 2:790
  See also specific zoonoses by name
Zoonotic diseases. *See* Zoonoses
Zyban. *See* Bupropion hydrochloride